Urology: A Clinical Approach

Urology: A Clinical Approach

Editor: Timothy Lawson

AMERICAN
MEDICAL PUBLISHERS
www.americanmedicalpublishers.com

AMERICAN
MEDICAL PUBLISHERS
www.americanmedicalpublishers.com

Cataloging-in-Publication Data

Urology : a clinical approach / edited by Timothy Lawson.
p. cm.
Includes bibliographical references and index.
ISBN 979-8-88740-548-3
1. Urology. 2. Urinary organs--Diseases--Diagnosis. 3. Urinary organs--Diseases--Treatment.
4. Genitourinary organs--Diseases--Diagnosis. 5. Genitourinary organs--Diseases--Treatment.
I. Lawson, Timothy.
RC871 .U76 2023
616.6--dc23

American Medical Publishers,
41 Flatbush Avenue,
1st Floor, New York,
NY 11217, USA

ISBN 979-8-88740-548-3 (Hardback)

Contents

Preface

In my initial years as a student, I used to run to the library at every possible instance to grab a book and learn something new. Books were my primary source of knowledge and I would not have come such a long way without all that I learnt from them. Thus, when I was approached to edit this book; I became understandably nostalgic. It was an absolute honor to be considered worthy of guiding the current generation as well as those to come. I put all my knowledge and hard work into making this book most beneficial for its readers.

Urology refers to a specialty of medicine that focuses on diseases of the reproductive organs and urinary tract system that can be treated medically or surgically. It includes organs such as the urinary bladder, kidneys, ureters, urethra, adrenal glands, as well as male reproductive organs such as seminal vesicles, epididymis, penis, testes, vas deferens and prostate. The reproductive and urinary tracts are interconnected and problems with one have an impact on the other. In the field of urology, diseases including urinary tract infections and enlarged prostates are treated medically, whereas prostate cancer, stress incontinence, bladder cancer and kidney stones are treated surgically. Surgeries assisted by laser, minimally invasive laparoscopy and robotic surgery, and other scope-guided treatments are examples of urological techniques. Pediatric surgery, oncology, gynecology, colorectal surgery, endocrinology, nephrology, andrology and gastroenterology are closely associated to urology. This book explores all the important aspects of clinical urology in the present day. It includes contributions of experts and researchers which will provide innovative insights into this field. The extensive content of this book provides the readers with a thorough understanding of the subject.

I wish to thank my publisher for supporting me at every step. I would also like to thank all the authors who have contributed their researches in this book. I hope this book will be a valuable contribution to the progress of the field.

Editor

1

Histological Inflammation in Human Ureter either Healthy or Fitted with Double-Pigtail Stent or a Thin 0.3 F Suture Thread

Benoît Vogt[1] **and Ilham Chokri**[2]

[1]*Department of Urology, Polyclinique De Blois, 1 Rue Robert Debré, 41260 La Chaussée Saint-Victor, France*
[2]*Laboratory of Anatomocytopathology, 1 Av Prof Alexandre Minkowski, 37170 Chambray-Lès-Tours, France*

Correspondence should be addressed to Benoît Vogt; message@benoitvogt.fr

Academic Editor: Kostis Gyftopoulos

Background. Ureteral stent intolerance reduces patients' quality of life. It has been suggested that changes in the shape of stents could decrease discomfort. In previous studies, the innovative pigtail-suture stent (i.e., JFil® or MiniJFil®) with a thin 0.3 F suture thread significantly decreased stent-related symptoms. Fortuitously, a dilation of the ureter containing the sutures was discovered. In addition, no inflammation was seen on the ureter wall around the suture in endoscopy. In this preliminary study, we assessed ureteral inflammation in the human ureter when it was healthy or when fitted with a double-pigtail stent or a thread. *Materials and Methods.* After consent and inclusion of patients in the protocol, fifteen segments of ureters were collected during cystectomy procedures for bladder tumors. Ureteral inflammation was assessed on the histological section stained with hematoxylin-eosin. Histological grading (cumulative range of 0 to 6) assessing inflammation was performed on the ureter section for mucosa inflammation and inflammation in the muscle layer. *Results.* A marked ureteral inflammatory reaction was observed in all cases of ureters fitted with a double-pigtail stent with a mean inflammation score of 4.8 ± 0.4. The ureter fitted with the thin suture thread showed inflammation in only one case with a mean inflammation score of 1.8 ± 1.3 ($p = 0.001$). *Conclusion.* Although the study was limited by the small number of patients, it confirmed that the double-pigtail stent induced ureteral inflammation in all cases and the thin 0.3 F suture thread caused less ureteral inflammation than the double-pigtail stent. The concept of material reduction within the urinary tract seems necessary in order to decrease mucosal irritation. The JFil® or the MiniJFil® thread could meet this requirement.

1. Introduction

Double-pigtail stents are frequently implanted in the ureter in urological practice, but ureteral stent intolerance reduces patients' quality of life. The symptoms may be largely due to bladder irritation caused by the stent and by the reflux during bladder voiding [1].

By decreasing the amount of material within the bladder, it should be possible to attenuate the stent-related symptoms [2–4].

To minimize the amount of material left in the bladder, a pigtail-suture stent (i.e., JFil® or MiniJFil®) was evaluated [2, 5]. With these innovative stents, the bladder loop is replaced with a thin suture thread (not more than 0.3 French). The suture thread results in the presence of only small amounts of material in the bladder. Moreover, the absence of an internal channel probably also limits renal reflux. With the pigtail-suture stent, the patients were improved [2, 5].

Fortuitously, a clear dilation of the ureter containing the sutures was discovered. We observed a ureteral diameter two to three times larger than the contralateral ureter on CT. In addition, no inflammation was seen on the ureter wall around the suture in endoscopy [2, 5]. These surprising properties led us to create the MiniJFil®, which is reduced to a thread attached to a simple loop of a pigtail stent [5, 6].

With the suture thread, the entire ureter can be dilated without inflammation, and the luminal vacuity of the ureter is preserved. Thus, the MiniJFil® may facilitate insertion of the ureteral access sheath and accelerate removal of stone fragments, and finally, MiniJFil® may improve outcome [6].

There are few studies on the interactions between the ureteral stent and the ureter, especially the human one. Several studies showed a marked ureteral inflammatory reaction when pigs were fitted with double-pigtail stents [7–9]. With the MiniJFil®, the absence of the inflammation of the ureteral mucosa in endoscopy motivated the decision to explore the ureteral histology. In this preliminary study, the objective was to determine if the thin 0.3 F suture thread caused less ureteral inflammation than the double-pigtail stent as suggested by the endoscopic appearance of previous studies [2, 5].

2. Materials and Methods

The study design has been approved by the French Ethical Committee (2017.09.02 bis). From September 2017 to September 2019 in a single institution, fifteen patients about to have a cystectomy with ileal conduit urinary diversion agreed to be included in the protocol and signed an informed consent form. There was no selection or exclusion, and all patients were included, even those with large tumors. Fifteen segments of ureters were gathered during cystectomy.

If gathering a human ureteral segment fitted with a double-pigtail stent is feasible, it is exceptionally rare for a ureter with a thin thread. In urological practice, cystectomy with removal of a part of the ureter is the only pathology to obtain a healthy ureteral segment fitted with a thread. The analysis of the ureters fitted with a thread can be altered by the presence of a pelvic tumor. To avoid a bias, the comparison with unstented or stented ureters was made with patients who also had a pelvic tumor.

Patients requiring no ureteral drainage served as unstented ureter controls. Patients requiring ureteral drainage for obstructive ureteral orifice were fitted with a 7 F double-pigtail stent. Patients without ureteral stents but requiring cystoscopic control before cystectomy were fitted with a MiniJFil® with the aim of facilitating the suture of the ureter in the ileal conduit urinary diversion.

The MiniJFil® stent was previously used in another study [5, 6]. In the procedure, a polyurethane double-pigtail stent (double-loop ureteral stents, 4.8 F, 26 cm, Coloplast) was sectioned perpendicularly to the main axis, just outside of the renal loop. The sectioned part is then cut parallel to the main axis to form a beveled tail that is 2 cm long. A polypropylene suture (Ethicon monofilament polypropylene suture; gauge size U.S.P.1; 0.1 to 0.15 mm; 5–0) perforates the loop and the end of the tail. The distal end of the MiniJFil® consists of two 0.3 F sutures, and each suture is approximately 36 cm long.

Ureters were fixed in 4% formalin, embedded in paraffin, serially cut, and stained with hematoxylin-eosin. As suggested by the endoscopic appearance, the ureteral mucosa looked normal in patients with a thread [2, 5]. The histological analysis was, therefore, focused on the inflammation of mucosa. Analysis of the muscular layer helped evaluate the wall of the ureter in depth. Histological grading assessing inflammation was performed on the ureter section. Following a standard evaluation protocol [9], each section was inspected for 2 characteristics: mucosa inflammation and inflammation in the muscle layer. A 4-point scale assessed the degree of change, with 0 indicating no change and 3 indicating severe changes, for each of the above characteristics (cumulative range of 0 to 6). A score was assigned by an experienced histopathologist (I.C.) blinded to the source of each specimen. The data were presented as mean ± SD and were analyzed using the Mann–Whitney test. Values of $p < 0.05$ were considered significant.

3. Results

Fifteen patients had bladder cancer, and three of which were sarcomas (5 women and 10 men, mean age 69.7 ± 9.6 years). Nine patients had preoperative chemotherapy, and 1 patient had surgery, chemotherapy, and radiotherapy for rectal cancer. Each group included at least a large tumor.

Five patients had no ureteral obstruction and did not require drainage with a stent. In five patients, an obstruction was located in the ureteral orifice, and these patients were fitted with an indwelling 7 F double-pigtail stent 1 to 2 months before and until cystectomy. Five patients were fitted with the MiniJFil® at least two weeks before and until cystectomy.

All ureteral segments of ureters were iliac and were gathered about 10 cm above the ureteral orifice during cystectomy. No tumor was observed on these ureteral segments.

Of the five unstented control segments, four showed no inflammation (Figures 1(a) and 1(d)). A marked ureteral inflammatory reaction was observed in all cases of ureter fitted with a double-pigtail stent (Figures 1(b) and 1(e)). In the ureter fitted with the thin 0.3 F suture thread, inflammation was observed in one case only (Figures 1(c) and 1(f)).

In cases of the ureter fitted with a double-pigtail stent, the mean inflammation score (4.8 ± 0.4) was significantly different from that of unstented control segments (1.4 ± 1.1; $p = 0.009$) or that of the ureter fitted with the thin 0.3 F suture thread (1.8 ± 1.3; $p = 0.001$).

In the ureter fitted with the thin 0.3 F suture thread, the mean inflammation score was not significantly different from that of unstented control segments ($p = 0.73$).

4. Discussion

There are few studies on the interactions between the ureteral stent and the ureter, especially the human one. Janssen at al. described severe intraluminal dilation, scuffed epithelium, and pronounced submucosal edema and inflammation in all ureters when the pigs were fitted with a 6 F double-pigtail stent [8]. Olweny et al. observed important edema of the bladder mucosa and fibrosis in the lamina propria at 1 week when Yucatan minipigs were fitted with a 7 F double-pigtail stent [9]. Natalin et al. found that histological grading scores for inflammation and fibrosis were

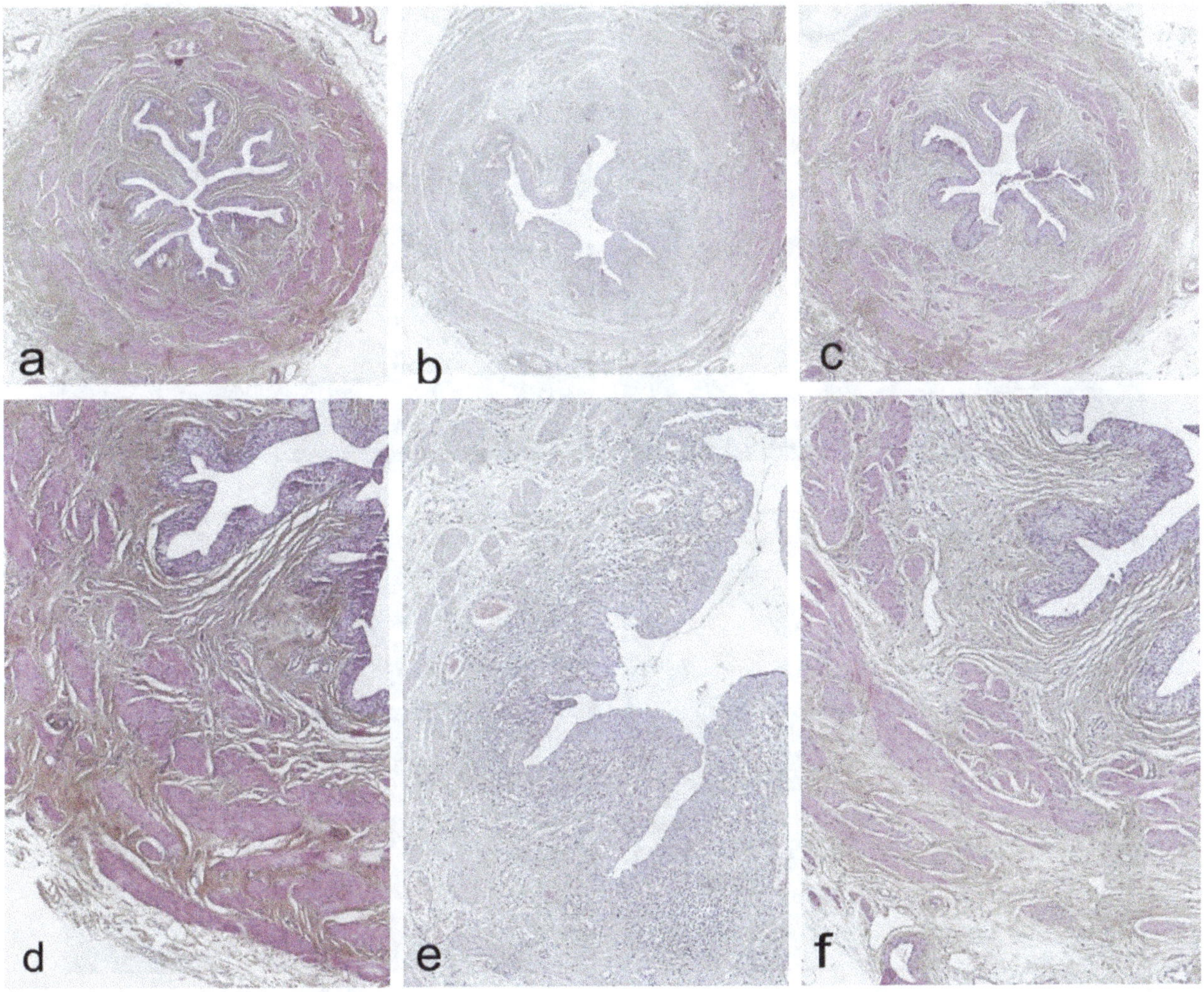

FIGURE 1: Histological appearance with hematoxylin-eosin staining. (a–c) Original magnification x3. (d–f) Original magnification x7. (a, d) Unstented control ureter showing no inflammation. (b, e) Ureter with the double-pigtail stent showing a marked ureteral inflammatory reaction. (c, f) Ureter with 0.3 F suture thread showing no inflammation.

more pronounced when the ureter or the ureteral orifice of pigs was fitted with a 6 F double-pigtail stent [7].

Natalin noted the interaction between stent material and the ureter as a mechanism of inflammation and aperistalsis. With a particular shape of stents, the authors observed a smaller reduction in peristalsis, possibly reflecting its lesser interaction with ureteral tissue [7]. As suggested by endoscopic appearance of previous studies (Figure 2) [2, 5], the thin thread is expected to decrease interactions with the ureteral and bladder mucosa, and histological inflammation.

Although the study was limited by the small number of patients, the use of a semiquantitative scale made it possible to specify the alterations of the ureteral wall less subjectively. In the preliminary study, the thin 0.3 F suture thread caused less ureteral inflammation than the double-pigtail stent. With the MiniJFil®, a healthy ureter in its entirety can be dilated without inflammation and the ureteral dilation could reduce ureteral stenosis. Further studies could explore the possibility of reducing postoperative ureteroileal stenosis using MiniJFil®.

In the ureter fitted with the thin 0.3 F suture thread or in the unstented control segments, inflammation was observed in only one case. The patient with a history of rectal cancer was fitted with a MiniJFil®. Radiotherapy could explain the ureteral inflammatory reaction observed in that particular case. However, no explanation was found for the control group patient with ureteral inflammation. There was considerable heterogeneity in patients due to tumor volume, treatments, and ureteral obstructions. Lymphatic obstruction and edematous infiltration due to the tumor mass burden may explain the heterogeneity of these results. Moreover, Janssen et al. already suggested some level of cross talk between the two sides that requires further investigation [8]. However, this apparent good result contrasts with the ureteral inflammation with double-pigtail stents and confirms that thinner material is in favour of good mucosa ureteral tolerance.

The concept of material reduction within the bladder seems necessary in order to decrease bladder mucosal irritation and stent-related symptoms [2–4]. However, the

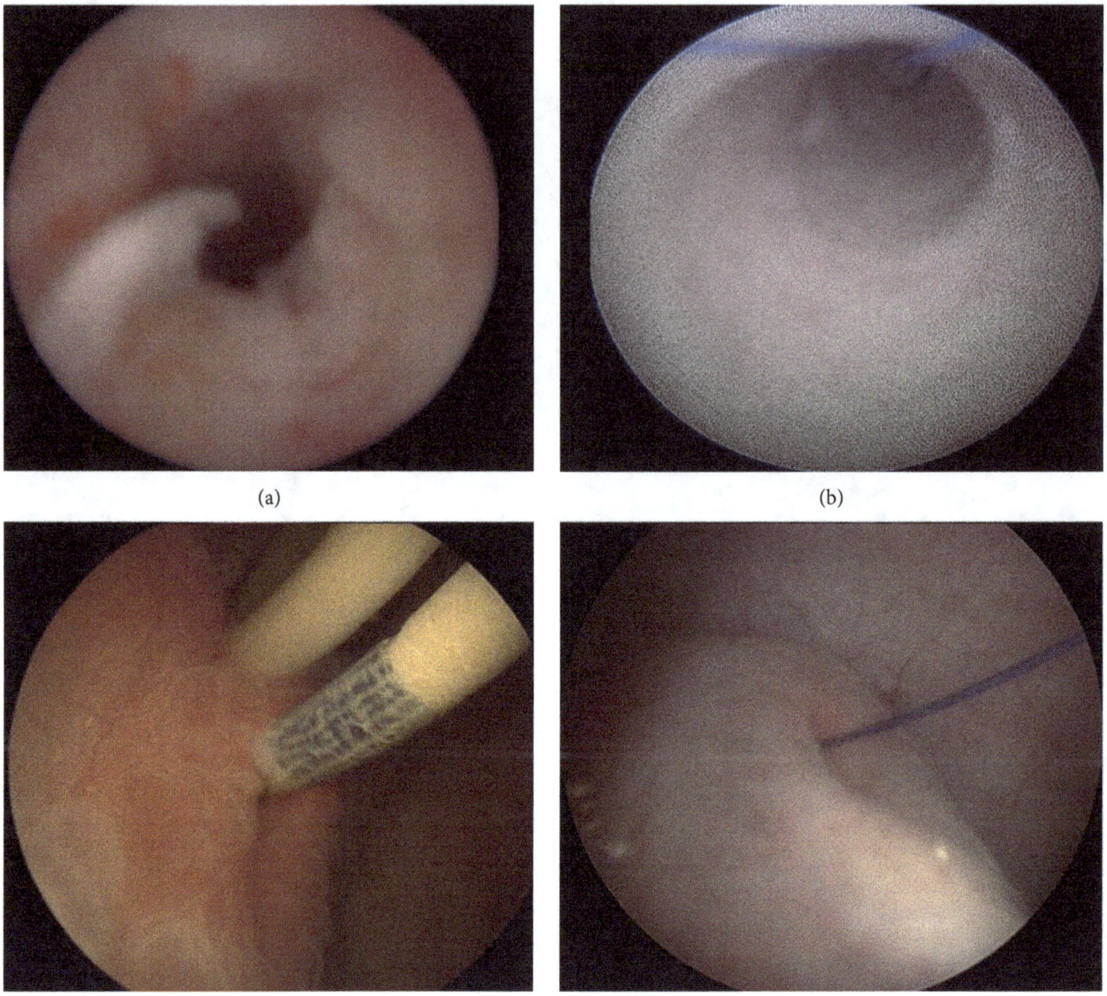

(a) (b) (c) (d)

Figure 2: Endoscopic appearance. (a) Appearance of the inflamed ureter around the double-pigtail stent after stent removal. (b) Dilation of the ureter without inflammation after pigtail-suture stent implantation. (c) Inflamed ureteral orifice around the double-pigtail stent. (d) Dilated ureteral orifice without inflammation after pigtail-suture stent implantation.

concept of material reduction within the ureter should focus attention in order to improve outcome. Sfoungaristos et al. showed that ureteral stents, even if they were removed just before extracorporeal shock wave lithotripsy, decreased the stone free rate. Edema formation with decreasing functional ureteral lumen diameter and low ureteral peristalsis may minimize the likelihood of stone passage [10]. Kuebker et al. noted that the overall rate of stone passage around the 6 F double-pigtail stent was 8% and the passage rate for ≥7 mm stones was 0% [11]. In comparison with the double-pigtail stent, the luminal burden of the ureter only fitted with a pigtail-suture stent was reduced to the threads (i.e., Mini-JFil®). The absence of edema around the suture and the luminal freedom may facilitate the elimination of stone fragments [6].

If the thinness of the thread is expected to limit the irritation of the ureter as suggested by the endoscopic appearance, the mechanisms or the local factors involved in the ureteral dilation are still unknown. As Janssen et al. suggested, improving our understanding of specific molecular mechanisms leading to stent-associated ureteral dysfunction may identify targets for future therapeutic agents [8].

There were several limitations to the present study. First, the small number of patients requires more targeted studies but, if gathering the ureteral segment fitted with a double-pigtail stent is feasible, it is exceptionally rare for a ureter with a thin thread because cystectomy is the only indication. Second, the heterogeneity of the bladder diseases and edematous infiltration due to the tumor mass burden may explain the heterogeneity of results.

5. Conclusion

Although the study was limited by the small number of patients, it confirmed that the double-pigtail stent induced ureteral inflammation in all cases and the thin 0.3 F suture thread caused less ureteral inflammation than the double-pigtail stent.

The concept of material reduction within the urinary tract seems necessary in order to decrease mucosal irritation.

The search for the ideal ureteral stent could focus on the shortening and the thinning of the intraureteral and bladder material at least in the healthy segments of the ureter. The JFil® or the MiniJFil® thread could meet this requirement.

Ethical Approval

All procedures performed in studies involving human participants were in accordance with the ethical standards of the institutional and/or national research committee (the French Ethical Committee: 2017.09.02 bis) and with the 1964 Declaration of Helsinki and its later amendments or comparable ethical standards.

Consent

Written informed consent and accompanying images published were obtained from all human participants included in the study.

Authors' Contributions

Benoît Vogt performed the protocol development and the data collection and analyzed and interpreted the data and wrote the manuscript. Ilham Chokri performed the histological examination. All authors read and approved the final manuscript.

Acknowledgments

The authors would like to thank Professor Janine Dove-Rumé, English Department, the University of Tours, for rereading the text.

References

[1] B. H. Chew and D. Lange, "Advances in ureteral stent development," *Current Opinion in Urology*, vol. 26, no. 3, pp. 277–282, 2016.

[2] B. Vogt, A. Desgrippes, and F.-N. Desfemmes, "Changing the double-pigtail stent by a new suture stent to improve patient's quality of life: a prospective study," *World Journal of Urology*, vol. 33, no. 8, pp. 1061–1068, 2015.

[3] S. Nestler, B. Witte, L. Schilchegger, and J. Jones, "Size does matter: ureteral stents with a smaller diameter show advantages regarding urinary symptoms, pain levels and general health," *World Journal of Urology*, vol. 38, no. 4, 2020.

[4] B. Vogt, "A new customized ureteral stent with nonrefluxing silicone end-piece to alleviate stent-related symptoms in malignant diseases," *Urology*, vol. 137, pp. 45–49, 2020.

[5] B. Vogt, A. Desgrippes, and F.-N. Desfemmes, "Sondes JFil et MiniJFil: progrès décisifs dans la tolérance des sondes urétérales et propriétés inattendues du fil urétéral," *Progrès en Urologie*, vol. 24, no. 7, pp. 441–450, 2014.

[6] B. Vogt, F. N. Desfemmes, A. Desgrippes et al., "MiniJFil®: a new safe and effective stent for well-tolerated repeated extracorporeal shockwave lithotripsy or ureteroscopy for medium-to-large kidney stones?" *Nephro-Urology Monthly*, vol. 8, no. 5, Article ID e40788, 2016.

[7] R. A. Natalin, G. W. Hruby, Z. Okhunov et al., "Pilot study evaluating ureteric physiological changes with a novel "ribbon stent" design using electromyographic and giant magnetoresistive sensors," *BJU International*, vol. 103, no. 8, pp. 1128–1131, 2009.

[8] C. Janssen, R. Buttyan, C. Y. Seow et al., "A role for the hedgehog effector Gli1 in mediating stent-induced ureteral smooth muscle dysfunction and aperistalsis," *Urology*, vol. 104, pp. 242.e1–242.e8, 2017.

[9] E. O. Olweny, A. J. Portis, C. P. Sundaram et al., "Evaluation of a chronic indwelling prototype mesh ureteral stent in a porcine model," *Urology*, vol. 56, no. 5, pp. 857–862, 2000.

[10] S. Sfoungaristos, O. N. Gofrit, D. Pode et al., "History of ureteral stenting negatively affects the outcomes of extracorporeal shockwave lithotripsy. results of a matched-pair analysis," *Prague Medical Report*, vol. 116, no. 3, pp. 225–232, 2015.

[11] J. M. Kuebker, J. Robles, J. J. Kramer, N. L. Miller, S. D. Herrell, and R. S. Hsi, "Predictors of spontaneous ureteral stone passage in the presence of an indwelling ureteral stent," *Urolithiasis*, vol. 47, no. 4, pp. 395–400, 2019.

2

The Current Role of Osteoclast Inhibitors in Patients with Prostate Cancer

Diomidis Kozyrakis,[1] **Dionyssios Paridis,**[2] **Stefanos Perikleous,**[1] **Konstantinos Malizos,**[3] **Anastasios Zarkadas,**[1] **and Antonios Tsagkalis**[2]

[1]*Department of Urology, "Achillopouleio" General Hospital of Volos, Magnesia, Greece*
[2]*Department of Orthopaedics, Animus-Kyanous Hospital, Larisa, Greece*
[3]*Department of Orthopaedics, Faculty of Medicine, School of Health Sciences, University of Thessaly, Larissa, Greece*

Correspondence should be addressed to Diomidis Kozyrakis; dkozirakis@yahoo.gr

Academic Editor: Kostis Gyftopoulos

Purpose. Prostate cancer (PCa) is one of the most frequently diagnosed malignancies worldwide. Hormonal deprivation therapy is a well-established treatment for locally advanced or metastatic diseases but exposes patients to the risk of osteoporosis and fragility fractures. Furthermore, the tropism of the PCa cells to osseous metastases increases the incidence of skeletal-related events (SREs). *Methods.* A nonsystematic review of the international literature was performed in respect to the use of osteoclast inhibitors zoledronic acid (ZA) and denosumab (DEN) in PCa patients. *Results.* DEN and ZA have proved their efficacy in preventing osteoporosis and bone mass loss in patients treated with hormonal therapy with no proven superiority of one agent over the other. However, the effectiveness in reducing fragility fractures has been proved only for DEN so far. In metastatic-free castrate-sensitive high-risk PCa patients, ZA has not shown any efficacy in preventing osseous metastasis, and evidence is lacking in favor or against the use of DEN. The use of osteoclasts inhibitors had no evident positive effect in overall and disease-specific survival in this group of patients. In advanced castrate-refractory malignancy, DEN has shown clinical superiority over ZA in preventing new SRE but not in overall survival. *Conclusion.* Superiority of DEN over ZA has been proved only in advanced castrate refractory disease in terms of preventing new SRE. In the rest of the cases, the selection of either agent should be based on the clinical condition of each patient and the cost of the treatment.

1. Introduction

Prostate cancer (PCa) is the second most prevalent malignancy worldwide [1, 2]. According to the US Cancer Statistics, during the year 2014, 172,258 new cases were diagnosed and 28,343 deaths were attributed to the disease in this country [1]. Despite the efforts for cancer control, about 6% patients will eventually develop skeletal metastasis during follow-up. This rate climbs up to 80%, should a poorly differentiated PCA is left untreated [3–7].

One of the characteristics of the PCa cells is their tropism to osseous metastases. Bone metastasis is a major factor of morbidity and mortality, causing a plethora of symptoms, such as persistent skeletal pain, bone fractures, spinal cord compression, and severe disability [3, 8, 9] thus, jeopardizing the patients' quality of life (QoL). The term *skeletal-related events* (SREs) has been used as a clinical endpoint which include the detection of pathologic bone fractures, the spinal cord compression, and the need for orthopedic surgery intervention or for palliative radiation to the bone [10].

Not only it is the malignancy itself but also the relevant therapy that may have a negative impact to the skeletal health. Osteopenia and osteoporosis are potential side-effects of pharmaceutical or surgical castration, which pose a threat to the skeletal health. The risk of therapeutic-induced bone fracture is directly related to the duration of treatment [8, 11, 12].

The phenotype of the metastatic PCa is characterized by intense osteoblastic activity. However, recent evidence suggests that a sequence of osteoblastic and osteoclastic activity takes place. At early stages, skeletal metastases with osteolytic lesions are detected but later on, the osteoblastic phenotype prevails at a rate up to 90% [9]. The tumor-induced disruption of the normal bone structure leads to the debulking of the osseous tissue, which explains the fragility of the bones with metastatic sites and the high fracture rates. [9].

Patients with metastatic disease describe episodes of extreme pain as a result of metastatic tumor invasion into the periosteum, the bone marrow cavity, and the bone matrix, which are innervated by sensory and sympathetic fibers. The bone sites affected by the tumor produce and release a plethora of stimuli to the peripheral nerve endings (for example, TNFα, prostaglandins (PGs), interleukin-1 (Il-1), and nerve growth factor). The stimuli activate the afferent nerve terminals inducing the phosphorylation of afferent sensory pathways and the generation of action potential. The action potential is transmitted via the primary afferent sensory nerves to the dorsal horn of the spinal cord, which subsequently activates the second-order neurons, thus transmitting the noxious signal up to the somatosensory cortex of the brain. In chronic pain conditions, the peripheral nerves along with other sites in the afferent pathways are shifted to a hypersensitive state and pain is perceived at a lower threshold of noxious stimuli [9].

For addressing the metastatic lesions to the bones and the relevant complications, several therapeutic options have been proposed. These comprise the delivery of external radiation therapy, radiation emitting isotopes (Str-89, Sa-153, and recently Ra-223), chemotherapy, new generation hormonal agents (e.g, enzalutamide), CYP17A1 inhibitor (abiraterone), and bone-targeted agents against osteoclast activity (bisphosphonates and denosumab (DEN)) [3, 13].

It is considered that the bisphosphonates and the RANK-L inhibitors play an important role in preserving the bone health and in inducing the osteoclasts' apoptosis. The rationale behind the use of these agents in osseous metastases is that, by remodeling the osseous tissue, the production of stimuli of the peripheral nerves (TNF, Il, PG, etc.) is controlled and the activation of afferent pathways is minimized [9].

The aim of this review article is to present the contemporary role of bisphosphonates and DEN not only in preventing drug-related osteoporosis and osteopenia but also in alleviating the metastatic pain and in treating the SRE in patients with prostate cancer.

2. Materials and Methods

A search in Medline/PubMed and Scopus databases from 1980 till now was performed using the following key words: *prostate cancer*, *bone metastasis*, *zoledronic acid*, *denosumab*, and *bisphosphonates*. Additional articles were identified by using the "similar articles" search tool of the Medline electronic platform, as well as by reviewing the list of references of related articles. A list of 2133 titles of articles and 24 additional records were initially evaluated by 2 authors DK and DP for relevance, and 102 abstracts of all types of articles (reviews, randomized controlled trials, and case series) were further examined. Full texts were retrieved by 57/102 articles and, after having the consensus of all the co-authors, 31 of them were included in the study (Figure 1). The clinical effects of osteoclast inhibitors were examined in various prostate cancer subpopulations (for example, castration-sensitive, castration refractory, and with or without skeletal metastasis), and the relevant results are presented herein.

3. Results

3.1. Bisphosphonates

3.1.1. Pathophysiology. Pyrophosphates are natural anions produced by the hydrolysis of ATP in cells. The biochemical role of these unstable anions is to inhibit the cascade of cholesterol biosynthesis in the osteoclasts' cytoskeleton, promoting changes in its function which induce the apoptosis of the cells [14]. It is estimated that the clinical role of this action is to maintain the integrity and correct the bone mass loss in sites affected by neoplasmatic cells [8]. By substituting oxygen with carbon, a stable compound is generated named bisphosphonate. First generation bisphosphonates are etidronate and clodronate, while pamidronate and zoledronic acid (ZA) are second and third generations respectively [3].

3.1.2. Bisphosphonates (excluding ZA), Castration-Sensitive M1. In older studies performed in castration-sensitive patients with osseous metastases, oral clodronate may marginally (not statistical significantly) prolong the onset of new skeletal symptoms and marginally increase survival compared to placebo. The drug is likely to prevent the worsening of the performance status but with a cost of high incidence of gastrointestinal side-effects, increased lactate dehydrogenase serum levels, and need for frequent dose adjustments [15]. An update of the original paper published six years later, denoted that first generation bisphosphonates compared to placebo could have a positive impact on overall survival among patients with metastatic disease (HR: 0.77, 95% CI: 0.60–0.98, $p = 0.032$). On the contrary, metastases-free patients do not experience prolonged survival (HR: 1.12 95% CI: 0.89–1.42, $p = 0.94$) [16].

Other reports revealed that clodronate failed to show clinical efficacy in alleviating pain and improving QoL in patients with castration-resistant disease and osseous metastasis [17]. Administration of 1400 mg clodronate once daily was recently compared with 4 mg of ZA iv once a month. In this prospective randomized trial conducted in castration-sensitive PCa patients with bone metastasis, ZA showed longer bone progression-free survival, improved control of skeletal pain, and significant increase of bone mineral density of the lumbar spine compared with clodronate. However, no benefit in overall survival between the two agents was recorded [18].

Older studies have tested low (30 mg every 2 weeks and 60 mg every 4 weeks) versus high (60 mg every 2 weeks or 90 mg every 4 weeks) dosages of pamidronate, a second

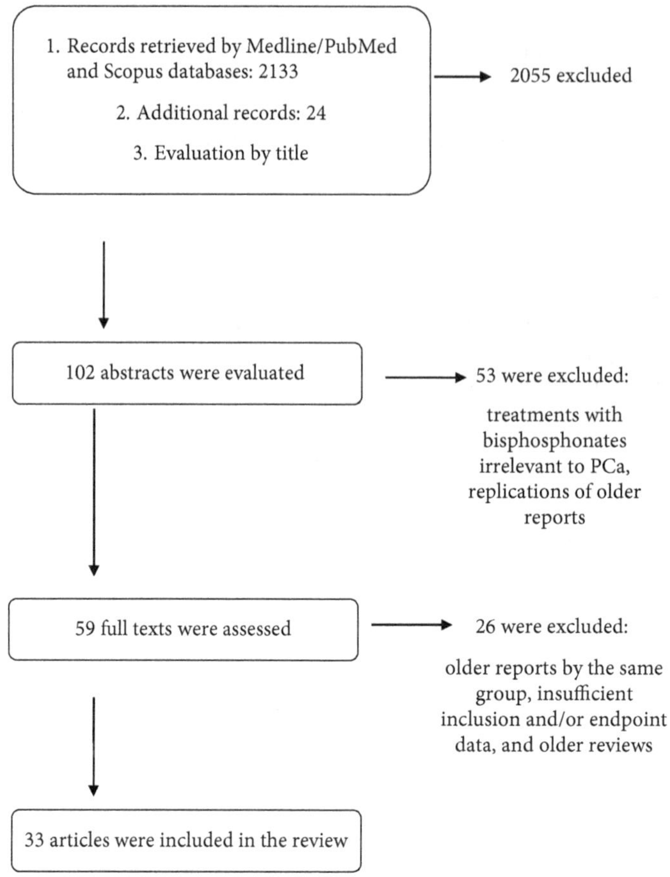

Figure 1: Flowchart of the review process.

generation bisphosphonate, in palliative treatment of metastatic prostate and breast cancer patients. In breast cancer population, a 25% healing of metastatic lesions was observed but only for high dose of pamidronate. In PCa patients, however, none of the tested dosages was effective. It could be assumed that these two malignancies may have a different degree of metastatic potential to the bones at least at baseline [19]. Likewise, Coleman et al. did not reveal any clinical efficacy in high-dose pamidronate in patients with as high bone resorption rates as those encountered in prostate cancer [20].

More recently, in a pooled analysis of 2 randomized controlled trials, Small et al. failed to show any significant improvement of pamidronate in alleviating bone pain and preventing the onset of new SRE in patients with osseous metastasis compared to placebo [21].

3.1.3. ZA, Castration-Sensitive M0. The third generation of bisphosphonates has been extensively examined in several clinical scenarios. In RTOG 0518 phase III clinical trial conducted in castration-sensitive nonmetastatic PCa patients, ZA showed a protective role in preventing hormonal deprivation-induced osteoporotic events compared to placebo but no difference in prevention of bone fractures or in improving QoL [22]. In another study, in which patients exposed to castration treatment for up to one year were recruited, the authors concluded that 4 mg of ZA iv every 3 months statistically significantly increased the bone mineral density by 3.6% in the femoral neck, 3.8% in the total hip, and 6.7% in the lumbar spine over placebo [23]. However, the authors provide no data in respect to fragility fracture rates, and the effects of ZA in fracture risk cannot be estimated.

In the Zometa European Study (ZEUS, 2015), the role of ZA in the prevention of skeletal metastasis in high-risk patients was examined. High risk was defined as PSA equal to or greater than 20 ng/ml and/or positive lymph nodes and/or Gleason score 8–10. Following the administration of the agent every three months for 4.8 years along with the standard therapy, no protective role against bone metastasis was revealed compared to the standard care alone (bone metastases rates: 14.7 and 13.2% for ZA and control group, respectively, $p = 0.65$) [24].

3.1.4. ZA, Castration-Sensitive M+. In the STAMPEDE trial (2016), high-risk PCa patients with and without osseous metastases were enrolled. The addition of ZA to the standard care also failed to improve overall survival (OS), and the authors concluded the agent has no role in delaying the onset of metastases in high-risk population [25].

The GALGB 90202 trial studied the effect of early administration (before the onset of castration resistance) of 4 mg of ZA every 4 weeks versus placebo in castration-sensitive metastatic PCa. Similar to the STAMPEDE trial, ZA was associated neither with a prolonged time before the onset of SRE (HR: 0.97, 95% CI: 0–1.17, $p = 0.39$) nor with an improved survival (HR: 0.88, 95% CI: 0.70–1.12, $p = 0.29$) [26]. In another multicenter randomized phase III trial (ZAPCA), no benefit was demonstrated in respect to the time of treatment failure, the time to new SRE, and OS. However, in patients with low baseline PSA (<200 ng/ml), a beneficial role of ZA in delaying the treatment failure was revealed (HR: 0.58, 95% CI: 035–0.93, $p = 0.023$) [27]. In another paper, an improvement in progression-free survival, skeletal pain, and SRE was recorded only in patients with Gleason score equal or greater than 8 [28], while others revealed a beneficial role of ZA only in time to PSA failure [29].

3.1.5. ZA, Castration-Resistant M+. Older studies have demonstrated the beneficial role of the agent in metastatic castration-resistant patients. Saad et al. showed that the administration of 4 mg every three weeks significantly reduced the incidence of SRE (33.2% versus 44.2% of placebo, 95% CI; −20.3% to −1.8%, $p = 0.021$), increased time prior to the onset of skeletal events (not reached for ZA 4 mg, 321 days for placebo, $p = 0.011$), and reduced the pain scores as well as the need for analgesic consumption compared to placebo. On the contrary, no difference was noted in disease progression, performance status, or QoL. This study also defined that due to the better tolerance profile and fewer side effects, 4 mg is the optimal dose compared to 8 mg [30]. Two years later, an update of the original paper was published, evaluating the long-term results of the agent. Compared with placebo, the administration of 4 mg of ZA was associated with fewer patients with (at least one) SRE (38% vs 49%, 95% CI: −20.2% to −1.3%, $p = 0.28$), increased time to first SRE (448 for ZA vs 321 for placebo, $p = 0.009$), and reduced the total risk for SRE by 36% (risk ratio 0.64, 95% CI: 0.485–0.845, $p = 0.002$), proving the effectiveness of ZA on a long-term basis [31].

Recent evidence suggests that ZA can be effectively combined with docetaxel-containing chemotherapy. Data from the TRAPEZE trial revealed that although no improvement in progression-free survival (PFS) and OS was noted, ZA increased the time interval before the onset of new SRE and diminished the incidence of SRE by approximately one third. The authors concluded that ZA might play a role in maintenance therapy following the chemotherapy [32].

In a recent systematic review based on the Cochrane Controlled Trials Registry and the Medline database, the authors extracted results from 18 randomized controlled trials about the role of bisphosphonates in patients with bone metastasis. They concluded that they had no benefit in pain response and that they probably decreased the disease progression and the number of SRE compared to the control group. However, the clinical benefit should be weighed against the potential complications of the therapy before decision-making [33]. An overview of the main publications regarding ZA is presented in Table 1.

3.1.6. Complications. In respect to the drug-related complications, bisphosphonates, particularly ZA, have been associated with renal failure and jaw osteonecrosis. It was estimated that the rate of renal failure was approximately 15% and 21% for the dose of 4 and 8 mg of ZA, respectively. By adjusting the dose in 4 mg and lowering the infusion rate, the incidence of renal failure reached the corresponding rate of placebo group [30]. The osteonecrosis of the jaw, which is defined as "the presence of exposed bone in the oral cavity despite the appropriate management for 8 weeks," represents a rare complication with an incidence up to 1.3%. It has been correlated with a history of tooth extraction, poor oral hygiene and perhaps smoking, diabetes mellitus, anemia, and the use of antiproliferative agents [12]. Improving the patients' dental health may diminish the jaw osteonecrosis events. Hypocalcemia is rarely encountered and should be corrected with administration of calcium supplements and vitamin D. Other potential complications are nausea, vomiting, fatigue, hyperpyrexia, anemia, and myalgia [12, 33].

3.2. Denosumab

3.2.1. Pathophysiology. Osteoblasts are bone cells that produce new osseous tissue and also express the receptor activator of nuclear factor-κB ligand (RANK-L). This molecule binds to the corresponding receptor (RANK) carried by the premature osteoclasts (preosteoclasts). The activation of this receptor promotes the maturation of the cells towards multinucleated osteoclasts. In high turnover conditions, such as in metastatic sites of prostatic malignancy, the RANK-L is highly expressed leading to bone resorption [9, 11]. Denosumab (DEN) a fully human monoclonal antibody IgG2 against RANK-L. It is estimated that the inhibition of osteoclasts' activity promoted by this agent may prevent the bone destruction process and the SRE caused by the deposition and activation of malignant cells on the bone tissue [9].

3.2.2. Castration-Sensitive M0. In 1,468 patients with castration-sensitive PCa without skeletal metastasis, it has been shown that the administration of 60 mg DEN subcutaneously every 6 months for 36 months increased the bone mineral density in multiple skeletal sites (lumbar spine, total hip, and distal radius) [11]. In a comparative study with similar population, the administration of 60 mg DEN statistically significantly decreased the likelihood of new vertebral fractures (RR: 0.38, 95% CI 0.19–0.78; $p = 0.006$) compared to placebo [34].

These studies indicate that DEN plays a protective role in preventing osteoporosis and osteopenia, which is frequently diagnosed in patients treated with hormonal deprivation agents. A recent meta-analysis compared the efficacy of antiosteoporotic medications in metastatic-free castration-sensitive patients. DEN and ZA showed equivalent efficacy in terms of improvement of bone mass density [35]. In this meta-analysis, the bone mass density was used as a surrogate

Table 1: Main publications regarding ZA.

Reference	Study population	Treatment	End points
[22] RTOG 0518	CS M0	ZA 4 mg vs placebo	↑ BMD in lumbar spine (6% vs −5%, $p < 0.0001$), left total hip (1% vs −8%, $p < 0.0002$), and femoral neck (3% vs −8%, $p = 0.0007$) No prevention of bone fractures or QoL
[23]	CS M0, <1 year ADT	ZA vs placebo	↑ BMD in femoral neck by 3.6% ($p = 0.0004$), hip by 3.8% ($p < 0.0001$), and spine bone by 6.7% ($p < 0.0001$)
[24] ZEUS 2015	PSA>20 ± LN+ ± gleason 8–10	ZA 4 mg + SOC vs SOC	Bone metastases: 14.7% in ZA vs 13.2% in placebo ($p = 0.65$); no protection from skeletal metastases
[25] STAMPEDE	CS, high-risk PCa (61% M1, 15% N+/M0, 24% N0M0,	ZA 4 mg + SOC vs SOC vs SOC + Doc vs SOC+ ZA +Doc	Median OS: NR for ZA + SOC vs 71 m for SOC vs 81 m for Doc + SOC vs 76 m for SOC + Doc + ZA No increased survival for ZA No delay of metastases for ZA
[26] GALBG 90202	CS M+	ZA 4 mg vs placebo	Similar time for new SRE: median time: 31.9 m for ZA vs 29.8 m for placebo ($p = 0.39$); no increased OS (HR: 0.88; 95% CI: 0.70–1.12, $p = 0.29$)
[27] ZAPCA	CS M+	ZA 4 mg + complete androgen blockade (CAB) vs CAB alone	Similar time to failure: 12.4 m vs 9.7 m (HR: 0.75, 95% CI: 0.57–1; $p = 0.051$); ↑ time to new SRE for ZA + CAB (64.7 vs 45.9 m, HR: 0.58; 95 % CI 0.38–0.88; $p = 0.009$) For PSA < 200, delay in treatment failure for ZA + CAB: 23.7 m vs 9.8 m (HR: 0.58, 95% CI: 0.35–0.93; $p = 0.023$)
[30]	CR M+	ZA 8 mg vs ZA 4 mg vs placebo	SRE for 4 mg ZA: 33.2% vs 44.2% placebo, 95% CI; −20.3% to −1.8%, $p = 0.021$; SRE for 8 mg ZA: 38.5% vs 32.74% placebo, 95% CI; −15.1% to 3.6%, $p = 0.222$. ZA 4 (but not 8) mg: ↓ incidence of SRE, ↑ time to new SRE, ↓ pain score No difference in PCa progression, PS & QoL
[31] (long term results of [30])	CR M+	ZA 4 mg vs placebo	↓ pts with SRE (38% for ZA vs 49%, 95% CI: −20.2% to −1.3%, p=0.28), ↑ time to first SRE (448d for ZA vs 321, p=0.009), ↓ risk for SRE by 36% (risk ratio: 0.64, 95% CI: 0.485–0.845, p=0.002)
[32] TRAPEZE	CR M+/45% radiation therapy, median PSA: 146 mg/ml	Doc vs Doc + ZA 4 mg vs Doc + ZA + Strontium-89 (Sr)	Similar CPFS for Doc vs Doc + ZA: HR, 0.98; 95% CI, 0.85–1.14; $p = 0.81$; similar OS for Doc vs Doc + ZA: HR, 0.99; 95% CI, 0.84–1.16; $p = 0.91$
[33] meta-analysis	18 RCT, CR M+	ZA vs control	Probably ↓ disease progression and ↓ SRE, with ZA, no effect in mortality, no effect in pair response Concern for potential complications

of the fracture risk. However, the clinical effectiveness of DEN and ZA in reducing the fragility fracture rates cannot be actually evaluated in this meta-analysis.

3.2.3. Castration-Resistant M0. In a multicenter, randomized double-blind placebo-controlled trial, the role of DEN was evaluated in the prevention of skeletal metastasis in castration-resistant PCa. Compared to placebo, 120 mg DEN administered subcutaneously increased significantly the bone metastasis-free survival by 4.2 months (HR: 0.85, 95% CI: 0.73–0.98, $p = 0.028$) and the time to first SRE (HR: 0.84, 95% CI: 0.71–0.98, $p = 0.032$) but not the overall survival (HR: 1.01, 95% CI: 0.85–1.20, $p = 0.91$) [36]. This study was one of the 6 RCTs included in a recent meta-analysis conducted in nonmetastatic patients. In the rest 5 trials, bisphosphonates were compared with the standard of care and a total of 5,974 cases were analyzed. The polled analysis showed that the bisphosphonates do not alter the incidence of skeletal metastases (HR: 1.09, 95% CI: 0.84–1.41, $p = 0.51$). In contrast, the aforementioned DEN trial [36] proved the effectiveness of RANK-L agents in delaying the onset of skeletal lesions in castration-resistant patients. It was also reconfirmed that the use of osteoclasts inhibitors of either group had no effect in overall and disease-specific survival [10].

It should be noted that evidence is lacking regarding the role of DEN in preventing the skeletal metastases castration-sensitive patients. In this group, it has already been shown that ZA does not improve time to SRE and overall survival and cannot be considered as an adjunct to the standard treatment [24, 25]. DEN plays a protective role in the prevention of osteoporosis and in the elimination of vertebral fracture events attributed to the castration. However the role of RANK-L agents in the prevention of skeletal dissemination of malignancy in castration-sensitive high-risk for metastases patients is still unknown and should be addressed in future studies.

3.2.4. Castration-Resistant M+. Other studies have directly compared the clinical effectiveness of bisphosphonates (specifically of ZA) with DEN in castration-refractory PCa patients. In a phase 3 multicenter randomized double-blind study, DEN was superior to ZA in preventing new SRE. The mean time to new (on study) SRE was 20.7 and 17.1 months for DEN and ZA, respectively (HR: 0.82, 95% CI: 0.71–0.95, $p = 0.0002$) [37]. In another phase 3 study published in 2015, it was reconfirmed that DEN is superior to ZA in reducing the risk of the first and any subsequent adverse event ($p = 0.005$ and $p = 0.004$, respectively) associated with the skeletal system, including skeletal pain and subclinical fractures [38].

Others have evaluated the value-for-money of DEN with that of ZA. DEN administration is related to fewer SRE and lower SRE cost. However, the estimated drug-related cost in the US was more than 10,000$ over that of ZA. Likewise, despite the fewer SRE attributed to DEN, the total cost per patient was more than 7,000$ higher than that of bisphosphonates, raising severe questions in respect to the cost-effectiveness of DEN [39]. Publications regarding the use of DEN in prostate cancer patients are provided in Table 2.

3.2.5. Complications. The safety profile of DEN is different from that of bisphosphonates. RANK-L agents have no detrimental effect on the renal function, should GFR is greater than 30 ml/min. Dose adjustment and monitoring of renal function is necessary only in patients with severe renal impairment [14]. Jaw osteonecrosis and hypocalcemia are rare but well-recognized side-effects of DEN encountered at rates up to 5% and 2%, respectively [36]. The risk for osteonecrosis is related to the duration of treatment [12, 14]. Correction of dental pathology and improvement of oral hygiene prior to the initiation of antiresorptive treatment may eliminate the osteonecrosis events. The hypocalcemia is more frequently diagnosed with DEN than with ZA (13% vs 6% in metastatic castration-resistant patients). Administration of oral calcium supplements with vitamin D is recommended for the correction of low calcium levels [12]. Acute phase reactions (e.g., fever, chills, and myalgia) may be encountered in patients under any antiresorptive treatment, but the corresponding rates are lower for DEN (8%) versus ZA (18%). Ocular side-effects, including eyelid edema, cataract, scleritis, and conjunctivitis, attributed to DEN, are very rare and respond well to treatment with cortisone. Cataract has been associated with disorders in calcium homeostasis [14].

4. Conclusions

Both main antiresorptive agents have proven their safety and effectiveness in preventing bone mass loss and osteoporosis in patients treated with hormonal therapy. In this population, a face to face comparison of DEN with ZA did not reveal superiority of any regimen over the other. However, effectiveness in reducing fragility fracture risks has been proven only for DEN. In castration-sensitive high risk for metastases PCa patients, ZA has not shown any efficacy in preventing osseous metastasis but DEN has not been extensively evaluated in these patients. Regarding cases with advanced disease in castration-resistant malignancy, DEN has shown clinical superiority over ZA in preventing new skeletal events and complications, but not in overall survival. One study indicates that clodronate may prolong survival in metastatic PCa, but before any generalization, the results should be replicated by others in comparative studies.

Chemotherapy has now emerged as a first-line treatment in patients with metastasic disease, but the combined treatment with docetaxel and ZA did not show any benefit in clinical progression and in overall survival compared to chemotherapy alone. However, the results of the addition of RANK-L agents to chemotherapy have not been examined so far. Furthermore, because none of the osteoclasts inhibitors has been coadministered with the newer hormonal agents, such as enzalutamide or abiraterone acetate in PCa patients, future trials could investigate the clinical outcomes of the combined therapy in metastatic population.

The cost of RANK-L agents, which is very high compared to that of bisphosphonates, should be considered prior to initiation of treatment. In patients with renal impairment, DEN should be preferred over ZA due to better safety profile. There some evidence that jaw osteonecrosis rates are comparable between these two agents and increase with the

Table 2: Main publications regarding DEN.

Reference	Study population	Treatment	End points
[11]	CS M0	DEN 60 mg vs placebo	↑ BMD in lumbar spine by 7.9%, total hip 5.7%, and distal radius 6.9% ($p < 0.0001$ for all sites)
[34] HALT	CS M0	DEN 60 mg vs placebo	↓ incidence of vertebral fractures at 36 months (1.5% vs. 3.9%) (RR: 0.38; 95% CC, 0.19 to 0.78; $p = 0.006$)
[35] meta-analysis	CS M0	DEN vs ZA vs others	Similar improvement in BMD for DEN and ZA (3% hip, 3% femoral, 6% lumbar)
[36]	CR M0/high risk (PSA > 8 mg/ml or and PSA DT < 10 m)	DEN 120 mg vs placebo	↑ median bone metastasis-free survival by 4.2 m with DEN (29. 5 vs 25.2, HR: 0.85, 95% CI 0.73–0.98, $p = 0.028$) ↑ time to first SRE (median 33.2 vs 29.5 m; HR 0·84, 95% CI: 0.71–0.98, $p = 0.032$) No improvement of survival (43.9 m vs 44.8, HR: 1.01, 95% CI: 0.85–1.20, $p = 0.91$)
[37]	CR M+/SRE	DEN 120 mg vs ZA 40 mg	↑ time to new SRE by 20.7 m with DEN vs 17.1 m with ZA (HR: 0.82, 95% CI 0.71–0·95; $p = 0.008$)
[38]	CR M+/symptomatic skeletal events	DEN 120 mg vs ZA 4 mg	↓ risk for new SRE for DEN (HR, 0.78; 95% CI: 0.66–0.93; $p = 0.005$) ↓ risk for any SRE for DEN (rate ratio: 0.78; 95% CI: 0.65–0.92; $p = 0.004$)

duration of treatment, but the incidence of hypocalcemia is higher in DEN and acute phase reactions are more frequent with ZA.

Abbreviations

BMD: bone mass density
FU: follow-up
NR: not reached
Doc: docetaxel
CS: castration-sensitive
ZA: zometa
HR: hazard ratio
CI: confidence interval
CPFS: clinical progression-free survival
QoL: quality of life
ADT: androgen-deprivation therapy
LN: lymph nodes
SOC: standard of care
SREs: skeletal-related events
CS: castration-resistant
OS: overall survival
PS: performance status
RTC: randomized control trials
DEN: denosumab
DT: doubling time.

Acknowledgments

The authors would like to express their sincere thanks to Miss Martha Mantakou, Msc, in Translation and English Studies, for her kind support in the grammatical editing of the manuscript.

References

[1] United States Cancer Statistics, *1999–2014 Incidence and Mortality Web-based Report*, U.S. Department of Health and Human Services, Centers for Disease Control and Prevention and National Cancer Institute, Atlanta, Georgia, 2017.

[2] J. Ferlay, I. Soerjomataram, R. Dikshit et al., "Cancer incidence and mortality worldwide: sources, methods and major patterns in GLOBOCAN 2012," *International Journal of Cancer*, vol. 136, no. 5, pp. E359–E386, 2014.

[3] B. I. Carlin and G. L. Andriole, "The natural history, skeletal complications, and management of bone metastases in patients with prostate carcinoma," *Cancer*, vol. 88, no. 12, pp. 2989–2994, 2000.

[4] A. Briganti, R. J. Karnes, G. Gandaglia et al., "Natural history of surgically treated high-risk prostate cancer," *Urologic Oncology: Seminars and Original Investigations*, vol. 33, no. 4, pp. 163.e7–163.e13, 2015.

[5] A. J. Katz and J. Kang, "Quality of life and toxicity after SBRT for organ-confined prostate cancer, a 7-year study," *Frontiers in Oncology*, vol. 4, p. 301, 2014.

[6] R. Siegel, J. Ma, Z. Zou, and A. Jemal, "Cancer statistics, 2014," *CA: A Cancer Journal for Clinicians*, vol. 64, no. 1, pp. 9–29, 2014.

[7] V. Beckendorf, S. Guerif, E. Le Prisé et al., "70 Gy versus 80 Gy in localized prostate cancer: 5-year results of GETUG 06 randomized trial," *International Journal of Radiation Oncology Biology Physics*, vol. 80, no. 4, pp. 1056–1063, 2011.

[8] M. Iranikhah, S. Stricker, and M. K. Freeman, "Future of bisphosphonates and denosumab for men with advanced prostate cancer," *Cancer Management and Research*, vol. 6, pp. 217–224, 2014.

[9] A. Muralidharan and M. T. Smith, "Pathobiology and management of prostate cancer-induced bone pain: recent

insights and future treatments," *Inflammopharmacology*, vol. 21, no. 5, pp. 339–363, 2013.

[10] A. R. Hayes, D. Brungs, and N. Pavlakis, "Osteoclast inhibitors to prevent bone metastases in men with high-risk, non-metastatic prostate cancer: a systematic review and meta-analysis," *PLoS ONE*, vol. 13, no. 1, Article ID e0191455, 2018.

[11] M. R. Smith, F. Saad, B. Egerdie et al., "Effects of denosumab on bone mineral density in men receiving androgen deprivation therapy for prostate cancer," *The Journal of Urology*, vol. 182, no. 6, pp. 2670–2676, 2009.

[12] B. A. Gartrell, R. E. Coleman, K. Fizazi, K. Miller, F. Saad, and C. N. Sternberg, "Toxicities following treatment with bisphosphonates and receptor activator of nuclear factor-κb ligand inhibitors in patients with advanced prostate cancer," *European Urology*, vol. 65, no. 2, pp. 278–286, 2014.

[13] F. Vignani, V. Bertaglia, C. Buttigliero, M. Tucci, G. V. Scagliotti, and M. Di Maio, "Skeletal metastases and impact of anticancer and bone-targeted agents in patients with castration-resistant prostate cancer," *Cancer Treatment Reviews*, vol. 44, pp. 61–73, 2016.

[14] R. Cathomas, Z. Bajory, M. Bouzid et al., "Management of bone metastases in patients with castration-resistant prostate cancer," *Urologia Internationalis*, vol. 92, no. 4, pp. 377–386, 2014.

[15] D. P. Dearnaley, M. R. Sydes, M. D. Mason et al., "A double-blind, placebo-controlled, randomized trial of oral sodium clodronate for metastatic prostate cancer (MRC PR05 trial)," *CancerSpectrum Knowledge Environment*, vol. 95, no. 17, pp. 1300–1311, 2003.

[16] D. P. Dearnaley, M. D. Mason, M. K. Parmar, K. Sanders, and M. R. Sydes, "Adjuvant therapy with oral sodium clodronate in locally advanced and metastatic prostate cancer: long-term overall survival results from the MRC PR04 and PR05 randomised controlled trials," *The Lancet Oncology*, vol. 10, no. 9, pp. 872–876, 2009.

[17] D. S. Ernst, I. F. Tannock, E. W. Winquist et al., "Randomized, double-blind, controlled trial of mitoxantrone/prednisone and clodronate versus mitoxantrone/prednisone and placebo in patients with hormone-refractory prostate cancer and pain," *Journal of Clinical Oncology*, vol. 21, no. 17, pp. 3335–3342, 2003.

[18] F. Wang, W. Chen, H. Chen et al., "Comparison between zoledronic acid and clodronate in the treatment of prostate cancer patients with bone metastases," *Medical Oncology*, vol. 30, no. 3, p. 657, 2013.

[19] A. Lipton, D. Glover, H. Harvey et al., "Pamidronate in the treatment of bone metastases: results of 2 dose-ranging trials in patients with breast or prostate cancer," *Annals of oncology: official journal of the European Society for Medical Oncology/ ESMO*, vol. 5, no. 7, pp. S31–S35, 1994.

[20] R. E. Coleman, O. P. Purohit, J. J. Vinholes, and J. Zekri, "High dose pamidronate," *Cancer*, vol. 80, no. 8, pp. 1686–1690, 1997.

[21] E. J. Small, M. R. Smith, J. J. Seaman, S. Petrone, and M. O. Kowalski, "Combined analysis of two multicenter, randomized, placebo-controlled studies of pamidronate disodium for the palliation of bone pain in men with metastatic prostate cancer," *Journal of Clinical Oncology*, vol. 21, no. 23, pp. 4277–4284, 2003.

[22] L. A. Kachnic, S. L. Pugh, P. Tai et al., "RTOG 0518: randomized phase III trial to evaluate zoledronic acid for prevention of osteoporosis and associated fractures in prostate cancer patients," *Prostate Cancer and Prostatic Diseases*, vol. 16, no. 4, pp. 382–386, 2013.

[23] C. W. Ryan, D. Huo, L. M. Demers, T. M. Beer, and L. V. Lacerna, "Zoledronic acid initiated during the first year of androgen deprivation therapy increases bone mineral density in patients with prostate cancer," *The Journal of Urology*, vol. 176, no. 3, pp. 972–978, 2006.

[24] M. Wirth, T. Tammela, V. Cicalese et al., "Prevention of bone metastases in patients with high-risk nonmetastatic prostate cancer treated with zoledronic acid: efficacy and safety results of the Zometa European Study (ZEUS)," *European Urology*, vol. 67, no. 3, pp. 482–491, 2015.

[25] N. D. James, M. R. Sydes, N. W. Clarke et al., "Addition of docetaxel, zoledronic acid, or both to first-line long-term hormone therapy in prostate cancer (STAMPEDE): survival results from an adaptive, multiarm, multistage, platform randomised controlled trial," *The Lancet*, vol. 387, no. 1024, pp. 1163–1177, 2016.

[26] M. R. Smith, S. Halabi, C. J. Ryan et al., "Randomized controlled trial of early zoledronic acid in men with castration-sensitive prostate cancer and bone metastases: results of CALGB 90202 (alliance)," *Journal of Clinical Oncology*, vol. 32, no. 11, pp. 1143–1150, 2014.

[27] T. Kamba, T. Lingua::EN::Titlecase, T. Kamoto et al., "A phase III multicenter, randomized, controlled study of combined androgen blockade with versus without zoledronic acid in prostate cancer patients with metastatic bone disease: results of the ZAPCA trial," *International Journal of Clinical Oncology*, vol. 22, no. 1, pp. 166–173, 2016.

[28] S. Ueno, A. Mizokami, T. Fukagai et al., "Efficacy of combined androgen blockade with zoledronic acid treatment in prostate cancer with bone metastasis: the ZABTON-PC (zoledronic acid/androgen blockade trial on prostate cancer) study," *Anticancer Research*, vol. 33, no. 9, pp. 3837–3844, 2013.

[29] T. Okegawa, M. Higaki, T. Matsumoto, H. Kase et al., "Bone Metastasis Prostate Cancer Group. Zoledronic acid improves clinical outcomes in patients with bone metastatic hormone-naïve prostate cancer in a multicenter clinical trial," *Anticancer Researchs*, vol. 34, no. 8, pp. 4415–4420, 2014.

[30] F. Saad, D. M. Gleason, R. Murray et al., "A randomized, placebo-controlled trial of zoledronic acid in patients with hormone-refractory metastatic prostate carcinoma," *JNCI Journal of the National Cancer Institute*, vol. 94, no. 19, pp. 1458–1468, 2002.

[31] F. Saad, D. M. Gleason, R. Murray et al., "Long-term efficacy of zoledronic acid for the prevention of skeletal complications in patients with metastatic hormone-refractory prostate cancer," *JNCI Journal of the National Cancer Institute*, vol. 96, no. 11, pp. 879–882, 2004.

[32] N. D. James, S. J. Pirrie, A. M. Pope et al., "Clinical outcomes and survival following treatment of metastatic castrate-refractory prostate cancer with docetaxel alone or with strontium-89, zoledronic acid, or both," *JAMA Oncology*, vol. 2, no. 4, pp. 493–499, 2016.

[33] S. Macherey, I. Monsef, F. Jahn et al., "Bisphosphonates for advanced prostate cancer," *Cochrane Database of Systematic Reviews*, vol. 12, article CD006250, 2017.

[34] M. R. Smith, B. Egerdie, N. H. Toriz et al., "Denosumab in men receiving androgen-deprivation therapy for prostate cancer," *New England Journal of Medicine*, vol. 361, no. 8, pp. 745–755, 2009.

[35] Y. Poon, P. Pechlivanoglou, S. M. H. Alibhai et al., "Systematic review and network meta-analysis on the relative efficacy of osteoporotic medications: men with prostate cancer on continuous androgen-deprivation therapy to reduce risk of

fragility fractures," *BJU International*, vol. 121, no. 1, pp. 17–28, 2017.

[36] M. R. Smith, F. Saad, R. Coleman et al., "Denosumab and bone-metastasis-free survival in men with castration-resistant prostate cancer: results of a phase 3, randomised, placebo-controlled trial," *The Lancet*, vol. 379, no. 9810, pp. 39–46, 2012.

[37] K. Fizazi, M. Carducci, M. Smith et al., "Denosumab versus zoledronic acid for treatment of bone metastases in men with castration-resistant prostate cancer: a randomised, double-blind study," *The Lancet*, vol. 377, no. 9768, pp. 813–822, 2011.

[38] M. R. Smith, R. E. Coleman, L. Klotz et al., "Denosumab for the prevention of skeletal complications in metastatic castration-resistant prostate cancer: comparison of skeletal-related events and symptomatic skeletal events," *Annals of Oncology*, vol. 26, no. 2, pp. 368–374, 2014.

[39] S. J. Snedecor, J. A. Carter, S. Kaura, and M. F. Botteman, "Denosumab versus zoledronic acid for treatment of bone metastases in men with castration-resistant prostate cancer: a cost-effectiveness analysis," *Journal of Medical Economics*, vol. 16, no. 1, pp. 19–29, 2012.

3

Combined Dorsal and Ventral Onlay Buccal Graft Technique for Large and Complex Penile Strictures

Nikolaos Mertziotis, Andreas Konandreas, and Christos Kyratsas

IASO General Hospital, Athens, Greece

Correspondence should be addressed to Nikolaos Mertziotis; mertz@hol.gr

Academic Editor: Matthew Rutman

Purpose. To present a modified technique of managing extensive penile urethral strictures with dorsal and ventral onlay buccal mucosa grafts. *Patients and Methods.* From October 2014 to January 2016, a total of 12 patients underwent urethroplasty for penile urethral strictures, using dorsal and ventral onlay grafts from buccal mucosa. The mean age was 42.75 (17–71). All patients completed the IPSS and QoL questionnaire, and uroflowmetry was done preoperatively. After surgery, the follow-up included completion of IPSS and QoL questionnaire and measuring of uroflow at 1, 3, 6, and 12 months. Postoperative urethrography was performed in complex cases or in the event of deterioration of voiding symptoms. *Results.* The mean length of the strictures was 5.45 (2, 2–16) cm. Mean Qmax changed from 3.45 ml/sec preoperatively to 18.33 postoperatively, and mean IPS score significantly decreased from 20.1 preoperatively to 8.98 postoperatively. All values were statistically significant ($p < 0.001$). No intraoperative or immediate postoperative complications were recorded. Overall, at 12 months, 11 out of 12 patients (91.6%) had a marked improvement in quality of life and uroflowmetry parameters. *Conclusions.* In the properly selected patient, the combined use of double graft for penile urethral strictures can be successful with minimal morbidity, at short-term follow-up.

1. Introduction

Urethroplasty is the treatment of choice for penile and bulbar urethral strictures, offering the best long-term results [1]. Although anastomotic urethroplasty is widely used for strictures up to 2 cm in length, more extensive strictures usually require some kind of graft augmentation, usually from buccal mucosa [2, 3]. Very often, the placement of a single graft, either ventrally or dorsally, is not sufficient to achieve adequate urethral caliber. The concurrent use of two grafts, on both the dorsal and ventral urethra (the "Palminteri" technique) has been proposed for extensive bulbar urethral strictures, with very satisfactory results [4]. Up to now, this technique has not been extensively studied for penile urethral strictures. Such strictures usually develop in men as a result of iatrogenic trauma [5]. Before the double graft, guidelines recommended a two-stage urethroplasty to achieve better results and reduce the possibility of graft rejection [6, 7]. The use of double graft could be a good alternative, as it could reduce the time to recovery of such patients. The aim of this study is to present the use of a modified Palminteri technique for patients with complex and/or extensive penile urethral strictures in a single procedure.

2. Materials and Methods

From October 2014 until January 2016, 12 patients aged 17–71 years (mean age 42.75 years) underwent urethroplasty with the use and application of free autologous graft on the dorsal and ventral surface of the urethra in one step by the same surgeon.

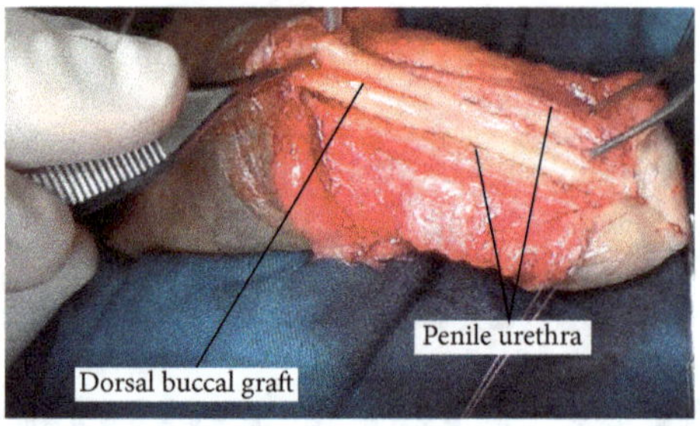

(a)

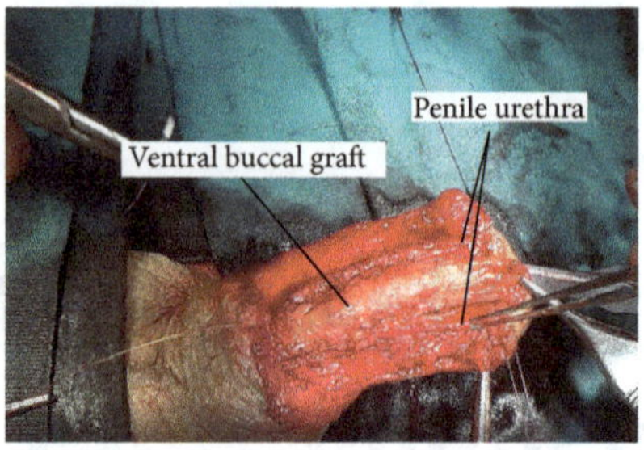

(b)

FIGURE 1: (a) Suturing the dorsal buccal graft on the tunica albuginea. (b) Placement and suturing in the urethra of the ventral buccal graft.

Preoperatively, all patients, besides the detailed history and physical examination, completed the IPSS questionnaire including the quality of life (QoL) domain and were evaluated with urine flow measurement, urethrogram (retrograde and during urination), and in some cases endoscopy and transabdominal ultrasound, in order to determine the nature and length of the stricture. 4 patients had a suprapubic catheter, while 6 of them had already been treated unsuccessfully for strictures caused by traffic accidents or correction of congenital hypospadias. 4 strictures were posttraumatic, 3 were iatrogenic, 2 were caused by lichen sclerosus (former balanitis xerotica obliterans), 2 were related to congenital hypospadias while 1 case was considered idiopathic. 2 patients had concurrent penile and bulbar urethral strictures.

2.1. Surgical Technique. Patients were advised to start mouth washouts with hexetidine solution 5 days before the operation. Preoperative antibiotics were usually used in the form of a fluoroquinolone 1 hour before the operation. Skin shaving of the scrotum and perineum was performed in the operating theater to reduce infection risk. General anesthesia was administered. Mouth exposure was achieved with the use of the Kilner–Doughty retractor, and the harvesting of the graft was always performed first. We prefer to use a single wide graft (from 6 to 10 centimeters long and 1.5 centimeters wide) which we then divide in two longitudinal halves, instead of harvesting from both cheeks. Oral mucosa was closed with a running 3-0 monocryl suture.

The rest of the procedure was usually performed with the patient in the supine position. A longitudinal penile skin incision was used to access the urethra, which was then mobilized with careful dissection through the dartos and Buck's fascia. A 16 or 18 Fr Nelaton catheter helped to identify the distal margin of the stricture. A longitudinal incision was then performed over the stenotic part of the ventral penile urethra and was extended up to the proximal margin of the stricture. A second incision was also performed on the dorsal surface of the urethral plate, involving the strictured area at its full length. Half strip of buccal graft was then sutured in dorsal inlay according to Asopa technique while the other half strip of the graft was placed as a ventral onlay (Figure 1). The corpus spongiosum, subcutaneous tissue, and skin were then closed with interrupted sutures. Care was taken to develop at least three subcutaneous layers without suture lines overlapping in order to minimize the risk of fistula formation.

The use of antibiotics was resumed immediately following the operation; patients were advised to have cold drinks and/or ice cream, as well as to follow a soft diet. Patients usually stayed in hospital for 48–72 hours. They completed a 10-day antibiotics course or continued taking antibiotics until the removal of the catheter, which was planned in 3 weeks postoperatively.

Follow-up included uroflowmetry at 1, 3, 6, and 12 months and urethrogram (when recurrence was suspected) and completion of the IPSS questionnaire. Surgical correction was considered successful when there was statistically significant improvement in Qmax, IPSS, and QoL score. The study also recorded operative time, catheterization period, and duration of hospitalization.

Statistical analysis was performed with the Stata MP Program 10.1® (StataCorp LP, Texas, USA). The regularity was tested using the Shapiro–Wilk test. The comparison with the Wilcoxon rank-sum test and the *t*-test was used for abnormal and normal distribution of values, respectively. Statistical significance was defined as $p < 0.05$.

3. Results

The mean stricture length was 5.45 cm (2.2–16) while the average follow-up was 8.91 months (3–14). The mean preoperative IPS score and QoL were 20.1 (9–32) and 3.26 (2–6), respectively, while mean preoperative Qmax was 3.45 ml/sec.

Postoperatively, the mean values for IPSS, QoL, and Qmax were 8.98, 1.35, and 18.33 ml/sec, respectively. The IPSS, QoL, and Qmax difference was −56.45%, −66.75%, and 158.16%, respectively, which was statistically significant for all three parameters ($p < 0.001$) (Table 1). Mean operative time was 186.25 minutes (90–270), mean duration of catheterization was 24.06 days (21–31), and mean hospitalization time was 2.81 days (2–4.5). The graft was harvested from buccal mucosa in 10 patients and from the penile foreskin in 1 patient, while in 1 patient there was a combination of both, because of extensive stenosis.

There were no intraoperative or immediate postoperative complications (Table 2), but only late adverse events. 2 out of the 4 patients with suprapubic catheter suffered from urinary tract infection (16.7%) after catheter

Table 1: Presentation of results.

Parameter	Mean		Difference (%)	p value
	Preoperative	Postoperative		
QoL	3.26	1.35	56.45	0.001
Qmax (ml/sec)	3.45	18.33	66.75	0.001
IPSS	20.1	8.98	158.16	0.001

Table 2: Presentation of complications.

Complications	Number patients	Percentage (%)	Clavien–Dindo classification
Fistula	0	0	—
Blood transfusion	0	0	—
UTI	2	16.7	II
Recurrence	1	8.3	IIIa

removal (Grade II complication, according to the Clavien–Dindo classification system of surgical complications). Only 1 patient (8.3%) with a complex and extensive penile and bulbar urethral stricture (~16 cm) developed a bulbar urethral stenosis in the anastomosis area with the membranous urethra, and he is currently managed by self-dilation (Grade IIIa complication, according to the Clavien–Dindo classification of surgical complications) [8]. This particular patient was one of four with suprapubic catheter due to urinary retention preoperatively. None of the patients developed a fistula or needed a blood transfusion.

4. Discussion

The use of double buccal mucosa grafts on the ventral and dorsal bulbar urethra, first described by Palminteri in 2008, since then had been applied only in small series to penile urethral strictures [4]. Our department has used the Palminteri technique with slight modifications (mainly as regarding the graft thickness) for penile urethral strictures. EAU Guidelines recommend a two-stage urethroplasty for better long-term results [6, 7]. We used not only buccal mucosa grafts but preputial grafts as well, in a single procedure. Although this is a retrospective study with few patients and a short follow-up, the technique looks very promising as it can provide adequate width of the urethra, and it can reduce the recurrence rate to minimum, even in complicated cases. The single patient who developed a recurrence had the longest stricture length, involving the largest part of the urethra, which was the result of a previous transurethral prostatectomy. The recurrence occurred in the area of the anastomosis of the graft with the membranous but not with the penile urethra.

One of our major concerns was the meticulous dissection through the scrotal layers of dartos and Buck's fascia so as to prevent the formation of urethrocutaneous fistula [9]. As a result, we did not experience any fistulae in our patients.

We regard the urinary tract infections that two patients developed as a result of the previously indwelling suprapubic catheters and the many courses of antibiotics that they had taken.

The high success rate of our series and the statistically significant improvement of uroflowmetry and IPS score are in concordance with the improvement in their quality of life scores, even in the patient who developed the restricture and eventually had to self-dilate every second week. This was not unexpected, given that this patient (who was the eldest in our series) had a long-term suprapubic catheter before the operation.

In conclusion, the concurrent use of double buccal mucosa from a single graft or preputial grafts in complex penile urethral strictures is a new technique, with excellent results as regards voiding parameters and quality of life. It can also reduce the recurrence and fistula formation rates common to older techniques. The outcome from its use in penile urethral strictures is encouraging but more extensive, prospective studies with larger series of patients and longer follow-up are needed.

Authors' Contributions

Nikolaos Mertziotis was responsible for the concept, the design, and the data analysis of the study. He was the supervisor and gave the approval of the final version of the manuscript. Andreas Konandreas was involved in the retrieval of the data and writing of the manuscript. Christos Kyratsas was involved in the writing of the manuscript, analysis of the data, and performed grammar and spelling modifications of the manuscript. All authors have read and approved the final version of the manuscript and agree with the order of presentation of the authors.

Acknowledgments

The authors would like to thank interpreter and translator Dr. Villy Rouchotas for her contribution in proofreading and translation of the manuscript.

References

[1] A. Mangera and C. Chapple, "Management of anterior urethral stricture: an evidence-based approach," *Current Opinion in Urology*, vol. 20, no. 6, pp. 453–458, 2010.

[2] R. A. Santucci, L. A. Mario, and J. W. McAninch, "Anastomotic urethroplasty for bulbar urethral stricture: analysis of 168 patients," *The Journal of Urology*, vol. 167, no. 4, pp. 1715–1719, 2002.

[3] G. Barbagli, G. Guazzoni, and M. Lazzeri, "One-stage bulbar urethroplasty: retrospective analysis of the results in 375 patients," *European Urology*, vol. 53, no. 4, pp. 828–833, 2008.

[4] E. Palminteri, G. Manzoni, E. Berdondini et al., "Combined dorsal plus ventral double buccal mucosa graft in bulbar urethral reconstruction," *European Urology*, vol. 53, no. 1, pp. 81–90, 2008.

[5] A. P. Berger, M. Deibl, G. Bartsch, H. Steiner, J. Varkarakis, and C. Gozzi, "A comparison of one-stage procedures for post-

traumatic urethral stricture repair," *BJU International*, vol. 95, no. 9, pp. 1299–1302, 2005.

[6] A. Mangeralowast, J. M. Patterson, and C. R. Chapple, "A systematic review of graft augmentation urethroplasty techniques for the treatment of anterior urethral strictures," *European Urology*, vol. 59, no. 5, pp. 797–814, 2011.

[7] D. E. Andrich, T. J. Greenwell, and A. R. Mundy, "The problems of penile urethroplasty with particular reference to 2-stage reconstructions," *The Journal of Urology*, vol. 170, no. 1, pp. 87–89, 2003.

[8] D. Dindo, N. Demartines, and P. A. Clavien, "Classification of surgical complications: a new proposal with evaluation in a cohort of 6336 patients and results of a survey," *Annals of Surgery*, vol. 240, no. 2, pp. 205–213, 2004.

[9] G. H. Jordan, S. M. Schlossberg, and C. J. Devine, "Surgery of the Penis and Urethra," in *Campbell's Urology*, P. C. Walsh, A. B. Retik, E. Darracott-Vaughan, and A. J. Wein, Eds., pp. 3316–3394, Saunders, Philadelphia, PA, USA, 7th edition, 1998.

4

Adult Neurogenic Lower Urinary Tract Dysfunction and Intermittent Catheterisation in a Community Setting: Risk Factors Model for Urinary Tract Infections

Michael Kennelly,[1] **Nikesh Thiruchelvam**,[2] **Márcio Augusto Averbeck**,[3] **Charalampos Konstatinidis**,[4] **Emmanuel Chartier-Kastler**,[5] **Pernille Trøjgaard**,[6] **Rikke Vaabengaard**,[6] **Andrei Krassioukov**,[7,8] **and Birte Petersen Jakobsen**[9]

[1]*Department of Urology, Carolinas Medical Center, Charlotte, NC, USA*
[2]*Department of Urology, Addenbrooke's Hospital, Cambridge, UK*
[3]*Moinhos de Vento Hospital, Porto Alegre, Brazil*
[4]*Urology & Neuro-urology Unit, National Rehabilitation Center, Athens, Greece*
[5]*Urology Clinic, Hôpital Raymond Poincaré, Paris, France*
[6]*Coloplast A/S, Humlebaek, Denmark*
[7]*Division of Physical Medicine and Rehabilitation, Department of Medicine, Faculty of Medicine, University of British Columbia, Vancouver, British Columbia, Canada*
[8]*G.F. Strong Rehabilitation Centre, Vancouver, British Columbia, Canada*
[9]*Independent Medical Consultant, MD, MedDevHealth, Copenhagen, Denmark*

Correspondence should be addressed to Michael Kennelly; michael.kennelly@atriumhealth.org

Academic Editor: Walid A. Farhat

A risk factor model for urinary tract infections in patients with adult neurogenic lower urinary tract dysfunction performing clean intermittent catheterisation was developed; it consists of four domains, namely, (1) general (systemic) conditions in the patient, (2) individual urinary tract conditions in the patient, (3) routine aspects related to the patient, and (4) factors related to intermittent catheters *per se*. The conceptual model primarily concerns patients with spinal cord injury, spina bifida, multiple sclerosis, or cauda equina where intermittent catheterisation is a normal part of the bladder management. On basis of several literature searches and author consensus in case of lacking evidence, the model intends to provide an overview of the risk factors involved in urinary tract infections, with specific emphasis to describe those that in daily practice can be handled and modified by the clinician and so come to the benefit of the individual catheter user in terms of fewer urinary tract infections.

1. Introduction

Adult neurogenic lower urinary tract dysfunction (ANLUTD) refers to "abnormal or difficult function of the bladder, urethra (and/or prostate in men) in mature individuals in the context of clinically confirmed relevant neurologic disorder" [1] (Appendix).

For community, residing ANLUTD subjects, clean intermittent catheterisation (CIC) is the gold standard for bladder emptying, as CIC is the safest method (voluntary, complete, low pressure emptying procedure) in terms of having the lowest potential for urological complications [2]. Indwelling transurethral catheterisation and, to a lesser extent, suprapubic cystostomy should be avoided due to high risk of UTIs and for significant long-term complications [2–4].

CIC is carried out between 16 and 56% of a spinal cord injury (SCI) population, depending on age and severity [5, 6]. In multiple sclerosis (MS) of longer duration, 68%–75% have urinary dysfunction [7, 8]; continuous use of CIC is dependent on the individual's perception of improvement in symptoms versus the burden of use and the appearance of a urinary tract infection (UTI) may also negatively influence the use of CIC [9]. In (adult) spina bifida (SB) patients CIC is a cornerstone in bladder treatment [10].

From daily clinical experience, clinical studies, and surveys, it is evident that UTIs are the commonest complication to intermittent catheterisation (IC) and constitutes a major reason for concern in patients and their clinicians and care givers [11]. The reported UTI incidence rates varies; during the rehabilitation phase of a SCI patient, UTI incidence rates were between 2 and 10 per year [12–19], whereas the UTI rates in the community-based population (>12 months after injury) ranged from 0.8–3.5 per year [20–27]. The present review focusses on community related data.

Several models have been used to describe risk factors for UTI in ANLUTD; Shekelle et al. [28] looked at three domains, the person and their functional level, balanced storage phase, and method of bladder drainage. Bladder emptying methods and residual urine were determined as clear risk factors, whereas reliable evidence was insufficient or missing for other factors. The model presented by Vasudeva and Madersbacher [29] identified intrinsic defence mechanisms, impaired washout, and catheterisation as culprits and concluded that further research is needed to understand the complex interplay between these mechanisms.

In a community-based setting of the ANLUTD population, the authors developed a simple, holistic clinical model (Figure 1) that encompasses four main areas of risk factors related to the neurogenic bladder patients performing IC, general (systemic) conditions, local urinary tract conditions, compliance, and intermittent catheters *per se*. The model should provide a useful tool to identify risk factors in the individual IC user.

2. Methods

At an initial workshop, upon a discussion of common risk factors for UTI in the IC users, the five experts, representing neurourology, rehabilitation medicine, and urology, expressed a need for a paper describing risk factors for UTI in the ANLUTD population; the model should aim, in a holistic and simple way, to visualise and describe the most common risk factors in this population and thereby provide a useful tool for health-care personal in the daily evaluation management of UTIs in connection with IC.

In a following workshop, inspired by the models of Shekelle et al. [28] and Vasudeva and Madersbacher [29], it was agreed that risk factors logically could be classified as belonging to one of four domains, namely, (1) general (systemic) conditions in the patient, (2) individual urinary tract conditions in the patient, (3) routine aspects related to the patient, and (4) factors related to intermittent catheters *per se* (Figure 1). The model should consider patients with SCI, SB, MS, and cauda equina (CE) where IC is a normal part of the bladder management. It was decided to describe the model in terms of a narrative review (position paper), as this approach appeared most relevant for the model in question.

Based on this workshop, two basic searches were performed; one search was performed in PubMed, Embase, and Cinahl using the same terms as in the original 1999 Shekelle et al.'s [28] review. Search: urinary tract, urinary tract infection, bacteriuria, paraplegia, quadriplegia, spinal cord injury, multiple sclerosis, neurogenic bladder, neuropathic bladder. Filters: Comparative Study, Controlled Clinical Trial, Meta-Analysis, Multicenter Study, Systematic Reviews, from 1999/08/01 to 2018/08/01, Humans, English, French, German, Adult: 19+ years. This retrieved 166, 37, and 3 citations in PubMed, Embase, and Cinahl, respectively. The citations in Cinahl and Embase were all included in the PubMed search. Nine relevant publications were identified [14, 17, 18, 20, 24, 30–33].

A further PubMed search was based on a modified Vasudeva search strategy: urinary tract infection, neurogenic bladder, spinal cord injury, spina bifida, multiple scleroses, cauda equina, bacterial flora, postvoid residual urine, reflux, intermittent catheterisation. Filters: from 1999/08/01 to 2018/08/01, Humans, English, French, German, Adult: 19+ years. This retrieved 8 citations, of which none described risk factors for UTIs. Additional literature searches for each specific risk factor (risk factor and UTI) were performed if deemed necessary.

All potential risk factors detected were presented at a third workshop. Using a modified Delphi approach, each risk factor was evaluated and discussed by the experts and, if found relevant for the model, classified to one of the four domains described above; in case of lacking or inconclusive evidence, the authors concluded by consensus. During this process, the model was finalised. The model intends to provide an overview of the risk factors involved, with specific emphasis to describe those that in daily practice can be handled and modified by the clinician and so come to the benefit of the individual IC user.

3. UTI: Definitions, Diagnoses, and Perceptions

3.1. UTI Definitions and Diagnoses. Uncomplicated UTI is a bacterial presence within the bladder and associated structures in patients with no structural abnormality and no comorbidities, whereas every UTI in patients with ANLUTD per definition are complicated. A key factor complicating the study of UTIs is the lack of consensus regarding its definition [33–35]. Different definitions of UTI for patients relying on IC not only consider laboratory parameters, but also signs and symptoms (Table 1). Among patients with neurourological diseases some present with impaired sensations in the lower urinary tract, like SCI subjects. They may find it difficult to report UTI-related symptoms accurately [36], which imposes a limitation to differentiate asymptomatic bacteriuria (AB) and UTI in the clinical practice. AB is a frequent finding in neurourological patients who perform IC, and it is a constant challenge to distinguish harmless colonization from pathogenic infection. According to international guidelines, prophylactic antibiotics should not be routinely prescribed to neurourological patients with AB, as this treatment might result in significantly more resistant bacterial strains without improving patient outcome

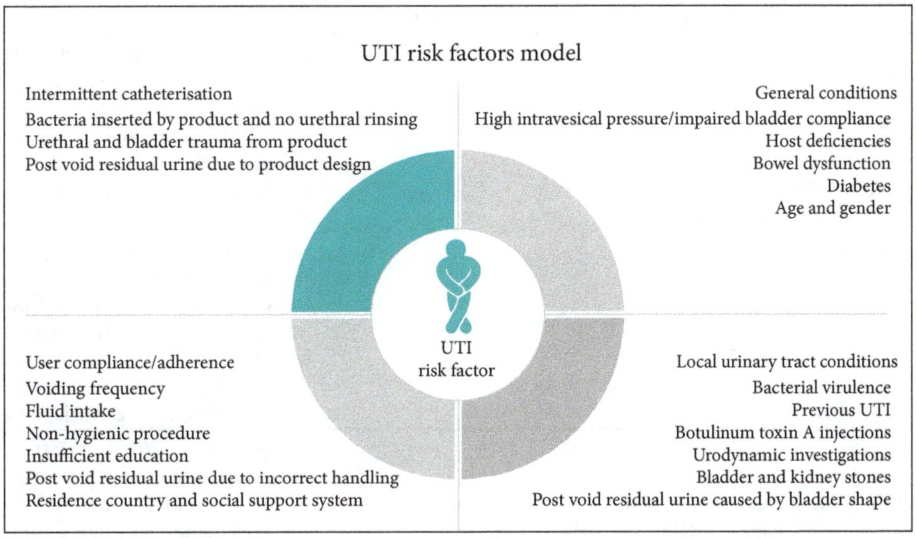

Figure 1: The UTI risk factors model with its four domains.

[37, 38]. However, some studies have reported beneficial effect of prophylactic intervention [26, 39].

The controversy regarding UTI definitions was also described in a systematic review trying to more accurately examine the UTI rate following botulinum injections; they found that amongst 50 selected publications, only 27 had defined the UTI with a total of 10 different definitions [43]. Two studies used the National Institute on Disability and Rehabilitation Research [44] UTI definition, whereas no studies used a definition which met the European Association of Urology [4] or Infectious Diseases Society of America [41] criteria.

Biomarkers for UTI have been assessed in a limited number of trials assessed the role of biomarkers, such as interleukins 6 and 8, C-reactive protein, and erythrocyte sedimentation rate, for predicting UTI in humans. Whilst detection of urinary tract infection appears more sensitive with the use of urinary interleukins than that with traditional culture or dipstick techniques, the test is not widely available, is not a simple bedside test, and is more costly than a standard urine dipstick and urine culture testing [35].

Another aspect is the variability regarding definition of recurrent UTIs. Some studies consider 0-1 UTI/year representing no infection problems [45, 46], some differentiate between 0, 1-2 (infrequent), and 3 or more (recurrent) UTIs per year [25] and other consider 0–2 and 3 or more UTIs per year as sporadic and recurrent UTIs, respectively [47]. Whatever definition, a subpart of the population does consistently not experience UTIs when reported on a yearly basis. There may also be a difference in incidence rates between self-reported UTIs and those medically documented in retrospective and prospective studies [17, 20, 25]. Altogether, such heterogeneous UTI definitions seriously hamper the clinical and research efforts and may over- or underscore the importance of various risk factors.

3.2. Patient Perspective on UTIs. CIC is widely used for the urological management of neurogenic bladders, and UTI is the most frequently reported and challenging complication [48]. The diagnosis of UTI in the general population is not generally applicable to individuals with SCI, SB, or CE due to loss of sensation and a neurogenic bladder requiring alternative bladder emptying like CIC. The common symptoms include increased bladder spasticity, new or worsening urinary incontinence, autonomic dysreflexia, and foul-smelling urine.

The NIDRR consensus statement on the prevention and management of UTI among people with SCI listed a set of signs and symptoms as suggestive of UTI [44]. The validity, accuracy, and predictive value of these signs and symptoms were evaluated during the first 3 months of a 1-year-long randomised controlled CIC-catheter trial (RCT) in chronic SCI patients [20, 49]. Subjects were able to predict their own UTI with an accuracy of 66%, and with positive and negative predictive values of 33% and 83%, respectively. Okamoto [50], evaluating CIC-users in general, presented findings along the same line, underlining the CIC-user's insecurity regarding the interpretation of their UTI signs and symptoms. Self-reported UTIs should hence be interpreted with care.

3.3. Rehabilitation Centres' Perspective on UTIs. A questionnaire-based survey of 13 German-speaking SCI rehabilitation centres sheds light on the variability of handling the UTIs in SCI patients (irrespective of bladder management), both with respect to diagnosing as well as treating a UTI [51]. The criteria for accepting a UTI urine analysis as positive differed and the symptomatic treatment was started with "fever without other causes" as the most frequently symptom irrespective of leucocyte count. These finding underlines both the impact of the personal experience of the treating physician and the paucity of published evidence.

When evaluating the evidence on UTI risk factors in neurogenic CIC-users, issues like heterogenic UTI definitions, uncertainty of patients' self-reported data, and significant differences between medical evaluation and treatment of UTIs could profoundly influence the level of

Table 1: Definitions for catheter-associated urinary tract infection.

2017/18 Guidelines on Neuro-Urology of the European Association of Urology (EAU) [4]. +* Blok et al. EAU guidelines on Neuro-Urology 2015 [40]	Signs and/or symptoms accompanied by laboratory findings of a UTI (bacteriuria, leucocyturia[a], and positive urine culture). Significant bacteriuria in persons performing IC is present with $>10^2$ colony-forming units (cfu)/mL, $>10^4$ cfu/mL in clean-void specimens*, and any detectable concentration in suprapubic aspirates. The most common signs and symptoms in those with neuro-urological disorders are fever, new onset or increase in incontinence, including leaking around an indwelling catheter, increased spasticity, malaise, lethargy or sense of unease, cloudy urine with increased urine odour, discomfort or pain over the kidney or bladder, dysuria, or autonomic dysreflexia
2009 International Clinical Practice Guidelines from the Infectious Diseases Society of America (IDSA) [41].	Symptoms or signs compatible with UTI with no other identified source of infection along with $\geq 10^3$ cfu/mL of ≥1 bacterial species in a single catheter urine specimen or in a midstream voided urine specimen from a patient whose urethral, suprapubic, or condom catheter has been removed within the previous 48 h[b]
ISCoS Urinary Tract Infection Basic Dataset [42].	(i) New onset of symptoms accompanied by laboratory findings (bacteriuria, leukocyturia and positive urine culture) of a UTI. (ii) Symptoms: fever, urinary incontinence/failure of control or leaking around the catheter, spasticity, malaise, lethargy or sense of unease, cloudy urine, malodorous urine, pyuria/leukocyturia, back pain, bladder pain, dysuria, autonomic dysrreflexia (AD). (iii) A clean-catch midstream technique from an immediately installed urine catheter. Any positive culture should be reported. The clinical Microbiological Laboratory (CML), 10^3 CFU ml^{-1} is a reliable finding with standardized inoculation with 10 μl urine.

[a]Leucocyturia is defined as 10 or more leucocytes in centrifuged urine samples per microscopic field (400×). [b]In the catheterised patient, pyuria is not diagnostic of CA-bacteriuria or CAUTI, and the presence, absence, or degree of pyuria alone does not, by itself, differentiate catheter-associated asymptomatic bacteriuria from CAUTI. However, the absence of pyuria in a symptomatic catheterised patient suggests a diagnosis other than CAUTI.

importance of the separate risk factors. Additionally, the importance of specific risk factors may differ between individual patients.

4. The Model: General Conditions

4.1. High Intravesical Pressure/Impaired Bladder Compliance. With any spinal cord injury, the disruption of the normal somatic and autonomic neurological control of bladder causes bladder dysfunction; in higher suprasacral injuries, a micturition reflex may emerge after the acute phase to cause detrusor overactivity and sometimes detrusor-sphincter dyssynergia (DSD) with ineffective bladder emptying and clinical significant large postvoid residual volumes. Lesions in the lumbosacral area affecting the autonomic nuclei may cause detrusor hypocontractility with bladder over-filling and voiding inability. All SCI and most of the SB patients have bladder dysfunction; it is common in MS, and if disease duration is above 10 years, up to 80% of the MS patients have bladder symptoms [11].

Individuals with high intravesical pressures and impaired bladder compliance are more prone to UTI's than those with low intravesical pressure and high capacity bladder that it is emptied periodically by IC. The risk factors are the high intravesical pressures in the first case and the risk of bladder over-distention in the other case [52].

The degree of bladder dysfunction (compliance, storage pressure), assessed through urodynamic parameters, appears to correlate to increased UTI incidence rates. In a retrospective study, low bladder compliance (<10 ml/cm H_2O), detrusor overactivity, and vesicoureteral reflux correlated with increased UTI incidence rates in 76 spina bifida patients performing CIC [53]. In contrast, a recent retrospective study could not verify a correlation in 194 SB children [46]. Experience from clinical practice supports a correlation between UTIs and poorly compliant bladder.

It has been speculated that Bladder ischemia due to decreased blood flow predisposes to UTI [54, 55]. In the neurogenic bladder, this may happen in relation to (untreated) increased intravesical pressure and overdistension due to large urine volumes [29]. Lapides suggested that "it was logical to assume that maintenance of a good blood supply by prevention of vesical overdistension and elevated intravesical pressures would combat infection" [54]. A 7-year prospective study showed that a mean volume of each catheterisation >400 ml is linked UTI [45].

4.2. Host Deficiencies (Impaired Immune System). Altered intrinsic defence mechanisms and immune suppression after spinal injuries augment the risk for UTIs possibly due to changes in the microbial flora, immunological deficiencies [56], and alterations in the bladder wall and its urothelium [29, 57]. Such conditions are presently not readily modifiable in daily clinical practice. Apart from the local injury in the spinal cord, patients may develop a variety of complications characterized by multiple-organ dysfunction such as lung injury, cardiovascular disease, liver and kidney damage, and increased susceptibility to infection. The damage to the autonomic nerve system (ANS) leads to a general immune dysfunction through the loss of neural innervation of lymphoid organs.

4.3. Bowel Dysfunction. The distal colon and urinary bladder have a similar function of the storage and evacuation of faeces and urine, and there is a joint peripheral innervation of both viscera, through the hypogastric, pelvic, and pudendal nerves [58]. It is therefore not unexpected that spinal cord injuries also affect colorectal motility, transit times, and bowel emptying, leading to constipation, faecal incontinence, or a combination of both. When treating neurogenic bowel dysfunction in terms of faecal incontinence and constipation with transanal irrigation, a more than three-fold reduction of UTI incidence rates was documented [59, 60]. The reason for this UTI reduction is unknown; it could be speculated that fewer episodes of faecal incontinence causes less genitourinary bacterial contamination or, given the role of the kidneys and bladder in filtration and storage of waste, respectively, microbial profiles and microbial metabolites of the gut might influence the urinary microbiota, and alterations might affect urinary homeostasis [61]. Further, rectal impaction has been suggested to cause lower urinary tract symptoms (LUTSs) by mechanically to impede bladder emptying [62]. Hence, an optimal bowel treatment of constipation and incontinence should go hand in hand with bladder management.

4.4. Diabetes. Diabetes *per se* bears a 2- to 3-fold risk for UTI compared to nondiabetic controls, and the severity is usually more severe and carries worse outcomes [63, 64]. A large cross-sectional Canadian Community Health Survey compared the prevalence of type 2 diabetes in the SCI population with that of a nonSCI population [65]. They found, regardless of the variables included in the models, an approximately 2-fold increased odd for type 2 diabetes in the SCI population, which is not explained by known risk factors for type 2 diabetes. In other words, unexplained occurrences of UTI may be related to undiagnosed diabetes.

4.5. Age and Gender. It is inconclusive whether age or gender plays a major role for the UTI risk in the neurogenic population; some studies suggest a slightly higher UTI rate for females [25, 45], whereas older studies reported conflicting results [28]. A recent, retrospective chart review of 194 SB patients (median age 22 years, range 8 months–58 years) found that increasing age was associated with decreasing odds of UTI by 7% per year, independent of gender [46]. As the authors could not verify compliance with the recommended CIC frequency or technique, age and maturity may have impacted the patient's ability to manage their bladder emptying and hence risk of UTI.

5. The Model: Local Urinary Tract Conditions

5.1. Bacterial Virulence. The development of UTIs in the neurogenic bladder relays on a balance between bacterial virulence and local host factors. When the ability to locally fight the infection is compromised, the uropathogens have better access to the urinary tract and their washout of the bladder is lost [29]. Further, upon alteration of protective flora and changes in the urothelium and bladder wall after injury may let the uropathogens inside the urinary tract more easily adhere to the urothelium and invade the bladder wall [57, 66]. All such events may end up in UTIs; however, investigation and treatment of these factors are at present on an experimental level.

Antibiotics may also interfere with the protective flora. A study in 70 women with UTIs showed that the original lactobacillus population had not been restored after treatment in most patients; rather, the uropathogenics dominated the flora [67]. A similar condition could be relevant for the microbiome in the bladder.

The strategy of supporting the host bacterial flora by adding nonpathogenic bacteria have been investigated in a couple of small studies [68, 69]. Inoculation of nonpathogenic bacteria (mostly *E. Coli*) into the bladder showed sufficient colonization rates of the inoculated pathogenic bacteria and significant reductions in UTI frequency. It appears that this approach could be useful, although there is still insufficient evidence to support the use of bacterial interference for UTI prevention in daily practice [4, 42].

5.2. Previous UTIs. Previous UTIs are accepted as a risk factor because they render the bladder urothelium into a chronic, inflammatory condition more susceptible to reinfection. A 7-year prospective study of CIC-users found two predictive factors; patients with high UTIs at the start of the study also had high UTI rates at the end of the follow-up period and high UTI rates were linked to development of high catheterisation volumes [45].

5.3. Botulinum Toxin A Injections. Detrusor treatment with Botulinum Toxin A injections efficiently combats neurogenic detrusor overactivity [70] but there is controversy about the UTI rates postinjection [43] and whether there should be antibiotic coverage for the therapeutic sessions [71]. Data from a single SCI rehabilitation centre, comprising 1104 patients with at least 3 years follow-up, found that the odds of a UTI increased 10-fold for those receiving botulinum detrusor injections [6].

5.4. Urodynamic Investigations. Urodynamic investigations are by far the most commonly used method for bladder evaluation, it is believed to increase the risk for UTIs, and therefore, the American Urological association suggests that high risk patients with neurogenic lower urinary tract dysfunction should receive antibiotic prophylaxis for UTI prophylaxis [72]. Data from a recent SCI study found that a history of UTI within the past 4 weeks prior to the urodynamic investigation increased the risk for a new UTI [73].

5.5. Bladder and Kidney Stones. Bladder and kidney stones are well-known risk factors for UTIs and evolve through two mechanisms; infection stones caused by urease-producing Gram-negative organisms and metabolic stones that passively trap bacteria from coexistent UTIs [74, 75]. By clinical experience, stones may stimulate the detrusor overactivity and hence the intravesical pressures, related to recurrent UTI's. In very rare occasion a foreign body, e.g. a hair, inserted through catheterisation, provides the basis for stone formation [76].

5.6. Postvoid Residual Urine Caused by Bladder Shapes. Merrit [77] originally described a correlation between postvoid residual volume and UTI frequency based on 105 SCI patients, which, however, could not be reproduced in a small-scale study in 12 SCI subjects [78]. Smaller volumes (<50 ml) in CIC-users did not predispose to UTIs [47]. Despite lack of clear evidence for a cut-off level, increased amounts of postvoid residual urine (>100 ml) is an accepted risk factor for UTI in the neurogenic population [62]. The reasons for experience residual urine could be many including anatomical bladder abnormalities, not proper education of patient, handling of IC catheter, and product choice (IC catheter).

Anatomical abnormalities that limit complete bladder emptying (e.g., prostatic impression, bladder diverticulum or trabeculated "Christmas tree bladders") are conditions in which lagoons of urine are difficult to empty during catheterisation and so potentially provide a nidus for bacterial proliferation. There are no studies addressing these conditions, but it appears logical to accept such as risk factors. Such bladders may also have altered compliance, contributing to the UTI risk.

6. The Model: User Compliance/Adherence

In relation to UTI, compliance in this article describes the extent to which a CIC-catheter user adheres to the medical advice given by their treating health-care provider as to prevent UTIs [79] (compliance in this review does not consider reasons for discontinuing CIC management). As noted by Shekelle et al. [28], there was at that time a "paucity of data on the independent effect of psychosocial, behavioural, or hygienic factors on the risk of UTI in people with SCI". Nothing seems to have changed substantially with respect to the evidence base of these factors, but it is generally recognized that factors like misconceptions, anxiety, embarrassment, and poor confidence can be barriers to CIC, which can be worsened by physical disabilities, e.g., dexterity or visual impairment [80, 81].

In the context of performing CIC it should also be taken into account that: (1) patients with neurodegenerative disorders often present with various levels of cognitive dysfunction; (2) psychiatric diagnoses, including depression and anxiety, are not unusual among individuals with relevant neurological diseases; (3) polypharmacy is not unusual in these patients and some medicines do impose a high anticholinergic burden. Cognitive function should be routinely assessed in neurourological patients to provide individualized counselling on IC technique.

6.1. Voiding Frequency. Voiding frequency and urine volume (two sides of the same coin) as infrequent voiding, result in larger bladder volumes that may over distend the bladder and so increase the risk for UTI. A survey of Canadian SCI patients found that voiding frequency was inversely related to number of UTIs, with one daily catheterisation having the highest UTI rate in a univariable analysis [25]. In a study of Paralympic athletes who catheterised from 1 to 10 per day (average 6 ± 2 times), the frequency of daily catheterisations was not related to the frequency of UTIs, $p = 0.07$ [21]. As mentioned above, the catheterisation volume must be kept below 400 ml [45].

6.2. Fluid Intake. Poor fluid intake is generally considered as a risk [82] for UTIs in neurogenic bladder disease, and a low fluid intake has been associated with an increase in urine osmolality and acidity, which may predispose to UTIs [83]. In this context, the absence of diurnal variation of antidiuretic hormone levels in spinal cord injured subjects could play a role for adequate fluid intake [84]. All in all, empirical evidence for role of fluid intake for UTI prevention in the neurogenic population is scarce, and therefore, it is not possible to draw any firm evidence-based conclusions about daily fluid intake [83]. However, general medical experience supports the intake of daily adequate amounts of fluids, which recently was supported by a clinical study showing that increased water intake prevents recurrent cystitis in premenopausal women [85].

6.3. Nonhygienic Procedures. The Canadian survey of 935 SCI patients living in community determined CIC hygienic practices found, based on a univariate model, that genital and peritoneal cleaning was associated with reduced UTI rate as was self-catheterisation compared to catheterisation by others [25]. Wyndaele et al. [86] compared the results in 25 paraplegic patients started on CIC 35 days postinjury with 48 paraplegic patients catheterised postinjury by nurses with a nontouch technique and found comparable UTI rates in the two groups. The EAUN guidelines strictly encourages the no-touch techniques; however, no evidence for the no-touch technique on the UTI rate is given [81]. For comparison, a study was carried out on simulation models, evaluating the difference between classical sterile procedure and a no-touch procedure in hospital settings [87]. The no-touch procedure caused a lower amount of sterility errors and shorter duration of the intervention compared with the classical method. Whether less sterility errors translates into a lower rate of UTIs remains to be shown.

The basic importance of hand washing for prevention of infection was already emphasised by Semmelweis and Koch [88, 89]. The various guidelines also underline that patients who self-catheterise should disinfect or wash hands thoroughly with water and soap before catheterisation [82, 90–92]; however, it appears that the recommendations are based on experience from hospital setting and not on clinical evidence form community settings. A recent survey of self-reported habits amongst community dwelling SCI subjects showed that only half of the subjects washed hands as recommended, but no relationship was found with either occurrence or frequency of UTIs [93].

Obesity may be independently associated with UTIs [94, 95], particularly prominent in very obese men (BMI > 50) but less so for women. No data specific for the neurogenic population are available. It could be speculated that obese subjects have difficulty with bowel hygiene and as such are at increased risk of vulvovaginal symptoms and UTI.

Self-catheterisation versus catheterisation by others was associated with a significantly reduced UTI rate in a Canadian national survey of intermittent catheterisation practices following SCI [25]. Similar, after commencement of IC in a SB population, it appeared that IC self-catheterisation prompted a greater reduction of UTI than assisted IC [96].

6.4. Insufficient Education. Guidelines to IC recommend that comprehensive training on IC technique should be provided to neurourological patients [4, 78, 82], but adherence to CIC technique as recommended by health-care personal was just followed by 76% of responders [93]. A RCT examined the impact of an educational program on UTI frequencies [32]; the educational intervention resulted in less bacteriuria and a nonsignificant trend toward fewer symptom reports and antibiotic treatment episodes as well as decreased UTIs. However, for individuals with recurrent UTIs, increased knowledge may lead to increased perceptions of the severity of UTIs. Education for spinal cord injured athletes suggests that education may be advantageous [92] but a systematic review of educational programs did not detect a substantial beneficial effect [97]. A shortcome of the previous studies did not assess quality of educational initiatives, as no objective feedback was obtained from the patients. In a European initiative undertaken by eight rehabilitation centres in Norway, France, and Italy, it was shown that a good education programme can improve adherence to IC during the first year at home (99 vs. 83% for the Education Programme and control groups, respectively; $p < 0.05$) [98]. From a clinical point of view, comprehensive training on IC technique should be provided to neurourological patients. Whenever a patient presents with UTI, IC technique and frequency must be reviewed [82].

6.5. Postvoid Residual Urine due to Incorrect Handling. The causes for residual urine could be many fold, as described previously. In particular, removal of the intermittent catheter before complete bladder emptying is frequently encountered in clinical practice and is considered as a risk for UTIs. This procedure should be included in the training of patients.

6.6. Residence Country and Social Support System (Reimbursement). The differences in patterns of care are closely related to socioeconomic status and resources of the geographic area [44, 99]. CIC is well established in developed countries and seems to be part of standard patient care in the larger Asian and South American countries [100]. In the same way, low UTI incidence rates are related to developed countries, whereas higher rates are detected in less developed areas [21]. These findings underline the unmet needs present in many countries.

The importance of compliance and lifestyle for UTI prevention in community living subjects is not based on solid clinical evidence but rather driven by economic conditions, guideline recommendations, health-care personnel directions and patients own habits based on their individual disabilities and physical surroundings. The guidance given varies between institutions, regions, and countries, heavily influenced by social security systems and reimbursement schedules. Evaluation of IC regimen and individual costs related to IC should be done to improve nationwide control of cost. However, feasibility is difficult to evaluate and as cost.

7. The Model: Intermittent Catheters

7.1. Bacteria Inserted by Product and No Urethral Rinsing. Intermittent catheterisation *per se* is an important etiological risk factor for UTI in the neurogenic bladder [29]. It allows bacteria from the lower urethral region to be deposited directly into the bladder and cannot create the mechanical rinsing of the bladder that occurs during normal voiding. Additionally, nonhygienic intermittent catheterisation practices can introduce bacteria into the urinary tract. The use of no-touch catheter technique, which includes use of a urinary catheters without touch by the user's hand, like a nontouch sleeve and insertion tip has been shown to reduce the risk. Clinical studies suggest that use of a no-touch catheter is associated with a 30% reduction in bacteriuria and general low bacteriuria levels [16, 101]; however, data are based on few patients and bacterial counts only.

A hospital study reported on a no-touch catheter and technique with 35% less infection (UTIs not defined) per admission when compared to a retrospective, very different control group [102]. Both studies are therefore not providing clinical evidence for the benefit of a no-touch catheter system. In a 2×2 weeks crossover study of a new no-touch sleeve system compared to a conventional catheter, five UTIs were reported, but without information about in which group they occurred [103]. Interestingly, in the Canadian survey, there was no difference in UTI incidence rate if catheters were disinfected between use or not [25].

In summary, the positive influence of catheter design is controversial, but overall, the present evidence suggests beneficial use of hydrophilic catheters for CIC management.

7.2. Urethral and Bladder Trauma from Product. Chemical and physical properties of the catheter surface are important when looking at risk for creating trauma from product. Compared to gel lubrication, catheters with hydrophilic coatings caused significantly less urethral trauma (haematuria), less removal friction, and less pain [104]. This could be related to the clinical experience that lubricating catheters with a gel is insufficient to protect the urethra from injury, as the lubricant is lost upon entering the urethral meatus [105]. The osmolality of hydrophilic catheter coatings was found to reduce both removal friction and urethral trauma (haematuria) during catheterisation since a hyperosmolar coating appears gentler to the urethral mucosa due to its higher water content [106]. A study of urethral cytology in SCI patients performing CIC demonstrated a significantly lower inflammatory response in patients using hydrophilic catheters compared to uncoated catheters [107]. The data demonstrates that single-use hydrophilic catheters have properties that minimize urethral trauma.

Urethral strictures are a consequence of long-term use of CIC [6, 108]. The authors found during an observation period of 5-6 years a stricture rate of 25% and 19%, of which 36% and 21% required urethrotomy, respectively. Difficult and traumatic catheterisations may cause injuries ranging from a mucosal tear to more serious false passages, which are associated with UTIs and strictures and subsequently may require surgical management [109]; strictures may make future catheterisations difficult and cause repeated injury and UTIs [110]. Careful education of catheterisation technique and selection of the proper catheter is fundamental [111].

Patterns of use. The 2014 Cochrane review by Prieto et al. [112] "Intermittent catheterisation for long-term bladder management" was one of the leading documents concerning bladder management in the neurogenic population. The opinion expressed in the paper however concerned many clinicians and led to an independent reanalysis of the Cochrane data [113]; consequently, the Cochrane publication was withdrawn due to their erroneous data selection, data extraction, data analysis, and use of outdated UTI definition. The reanalysis could not detect any significant differences in the UTI incidence rates between aseptic vs. other techniques and single vs. multiple use of catheters due to the small number of participants and short or unclear duration of trials; it was not possible to draw final conclusions. In contrast to the Cochrane review, a significant difference favouring use of hydrophilic catheters vs. other catheters was detected.

The studies that were eligible for inclusion in the meta-analyses were executed in in-patient hospital/rehabilitation centres and/or community environments and included in total 502 patients, essentially evaluated over a few months (hospital/rehab centres: 209 patients during a median study period of 12 weeks; hospital/rehab and subsequent community residence: 123 SCI patients SCI during a 52-week study period; community: 56 SCI patients during 52 weeks and 82 SB children during a median study period of 16 weeks; 32 male patients with enlarged prostates were studied during a 6-week period). The two long-term trials of 52 weeks in SCI patients showed comparable results. De Ridder et al. [17] performed the trial in 123 patients during rehabilitation and subsequent community residence and found significantly less UTIs associated with hydrophilic catheters than with uncoated (single use). Cardenas et al. [20] in 56 community dwelling patients also documented significantly less UTIs associated with hydrophilic than with uncoated catheters (single use).

As stated by the authors of the meta-analysis, due to the inadequate numbers of participants and the predominantly short trial duration, additional trials are necessary to conclude about catheterisation technique and catheter usage. Based on the present level of evidence, the authors recommended single use hydrophilic catheters.

Since the analyses, based on data collected until 2014, several new studies have emerged. Rognoni et al. [114] also challenged the outcome of previously published meta-analyses and compared complication rates in terms of UTI and urethral trauma/haematuria related to hydrophilic coated catheters vs. nonhydrophilic urinary catheters. The meta-analyses exploring UTI frequencies showed a 16% lower risk ratio associated with hydrophilic catheters in comparison to standard ones (95% CI, 6–25%, $p = 0.003$) and so corroborate the benefits of hydrophilic catheters.

Kiddoo et al. [115] studied the UTI incidence rate in a crossover trial (2×24 weeks) of single use hydrophilic catheters vs. multiple use polyvinylchloride catheters in 66 SP children. They found a statistically significant lower person week of UTI (defined as positive leucocyte dipstick and self-reported fever/pain/increased incontinence or cloudy/odorous urine) in multiple use, but no differences with respect to fever, antibiotic use visits to physicians, missed activities, and positive dipstick for leucocytes and haematuria. In other words, there was no difference in febrile or antibiotic-treated UTIs between use of these two catheter types.

7.3. Postvoid Residual Urine due to Product Design. Choosing the appropriate intermittent catheter tailored to the patient is important to avoid residual urine; this includes, e.g., choosing a catheter of a proper length with proper placement of the eyelets, considering catheter stiffness, and adapting catheter handling to this features.

8. Discussion

The purpose of this review was several folds: to remind clinicians that the correct diagnosis and thereby treatment/ management of UTI/bacterial contamination in the

ANLUTD patient population is challenging and far from simple; to update and discuss the UTI risk factors associated to IC in community settings; and to provide a simple, holistic, and useful risk factors model that can be used by the clinician for daily practice and thereby optimise the modification of these risk factors to the benefit of these patients.

A basic prerequisite is the alignment on the definition of a UTI. As described, many definitions are used in the real-world setting and complicate the understanding and comparability of results. Various medical societies have suggested their UTI definition, but it is imperative from a research perspective that a unified global UTI definition be agreed upon in order to objectively study current and future diagnostic and therapeutic treatment options for UTI.

Overall, the evidence for many of these risk factors role for the development of UTIs are limited and the impact of the personal experience of the clinicians may affect the handling of these risk factors, which should not prevent deciding on specific diagnosis, like UTI, based on available guidelines.

Some of the risk factors have with relative certainty causality roles for UTIs, like high intravesical pressure, the coexistence of a detrusor external-sphincter system dysfunction, catheter and catheterisation procedures, and nonadherence to CIC recommendations. Other proposed risk factors, like Botox injections, urodynamic investigations, or patient education, may to a higher degree be based on expert opinions. Future research is clearly necessary for a better understanding of the impact of a specific risk, both in terms of evaluating a direct causality as well as estimating their importance in real-life situations, where other factors additionally can modify the risk.

Individual conditions for each patient also play an important role and the clinicians should take all this individual variability into account. Each new UTI should trigger a holistic assessment of the patient's situation including overall health, mobility, bladder urodynamic situation, and bowel function. Further, the patients' cognitive function should be assessed to determine the correct understanding of IC procedures and compliance issues. Recurrent UTIs warrant additional investigation and assessment, which may involve imaging, flexible cystoscopy, and video-urodynamic assessment. In case of carer-assisted IC, procedure-related and educational approaches may be necessary.

The importance of catheter properties appears to be of relevance. The risk related to different IC-catheter types, like uncoated catheters, reuse catheters, or single use, hydrophilic ready-to-use catheters have been thoroughly discussed in the recent years; meta-analyses have provided some indications that hydrophilic catheters appear to be linked to the lowest UTI risk [113, 114]. This reflects the physiological common sense that less trauma to urethra and bladder is likely to leads to less UTI. Catheters ready-to-use (hydrophilic coated catheter) appear to cause less constraints for daily use in patients suffering from debilitating conditions like SCI, SB, or MS. Due to the heterogeneity of catheter-users, it can be anticipated, that a hydrophilic, ready-to-use catheter takes away the user's variability in use of the product. This product safety feature of ready-to-use catheters in essence improves product safety by decreasing individual variability in its use.

9. Conclusion

There is a need for alignment of the definition and diagnosis of UTI. It may be done disease per disease or more generally. Even with less complications than other bladder management methods, CIC still expose ANLUTD patients with a high risk of UTIs, a condition associated with increased morbidity and mortality in this patient group. There is a paucity of evidence describing the UTI risk profile, and well-designed clinical trials are warranted to provide the clinician a better platform for adequate management of the UTI risk profile to the benefit of these patients. Guidelines, when available, should be adhered to.

Appendix

Intermittent catheterisation (IC) is defined as drainage of the bladder or a urinary reservoir with subsequent removal of the catheter mostly at regular intervals. Clean IC (CIC): this involves use of a clean technique. This implies ordinary hand and genital washing techniques and use of disposable or cleansed reusable catheters [1].

Aseptic IC: this implies genital antiseptic preparation and the use of sterile (single use) catheters and instruments/gloves in a designated clean area.

Sterile IC: complete sterile setting, including genital skin antisepsis, sterile gloves, forceps, gown, and mask.

No-touch technique IC: this was introduced as an easier way for the patient to perform self-intermittent catheterisation with a ready-to-use catheter (prelubricated catheter, usually a hydrophilic catheter).

Acknowledgments

This study was financially supported by Coloplast A/S, Denmark, by a fee to Birte Petersen Jakobsen for manuscript writing and editing. Article processing charges was also covered by Coloplast A/S, Denmark.

References

[1] J. B. Gajewski, B. Schurch, R. Hamid et al., "An International Continence Society (ICS) report on the terminology for adult neurogenic lower urinary tract dysfunction (ANLUTD)," *Neurourology and Urodynamics*, vol. 37, no. 3, pp. 1152–1161, 2018.

[2] K. J. Weld and R. R. Dmochowski, "Effect of bladder management on urological complications in spinal cord

injured patients," *Journal of Urology*, vol. 163, no. 3, pp. 768–772, 2000.
[3] M. Stöhrer, B. Blok, D. Castro-Diaz et al., "EAU guidelines on neurogenic lower urinary tract dysfunction," *European Urology*, vol. 56, no. 1, pp. 81–88, 2009.
[4] B. Blok, D. Castro-Diaz, G. del Popolo et al., *EAU Guidelines on Neuro-Urology*, European Association of Urology, Arnhem, Netherlands, 2017, https://uroweb.org/guideline/neuro-urology/.
[5] J. J. E. Adriaansen, F. W. A. van Asbeck, M. Tepper et al., "Bladder-emptying methods, neurogenic lower urinary tract dysfunction and impact on quality of life in people with long-term spinal cord injury," *Journal of Spinal Cord Medicine*, vol. 40, no. 1, pp. 43–53, 2017.
[6] J. Krebs, J. Wöllner, and J. Pannek, "Urethral strictures in men with neurogenic lower urinary tract dysfunction using intermittent catheterization for bladder evacuation," *Spinal Cord*, vol. 53, no. 4, pp. 310–313, 2015.
[7] C. R. de Almeida, K. Carneiro, R. Fiorelli, M. Orsini, and R. M. P. Alvarenga, "Urinary dysfunction in women with multiple sclerosis: analysis of 61 patients from rio de janeiro, Brazil," *Neurology International*, vol. 5, no. 4, p. 23, 2013.
[8] V. Kalsi and C. J. Fowler, "Therapy insight: bladder dysfunction associated with multiple sclerosis," *Nature Clinical Practice Urology*, vol. 2, no. 10, pp. 492–501, 2005.
[9] D. McClurg, C. Bugge, C Elders et al., "Factors affecting continuation of clean intermittent catheterisation in people with multiple sclerosis: results of the COSMOS mixed-methods study," *Multiple Sclerosis Journal*, vol. 27, no. 3, pp. 231–237, 2018.
[10] D. B. Clayton, J. W. Brock 3rd, and D. B. Joseph, "Urologic management of spina bifida," *Developmental Disabilities Research Reviews*, vol. 16, no. 1, pp. 88–95, 2010.
[11] X. Gamé, C. J. Fowler, and J. N. Panicker, "Neuropathic bladder dysfunction," *Trends in Urology, Gynaecology & Sexual Health*, vol. 15, no. 1, pp. 23–28, 2010.
[12] S. Sarica, Y. Akkoc, H. Karapolat, and H. Aktug, "Comparison of the use of conventional, hydrophilic and gel-lubricated catheters with regard to urethral micro trauma, urinary system infection, and patient satisfaction in patients with spinal cord injury: a randomized controlled study," *European Journal of Physical and Rehabilitation Medicine*, vol. 46, no. 4, pp. 473–479, 2010.
[13] R. B. King, C. E. Carlson, J. Mervine, Y. Wu, and G. M. Yarkony, "Clean and sterile intermittent catheterization methods in hospitalized patients with spinal cord injury," *Archives of Physical Medicine and Rehabilitation*, vol. 73, no. 9, pp. 798–802, 1992.
[14] A. Giannantoni, S. M. Di Stasi, G. Scivoletto, G. Virgili, S. Dolci, and M. Porena, "Intermittent catheterization with a prelubricated catheter in spinal cord injured patients: a prospective randomized crossover study," *Journal of Urology*, vol. 166, no. 1, pp. 130–133, 2001.
[15] L. M. Duffy, J. Cleary, S. Ahern et al., "Clean intermittent catheterization: safe, cost-effective bladder management for male residents of VA nursing homes," *Journal of the American Geriatrics Society*, vol. 43, no. 8, pp. 865–870, 1995.
[16] C. J. Bennett, M. N. Young, and H. Darrington, "Differences in urinary tract infections in male and female spinal cord injury patients on intermittent catheterization," *Spinal Cord*, vol. 33, no. 2, pp. 69–72, 1995.
[17] D. J. M. K. De Ridder, K. Everaert, L. G. Fernández et al., "Intermittent catheterisation with hydrophilic-coated catheters (SpeediCath) reduces the risk of clinical urinary tract infection in spinal cord injured patients: a prospective randomised parallel comparative trial," *European Urology*, vol. 48, no. 6, pp. 991–995, 2005.
[18] D. D. Cardenas, K. N. Moore, A. Dannels-McClure et al., "Intermittent catheterization with a hydrophilic-coated catheter delays urinary tract infections in acute spinal cord injury: a prospective, randomized, multicenter trial," *PM&R*, vol. 3, no. 5, pp. 408–417, 2011.
[19] C. E. Anderson, "Bladder emptying method is the primary determinant of urinary tract infections in patients with spinal cord injury: results from a prospective rehabilitation cohort study," *BJU International*, vol. 123, no. 2, pp. 342–352, 2018.
[20] D. D. Cardenas, J. M. Hoffman, and Hoffman, "Hydrophilic catheters versus noncoated catheters for reducing the incidence of urinary tract infections: a randomized controlled trial," *Archives of Physical Medicine and Rehabilitation*, vol. 90, no. 10, pp. 1668–1671, 2009.
[21] A. Krassioukov, J. J. Cragg, C. West, C. Voss, and D. Krassioukov-Enns, "The good, the bad and the ugly of catheterization practices among elite athletes with spinal cord injury: a global perspective," *Spinal Cord*, vol. 53, no. 1, pp. 78–82, 2015.
[22] K. N. Moore, D. Kiddoo, B. Sawatzky et al., "Randomised crossover trial of hydrophilic single use versus PVC multiuse catheters for CIC in children with neural tube defects (spina bifida) (Abstract number 171)," *Neurourology and Urodynamics*, vol. 32, no. 6, pp. 760-761, 2013.
[23] A. E. De Ruz, E. G. Leoni, and R. H. Carrera, "Epidemiology and risk factors for urinary tract infections in patients with spinal cord injury," *Journal of Urology*, vol. 164, pp. 1285–1289, 2000.
[24] J. M. Vapnek, F. M. Maynard, and J. Kim, "A prospective randomized trial of the LoFric hydrophilic coated catheter versus conventional plastic catheter for clean intermittent catheterization," *Journal of Urology*, vol. 169, no. 3, pp. 994–998, 2003.
[25] M. G. Woodbury, K. C. Hayes, and H. K. Askes, "Intermittent catheterization practices following spinal cord injury: a national survey," *Canadian Journal of Urology*, vol. 15, no. 3, pp. 4065–4071, 2008.
[26] H. Fisher, Y. Oluboyede, T. Chadwick et al., "Continuous low-dose antibiotic prophylaxis for adults with repeated urinary tract infections (AnTIC): a randomised, open-label trial," *Lancet Infectious Diseases*, vol. 18, no. 9, pp. 957–968, 2018.
[27] J. Krebs, J. Wöllner, and J. Pannek, "Risk factors for symptomatic urinary tract infections in individuals with chronic neurogenic lower urinary tract dysfunction," *Spinal Cord*, vol. 54, no. 9, pp. 682–686, 2016.
[28] P. G. Shekelle, S. C. Morton, K. A. Clark, M. Pathak, and B. G. Vickrey, "Systematic review of risk factors for urinary tract infection in adults with spinal cord dysfunction," *Journal of Spinal Cord Medicine*, vol. 22, no. 4, pp. 258–272, 1999.
[29] P. Vasudeva and H. Madersbacher, "Factors implicated in pathogenesis of urinary tract infections in neurogenic bladders: some revered, few forgotten, others ignored," *Neurourology and Urodynamics*, vol. 33, no. 1, pp. 95–100, 2014.
[30] E. J. Lucas, C. Baxter, C Singh et al., "Comparison of the microbiological milieu of patients randomized to either hydrophilic or conventional PVC catheters for clean intermittent catheterization," *Journal of Pediatric Urology*, vol. 12, no. 3, pp. 172.e1–178.e8, 2016.

[31] K. N. Moore, J. Burt, and D. C. Voaklander, "Itermittent catheterization in the rehabilitation setting: a comparison of clean and sterile technique," *Clinical Rehabilitation*, vol. 20, no. 6, pp. 461–468, 2006.

[32] D. D. Cardenas, J. M. Hoffman, E. Kelly, and M. E. Mayo, "Impact of a urinary tract infection educational program in persons with spinal cord injury," *Journal of Spinal Cord Medicine*, vol. 27, no. 1, pp. 47–54, 2004.

[33] A. P. Cameron, G. M. Rodriguez, A. Gursky, C. He, J. Q. Clemens, and J. T. Stoffel, "The severity of bowel dysfunction in patients with neurogenic bladder," *Journal of Urology*, vol. 194, no. 5, pp. 1336–1341, 2015.

[34] R. J. Madden-Fuentes, E. R. McNamara, J. C. Lloyd et al., "Variation in definitions of urinary tract infections in spina bifida patients: a systematic review," *Pediatrics*, vol. 132, no. 1, pp. 132–139, 2013.

[35] M. A. Averbeck, A. Rantell, A. Ford et al., "Current controversies in urinary tract infections: ICI-RS 2017," *Neurourology and Urodynamics*, vol. 37, no. S4, pp. S86–S92, 2018.

[36] T. Linsenmeyer and A. Oakley, "Accuracy of individuals with spinal cord injury at predicting urinary tract infections based on their symptoms," *Journal of Spinal Cord Medicine*, vol. 26, no. 4, pp. 352–357, 2003.

[37] G. Bonkat, R. Pickard, R. Bartoletti et al., *EAU Guidelines on Urological Infections*, European Association of Urology, Arnhem, Netherlands, 2018.

[38] L. E. Nicolle, "Urinary tract infections in patients with spinal injuries," *Current Infectious Disease Reports*, vol. 16, no. 1, p. 390, 2014.

[39] J. Salomon, P. Denys, C. Merle et al., "Prevention of urinary tract infection in spinal cord-injured patients: safety and efficacy of a weekly oral cyclic antibiotic (WOCA) programme with a 2 year follow-up-an observational prospective study," *Journal of Antimicrobial Chemotherapy*, vol. 57, no. 4, pp. 784–788, 2006.

[40] B. Blok, D. Castro-Diaz, G del Popolo et al., *Guidelines on Neuro-Urology*, European Association of Urology, Arnhem, Netherlands, 2015.

[41] T. M. Hooton, S. F. Bradley, D. D. Cardenas et al., "Diagnosis, prevention, and treatment of catheter-associated urinary tract infection in adults: 2009 international clinical practice guidelines from the infectious diseases society of America," *Clinical Infectious Diseases*, vol. 50, no. 5, pp. 625–663, 2010.

[42] L. L. Goetz, D. D. Cardenas, M. Kennelly et al., "International spinal cord injury urinary tract infection basic data set," *Spinal Cord*, vol. 51, no. 9, pp. 700–704, 2013.

[43] A. W. Stamm, S. A. Adelstein, A. Chen, A. Lucioni, K. C. Kobashi, and U. J. Lee, "Inconsistency in the definition of urinary tract infection after intravesical botulinum toxin A injection: a systematic review," *Journal of Urology*, vol. 200, no. 4, pp. 809–814, 2018.

[44] NIDRR, "The prevention and management of urinary tract infections among people with spinal cord injuries," *Journal of the American Paraplegia Society*, vol. 15, no. 3, pp. 194–207, 1992.

[45] A. Bakke, A. Digranes, and P. A. Hoisoeter, "Physical predictors of infection in patients treated with clean intermittent catheterization: a prospective 7-year study," *BJU International*, vol. 79, no. 1, pp. 85–90, 1997.

[46] R. Chaudhry, Z. R. Balsara, R. J. Madden-Fuentes et al., "Risk factors associated with recurrent urinary tract infection in neurogenic bladders managed by clean intermittent catheterization," *Urology*, vol. 102, pp. 213–218, 2017.

[47] J. Krebs, P. Bartel, and J. Pannek, "Residual urine volumes after intermittent catheterization in men with spinal cord injury," *Spinal Cord*, vol. 51, no. 10, pp. 776–779, 2013.

[48] J.-J. Wyndaele, A. Brauner, S. E. Geerlings, K. Bela, T. Peter, and T. E. Bjerklund-Johanson, "Clean intermittent catheterization and urinary tract infection: review and guide for future research," *BJU International*, vol. 110, no. 11c, pp. E910–E917, 2012.

[49] L. M. Massa, J. M. Hoffman, and D. D. Cardenas, "Validity, accuracy, and predictive value of urinary tract infection signs and symptoms in individuals with spinal cord injury on intermittent catheterization," *Journal of Spinal Cord Medicine*, vol. 32, no. 5, pp. 568–573, 2009.

[50] I. Okamoto, J. Prieto, M. Avery et al., "Intermittent catheter users' symptom identification, description and management of urinary tract infection: a qualitative study," *BMJ Open*, vol. 7, no. 9, article e016453, 2017.

[51] J. Pannek, "Treatment of urinary tract infection in persons with spinal cord injury: guidelines, evidence, and clinical practice," *Journal of Spinal Cord Medicine*, vol. 34, no. 1, pp. 11–15, 2011.

[52] C. Konstantinidis and A. Karafotias, "Urinary tract infections in neuro-patients," in *Microbiology of Urinary Tract Infections-Microbial Agents and Predisposing Factors*, P. Behzadi, Ed., IntechOpen Open Access Publisher, London, UK, 2018, ISBN 978-1-78984-956-1.

[53] N. Seki, K. Masuda, N. Kinukawa, K. Senoh, and S. Naito, "Risk factors for febrile urinary tract infection in children with myelodysplasia treated by clean intermittent catheterization," *International Journal of Urology*, vol. 11, no. 11, pp. 973–977, 2004.

[54] J. Lapides, A. C. Diokno, S. J. Silber, and B. S. Lowe, "Clean, intermittent self-catheterization in the treatment of urinary tract disease," *Journal of Urology*, vol. 107, no. 3, pp. 458–461, 1972.

[55] J. Lapides, "Mechanisms of urinary tract infection," *Urology*, vol. 14, no. 3, pp. 217–225, 1979.

[56] H. Prüss, A. Tedeschi, A. Thiriot et al., "Spinal cord injury-induced immunodeficiency is mediated by a sympathetic-neuroendocrine adrenal reflex," *Nature Neuroscience*, vol. 20, no. 11, pp. 1549–1559, 2017.

[57] D. J. Allison and D. S. Ditor, "Immune dysfunction and chronic inflammation following spinal cord injury," *Spinal Cord*, vol. 53, no. 1, pp. 14–18, 2015.

[58] A. P. Malykhina, J.-J. Wyndaele, K.-E. Andersson, S. De Wachter, and R. R. Dmochowski, "Do the urinary bladder and large bowel interact, in sickness or in health?: ICI-RS 2011," *Neurourology and Urodynamics*, vol. 31, no. 3, pp. 352–358, 2012.

[59] P. Christensen, G. Bazzocchi, M. Coggrave et al., "A randomized, controlled trial of transanal irrigation versus conservative bowel management in spinal cord-injured patients," *Gastroenterology*, vol. 131, no. 3, pp. 738–747, 2006.

[60] M. Spinelli, L. Rizzato, J. Renard, and L. Frediana, "A simple morpho-functional evaluation leads to a high transanal irrigation success rate in neurogenic bowel management," *Pelviperineology*, vol. 34, no. 4, pp. 124–128, 2016.

[61] S. A. Whiteside, H. Razvi, S. Dave, G. Reid, and J. P. Burton, "The microbiome of the urinary tract-a role beyond infection," *Nature Reviews Urology*, vol. 12, no. 2, pp. 81–90, 2015.

[62] M. A. Averbeck and H. Madersbacher, "Follow-up of the neuro-urological patient: a systematic review," *BJU International*, vol. 115, no. 6, pp. 39–46, 2015.
[63] J. E. Patterson and V. T. Andriole, "Bacterial urinary tract infections in diabetes," *Infectious Disease Clinics of North America*, vol. 11, no. 3, pp. 735–750, 1997.
[64] O. Nitzan, M. Elias, B. Chazan, and W. Saliba, "Urinary tract infections in patients with type 2 diabetes mellitus: review of prevalence, diagnosis, and management," *Diabetes, Metabolic Syndrome and Obesity: Targets and Therapy*, vol. 8, pp. 129–136, 2015.
[65] J. J. Cragg, V. K. Noonan, M. Dvorak, A. Krassioukov, G. B. J. Mancini, and J. F. Borisoff, "Spinal cord injury and type 2 diabetes: results from a population health survey," *Neurology*, vol. 81, no. 21, pp. 1864–1868, 2013.
[66] X. Sun, Z. B. Jones, X. M. Chen, L. Zhou, K. F. So, and Y. Ren, "Multiple organ dysfunction and systemic inflammation after spinal cord injury: a complex relationship," *Journal of Neuroinflammation*, vol. 13, no. 1, p. 260, 2016.
[67] G. Reid, A. W. Bruce, R. L. Cook, and M. Llano, "Effect on urogenital flora of antibiotic therapy for urinary tract infection," *Scandinavian Journal of Infectious Diseases*, vol. 22, no. 1, pp. 43–47, 1990.
[68] F. Sundén, L. Håkansson, E. Ljunggren, and B. Wullt, "*Escherichia coli* 83972 bacteriuria protects against recurrent lower urinary tract infections in patients with incomplete bladder emptying," *Journal of Urology*, vol. 184, no. 1, pp. 179–185, 2010.
[69] R. O. Darouiche, B. G. Green, W. H. Donovan et al., "Multicenter randomized controlled trial of bacterial interference for prevention of urinary tract infection in patients with neurogenic bladder," *Urology*, vol. 78, no. 2, pp. 341–346, 2011.
[70] I. Soljanik, "Efficacy and safety of botulinum toxin A intradetrusor injections in adults with neurogenic detrusor overactivity/neurogenic overactive bladder: a systematic review," *Drugs*, vol. 73, no. 10, pp. 1055–1066, 2013.
[71] S. Mouttalib, S. Khan, E. Castel-Lacanal et al., "Risk of urinary tract infection after detrusor botulinum toxin A injections for refractory neurogenic detrusor overactivity in patients with no antibiotic treatment," *BJU International*, vol. 106, no. 11, pp. 1677–1680, 2010.
[72] A. P. Cameron, L. Campeau, B. M. Brucker et al., "Best practice policy statement on urodynamic antibiotic prophylaxis in the non-index patient," *Neurourology and Urodynamics*, vol. 36, no. 4, pp. 915–926, 2017.
[73] S.-I. Hwang, B.-S. Lee, Z.-A. Han, H.-J. Lee, S.-H. Han, and M.-O. Kim, "Factors related to the occurrence of urinary tract infection following a urodynamic study in patients with spinal cord injury," *Annals of Rehabilitation Medicine*, vol. 40, no. 4, pp. 718–724, 2016.
[74] R. Miano, S. Germani, and G. Vespasiani, "Stones and urinary tract infections," *Urologia Internationalis*, vol. 79, no. 1, pp. 32–36, 2007.
[75] B. Welk, A. Fuller, H. Razvi, and J. Denstedt, "Renal stone disease in spinal-cord-injured patients," *Journal of Endourology*, vol. 26, no. 8, pp. 954–959, 2012.
[76] M. Joshi and N. Mittal, "Bladder calculi formed over a hair nidus in spinal injury cases," *Journal of Spinal Cord Medicine*, vol. 37, no. 3, pp. 346–348, 2014.
[77] J. L. Merrit, "Residual urine volume: correlate of urinary tract infection in patients with spinal cord injury," *Archives of Physical Medicine and Rehabilitation*, vol. 62, no. 11, pp. 558–561, 1981.
[78] A. E. Jensen, N. Hjeltnes, J. Berstad et al., "Residual urine following intermittent catheterisation in patients with spinal cord injuries," *Spinal Cord*, vol. 33, no. 12, pp. 693–696, 1995.
[79] J. K. Aronson, "Compliance, concordance, adherence," *British Journal of Clinical Pharmacology*, vol. 63, no. 4, pp. 383-384, 2007.
[80] J. H. Seth, C. Haslam, and J. N. Panicker, "Ensuring patient adherence to clean intermittent self-catheterization," *Patient Preference and Adherence*, vol. 8, pp. 191–198, 2014.
[81] S. I. Afsar, O. U. Yemisci, S. N. S. Cosar, and N. Cetin, "Compliance with clean intermittent catheterization in spinal cord injury patients: a long-term follow-up study," *Spinal Cord*, vol. 51, no. 8, pp. 645–649, 2013.
[82] S. Vahr, H. Cobussen-Boekhorst, J. Eikenboom et al., "Evidence-based Guidelines for best practice in urological health care," in *Catheterisation; Urethral Intermittent in Adults; Dilatation, Urethral Intermittent in Adults*, European Association of Urology Nurses (EAUN), Arnhem, Netherlands, 2013.
[83] Y. Lotan, M. Daudon, F. Bruyère et al., "Impact of fluid intake in the prevention of urinary system diseases," *Current Opinion in Nephrology and Hypertension*, vol. 22, no. 1, pp. S1–S10, 2013.
[84] S. Kilinç, M. Akman, F. Levendoglu, and R. Özker, "Diurnal variation of antidiuretic hormone and urinary output in spinal cord injury," *Spinal Cord*, vol. 37, no. 5, pp. 332–335, 1999.
[85] T. M. Hooton, M. Vecchio, A. Iroz et al., "Effect of increased daily water intake in premenopausal women with recurrent urinary tract infections," *JAMA Internal Medicine*, vol. 178, no. 11, pp. 1509–1515, 2018.
[86] J.-J. Wyndaele and D. Maes, "Clean intermittent self-catheterization: a 12-year followup," *Journal of Urology*, vol. 143, no. 5, pp. 906–908, 1990.
[87] A.-S. Goessaert, S. Antoons, M. Van Den Driessche, A. Tourchi, R. Pieters, and K. Everaert, "No-touch intermittent catheterization: caregiver point of view on sterility errors, duration, comfort and costs," *Journal of Advanced Nursing*, vol. 69, no. 9, pp. 2000–2007, 2013.
[88] Semmelweis, http://history-of-handwashing.leadr.msu.edu/aftermath-of-the-germ-theory/.
[89] Koch, http://history-of-handwashing.leadr.msu.edu/aftermath-of-the-germ-theory/.
[90] P. Tenke, B. Kovacs, T. E. Bjerklund Johansen et al., "European and Asian guidelines on management and prevention of catheter-associated urinary tract infections," *International Journal of Antimicrobial Agents*, vol. 31, no. 1, pp. 68–78, 2008.
[91] N. Ghafoor, F. Stoffel, and M. Mader, "Clean intermittent catheterization (CIC) in spinal cord injury patients," *Journal fur Urologie und Urogynakologie*, vol. 8, no. 1, pp. 8–11, 2001.
[92] S. Compton, L. Trease, C. Cunningham, and D. Hughes, "Australian Institute of Sport and the Australian Paralympic Committee position statement: urinary tract infection in spinal cord injured athletes," *British Journal of Sports Medicine*, vol. 49, no. 19, pp. 1236–1240, 2015.
[93] M. Forchheimer, M. A. Meade, D. Tate, A. P. Cameron, G. Rodriguez, and L. DiPonio, "Self-report of behaviors to manage neurogenic bowel and bladder by individuals with chronic spinal cord injury: frequency and associated outcomes," *Topics in Spinal Cord Injury Rehabilitation*, vol. 22, no. 2, pp. 85–98, 2016.

[94] M. J. Semins, A. D. Shore, M. A. Makary, J. Weiner, and B. R. Matlaga, "The impact of obesity on urinary tract infection risk," *Urology*, vol. 79, no. 2, pp. 266–269, 2012.

[95] W. Saliba, O. Barnett-Griness, and G. Rennert, "The association between obesity and urinary tract infection," *European Journal of Internal Medicine*, vol. 24, no. 2, pp. 127–131, 2013.

[96] F. Faleiros, C. de Oliveira Käppler, T. Rosa, and F. R. E. Gimenes, "Intermittent catheterization and urinary tract infection: a comparative study between Germany and Brazil," *Journal of Wound, Ostomy and Continence Nursing*, vol. 45, no. 6, pp. 521–526, 2018.

[97] R. Mays, A. McIntyre, S. Mehta, D. Hill, D. Wolfe, and R. Teasell, "A review of educational programs to reduce UTIs among individuals with SCI," *Rehabilitation Nursing*, vol. 39, no. 5, pp. 240–249, 2014.

[98] L. G. Zanollo, G. C. Stensrød, J. Kerdraon et al., "Standardized intermittent catheterisation education improves catheterisation compliance in individuals with spinal cord injury," *International Journal of Urological Nursing*, vol. 9, no. 3, pp. 165–172, 2015.

[99] A. Gomelsky, G. E. Lemack, J. C Castano Botero et al., "Current and future international patterns of care of neurogenic bladder after spinal cord injury," *World Journal of Urology*, vol. 36, no. 10, pp. 1613–1619, 2018.

[100] M. Przydacz, P. Denys, and J. Corcos, "What do we know about neurogenic bladder prevalence and management in developing countries and emerging regions of the world?," *Annals of Physical and Rehabilitation Medicine*, vol. 60, no. 5, pp. 341–346, 2017.

[101] C. J. Bennett, M. N. Young, S. S. Razi, R. Adkins, F. Diaz, and A. McCrary, "The effect of urethral introducer tip catheters on the incidence of urinary tract infection outcomes in spinal cord injured patients," *Journal of Urology*, vol. 158, no. 2, pp. 519–521, 1997.

[102] R. Charbonneau-Smith, "No-touch catheterization and infection rates in a select spinal cord injured population," *Rehabilitation Nursing*, vol. 18, no. 5, pp. 296–299, 1993.

[103] P. Denys, VaPro Study Group in France, J. G. Prévinaire et al., "Intermittent self-catheterization habits and opinion on aseptic VaPro catheter in French neurogenic bladder population," *Spinal Cord*, vol. 50, no. 11, pp. 853–858, 2012.

[104] J. Stensballe, D. Looms, P. N. Nielsen, and M. Tvede, "Hydrophilic-coated catheters for intermittent catheterisation reduce urethral micro trauma: a prospective, randomised, participant-blinded, crossover study of three different types of catheters," *European Urology*, vol. 48, no. 6, pp. 978–983, 2005.

[105] S. Muctar, "The importance of a lubricant in transurethral interventions," *Urologe B*, vol. 31, pp. 153–155, 1991.

[106] J. Lundgren, O. Bengtsson, A. Israelsson, A.-C. Jönsson, A.-S. Lindh, and J. Utas, "The importance of osmolality for intermittent catheterization of the urethra," *Spinal Cord*, vol. 38, no. 1, pp. 45–50, 2000.

[107] S. Vaidyanathan, B. M. Soni, S. Dundas, and K. R. Krishnan, "Urethral cytology in spinal cord injury patients performing intermittent catheterisation," *Spinal Cord*, vol. 32, no. 7, pp. 493–500, 1994.

[108] J. Wyndaele, "Intermittent catheterization: which is the optimal technique?," *Spinal Cord*, vol. 40, no. 9, pp. 432–437, 2002.

[109] P. A. Willette and S. Coffield, "Current trends in the management of difficult urinary catheterizations," *Western Journal of Emergency Medicine*, vol. 13, no. 6, pp. 427–478, 2012.

[110] L. Hadfield-Law, "Male catheterization," *Accident and Emergency Nursing*, vol. 9, no. 4, pp. 257–263, 2001.

[111] I. Kurze, V. Geng, and R. Böthig, "S2k-Leitlinie der Deutschen Gesellschaft für Urologie," *Der Urologe*, vol. 54, no. 3, pp. 385–393, 2015.

[112] J. Prieto, C. L. Murphy, K. N. Moore, and M. Fader, "Intermittent catheterisation for long-term bladder management," *Cochrane Database of Systematic Reviews*, no. 9, p. CD006008, 2014.

[113] K. Christison, M. Walter, J.-J. J. M. Wyndaele et al., "Intermittent catheterization: the devil is in the details," *Journal of Neurotrauma*, vol. 35, no. 7, pp. 985–989, 2018.

[114] C. Rognoni and R. Tarricone, "Intermittent catheterisation with hydrophilic and non-hydrophilic urinary catheters: systematic literature review and meta-analyses," *BMC Urology*, vol. 17, no. 1, p. 4, 2017.

[115] D. Kiddoo, B. Sawatzky, C.-D. Bascu, N. Dharamsi, K. Afshar, and K. N. Moore, "Randomized crossover trial of single use hydrophilic coated vs multiple use polyvinylchloride catheters for intermittent catheterization to determine incidence of urinary infection," *Journal of Urology*, vol. 194, no. 1, pp. 174–179, 2015.

5

Critical Assessment of Single-Use Ureteroscopes in an *In Vivo* Porcine Model

Brian Ceballos,[1] **Charles U. Nottingham**,[1] **Seth K. Bechis**,[2] **Roger L. Sur**,[2] **Brian R. Matlaga**,[3] **and Amy E. Krambeck**[1]

[1]*Indiana University School of Medicine, Department of Urology, 1801 Senate Blvd. Suite 220, Indianapolis, IN 46202, USA*
[2]*University of California San Diego School of Medicine, Department of Urology, 200 West Arbor Drive #8897, San Diego, CA 92103, USA*
[3]*Johns Hopkins University School of Medicine, James Buchanan Brady Urological Institute, 600 North Wolfe Street Park 2 Room 221, Baltimore, MD 21287, USA*

Correspondence should be addressed to Charles U. Nottingham; cunottingham@gmail.com

Academic Editor: Matthew Rutman

Introduction and Objectives. In recent years, there has been increasing utilization of single-use ureteroscopes albeit with few studies comparing the performance characteristics between these devices. We compared two commonly utilized single-use ureteroscopes in a porcine model. *Methods.* A female pig was placed under general anesthesia and positioned supine, and retrograde access to the renal collecting system was obtained. The LithoVue (Boston Scientific) and Uscope (Pusen Medical) were evaluated by three experienced surgeons, and each surgeon started with a new scope. The following parameters were compared between each ureteroscope: time for navigation to upper and lower pole calyces with and without implements (1.9 F basket, 200 μm laser fiber, and 365 μm laser fiber for upper only) in the working channel and subjective evaluations of maneuverability, irrigant flow through the scope, lever force, ergonomics, and scope optics. *Results.* Navigation to the lower pole calyx was significantly faster with LithoVue compared to Uscope when the working channel was empty (24.3 vs. 49.4 seconds, $p < 0.01$) and with a 200 μm fiber (63.6 vs. 94.4 seconds, $p = 0.04$), but not with the 1.9 F basket. Navigation to the upper pole calyx was similar for all categories except faster with LithoVue containing the 365 μm fiber (67.1 vs. 99.7 seconds, $p = 0.02$). Subjective assessments of scope maneuverability to upper and lower pole calyces when the scope was empty and with implements favored LithoVue in all categories, as did assessments of irrigant flow, illumination, image quality, and field of view. Both scopes had similar scores of lever force and ergonomics. *Conclusions.* In an *in vivo* porcine model, the type of single-use ureteroscope employed affected the navigation times and subjective assessments of maneuverability and visualization. In all cases, LithoVue provided either equivalent or superior metrics than Uscope. Further clinical studies are necessary to determine the implications of these findings.

1. Introduction

Renal stone disease is a growing concern for patients in the United States, which makes optimal management increasingly important. Between 1994 and 2007, there was an increase in incidence in renal stones according to the National Health and Nutrition Examination Survey (NHANES) [1]. The increase was estimated to be from 6.3% to 10.6% in men and from 4.1% to 7.1% in women [2]. Despite the various methods of management for uncomplicated urolithiasis, ureteroscopy has become widely accepted as a desirable form of treatment owing to its efficacy, efficiency, ability to be performed in an outpatient setting, and minimal side effect profile [3].

A more recent advancement in the surgical treatment of urolithiasis has been the use of disposable (non-reusable) ureteroscopes as opposed to the traditional reusable ureteroscopes [4]. In October 2015, Boston Scientific introduced LithoVue, the first disposable flexible ureteroscope in efforts to avoid maintenance costs and loss of deflection with repeated use, as this was a central concern for the reusable ureteroscopes [5].

Looking forward, the difference in safety and efficacy between single-use and reusable ureteroscopy becomes essential to understand when considering the management of stone disease and cost of treatment. It is estimated that urolithiasis will cost the healthcare economy up to $3 billion by the year 2030 [6], and it is unclear exactly how integration of disposable ureteroscopes will impact costs going forward. To date, the studies between disposable ureteroscopes are limited, as only a handful of scopes are available for clinical use. The objective of this study is to compare maneuverability, navigation time, and visualization between two disposable ureteroscopes in a porcine model: the Boston Scientific LithoVue and Pusen Uscope.

2. Methods

The study was conducted at CBSET, Inc. (Lexington, MA), under IACUC protocol #I00240. A female pig weighing approximately 35 kg was placed under general anesthesia and positioned supine, and retrograde access to the renal collecting system was obtained cystoscopically. An 11/13 ureteral access sheath was placed under fluoroscopic guidance, with proximal positioning in the proximal ureter. Ureteroscopy was performed by three experienced endourologists (SB, RS, and AK) with both the LithoVue (Boston Scientific, Boston, MA) and the first-generation Uscope (Zhuhai Pusen Medical Co., Zhuhai, Guangdong, China). Each ureteroscope had a tip diameter of 9.5 French as well as a working channel that measured 3.6 French in size. Each surgeon started with a new scope, but they were not formally blinded due to the fact that they each had prior experience with the LithoVue ureteroscope. For all individual scopes, each surgeon completed seven total tasks five times each, for a total of 35 passes of a given scope.

The time required for navigation to upper and lower pole calyces was recorded in seconds. These tasks were assessed with and without implements placed through the working channel. The implements used were a 200 μm holmium:YAG laser fiber (Flexiva, Boston Scientific) and a 1.9 French nitinol basket (Zero Tip, Boston Scientific). An additional implement of a 365 μm holmium:YAG laser fiber (Flexiva, Boston Scientific) was also used, but the scopes were only passed to the upper pole with this fiber. Following completion of these tasks, each surgeon gave a subjective assessment of scope maneuverability on a 0–5 scale, with 0 being the lowest maneuverability score and 5 being the highest.

Upon completion of all 35 passes for a given scope, each surgeon then gave a subjective assessment of irrigant flow through the scope, lever force, ergonomics, and scope visualization at the completion of all passes of each scope, thereby representing visualization at only the very end of the scope's life span. The visualization included three categories: image quality, illumination, and field of view. These assessments were also graded on a 0–5 scale, with 0 being the lowest visualization score and 5 being the highest.

Mean times and scores were calculated and compared between the LithoVue and Uscope for each parameter using two-sided student's t-test. Statistical analysis was performed using SPSS version 25.0 (Armonk, NY).

3. Results

Each pass of the ureteroscope by each surgeon for all parameters was included for analysis. Each surgeon successfully performed a total of 35 passes with each ureteroscope.

The results of navigation times to upper and lower pole calyces are summarized in Table 1. Navigation to the lower pole calyx was significantly faster with LithoVue compared to Uscope when the working channel was empty (24.3 vs. 49.4 seconds, $p < 0.01$) and with a 200 μm fiber (63.6 vs. 94.4 seconds, $p = 0.04$), but not with the 1.9 F basket (58.2 vs. 70.1 seconds, $p = 0.18$). Navigation to the upper pole calyx was not significantly faster in either scope with the working channel was empty, with a 1.9 F basket, and with a 200 μm fiber. However, upper pole navigation was faster using LithoVue with a 365 μm fiber (67.1 vs. 99.7 seconds, $p = 0.02$).

Subjective maneuverability assessments of each ureteroscope are summarized in Table 2. LithoVue had significantly higher assessment scores than Uscope for navigation to both upper and lower poles when the working channel was empty and when it contained all three implements.

The subjective assessment of irrigant flow, lever force, ergonomics, and scope optics upon completion of scope usage is presented in Table 3. Both scopes had statistically similar scores for lever force and ergonomics. LithoVue had significantly higher ratings than Uscope in the categories of irrigant flow (5.0 vs. 3.3, $p = 0.01$), illumination (4.0 vs. 1.3, respectively; $p = 0.02$), image quality (4.0 vs. 1.3, respectively; $p = 0.02$), and field of view (4.7 vs. 1.3, respectively; $p < 0.01$).

Figure 1 shows representative photographs of the tip of each ureteroscope following completion of all 35 passes.

4. Discussion

The purpose of this study was to compare differences between the Boston Scientific LithoVue and Pusen Uscope, two commonly used disposable ureteroscopes in a porcine model. After 35 passes with each type of ureteroscope by all three surgeons, it was determined that the LithoVue provided either equivalent or faster navigation time to the renal calyces, and that the subjective visualization was superior when compared to the Uscope. To our knowledge, this is the first critical comparison between these two ureteroscopes in a porcine model.

In comparison to the current literature, our results regarding the disposable ureteroscopes appear similar in nature. Although we did not evaluate resolution at specified distances, Winship and colleagues reported superior resolution using the LithoVue in comparison to the Uscope when evaluated at 10 mm [7]. When the LithoVue was compared to the Uscope and the reusable Flex-X2 ureteroscope by Marchini et al, they found that the LithoVue was superior to both the Uscope and Flex-X2 in regards to optical resolution, field of view, deflection capacity, and irrigation when working with larger instruments in the working channel [8]. These studies

Table 1: Surgeon times (seconds) for navigation to upper and lower poles between LithoVue and Uscope when the working channel is empty, with a 1.9-French basket, a 200 μm laser fiber, and a 365 μm laser fiber (upper only).

Surgeon time in seconds	Empty working channel	1.9-French basket	200 μm laser fiber	365 μm laser fiber
Navigation to upper pole				
LithoVue	50.4 (31.5)	75.3 (32.7)	76.0 (37.6)	67.1 (23.7)
Uscope	35.7 (25.4)	106.8 (46.6)	90.1 (41.5)	99.7 (42.0)
p value	0.20	0.05	0.37	0.02
Navigation to lower pole				
LithoVue	24.3 (11.9)	58.2 (18.5)	63.6 (25.9)	—
Uscope	49.4 (31.4)	70.1 (27.4)	94.4 (47.8)	—
p value	0.01	0.18	0.04	—

The values are expressed as mean (SD).

Table 2: Subjective surgeon assessment of maneuverability between LithoVue and Uscope for navigation to upper and lower poles when the working channel is empty, with a 1.9-French basket, a 200 μm laser fiber, and a 365 μm laser fiber (upper only).

Subjective scope maneuverability assessment (0–5 rating, 5 = highest)	Empty working channel	1.9-French basket	200 μm laser fiber	365 μm laser fiber
Navigation to upper pole				
LithoVue	4.40 (0.51)	4.47 (0.52)	5.00 (0.00)	4.87 (0.35)
Uscope	3.80 (0.41)	3.47 (0.74)	3.00 (0.65)	2.23 (0.93)
p value	<0.01	<0.01	<0.01	<0.01
Navigation to lower pole				
LithoVue	4.33 (0.49)	4.67 (0.49)	5.00 (0.00)	
Uscope	3.40 (0.63)	3.60 (0.51)	3.00 (0.76)	—
p value	<0.01	<0.01	<0.01	—

The values are expressed as mean (SD).

Table 3: Subjective surgeon assessments of irrigant flow, lever force, ergonomics, and scope optics between LithoVue and Uscope after completion of 35 passes of the ureteroscope.

Subjective assessments (0–5 rating, 5 = highest)	LithoVue	Uscope	*p* value
Irrigant flow	5.0 (0.0)	3.3 (0.6)	0.01
Lever force	4.0 (1.0)	3.0 (1.7)	0.44
Ergonomics	4.7 (0.6)	3.0 (1.7)	0.19
Illumination	4.0 (1.0)	1.3 (0.6)	0.02
Image quality	4.0 (1.0)	1.3 (0.6)	0.02
Field of view	4.7 (0.6)	1.3 (0.6)	<0.01

The values are expressed as mean (SD).

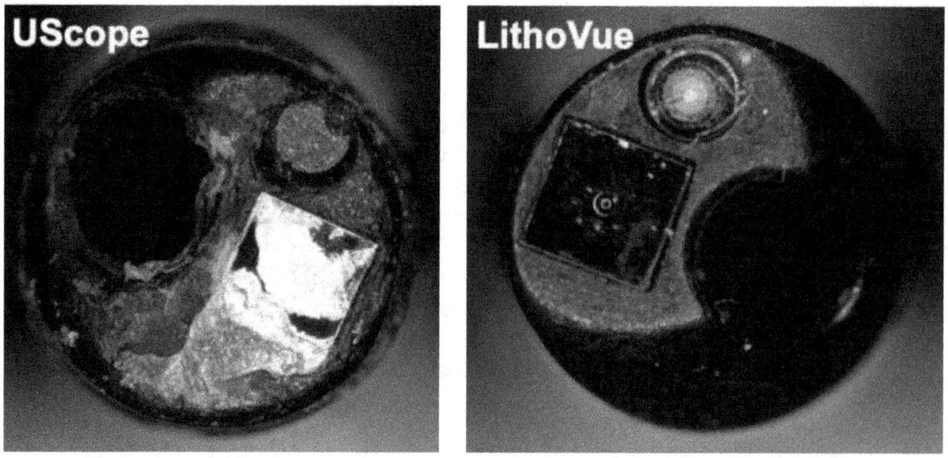

(a) (b)

Figure 1: Representative photographs of the tip of the Uscope (a) and LithoVue (b) following completion of all tasks (total of 36 passes per scope).

support the potential benefits of the disposable ureteroscopes, as optimal resolution plays an essential role in safety during ureteroscopy.

While costs often vary between regions and institutions, the price of ureteroscopy is an important factor that should be taken into account when comparing ureteroscopes. According to Salvadó et al., the disposable ureteroscopes are 32 times cheaper than the overall costs of a reusable ureteroscope in Chile [9]. Between disposable ureteroscopes, the Uscope is about 42% cheaper than the LithoVue [9]. However, the LithoVue is the only disposable ureteroscope that has a one-ureteroscope-per case guarantee, which ensures that Boston Scientific will replace the ureteroscope at no additional cost to the patient or care facility if a LithoVue ureteroscope breaks during a procedure [7].

Another factor to consider when comparing ureteroscopes is rates of malfunction. Because each disposable ureteroscope typically costs >$800 per case, rates of failure become an integral part in cost analysis [4]. In our study, we had no malfunction of either disposable ureteroscope that required replacement during a case, which is consistent with the experience of Salvadó et al. who did not experience malfunction of the Pusen Uscope in their series of 71 cases [9]. However, in regards to the LithoVue, our results appear to be slightly improved to that of Usawachintachit et al., who experienced a rate of malfunction of 4.4% among their 129 cases [10]. However, it is once again worth noting that the one-ureteroscope-per-case policy previously outlined is only supported by Boston Scientific [7].

While there are limitations to this study, our aim is to provide insight towards our experience with the LithoVue and Uscope disposable ureteroscopes. One limitation is the difficulty with blinding for the type of ureteroscope used by the urologist. The design, color, and interface of each scope may be enough to influence the user's analysis. Another possible limitation is the inability to control for variable experience with each scope. While one surgeon may have ease with one ureteroscope, their lack of experience with the other may influence their functional use and analysis of the product. The value in this study is in its *in vivo* nature as it takes on a more practical approach to the analysis as opposed to benchtop analysis. Another strength of our study is the analysis by three surgeons of different institutions, as this helps reduce the bias that could result from similar practices within the same care facility.

5. Conclusion

Using an *in vivo* porcine model, the type of disposable ureteroscope significantly affected the navigation times and subjective visualization among three experienced urologists. Overall, the LithoVue proved to be either equivalent or superior to the Pusen Uscope.

References

[1] K. K. Stamatelou, M. E. Francis, C. A. Jones, L. M. Nyberg, and G. C. Curhan, "Time trends in reported prevalence of kidney stones in the United States: 1976–199411. See editorial by Goldfarb, p. 1951," *Kidney International*, vol. 63, no. 5, pp. 1817–1823, 2003.

[2] C. D. Scales, A. C. Smith, J. M. Hanley, and C. S. Saigal, "Prevalence of kidney stones in the United States," *European Urology*, vol. 62, no. 1, pp. 160–165, 2012.

[3] T. Anagnostou and D. Tolley, "Management of ureteric stones," *European Urology*, vol. 45, no. 6, pp. 714–721, 2004.

[4] U. Boylu, M. Oommen, R. Thomas, and B. R. Lee, "In vitro comparison of a disposable flexible ureteroscope and conventional flexible ureteroscopes," *Journal of Urology*, vol. 182, no. 5, pp. 2347–2351, 2009.

[5] S. Butticè, T. E. Sener, C. Netsch, E. Emiliani, R. Pappalardo, and C. Magno, "LithoVue™: a new single-use digital flexible ureteroscope," *Central European Journal of Urology*, vol. 69, pp. 302–305, 2016.

[6] K. B. Scotland, J. Y. H. Chan, and B. H. Chew, "Single-use flexible ureteroscopes: how do they compare with reusable ureteroscopes?" *Journal of Endourology*, vol. 33, no. 2, pp. 71–78, 2019.

[7] B. Winship, D. Wollin, E. Carlos, J. Li, G. M. Preminger, and M. E. Lipkin, "Avoiding a lemon: performance consistency of single-use ureteroscopes," *Journal of Endourology*, vol. 33, no. 2, pp. 127–131, 2019.

[8] G. S. Marchini, C. A. Batagello, M. Monga et al., "In vitro evaluation of single-use digital flexible ureteroscopes: a practical comparison for a patient-centered approach," *Journal of Endourology*, vol. 32, no. 3, pp. 184–191, 2018.

[9] J. A. Salvadó, R. Olivares, J. M. Cabello et al., "Retrograde intrarenal surgery using the single-use flexible ureteroscope Uscope 3022 (PUSEN™): evaluation of clinical results," *Central European Journal of Urology*, vol. 71, pp. 202–207, 2018.

[10] M. Usawachintachit, D. S. Isaacson, K. Taguchi et al., "A prospective case-control study comparing LithoVue, a single-use, flexible disposable ureteroscope, with flexible, reusable fiber-optic ureteroscopes," *Journal of Endourology*, vol. 31, no. 5, pp. 468–475, 2017.

6

Epidemiological and Diagnostic Aspects of Bladder Bilharziomas in the Urology Department of Idrissa Pouye General Hospital (HOGIP)

Oumar Gaye,[1] Mohamed Jalloh,[1] Ngor M Thiam,[1] Medina Ndoye,[1] Khadidiatou Dansokho,[2] Youssef Bellamine,[1] Saint C. N Kouka,[3] Cherif Dial,[2] Mouhamadou M Mbodji,[1] Ayun Cassell,[1] Issa Labou,[1] Lamine Niang,[1] and Serigne Gueye[1]

[1]*Urology-andrology Department, Hôpital General Idrissa Pouye, Dakar, Senegal*
[2]*Pathological Anatomy Laboratory, Hôpital General Idrissa Pouye, Dakar, Senegal*
[3]*Urology-andrology Department, UFR Santé Université de Thies, Dakar, Senegal*

Correspondence should be addressed to Oumar Gaye; oumargaye-uro@outlook.fr

Academic Editor: Muhammad Shahid; muhammad.shahid@hsc.wvu.edu

Objective. The aim of our study is to assess the diagnostic aspects of bladder bilharzioma in the Urology Department of Idrissa Pouye General Hospital (Senegal). *Materials and Methods.* It is a descriptive study from January 2013 to December 2018. The patients included in the study were those who had anatomopathological examination of bladder biopsy that showed a schistosomiasis pseudotumor of the bladder. The variables studied were sociodemographic, clinical symptoms, imaging findings, histology, and treatment. The data have been saved and analyzed by the 2013 Excel software. *Results.* Thirteen patients were included in our study. The average age was 27 ± 12.1 years. Sex ratio was 1.6. The majority of the patients were from the northern part of Senegal. Hematuria was the main symptom for all the patients. Cystoscopy was performed for all the patients and showed 5 granulomas and 8 fibrocalcic polyps. A transurethral resection of the bladder was performed, and treatment with praziquantel (40 mg/kg of bodyweight) has been carried out. One patient presented precancerous lesions such as metaplasia and dysplasia of the bladder mucosa. After a median follow-up of 40 months (6–57 months), ten patients had a favorable clinical and endoscopic outcome. *Conclusion.* Granulomas and fibrocalcic polyps of the bladder mucosa are, respectively, confused with squamous cell carcinoma and bladder lithiasis in endemic areas of schistosomiasis. Good cystoscopy interpretation can provide the diagnosis of bladder bilharzioma and start the treatment.

1. Introduction

Schistosoma haematobium bilharziasis is responsible for urogenital bilharziasis. It reaches a hundred million people in sub-Saharan Africa [1]. In Senegal, it prevails in all regions with a prevalence reaching more than 50% in certain areas [2, 3]. Infection of humans with schistosomes occurs through contact with water contaminated with furcocercariae which actively penetrate through the skin. The breeding grounds for the disease are stagnant water, the banks of rivers, the banks of lakes, and irrigation canals. Children are the most affected age group [2, 4]. Fishermen, cultivators, rice farmers, and workers who maintain irrigation canals are the most exposed adults. Women, because of their daily frequentation in places at risk for household chores, are more affected than men [4].

As soon as they penetrate through the skin, the schistosomules reach the intrahepatic portal venules by circulatory route. They will continue their sexual development and maturation towards the venous plexuses of the bladder and other pelvic organs [5]. The involvement of the various urogenital organs varies according to the richness of their vascularization. This is how the bladder, seminal vesicles, and the end of the ureters are more affected by the disease, thanks to their rich vascular supply [6].

In the bladder plexus, the female leaves the male to enter the submucosa where she begins to lay eggs. Some eggs will be eliminated by the urine, but many of them will remain blocked in the bladder wall or will be embolized at a distance [4, 7].

The eggs blocked in the tissue will determine the formation of a bilharzian granuloma. Indeed, these eggs secrete an antigen that triggers a cell-mediated immune response. The cell infiltrate is characterized by the presence of eosinophils, histiocytes, fibroblasts, epithelioid, and giant cells [6].

Bladder bilharziomas can manifest clinically as hematuria, lower urinary tract symptoms, or acute retention of urine [8–10].

El-Badawi described three types of bladder bilharzioma: granulomatous polyps, fibrocalcic polyps, and villous polyps [8].

The granulomatous polyp and the fibrocalcic polyp pose, respectively, the problem of differential diagnosis with squamous cell carcinoma of the bladder and bladder stones in the area of bilharzian endemia. Nevertheless, a good exploration with cystoscopy makes it possible to differentiate them from the latter and to propose an adequate treatment. Villous polyps are more difficult to diagnose and require histological analysis [8].

The treatment of bladder bilharziomas is related to antibilharzian treatment. Praziquantel at a dose of 40 mg/kg is recommended. Transurethral resection of the bladder and bladder biopsy are indicated for residual masses or when the endoscopic diagnosis of bilharzioma is not obvious [6].

The objective of our study was to describe the diagnostic aspects of bladder bilharziomas in our center.

2. Materials and Methods

This is a descriptive study from January 2013 to December 2018. The patients included were those who underwent transurethral resection of the bladder indicated before a bladder tumor and whose results of the anatomopathological examination of the shavings of resection concluded in a bilharzian pseudotumor of the bladder. The parameters studied were age, sex, geographic origin, clinical signs, type, location and number of bilharziomas, results of anatomopathological examination of the resection chips, treatment, and course. The data were recorded and analyzed by Excel 2013 software.

3. Results

This study involved 13 patients. The mean age of the patients was 27 ± 12.1 years. The sex ratio was 1.6. Ten of our patients were from northern Senegal in the Senegal River region. A notion of swimming in fresh water had been clarified in eleven of the patients. Hematuria was the finding in all patients and was associated with dysuria in two patients (Table 1). A urine pellet was produced in two of our patients, one of whom isolated bilharzia eggs. The cystoscopy performed in all the patients objectified five granulomatous polyps (38.5%) and eight fibrocalcic polyps (61.5%). It also showed lesions of semolina vesical bilharziasis associated in the five granulomatous polyps (Figures 1 and 2) and in four of the fibrocalcic polyps (Figure 3). The granulomatous polyps were unique in three patients and were located mainly in the perimeatic regions. The fibrocalcic polyps were unique in six patients and were mainly located in the bladder dome (Table 2). An ultrasound of the urinary tree was performed in 2 patients and showed focal parietal thickening of the bladder without affecting the upper urinary tract. A URO-computed tomography (URO-CT) was performed in 2 patients and objectified a bladder tumor (Figure 3). Transurethral resection of the bladder tumor (TURBT) associated with medical treatment with praziquantel (40 mg/kg as a single dose) had been performed in all our patients. Pathological examination of the resection shavings showed an epitheliogigantocellular and polynuclear inflammatory eosinophilic granulomatous inflammatory reaction around bilharzian eggs belonging to the species *Schistosoma haematobium* (Figures 4 and 5). Precancerous lesions such as metaplasia and dysplasia of the bladder mucosa were objectified in one of our patients (Figure 6). After a median follow-up of 40 months (6–57 months), three patients were lost to follow-up. Good clinical and endoscopic improvement was noted in nine patients with disappearance of hematuria and cystoscopy images in nine patients. A recurrence in one patient required a second RTUV whose histology concluded with a bilharzioma.

4. Discussion

Bladder bilharziomas are inflammatory pseudotumors secondary to *Schistosoma haematobium* infection and results from chronic inflammation. The presence of such tumor poses a problem of differential diagnosis. Generally, the confirmation of the diagnosis is performed after TURBT. In spite of the controversies regarding the role of schistosomiasis as a risk factor for bladder cancer, any patient with hematuria or the diagnosis of bladder mass will be investigated for a history of bladder schistosomiasis.

Ten of our patients were from northern Senegal living next to Senegal river. This area is known for its high prevalence of bladder schistosomiasis (53%) [3, 11].

The mean age of our patients was 27 years which is in accordance to the higher prevalence of this infection in young adults [8] and children [5, 10].

The sex ratio of our patients was 1.6. This male predominance of bilharziasis has been objectified by several studies carried out in Africa [12–14] and is explained by professional exposure during farming and fishing. However, according to Guiguen et al., women are more exposed to schistosomiasis in areas that do not have access to running water because in such case, women are in contact with infesting water during domestic work [4].

Hematuria was the finding in all patients and was associated with difficulty passing urine in two patients. El-Badawi had also objectified hematuria as the main symptom (73.3%) associated with burning sensation when voiding (66.3%), dysuria (59.3%), frequency (58.1%), suprapubic pain (50%), pyuria (44.2%), or renal colic (30.2%). Renal colic was explained by the obstruction of the ureteral meatus by the mass or a stenosing fibrosis of the ureter [8].

Table 1: Clinical information of the patients.

	Age	Sex	Residence	Notion of swimming in fresh water	Clinical sign
Patient 1	42	F	Fouta	Yes	Hematuria
Patient 2	24	F	Fouta	Yes	Hematuria
Patient 3	16	F	Fouta	Yes	Hematuria
Patient 4	17	F	Dakar	Unspecified	Hematuria
Patient 5	17	F	Fouta	Yes	Hematuria + dysuria
Patient 6	45	M	Dakar	Yes	Hematuria
Patient 7	23	M	Mauritanie	Unspecified	Hematuria
Patient 8	32	M	Fouta	Yes	Hematuria
Patient 9	23	M	Fouta	Yes	Hematuria
Patient 10	12	M	Fouta	Yes	Hematuria
Patient 11	26	M	Fouta	Yes	Hematuria + dysuria
Patient 12	48	M	Fouta	Yes	Hematuria
Patient 13	26	M	Fouta	Yes	Hematuria

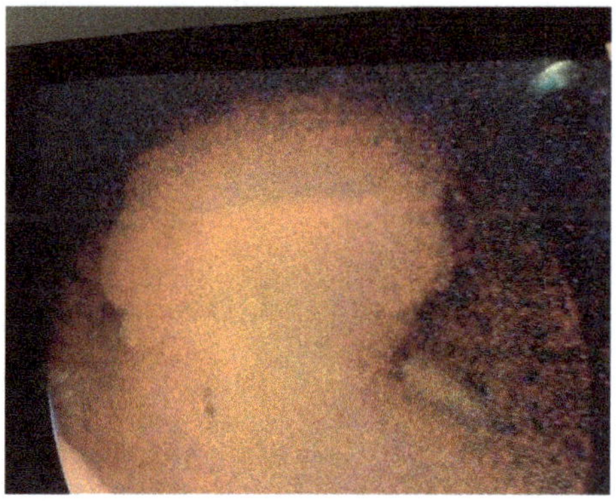

Figure 1: Polyp sitting around the left ureteral meatus viewed with cystoscopy.

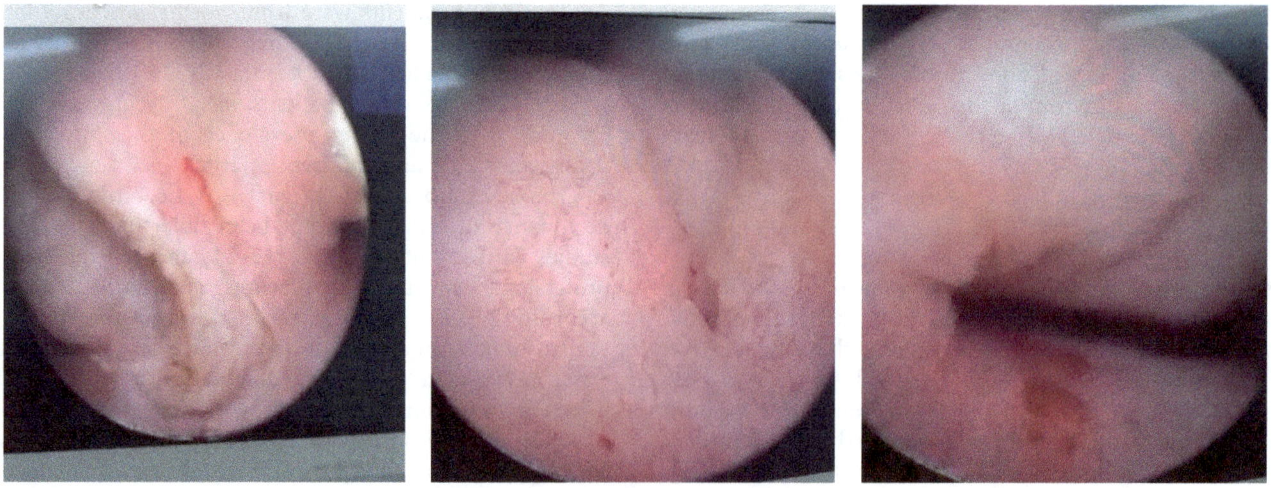

(a) (b) (c)

Figure 2: Continued.

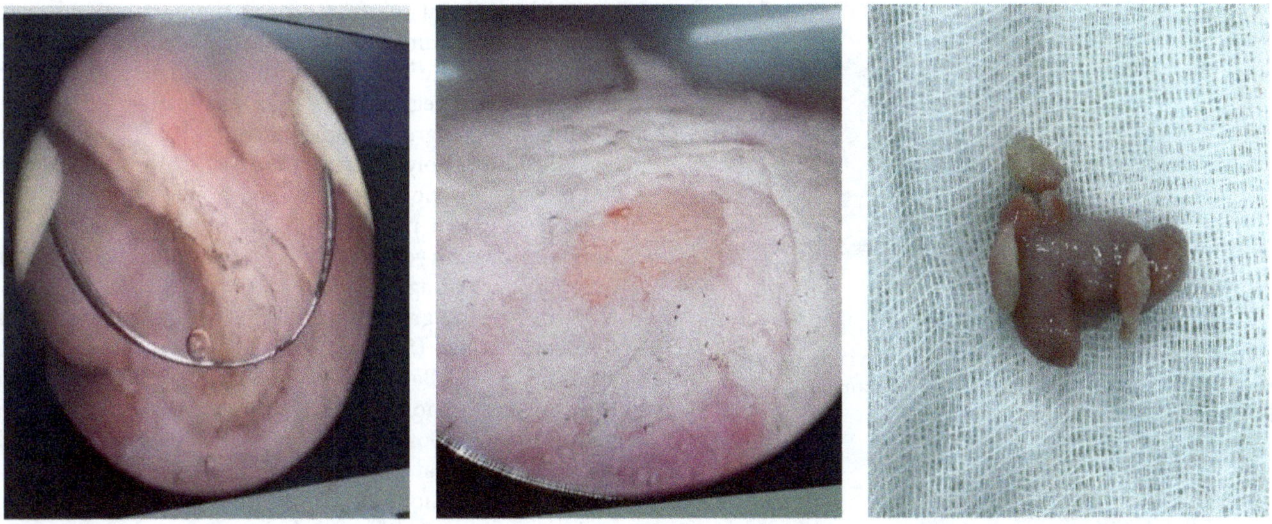

(d) (e) (f)

FIGURE 2: Polyp granulomatous sitting around the left ureteral meatus. (a) Granulomatous polyp developed on left ureteral meatus. (b) Left ureteral meatus. (c) Granulomatous polyp and its implantation base. (d) Resection of the granulomatous polyp. (e) Aspect of the left ureteral meatus after resection. (f) Resected granulomatous polyp.

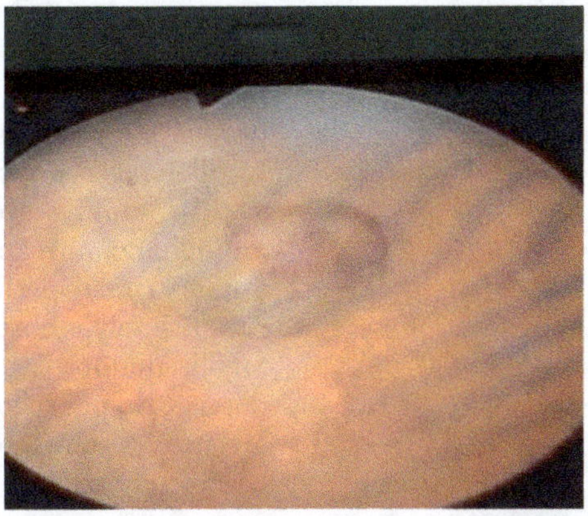

FIGURE 3: Fibrocalcic polyp located at the level of the bladder dome visible on cystoscopy.

TABLE 2: Distribution of polyps according to their characteristics.

Characteristics of bladder polyps	Granulomatous polyps	Fibrocalcium polyps	Polyps villous
Seat of polyps			
Right perimeatic	3	2	0
Left perimeatic	2	1	0
Trigone	0	0	0
Posterior side	0	1	0
Dome	0	4	0
Number of polyps			
Unique	2	6	0
Multiple	3	2	0

Abdel-Salam and Ehsan, on the other hand, reported difficulty passing urine as a predominant symptom in patients with a granulomatous polyp and in more than 50% of patients with a fibrocalcic polyp [9]. The other symptoms he described were hematuria and pyuria [9].

A urine analysis was performed in two of our patients and showed bilharzia eggs in one of them. According to Abdel-Salam, the presence of viable eggs is very sensitive for the diagnosis of granulomatous polyps (70%) and less sensitive in fibrocalcic polyps (16.5%) [9].

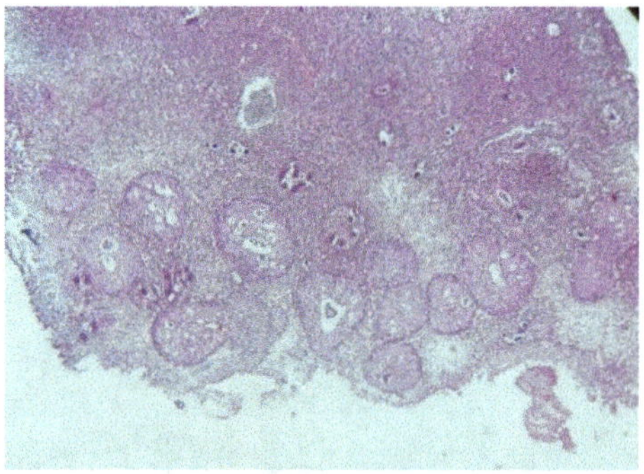

FIGURE 4: Giant cells phagocytizing eggs of viable bilharzia. Hematoxylin and eosin x 100 (image of Professor Dial, head of the pathological anatomy laboratory of HOGIP).

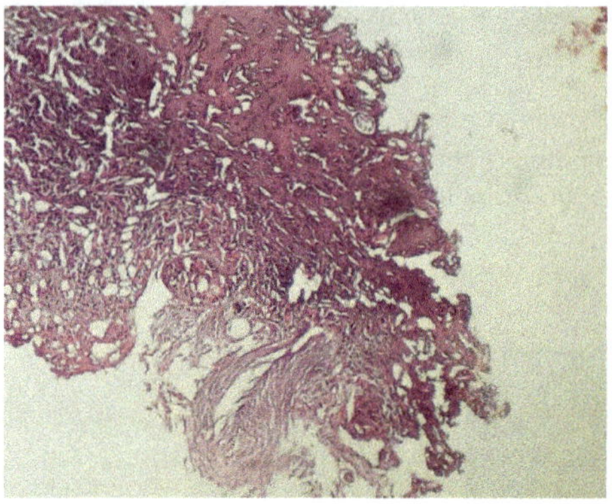

FIGURE 5: Granulomatous inflammatory reaction and not viable bilharzia egg. Hematoxylin and eosin x 100 (image of Professor Dial, head of the pathological anatomy laboratory of HOGIP).

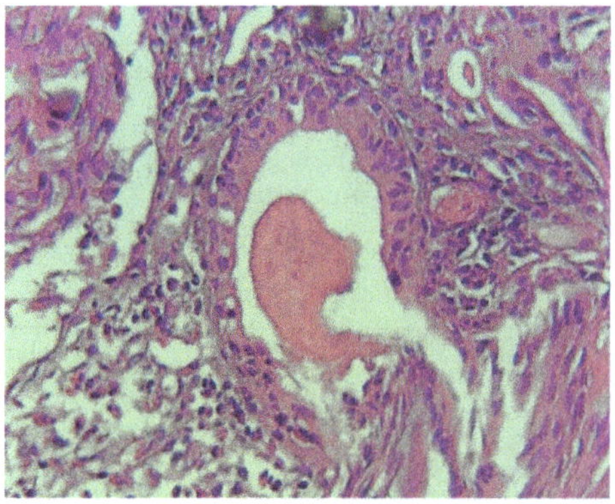

FIGURE 6: Dysplastic lesion associated with granulomatous inflammatory reaction due to *Schistosoma haematobium*. Hematoxylin and eosin x 100 (image of Professor Dial, head of the pathological anatomy laboratory of HOGIP).

We had reported 38.5% of granulomatous polyps and 61.5% of fibrocalcic polyps. El-Badawi [8], on the other hand, found a predominance of granulomatous polyps (60.5%), while Abdel-Salam and Ehsan [9] showed an equal proportion of granulomatous and fibrocalcic polyps.

In the area of schistosomiasis endemic, large granulomatous polyps can be confused with squamous cell carcinoma of the bladder. But they can be differentiated by their typical location at the trigone and the paraureteral region, their multiple numbers, the pedunculated aspect, red appearance, and the tendency to bleed when pressed by the cystoscope. The regression of such lesion after antibilharzian treatment has a great diagnostic value [8].

Fibrocalcic polyps can be confused with bladder stones, but they do not move freely like stones with the filling of the bladder or when pushed by the cystoscope. They are pedunculated, dull yellowish in color, and occur in patients over 20 years of age [8].

Three of the granulomatous polyps (60%) and 4 of the fibrocalcic polyps (50%) were associated with semolina grain appearance. El-Badawi [8] reported bilharzian lesions (bruises and semolina grains appearance) associated with granulomatous polyps in the majority of cases (96%). He also observed that fibrocalcic and villous polyps were associated with lesions of chronic bilharzian cystitis in the majority of cases and active lesions in a minority of cases (8.8%). Pinto et al. had also observed lesions of active bilharziasis associated with granulomatous polyps [5, 10].

In our series, patient who had pathologic features of dysplasia and metaplasia were lost to follow-up. Regular endoscopic monitoring of these patients would have made it possible to diagnose a possible evolution towards squamous cell carcinoma. Indeed, according to Berry et al. [15], the genesis of carcinoma follows the sequence hyperplasia-metaplasia-dysplasia-carcinoma. Amin et al. [16] also reported the diagnosis of squamous cell carcinoma of the bladder following bilharzioma.

The rapid regression of granulomatous polyps under antibilharzian treatment limited the indications for surgery. Surgery can be performed if medical treatment fails or when residual polyps obstruct the urethral orifices or bladder neck. Small, nonobstructing fibrocalcic polyps without further damage do not require treatment, unless there is evidence of an active schistosomiasis. The villous polyps must be completely excised to allow a careful histological examination [8].

Pinto et al. have successfully treated granulomatous polyps with medical treatment [5, 10].

We have associated transurethral resection of the bladder with praziquantel in all our patients. A good characterization of the lesions at cystoscopy would have allowed us to evoke the diagnosis of bladder bilharzioma and to reserve surgery for therapeutic failures. Indeed, the treatment of uncomplicated bladder bilharziomas falls under the antibilharzian treatment. Praziquantel at a dose of 40 mg/kg is recommended. Transurethral resection of the bladder and bladder biopsy are indicated for residual masses or when the endoscopic diagnosis of bilharzioma is not obvious [6].

Our study shows the importance of pathology in the diagnosis of bladder schistosomiasis lesions. It is important in our region to consider the diagnosis in spite of the compelling need to consider the possibility of neoplasm. While we acknowledge a limitation related to the small sample size, our study shed light in the endoscopic and pathologic feature of bilharzioma in the setting of schistosomiasis endemic.

5. Conclusion

Bladder bilharziomas pose the problem of differential diagnosis with squamous cell carcinoma and bladder stones in areas of bilharzian endemic. Nevertheless, a clever exploration with cystoscopy would allow to evoke the diagnosis and to initiate the antibilharzian treatment sometimes supplemented by an endoscopic resection of the bladder lesion.

Consent

Informed consent was obtained from all individual participants included in the study.

Acknowledgments

The authors would like to thank the Urology-Andrology Department, Idrissa Pouye General Hospital, Sénégal.

References

[1] P. J. Hotez and A. Kamath, "Neglected tropical diseases in sub-saharan Africa: review of their prevalence, distribution, and disease burden," *PLoS Neglected Tropical Diseases*, vol. 3, no. 8, p. e412, 2009.

[2] B. Senghor, A. Diallo, S. N. Sylla et al., "Prevalence and intensity of urinary schistosomiasis among school children in the district of Niakhar, region of Fatick, Senegal," *Parasites & Vectors*, vol. 7, no. 1, p. 5, 2014.

[3] M. Sene-Wade, B. Marchand, D. Rollinson, and B. L. Webster, "Urogenital schistosomiasis and hybridization between Schistosoma haematobium and Schistosoma bovis in adults living in Richard-Toll, Senegal," *Parasitology*, vol. 145, no. 13, pp. 1723–1726, 2018.

[4] C. Guiguen, S. Belaz, F. Robert-Gangneux, and J.-P. Gangneux, "Les bilharzioses: aspects épidémio-cliniques et diagnostiques," *Revue Francophone des Laboratoires*, vol. 2013, no. 457, pp. 75–85, 2013.

[5] S. Z. Pinto, R. Friedman, and E. J. Van Den Berg, "A case of paediatric bladder bilharzioma in Johannesburg, South Africa," *Clinical Case Reports*, vol. 7, no. 10, pp. 1890–1894, 2019.

[6] M. A. Ghoneim, "Bilharziasis of the genitourinary tract," *BJU International*, vol. 89, no. 1, pp. 22–30, 2002.

[7] P. T. Loverde and L. Chen, "Schistosome female reproductive development," *Parasitology Today*, vol. 7, no. 11, pp. 303–308, 1991.

[8] A. A. El-Badawi, "Bilharzial polypi of the urinary bladder," *British Journal of Urology*, vol. 38, no. 1, pp. 24–35, 1966.

[9] E. Abdel-Salam and A. Ehsan, "Cystoscopic picture of schistosoma haematobium in Egyptian children correlated to intensity of infection and morbidity," *The American Journal of Tropical Medicine and Hygiene*, vol. 27, no. 4, pp. 774–778, 1978.

[10] T. Merrot, K. Retornaz, K. Chaumoitre, J. M. Garnier, and P. Alessandrini, "Forme pseudotumorale de bilharziose vésicale de l'enfant: à propos de 2 observations récentes," *Archives de Pédiatrie*, vol. 10, no. 8, pp. 710–712, 2003.

[11] S. Frigerio, F. Bert, M. Clari et al., "Knowledge, attitudes, and practices related to Schistosomiasis among children in Northern Senegal," *Annals of Global Health*, vol. 92, no. 5, pp. 940–947, 2016.

[12] U. S. Ugbomoiko, I. E. Ofoezie, I. C. Okoye, and J. Heukelbach, "Factors associated with urinary schistosomiasis in two peri-urban communities in south-western Nigeria," *Annals of Tropical Medicine & Parasitology*, vol. 104, no. 5, pp. 409–419, 2010.

[13] T. N. Nanvya, D. A. Dakul, and G. S. Mwansat, "Schistosomiasis in ndinjor district of langtang, north local government area of plateau state, Nigeria," *Nigerian Journal of Parasitology*, vol. 32, pp. 209–214, 2011.

[14] D. Ndiaye, M. Diouf, Y. Diedhiou, M. Toure, M. Sembene, and O. Ndir, "Prevalence of urinary schistosomiasis in the school population in Senegal in 2002," *Dakar Medical*, vol. 50, no. 3, pp. 198–201, 2005.

[15] A. Berry, X. Iriart, J. Fillaux, and J.-F. Magnaval, "Schistosomose urogénitale et cancer," *Bulletin de la Société de pathologie exotique*, vol. 110, no. 1, pp. 68–75, 2017.

[16] H. A. A. Amin, M. H. Kobaisi, and R. M. Samir, "Schistosomiasis and bladder cancer in Egypt: truths and myths," *Open Access Macedonian Journal of Medical Sciences*, vol. 7, no. 23, pp. 4023–4029, 2019.

7

Pattern of Ureteric Pathology Presenting to a Fistula Centre in Western Kenya

Anthony Wanjala[1] **Henry Mwangi,**[2] **and Hillary Mabeya**[3]

[1]*Malava County Hospital, Kakamega, P.O. Box 1561-50200, Bungoma, Kenya*
[2]*Moi Teaching and Referral Hospital, P.O. Box 3-30100, Eldoret, Kenya*
[3]*Department of Reproductive Health, Moi University School of Medicine, P.O. Box 3900-30100, Eldoret, Kenya*

Correspondence should be addressed to Anthony Wanjala; anthonynakhisa@gmail.com

Academic Editor: Miroslav Djordjevic

Background. Ureteric pathology arises from surgical misadventures, trauma, and congenital anomalies. Early detection and treatment is of the essence. *Objectives.* To determine the types/etiology and outcome of ureteric pathology presenting to Gynocare Fistula Centre, Eldoret, Kenya. *Methods.* Descriptive retrospective study that evaluated patients presenting with ureteric pathology at Gynocare between 1st January 2012 and 31st December 2016. We pulled out patient charts and extracted and analyzed relevant data using STATA 13E statistical software. *Results.* We analyzed 33 charts, and their age ranged from 10 to 58 years. Annual proportion for 2012, 2013, 2014, 2015, and 2016 was 2.5%, 2.8%, 1.2%, 1.4%, and 3.0% respectively among all the fistula patients treated in the hospital. All the patients presented with urinary incontinence, and 7 (21.2%) had flank pain. Iatrogenic injuries contributed 84.8% (28), and 3 (9.1%) were congenital while trauma and infection had 1 each. Of those resulting from surgical misadventures, 17 (60.7%) were from obstetric while 11 (39.2%) were from gynecological surgery. All the injuries were in the distal third of the ureter; 5 were bilateral; and 11 were left sided while 17 were right-sided. Repair and/or reimplantation was successful in 31 (93.93%) of the patients. *Conclusion.* Highest proportion of ureteric pathologies was accounted for by iatrogenic causes and surgical repair and/or reimplantation has a high success rate.

1. Introduction

Ureteric pathology may arise from abdominal and pelvic surgery, trauma, congenital anomalies, malignancies, and radiation. Iatrogenic causes, though rare, account for most of the ureteric pathology [1]. The location of the ureter in the retroperitoneal space and its close proximity to the pelvic reproductive organs make it susceptible to injury during surgery [2]. Congenital anomalies of the ureter rarely occur alone and are likely to be accompanied by other anomalies on the urinary tree [3].

If not diagnosed and treated early, ureteric pathology is associated with worsening morbidity, including delayed hospital stay, risk of reoperation, compromise of the initial surgery, infection, ureterovaginal fistula, and loss of kidney function [4]. This is in addition to the psychological trauma felt by the patient and the possible risk of litigation. Patients may present with flank pain, urinary incontinence, fever, ascites, prolonged ileus, anuria, and even hydronephrosis and dysfunctional kidneys [5].

High index of suspicion and early diagnosis is of the essence in mitigating the effects of the resulting morbidities [6]. In the event of injury, several authors have demonstrated that early detection and treatment is associated with better short-term and long-term outcomes [2, 7].

In our set up, patients presenting with ureteric pathology are likely to be referred to a urologist if they are male, a fistula surgeon if they are female, and a pediatric surgeon in the event of children. Every so often, these subspecialties work together on select cases.

There exist gaps in published research on the extent of ureteric pathology in this region. The study set out to describe types/etiology and outcome of ureteric pathology presenting to a fistula centre in Western Kenya.

2. Methods

This was a descriptive retrospective study that evaluated all patients who presented with ureteric pathology at Gynocare Fistula Centre from 1st January 2012 to 31st December 2016. Located in Eldoret town on the Western part of Kenya, Gynocare is the biggest fistula referral centre in Kenya, with a bed capacity of 74. Every year the hospital performs over 300 fistula-related surgeries and manages many others conservatively. In 2014, the centre was accredited by WHO (World Health Organization) through FIGO (International Federation of Gynecology and Obstetrics) to train upcoming fistula surgeons. Since then, a total of 7 surgeons have been trained and certified while many others have visited to gain experience in specific areas.

The study population included all women with a diagnosis of ureteric pathology admitted at Gynocare center for a period of 5 years (from 1st January 2012 to 31st December 2016).

Patients' medical records were retrieved from the records department, and relevant data were extracted and entered on to chart review forms. This included information on bio-data, presenting symptoms, examination findings, diagnosis, presurgical evaluation, treatment offered, and condition at discharge. Presurgical evaluation included dye studies, kidney function tests, and abdominopelvic ultrasound. Where there was need, examination-under-anesthesia was done. Findings at surgery were also captured, including the type and location of ureteric pathology, comorbidities, and the surgical intervention chosen by the surgeon.

Data analysis was done using STATA 13E statistical software. Descriptive statistics were done to explore and summarize the data. Categorical data were summarized through frequency and proportions and presented in tables and charts, while numerical data were summarized using measures of central tendency and dispersion.

We sought approval from the Gynocare administration and scientific committee.

We used deidentifiers to code the review forms.

3. Results

3.1. Demographics. A total of 33 patients were admitted to Gynocare with ureteric pathology between 1st January 2012 to 31st December 2016. All were female, and their age ranged from 10 years to 58 years with a mean of 36.8 (SD 12) years and a median of 41 (IQR 14). Peak age incidence was in the age range 40–49 years (Figure 1). Slightly above half 18 (54.6%) were referrals, where majority 10 (58.8%) of these were referred by community health workers and 7 (41.2%) were referred from other health facilities (Table 1). Median duration of symptoms was 0.25 years (IQR 8.9) with minimum being 0.019 (1 week) and maximum 17 years.

3.2. Presentation, Annual Proportion, and Etiology. All the patients complained of urinary incontinence at presentation while only 7 (21.2%) presented with flank pain (Table 1). Other complains included abdominal pain, amenorrhea, and per vaginal discharge.

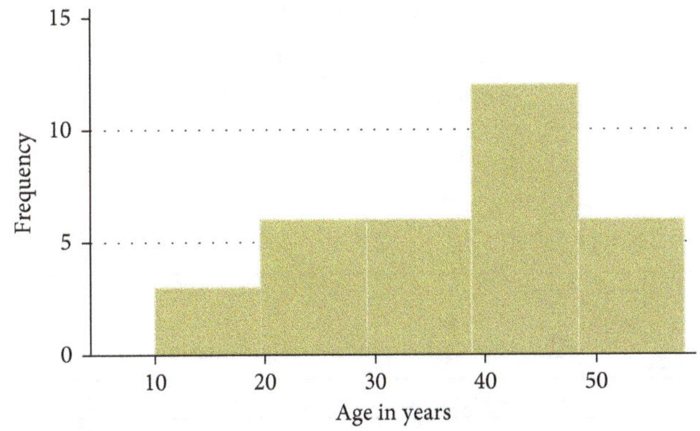

Figure 1: Age distribution.

Table 1: Age, referral status, and clinical presentation.

Variable	Categories	Frequency	Percentage
Age	<20 years	3	9.1
	≥20 years	30	90.9
Referral	No	15	45.5
	Yes	18	54.5
Referral from	Other health facilities	7	38.9
	Community health workers	10	55.6
	Self-referral	1	0.056
Incontinence	No	0	0
	Yes	33	100
Flank pain	No	26	78.8
	Yes	7	21.2

Table 2: Ureteric pathology annual proportion.

Year	Frequency	Total fistula	Proportion (%)
2012	5	200	2.5
2013	8	285	2.8
2014	4	325	1.2
2015	5	348	1.4
2016	11	372	3.0
Total	33		

The annual proportion of patients presenting with ureteric pathology against all the other fistula patients never exceeded 3% for the years 2012–2016, the highest, 3% coming in 2016 (Table 2). This is despite a steady rise in the number of fistula surgeries from 2012 to 2016.

At 84.8%, ureteric injuries from surgical misadventures contributed the highest percentage of pathologies, with obstetric accounting for 17 (60.7%) and gynecological surgeries accounting for 11 (39.3%) (Table 3). Of the remaining, 3 (9.1%) patients had congenital malformations while trauma and infection contributed 1 each. In the congenital malformation category, 2 had left sided double ureter with one opening through the vagina while the other had a normal right ureter opening into the urethra. All the pathologies were in the distal third of the ureter, 5 (15.2%) were bilateral, 11 (33.3%) left sided while 17 (51.5%) were right-sided.

3.3. Renal Function Tests. As a diagnostic and presurgical evaluation, all patients underwent a mandatory renal function

Table 3: Etiology of ureteric pathology.

Variable	Categories	Frequency	Percentage
Cause	Previous surgery	28	84.8
	Congenital	3	9.1
	Trauma	1	3.0
	PID	1	3.0
Surgery type	Gynecology	11	39.3
	Obstetric	17	60.7

Table 4: Renal function at admission.

Variable	Categories	Frequency	Percentage
Urea	<3.0	14	46.7
	3.00–8.39	15	50.0
	>8.39	1	3.3
K	3.40–5.10	29	96.7
	>5.10	1	3.3
Creatinine	44.00–133.00	28	93.3
	>133.00	2	6.7

and electrolyte test upon presentation. They were largely within the reference range, save for 1 (3.3%) who had elevated creatinine, urea and potassium and another who had elevated creatinine with normal urea and potassium (Table 4). Pre-surgical renal function tests for 3 patients could not be traced. Prior to discharge, the lab works were repeated and all were within reference ranges.

3.4. Management. Surgical intervention was the management of choice for all the 33 patients (Table 5). Slightly over half had ureteroneocystostomy while close to one-third had both ureteroneocystostomy and fistula repair. The remaining two patients had repair. Upon discharge, 2 patients still had urinary incontinence and were asked to come back for reoperation later. One presented to another fistula centre for repair while the other was lost to follow-up. Median time of hospitalization was 17 days (IQR 2), with minimum being 14 days and maximum 48 days. Postoperatively, there was no reported mortality or severe morbidity.

4. Discussion

Ureteric pathology can lead to serious morbidity and mortality if not detected early and treated. Among the leading causes of this is inadvertent ureteric injury during surgery [8, 9].

In the female pelvis, the ureter lies close to the uterus and the cervix making it susceptible to injury during either gynecological or obstetric surgeries [10]. As such, lower third ureteric injuries, just like in this study, are the commonest, probably from dissection of lower uterus and cervix or from injury during ligation of uterine vessels. It is thought that as high as 50–75% of these injuries arise from gynecological procedures [5], while the rest are largely from obstetric causes. This is well demonstrated in this study as about 89% of all ureteric pathology resulted from surgical misadventures, majority being obstetric (60%). Obstetric surgeries associated with ureteric injury include cesarean section, repair of uterine rupture, and cesarean hysterectomy. Advancement in labor

Table 5: Treatment offered.

Variable	Categories	Frequency	Percentage
Was surgery offered	No	0	0
	Yes	33	100
Type of surgery done	Repair	2	6.1
	Ureteroneocystostomy	21	63.6
	Repair + ureteroneocystostomy	10	30.3
Discharge condition	Leaking urine	2	6.1
	Not leaking urine	31	93.9

management and monitoring has led to an increase in the CS rate the world over. In Kenya, most of these are done by relatively junior doctors due to acute shortage of specialists. This may account for the cases of ureteric injury from obstetric causes as less surgical experience is a risk factor to injury [11]. Gynecological procedures associated with ureteric injury include total abdominal hysterectomy, vaginal hysterectomy, removal of pelvic masses, oophorectomy, suspension procedures, and so on.

The annual proportion of 3% or less cannot be easily compared with other studies because they have used total hospital surgeries as the baseline whereas this study uses total fistula surgeries as the baseline, an obvious bias. Nevertheless with such annual proportion at a referral centre it is safe to say ureteric pathology is not common.

The fact that all patients presented with urinary incontinence points to a likelyhood of ureterovaginal fistula which in this case is protective to the kidneys. This may explain why for most patients their renal function tests were within reference ranges despite some having had the pathology for a long duration. Ureteric injury without incontinence may lead to leakage of urine into the peritoneum with attendant peritonitis or loss of kidney function in the event of ureteric ligation [6].

The left ureter is more liable to injury due to slight uterine rotation [12, 13]. This contrasts somewhat with this study where slightly more than half of patients had right-sided pathology, majority of who were iatrogenic.

Surgical intervention has proven to be key in the treatment of patients with ureteric pathology [1]. In this, high index of suspicion, early diagnosis, and timely treatment offer patients the best chance of recovery. The surgical options available include ureteroneocystostomy with or without psoas hitch and/or boari flap, ureteroneocystostomy, end to end anastomosis, primary repair when there is partial resection, and suture removal in the event of ligation among others. Surgery offered cure for 31 (94%) of patients in this study.

5. Conclusion

Iatrogenic injury is the commonest cause of ureteric pathology, from either obstetric or gynecological surgeries. The close association between reproductive organs and the ureter makes it more liable to injury. Surgical intervention has a high success rate.

Acknowledgments

The authors wish to acknowledge the contribution of the research assistants Steve Katumo and Joan Migosi to the success of this study. The authors also wish to acknowledge the Gynocare administration for allowing them to carry out this research in their institution.

References

[1] H. A. Mahendran, P. Singam, C. Ho, G. E. Hong, T. G. Hee, and Z. M. Zainuddin, "Iatrogenic ureter injuries : eleven years experience in a tertiary hospital," *Medical Journal of Malaysia*, vol. 67, no. 2, pp. 169–172, 2012.

[2] M. Rafique and M. H. Arif, "Management of iatrogenic ureteric injuries associated with gynecological surgery," *International Urology and Nephrology*, vol. 34, no. 1, pp. 31–35, 2002.

[3] A. H. Al-Salem, "Congenital urological malformations," in *An Illustrated Guide to Pediatric Urology*, Springer International Publishing, Cham, Switzerland, 2017.

[4] J. D. Watterson, J. E. Mahoney, N. G. Futter, and J. Gaffield, "Iatrogenic ureteric injuries: approaches to etiology and management," *Canadian Journal of Surgery*, vol. 41, no. 5, pp. 379–382, 1998.

[5] P. L. Chalya, A. N. Massinde, A. Kihunrwa, and S. Simbila, "Iatrogenic ureteric injuries following abdomino-pelvic operations: a 10-year tertiary care hospital experience in Tanzania," *World Journal of Emergency Surgery*, vol. 10, no. 1, p. 17, 2015.

[6] J. Mensah, G. Klufio, F. Ahiaku, C. Osafo, and S. Gepi-Attee, "Delayed recognition of bilateral ureteral injury after gyneacological surgery," *Ghana Medical Journal*, vol. 42, no. 4, pp. 133–136, 2008.

[7] M. S. Anwar, M. Tariq, K. Saeed, T. Ghafoor, and G. M. Mustafa, "Causes of ureteric injuries and outcome of different surgical procedures for the repair of ureter," *Journal of Sheikh Zayed Medical College*, vol. 1, pp. 16–20, 2010.

[8] K. H. Tijani, K. I. Onwuzurigbo, R. W. Ojewola, B. B. Afolabi, and N. O. Akanmu, "Iatrogeni ureteric injuries in a nigerian teaching hospital-experience in the last decade," *East African Medical Journal*, vol. 88, no. 9, 2011.

[9] S. N. Durrani, A Ur Rehman, S. Khan, H. Ullah, M. K. Khan, and A. Ullah, "Ureteral trauma during open surgery: aetiology, presentation and management," *Journal of Ayub Medical College Abbottabad*, vol. 25, no. 3-4, pp. 3–43, 2013.

[10] R. Fröber, "Surgical anatomy of the ureter," *BJU International*, vol. 100, no. 4, pp. 949–965, 2007.

[11] F. T. Hammad, K. M. AlQaiwani, and S. S. Shirodkar, "The role of urologists in the management of urological injuries during obstetric and gynaecologic surgery," *International Urogynecology Journal*, vol. 21, no. 10, pp. 1237–1241, 2010.

[12] A. E. Aghaji and C. Odoemene, "Ureteric injuries in Enugu, Nigeria," *East African Medical Journal*, vol. 76, no. 4, pp. 184–188, 1999.

[13] I. Nnabugwu and O. Amu, "Iatrogenic ureteric injuries complicating open obstetric and gynaecologic operations in South East Nigeria-case series," *Journal of the West African College of Surgeons*, vol. 1, no. 3, pp. 98–108, 2011.

8

Prospective Multicenter Open-Label One-Arm Trial Investigating a Pumpkin Seed, Isoflavonoids and Cranberry Mix in Lower Urinary Tract Symptoms/Benign Prostatic Hyperplasia

Elie Nemr, Elie El Helou, Georges Mjaess, Albert Semaan, and Josselin Abi Chebel

Université Saint Joseph, Faculty of Medicine, Beirut, Lebanon

Correspondence should be addressed to Elie Nemr; elie.nemr@usj.edu.lb

Academic Editor: Kostis Gyftopoulos

Phytotherapy for lower urinary tract symptoms (LUTSs) due to benign prostate hyperplasia (BPH) is progressively demanded by patients and trusted by physicians. The aim was to assess the efficacy of a mix of pumpkin seed extract, soy germ isoflavonoids, and cranberry (Novex®) in the management of mild to moderate LUTS in BPH patients. Male patients aged ≥40 years, who had had mild to moderate LUTS for >6 months at screening, with no previous therapy or who are still symptomatic despite current use of alpha-blockers, were recruited. Exclusion criteria were an IPSS >19 and an age >80 years. The mixed compound was administered orally, daily, for 3 months. Patients were evaluated by means of IPSS, urological quality of life (uQoL) index, and International Index of Erectile Function (IIEF-5) at 3 visits: baseline (visit 1), 30 days (visit 2), and 90 days after treatment (visit 3). Among 163 screened patients, 128 patients (61.8 ± 9.9 years) were recruited. IPSS improved from 15 (Q1 : 12–Q3 : 17) in visit 1, to 11 (Q1 : 8–Q3 : 14) in visit 2, and to 9 (Q1 : 6–Q3 : 12) in visit 3 ($p < 0.001$). uQoL improved from 4 (3–4) in visit 1, to 3 (2–3) in visit 2, and to 2 (1–2) in visit 3 ($p < 0.001$). The patients had an IIEF-5 score of 15 (12–18.7) in visit 1, 15 (12–18) in visit 2, and 17 (13–19) in visit 3 ($p = 0.99$ visits 1 vs. 2, $p = 0.004$ visits 2 vs. 3, and $p = 0.001$ visits 1 vs. 3). Treating mild to moderate LUTS/BPH patients with Novex® might therefore relieve symptoms, improve the quality of life, and have a mild beneficial effect on erectile function.

1. Introduction

Phytotherapy for lower urinary tract symptoms (LUTSs) due to benign prostate hyperplasia (BPH) is being increasingly demanded by patients and trusted by physicians, reaching roughly 90% in some countries like Germany and Austria [1]. Phytotherapy is mainly used for mild to moderate LUTS while guidelines still advocate the use of alpha-blockers and phosphodiesterase 5 inhibitors for moderate to severe LUTS [2, 3].

Among many phytotherapeutic compounds available and studied in the literature, pumpkin seed extract, soy germ isoflavonoids, and cranberry have shown efficacy and safety in the treatment of LUTS. Pumpkin seed is the most studied nutraceutical and has shown a significant improvement in LUTS and in urological quality of life. Fewer studies evaluated the role of soy germ isoflavonoids and cranberry and showed a beneficial effect on LUTS.

BPH patients presenting with LUTS have a high rate of erectile dysfunction (ED) and LUTS is considered as an independent risk factor for ED [4, 5]. Treatment of LUTS with alpha-blockers has been associated with improvement of erectile function [6], but the effect of the nutraceuticals used to treat LUTS on erectile function remains elusive. To date, no studies have assessed the effect of a combination of the three compounds (pumpkin seed extract, soy germ isoflavonoids, and cranberry) on LUTS in BPH patients and their impact on the urological quality of life.

Therefore, the aim of the current study is to assess the efficacy and safety of a new complex containing pumpkin seed extract, soy germ isoflavonoids, and cranberry in the treatment of mild to moderate LUTS and erectile dysfunction in LUTS/BPH patients.

2. Materials and Methods

2.1. Study Design and Setting. This is a single-arm prospective open-label trial investigating a combination of pumpkin seed, isoflavonoids, and cranberry mix in improving LUTS, urological quality of life, and erectile function in BPH patients. The study took place in outpatient settings in several clinics across Lebanon. An Institutional Review Board approval was obtained, and patients signed a written informed consent form. The urology specialists in the outpatient clinics were introduced to the study protocol by the investigators and were invited to recruit the patients who satisfied the eligibility criteria. Recruitment started in April 2018 and lasted until October 2018 (last patient last visit). Recruited patients were seen at 3 visits: initial visit (visit 1), 1-month visit (visit 2), and 3-month visit (visit 3), and their data were collected in a dedicated case report form. The compound was administered orally, two tablets daily, for 3 months.

2.2. Investigational Drug. Novex® is a nutraceutical complex made of pumpkin seed extract 550 mg, soy germ isoflavonoids 50 mg, and cranberry 50 mg. The recommended dose is 2 tablets/day taken orally. Pumpkin seed, which is the main component in this complex, was produced through a proprietary PS990 HyperPure process that ensures highly selective removal of the fat-soluble components. The flowchart of the production process of each component is shown in Figure 1.

2.3. Participants. Male subjects seen at the outpatient clinics between January and October 2018 were eligible to participate in the study if they fulfilled the following criteria: (1) age ≥40 years; (2) with mild to moderate LUTS for at least 6 months at the initial visit; (3) and who have no previous therapy or are still symptomatic despite the current use of alpha-blockers. Exclusion criteria were as follows: (1) an International Prostate Symptom Score (IPSS) > 19, (2) an age >80 years, (3) prostate cancer, and (4) urethral stenosis. Enrolled patients were invited to an assessment visit at the 1-month and the 3-month visits.

2.4. Variables. The patients were evaluated using detailed urological history and a clinical examination, and the outcome was measured using the following validated scales:

(a) IPSS: International Prostate Symptom Score, with its subscores for voiding, storage, and nocturia

(b) Quality of life due to urinary symptoms (uQoL) index

(c) International Index of Erectile Function (IIEF-5)

The scales were used at baseline (visit 1) to derive baseline values for IPSS, uQoL, and IIEF-5. The scales were reused at 1-month (visit 2) and 3-month visit (visit 3) to derive follow-up values of the same score in a repeated-measures design. The data were recorded by the specialist during the scheduled visit.

The primary outcome was any change in the IPSS at 1- and 3-month visits. Secondary outcomes were any change in IPSS subscores, uQoL, IIEF-5, and the rate of ejaculatory dysfunction and orthostatic hypotension.

2.5. Study Size. Basing the calculations on F tests for within-factors ANOVA with repeated measures, the following assumptions were taken conservatively: effect size $f = 0.20$; error probability $\alpha = 0.05$; power (1-β error probability) = 0.90; number of groups = 1; number of measurements = 3; correlation among repeated measures = 0.3; and non-sphericity correction $\varepsilon = 0.5$. The total sample size satisfying these assumptions is 125 subjects.

2.6. Statistical Methods. The distribution of IPSS score (in addition to voiding, storage, and nocturia IPSS subscores), IIEF-5 score, QoL, and optional tests was checked for departure from normality assumptions using Kolmogorov–Smirnov test and visual inspection by quantile-quantile plots. The scores were expressed as median with its interquartile range (Q1–Q3). To take into account the repeated-measures design, for IPSS, uQoL, and IIEF-5 at the initial visit, 1-month visit, and 3-month visit, Friedman's nonparametric repeated-measures ANOVA by ranks was used. Post hoc pairwise comparisons were used, and p values were adjusted for multiplicity. Subscores of IPSS for nocturia, filling, and voiding were also analyzed in a similar fashion. Analyses were run using SPSS software (IBM Corp. Released 2013, SPSS Statistics for Windows version 22.0, Armonk, NY).

3. Results and Discussion

3.1. Patient Characteristics. 163 patients were screened, of whom 140 patients were enrolled in the study and 12 patients dropped out. The final number of patients included in the analysis was 128, aged 61.8 ± 9.9 years.

3.2. Main Results. Patients had a baseline median IPSS score of 15 (12–17), significantly decreasing to 11 (8–14) at 1-month visit and then to 9 (6–12) at 3-month visit ($p < 0.001$). Post hoc analysis using pairwise comparisons showed a significant difference between visit 1 and visit 2 ($p < 0.001$), visit 2 and visit 3 ($p < 0.001$), and visit 1 and visit 3 ($p < 0.001$) (Figure 2(a)).

As for the secondary outcomes, the same pattern of variation was observed when analyzing voiding, storage, and nocturia IPSS subscores. Median IPSS voiding symptom score significantly decreased from baseline 9 (7–10) to 7 (4.75–8) at 1-month visit and then to 5 (3–7) at 3-month visit ($p < 0.001$) (Figure 3(a)). Median IPSS storage symptoms score significantly decreased from baseline 6 (5–7) to 5 (3.75–6) at 1-month visit and then to 4 (3–5) at 3-month

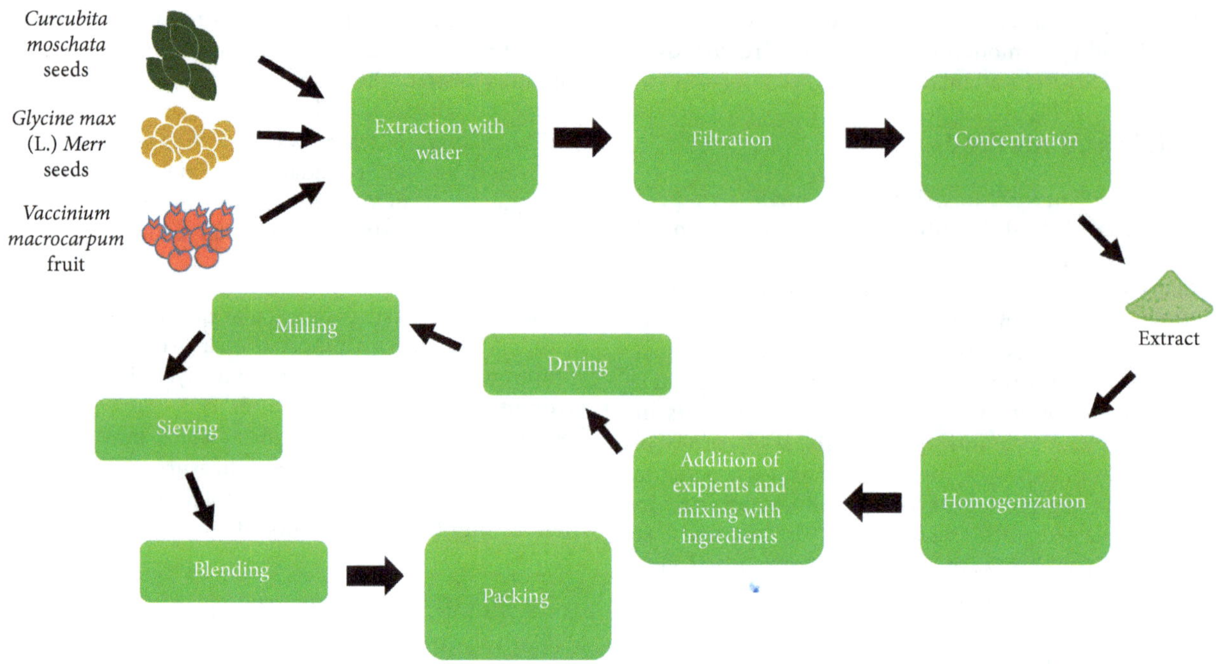

FIGURE 1: Process flowcharts of pumpkin seed extract, soy extract 40% isoflavones, and cranberry.

visit ($p < 0.001$) (Figure 3(b)). IPSS nocturia score significantly decreased from baseline 2 (2–3) to 2 (1–2) at 1-month visit and then to 1 (1–2) at 3-month visit ($p < 0.001$) (Figure 3(c)). Post hoc analyses of the subscores showed a significant difference between visit 1 and visit 2 ($p < 0.001$), visit 2 and visit 3 ($p < 0.001$), and visit 1 and visit 3 ($p < 0.001$ for voiding and storage symptoms, $p = 0.011$ for nocturia).

Regarding the quality of life related to urological symptoms (uQoL), 39.1% of the patients were mostly dissatisfied and 14.1% were unhappy, making a total of 53.2% having a low quality of life at baseline visit. At 1-month visit, 15.6% of the patients were mostly dissatisfied and 2.3% were unhappy, making a total of 17.9% having a low quality of life. At 3-month visit, 7.0% of the patients were mostly dissatisfied and 3.9% were unhappy, making a total of 10.9% having a low quality of life. uQoL significantly decreased from a median of 4 (3–4) at baseline to 3 (2–3) at 1-month visit and then to 2 (1–2) at 3-month visit (overall $p < 0.001$). The post hoc analyses showed that this difference also stemmed from the difference between all 3 visits (all p values <0.001) (Figure 2(b)).

At baseline, the International Index of Erectile Function (IIEF-5) score was 15 (12–18.75); it remained at a median of 15 (12–18) at 1-month visit and then increased to 17 (13.75–19) at 3-month visit (overall $p < 0.001$). The post hoc analysis showed no significant difference between visit 1 and visit 2, but the difference between visit 2 and visit 3 was significant ($p = 0.004$) (Figure 2(c)).

Neither ejaculatory dysfunction nor orthostatic hypotension was reported by the patients (0%).

3.3. Discussion. The use of nutraceuticals as phytotherapy for the relief of LUTS due to BPH seems to be gaining momentum worldwide and is being considered by clinicians as a treatment option in the management of mild to moderate LUTS/BPH patients. On the other hand, urological societies scarcely mention phytotherapy and do not recommend until now the use of phytotherapeutic agents due to the heterogeneity of their composition and clinical effects, as well as the lack of evidence regarding their benefit [2, 3].

The current study assessed the efficacy of a nutraceutical complex made of pumpkin seed extract, soy germ isoflavonoids, and cranberry, in the management of male patients suffering from mild to moderate LUTS/BPH. The results show that (1) the IPSS score decreased significantly at one and three months of treatment (for the voiding, storage, and nocturia subscores); (2) the uQoL score improved significantly after one and three months of treatment, and a significant inferior proportion of low quality of life was found among patients after one and three months of treatment; and (3) it took three months for the IIEF-5 score to improve significantly.

Several studies performed in the preclinical and clinical setting showed that the use of *Cucurbita pepo* (pumpkin seeds) in the management of patients affected by LUTS/BPH seems to be useful for improving symptoms and quality of life. In the preclinical setting, pumpkin seed showed an antioxidant, antiandrogen, and anti-inflammatory activity and had a positive effect on bladder contractility and reduction of prostate gland growth, while not having any side effects [7]. Tsai et al. showed that the use of pumpkin seed decreases the size of the prostate in testosterone/prazosin-induced prostatic growth [8]. Hong et al. showed, in a placebo-controlled study, a decrease of the IPSS score and an improvement in the urologic quality of life, in patients treated with pumpkin seed extract [9]. Vahlensieck et al. showed that treatment with pumpkin seed results in a significant improvement in BPH/LUTS and a clinically significant improvement in IPSS-related QoL [10].

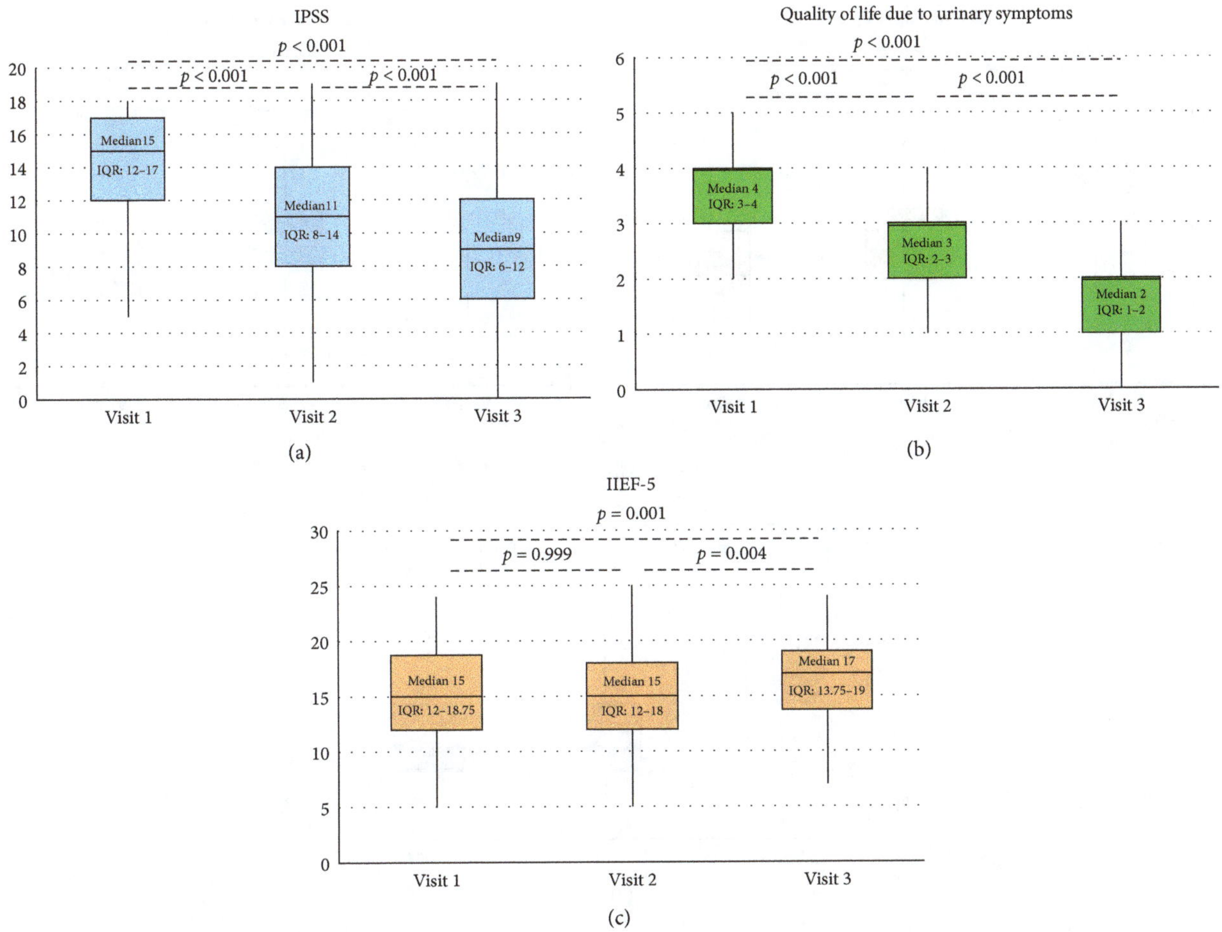

Figure 2: (a) International Prostate Symptoms Score (IPSS), (b) urological quality of life (uQoL), and (c) International Index of Erectile Function (IIEF-5) obtained at the three visits: median, Q1, Q3, minimum, and maximum.

The soy germ isoflavones showed good effect in treating BPH in men, via their antioxidative properties. In the preclinical setting, soybean isoflavones have been shown to decrease PSA expression when cultured with prostate cancer cells [11]. A significant reduction of PSA has been also reported using an isoflavone-rich supplement as part of an intensive diet and lifestyle intervention [12], and trends toward a reduction in PSA have been noted from some other small trials [13]. Bae et al. reported an amelioration of the IPSS score, storage symptoms, and quality of life in men taking Seoritae extract, a type of black soybean containing isoflavone, at 4 and 12 weeks of administration [14]. Wong et al. showed amelioration in Q_{max} and incomplete emptying in patients taking 40 mg of isoflavones daily compared to placebo [1]. Both studies showed excellent tolerability of isoflavones and no particular side effects.

Although cranberry has been evaluated thoroughly in recurrent urinary tract infection prophylaxis [15], its role in the treatment of LUTS in males with BPH has also been evaluated. The first trial evaluating cranberry in the treatment of LUTS, elevated PSA levels, and nonbacterial prostatitis was conducted by Vidlar et al. in 2010 [16]. In this trial, 42 patients were randomized equally to 1500 mg of cranberry fruit powder (*Vaccinium macrocarpon*) daily versus placebo. Six months later, patients who received cranberry had a statistically significant lower IPSS and QoL score than controls. All parameters of urination (Q_{max}, average urinary flow rate (Q_{ave}), and prostate bladder voiding and postvoid residual urine volumes) were significantly improved. Furthermore, in a 6-month, randomized, double-blind, placebo-controlled study, Vidlar et al. evaluated cranberry powder (Flowens™) 250 mg and 500 mg versus placebo showing a clinically relevant, dose-dependent, and significant reduction in LUTS in moderately symptomatic men over 45 [17].

Since each compound has been shown to act through a different mechanism of action, giving minor results in the studies abovementioned, the authors think that combining these effects altogether might give an additional clinical value. The combination of these three compounds seems to be promising as shown by this study: the median IPSS decreased by 6 points (15 to 9) after 3 months, which is higher than the predefined 3 points necessary for a patient to perceive a clinical benefit as described in the literature [18]. These results are comparable with those obtained by the use of alpha-blockers in moderate to severe LUTS as reported in the meta-analysis done by Yuan et al. with a decrease of IPSS of 5.4–7 points [19]. This improvement in the IPSS was due

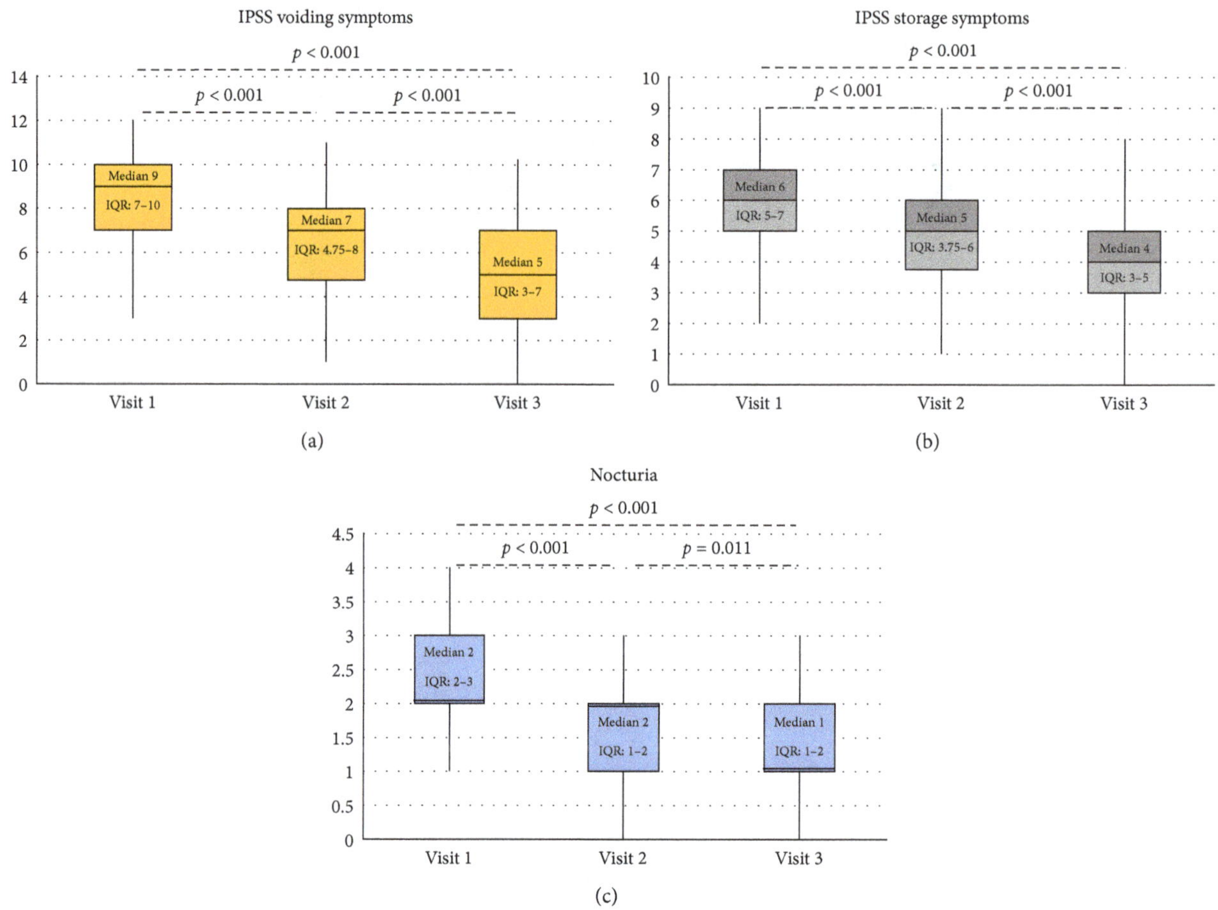

FIGURE 3: (a) IPSS voiding, (b) IPSS storage, and (c) nocturia subscores obtained at the three visits: median, Q1, Q3, minimum, and maximum.

to a decrease in voiding and storage subscores. Therefore, this phytotherapy could be beneficial for all mild to moderate LUTS/BPH patients independently of their LUTS type.

Patients with mild LUTS are usually treated with behavioral modifications and watchful waiting until their LUTS becomes moderate (until the benefit of medical treatment outweighs the side effects). Having no adverse events, Novex® may be a suitable choice for mild LUTS/BPH patients. Furthermore, it might be offered as a suitable treatment for patients with moderate LUTS, alone, or in combination with alpha-blockers, having an efficacy comparable to alpha-blockers in this category of patients. The role of nutraceuticals in the treatment of severe LUTS/BPH alone or as an add-on for alpha-blockers needs to be assessed in further studies.

This study is considered a pilot study and has limitations. First, it is a noncomparative study lacking a control arm and using a subjective outcome measure based on the patients' impression. Second, a follow-up of 3 months is relatively short. Therefore, a prospective controlled study with a longer follow-up, and using objective outcome measures (uroflowmetry, voiding diary, etc.), comparing the effect of this phytotherapeutic compound to a placebo group, is being planned.

4. Conclusions

This pilot study seems promising, demonstrating that an oral combination of pumpkin seed extract, soy germ isoflavonoids, and cranberry could be beneficial for BPH patients with mild to moderate LUTS, and to our knowledge, this is the first study to assess the beneficial effect of phytotherapy used primarily for LUTS/BPH patients on erectile function, which seems to take more time to occur when compared to the fast amelioration of LUTS. Future randomized placebo-controlled trials should be done in order to prove its efficacy alone or in combination with an alpha-blocker to improve urinary and sexual function.

Acknowledgments

This study was supported by Med-Vial Group.

References

[1] W. C. W. Wong, E. L. Y. Wong, H. Li et al., "Isoflavones in treating watchful waiting benign prostate hyperplasia: a double-blinded, randomized controlled trial," *The Journal of Alternative and Complementary Medicine*, vol. 18, no. 1, pp. 54–60, 2012.

[2] K. T. McVary, C. G. Roehrborn, A. L. Avins et al., *American Urological Association Guideline: Management of Benign Prostatic Hyperplasia (BPH)*, American Urological Association, Linthicum, MD, USA, 2010, http://www.auanet.org/education/guidelines/benign-prostatic-hyperplasia.cfm.

[3] C. Gratzke, A. Bachmann, A. Descazeaud et al., "EAU guidelines on the assessment of non-neurogenic male lower urinary tract symptoms including benign prostatic obstruction," *European Urology*, vol. 67, no. 6, pp. 1099–1109, 2015.

[4] M. H. Blanker, J. L. H. R. Bosch, F. P. M. J. Groeneveld et al., "Erectile and ejaculatory dysfunction in a community-based sample of men 50 to 78 years old: prevalence, concern, and relation to sexual activity," *Urology*, vol. 57, no. 4, pp. 763–768, 2001.

[5] J. C. Kaminetsky, "Comorbid LUTS and erectile dysfunction: optimizing their management," *Current Medical Research and Opinion*, vol. 22, no. 12, pp. 2497–2506, 2006.

[6] S. A. Kaplan, A. F. De Rose, R. S. Kirby, M. P. O'leary, and K. T. McVary, "Beneficial effects of extended-release doxazosin and doxazosin standard on sexual health," *BJU International*, vol. 97, no. 3, pp. 559–566, 2006.

[7] R. Damiano, T. Cai, P. Fornara, C. A. Franzese, R. Leonardi, and V. Mirone, "The role of Cucurbita pepo in the management of patients affected by lower urinary tract symptoms due to benign prostatic hyperplasia: a narrative review," *Archivio Italiano di Urologia e Andrologia*, vol. 88, no. 2, pp. 136–143, 2016.

[8] Y.-S. Tsai, Y.-C. Tong, J.-T. Cheng, C.-H. Lee, F.-S. Yang, and H.-Y. Lee, "Pumpkin seed oil and phytosterol-F can block testosterone/prazosin-induced prostate growth in rats," *Urologia Internationalis*, vol. 77, no. 3, pp. 269–274, 2006.

[9] H. Hong, C.-S. Kim, and S. Maeng, "Effects of pumpkin seed oil and saw palmetto oil in Korean men with symptomatic benign prostatic hyperplasia," *Nutrition Research and Practice*, vol. 3, no. 4, pp. 323–327, 2009.

[10] W. Vahlensieck, C. Theurer, E. Pfitzer, B. Patz, N. Banik, and U. Engelmann, "Effects of pumpkin seed in men with lower urinary tract symptoms due to benign prostatic hyperplasia in the one-year, randomized, placebo-controlled GRANU study," *Urologia Internationalis*, vol. 94, no. 3, pp. 286–295, 2015.

[11] M. Onozawa, K. Fukuda, M. Ohtani, H. Akaza, T. Sugimura, and K. Wakabayashi, "Effects of soybean isoflavones on cell growth and apoptosis of the human prostatic cancer cell line LNCaP," *Japanese Journal of Clinical Oncology*, vol. 28, no. 6, pp. 360–363, 1998.

[12] D. Ornish, G. Weidner, W. R. Fair et al., "Intensive lifestyle changes may affect the progression of prostate cancer," *Journal of Urology*, vol. 174, no. 3, pp. 1065–1070, 2005.

[13] F. H. Schröder, M. J. Roobol, E. R. Boevé et al., "Randomized, double-blind, placebo-controlled crossover study in men with prostate cancer and rising PSA: effectiveness of a dietary supplement," *European Urology*, vol. 48, no. 6, pp. 922–931, 2005.

[14] W. J. Bae, H. J. Park, H. C. Koo, D. R. Kim, U.-S. Ha et al., ""The effect of Seoritae extract in men with mild to moderate lower urinary tract symptoms suggestive of benign prostatic hyperplasia," evid.-based complement," *Evidence-Based Complementary and Alternative Medicine*, vol. 2016, Article ID 1960926, 6 pages, 2016.

[15] M. E. T. McMurdo, I. Argo, G. Phillips, F. Daly, and P. Davey, "Cranberry or trimethoprim for the prevention of recurrent urinary tract infections? A randomized controlled trial in older women," *Journal of Antimicrobial Chemotherapy*, vol. 63, no. 2, pp. 389–395, 2009.

[16] A. Vidlar, J. Vostalova, J. Ulrichova et al., "The effectiveness of dried cranberries (Vaccinium macrocarpon) in men with lower urinary tract symptoms," *British Journal of Nutrition*, vol. 104, no. 8, pp. 1181–1189, 2010.

[17] A. Vidlar, V. Student, J. Vostalova et al., "Cranberry fruit powder (Flowens) improves lower urinary tract symptoms in men: a double-blind, randomized, placebo-controlled study," *World Journal of Urology*, vol. 34, no. 3, pp. 419–424, 2016.

[18] Y. Dong, L. Hao, Z. Shi, G. Wang, Z. Zhang, and C. Han, "Efficacy and safety of tadalafil monotherapy for lower urinary tract symptoms secondary to benign prostatic hyperplasia: a meta-analysis," *Urologia Internationalis*, vol. 91, no. 1, pp. 10–18, 2013.

[19] J.-Q. Yuan, C. Mao, S. Y.-S. Wong et al., "Comparative effectiveness and safety of monodrug therapies for lower urinary tract symptoms associated with benign prostatic hyperplasia," *Medicine*, vol. 94, no. 27, p. e974, 2015.

9

Efficacy of Transdermal Oxybutynin in the Treatment of Overactive Bladder Syndrome: Does It Make Sense Using It in 2017?

Raúl Vozmediano-Chicharro ,[1] Blanca Madurga,[2] and Pedro Blasco[3]

[1]*Department of Urology, Hospital Regional de Málaga, Hospital Civil, University of Malaga, Plz Hospital Civil s/n, 29009 Malaga, Spain*
[2]*Department of Urology, Hospital Universitario Puerta del Mar, Av. Ana de Viya 21, 11009 Cadiz, Spain*
[3]*Department of Urology, Hospital Universitario de Valme, Ctra. de Cádiz Km. 548.9, 41014 Seville, Spain*

Correspondence should be addressed to Raúl Vozmediano-Chicharro; vozme@msn.com

Academic Editor: Matthew Rutman

Objectives. Evaluation of changes in symptoms among patients with overactive bladder syndrome treated with transdermal oxybutynin and tolerability after 12 months of follow-up. *Methods.* This was a multicenter, retrospective, single-cohort, observational study. Changes in symptoms were evaluated primarily with a 3-day voiding diary. Results were compared to baseline. Subgroup analyses were performed in patients previously treated for OAB or not and aged < 65 years versus ≥65 years. *Results.* Clinical records of 105 patients were examined; 92.4% were women. At 12 months, 58 patients continued to receive transdermal oxybutynin. Changes in symptoms according to the voiding diary were evaluated in 47 patients. Significant improvements from baseline were observed in urinary frequency (−2.6 voids/24 hours (95% CI: −3.5; −1.8), $p < 0.001$); daily number of urgent episodes (−4.7 episodes/day (95% CI: −6.1; −3.6), $p < 0.001$); and urge incontinence (−1.9 episodes/day (95% CI: −2.9; −1.3), $p < 0.001$). No statistically significant differences were found in subgroup analyses. In total, 38.1% of patients had adverse events, primarily in the application site (27.6%). No severe systemic adverse events occurred. Only 6 patients (5.7%) reported dry mouth. *Conclusions.* Improved symptoms and good tolerability observed after 1 year of treatment with transdermal oxybutynin shows that it currently has a place in the treatment of OAB patients.

1. Introduction

Overactive bladder syndrome (OAB) has been clinically defined as urinary urgency, with or without incontinence, generally accompanied by an increase in urinary frequency and nocturia, after any local disease or metabolic disorder that would explain these symptoms has been ruled out [1]. According to the EPIC study in 2009, the prevalence of overactive bladder and/or urinary incontinence in Spain reached 54% in subjects over the age of 65 [2]. The number of individuals with OAB is expected to increase in successive years as the population ages.

Despite the benefits of antimuscarinics in OAB treatment [3, 4], oral administration causes well-known side effects, in particular dry mouth, often leading patients to discontinue treatment and tolerate their incontinence [5]. Administration of transdermal oxybutynin (OXY-TDS) was approved by the Spanish Medicine Agency in 2004. Transdermal delivery has been shown to significantly reduce side effects by decreasing the active metabolite of oxybutynin (N-DEO) involved in their onset, thus possibly improving treatment adherence [6]. The efficacy and safety of OXY-TDS in the treatment of OAB have been established in several clinical trials [7–9].

Although randomized clinical trials are still the gold standard, generalization of results from these studies may be limited by widely varying mid- and long-term responses in real-world situations, lack of treatment adherence, or the use of drugs in patients with diverse morbidities. Therefore, the aim of this study was to ascertain if the improvement in symptoms and good tolerability shown in clinical trials are reproduced under clinical practice conditions.

2. Methods

The Oxybutynin-transdermal in Standard ClinicAl pRactice study (OSCAR study) was a retrospective cohort study in clinical practice conditions. Clinical records of patients with a diagnosis of OAB who received OXY-TDS in 3 centers in the same Spanish health-care region were reviewed. Data were collected at baseline, before starting treatment with OXY-TDS, and at 6 and 12 months of treatment. Adult patients of both sexes with a diagnosis of OAB according to their clinical records and a 3-day voiding diary (3 DVD) who had started treatment with OXY-TDS at least 12 months before inclusion in the study were enrolled. The study was conducted in accordance with the ethical requirements of the Declaration of Helsinki and Good Clinical Practice guidelines and approved by the Provincial Research Ethics Committee of Malaga.

The primary objective was to evaluate changes in symptoms in OAB patients receiving OXY-TDS after 12 months of treatment. Tolerability to OXY-TDS was also evaluated.

Changes in symptoms were evaluated using the 3 DVD as the primary tool. Parameters included in the 3 DVD are shown in Table 1. The urgency visual analogue scale (VAS) was a 10-point Likert-type scale, the OAB-V8 scale for detection of symptomatic OAB [10], and the Spanish validation of the International Consultation on Incontinence Questionnaire-Short Form (ICIQ-SF) [11] were also used. Tolerability was evaluated from adverse events recorded, percentage of treatment interruptions, and reasons for discontinuation.

Subgroup analyses were also performed to compare changes in 3 DVD parameters among patients treated (nonnaive) versus not previously treated (naive) with OXY-TDS for OAB and patients aged less than 65 years versus 65 years or more.

Sample size was based on an alpha risk of 5% and a statistical power of 80% for comparing 24-hour urinary frequency pre- and posttreatment with OXY-TDS. A minimum of 118 subjects were estimated to be necessary for detecting statistically significant differences around 10% between baseline and end of the treatment. A baseline voiding frequency of 11 was assumed, along with a standard deviation of 4.

The primary statistical analysis was based on a comparison of clinical outcomes between the OXY-TDS pre- and posttreatment periods (baseline versus 12 months) in patients who completed the study correctly (per protocol analysis). The baseline status was also compared with status after 6 months of OXY-TDS treatment to evaluate an interim response between the different study parameters.

Data were described by counts and percentages, mean and standard deviation, or median and minimum and maximum, as appropriate. Pre- to posttreatment results were compared by paired t-test, Wilcoxon's signed rank test, McNemar's test, or the McNemar-Bowker marginal homogeneity chi-squared test, as appropriate.

Statistical tests were performed using SPSS version 20.0 (IBM SPSS, Inc., Chicago, IL, USA) and Stats Direct software (V.2.s8).

3. Results

Clinical records of 105 patients who met the study selection criteria were evaluated. Figure 1 shows the study flow chart. All patients included in the study were Caucasian, 92.4% were women (7.62% men). Age was 59.4 (11.8) (mean and SD) years, and body mass index was 26.8 (4.4). Time since onset of OAB before treatment with OXY-TDS was 4.10 (4.9) years. The most common clinical antecedents were depression in 18 patients (17.1%) and surgical interventions for urinary incontinence in 19 patients (18.1%). Overall, of the patients for whom data was available, 66 patients (66.7%) had received previous treatment for OAB before starting OXY-TDS. Anticholinergics were the most common, followed by beta-3 agonists, and in both cases, the most common reason for discontinuation was lack of efficacy, although adverse events were also a very common cause of discontinuation of anticholinergics. All previous treatments were discontinued before the start of OXY-TDS except for 1 patient who was taking a beta-3 agonist.

After 6 months of treatment, 63 patients (60.0%) continued to receive OXY-TDS, 45 of whom provided 3 DVD data. Reductions were observed in the number of daytime, night-time, and 24-hour urinary episodes, number of episodes of urgency and urgency grade, and the number of changes of underwear or protective pads. All these changes were statistically significant.

Twelve months after initiating treatment, 58 patients (55.2%) continued to receive OXY-TDS. Complete 3 DVD data were available at 12 months from 47 of 58 patients (81.0%). Statistically significant improvements from baseline were observed in the number of voids, both during the day and at night, in the number of daily urinary urgency and urgent urinary episodes and in urinary urgency grade. Statistically significant changes were also observed in the number of times a patient needed a change of underwear or absorbent pads (Table 1). A total of 33 patients (70.2%) presented more than 4 episodes of urgency/day at baseline, and this proportion fell to 2 of 47 patients or 4.2% after 12 months of treatment with OXY-TDS ($p < 0.001$).

Although all patients completed the urgency VAS ($N = 58$) at 12 months, the evaluation of the 3 DVD completed by patients ($N = 47$) showed a statistically significant improvement from baseline (−4.50 points (95% CI: −5.50; −4.00), $p < 0.001$). The difference in the mean ICIQ-SF scale at baseline and after 12 months of treatment was −8 points (95% CI: −10.0; −6.5, $p = 0.000$) (Table 2), while on OAB-V8, the difference in score was −13.5 (95% CI: −16.0; −11.5, $p < 0.001$).

No statistically significant differences were observed in any of the 3 DVD variables at 12 months of treatment between patients who were not previously treated for OAB (naive) and patients who had been treated (nonnaive). Nor

Table 1: Changes from pre- to posttreatment in 3 DVD parameters after 12 months of OXY-TDS treatment.

3 DVD parameters	Pretreatment		Posttreatment		Change (95% CI)	p value
	N	M (SD)	N	M (SD)		
DUF (episodes/day)*	47	9.1 (3.1)	46	7.0 (1.6)	−1.7 (−2.55;−1.15)	<0.001
NUF (episodes/night)*	47	1.6 (1.4)	44	0.8 (0.8)	−0.9 (−1.12;−0.45)	<0.001
UF/24 h (episodes/day)*	47	10.7 (3.9)	47	7.7 (1.8)	−2.6 (−3.50;−1.80)	<0.001
Maximum UV (ml)*	38	250.7 (107.8)	39	346.0 (278.5)	63.3 (19.95; 105.85)	0.006
Nocturnal UV (ml)	38	146.6 (134.1)	39	134.2 (147.7)	−16.2 (−81.65; 48.35)	0.651
Mean UV (ml)	5	134.8 (83.4)	5	202.6 (47.9)	0.8 (−22.30; 20.70)	0.976
Urgency (episodes/day)	47	7.0 (4.7)	47	1.5 (1.5)	−4.7 (−6.05;−3.55)	<0.001
Urgency grade*	47	3.7 (0.5)	44	2.3 (1.3)	−1.4 (−1.85; −0.85)	<0.001
UUI (episodes/day)*	46	2.7 (2.7)	43	0.5 (0.9)	−1.9 (−2.85; −1.30)	<0.001
SUI (episodes/day)*	47	0.7 (1.2)	47	0.2 (0.5)	0.0 (−0.85; 0.00)	0.007
Pad/underwear changes (number/day)*	40	3.4 (4.1)	45	0.7 (1.1)	−2.2 (−2.80; −1.50)	<0.001
Liquid intake/24 h (ml)	38	1435.1 (406.1)	38	1453.5 (518.9)	15.8 (−134.15; 179.95)	0.698
Urine output/24 h (ml)	38	1385.9 (381.2)	39	1504.4 (381.1)	115.9 (0.00; 223.35)	0.054**
Nocturnal urine output (ml)	37	200.8 (161.5)	38	174.7 (202.4)	−30.9 (−107.50; 34.20)	0.51

3 DVD: 3-day voiding diary; DUF: daytime urinary frequency; NUF: night-time urinary frequency; UF/24 h: 24-hour urinary frequency (total number of episodes/24 hours); SUI: stress urinary frequency; UV: urinary volume; UUI: urge urinary frequency. p values: Student's t-test or *Wilcoxon signed rank test. Change: mean difference or *Hodges-Lehman estimator of location shift. **This variable was not reported in the 6-month visit in any of the evaluable cases. For this reason, no statistical comparisons were performed.

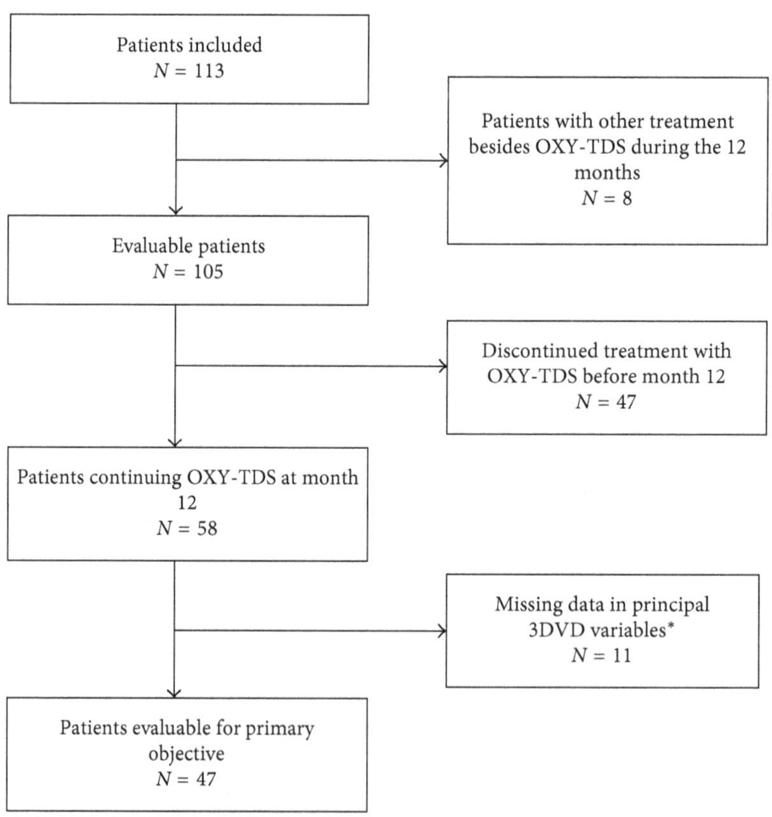

Figure 1: Study flow chart. Patients evaluated for study objectives according to data collected in clinical records. *Frequency, urgency, and urge incontinence. OXY-TDS: transdermal oxybutynin. 3 DVD: 3-day voiding diary.

were statistically significant differences observed between patients who were younger than 65 years and those who were 65 and older (Tables 3 and 4).

Twelve months after starting treatment, 47 patients (44.8%) had discontinued treatment. Reasons for discontinuation were adverse events in 18 patients (38.3%), lack of response in 17 (36.2%), and lack of treatment compliance in 4 (8.5%); another reason or no reason was given for 8 (17.0%) patients.

Regarding tolerability, 40 patients (38.1%) had some kind of adverse event at 12 months, mainly at the site of application of the patch (29 patients, 27.6%), 16 (15.2%) in the form of pruritus, 4 (3.8%) with erythema, and 13 (12.4%) with irritated skin. Two of the local adverse events (skin irritation)

TABLE 2: ICIQ-SF questionnaire. Changes from baseline after 12 months of treatment with OXY-TDS.

ICIQ-SF questionnaire	Pretreatment patients $N = 47$ n	Posttreatment patients $N = 47$ n	p value**
No urine leaks	2 (4.3%)	18 (38.3%)	<0.001
Leaks before you can get to the toilet	41 (87.2%)	22 (46.81%)	<0.001
Leaks when you cough or sneeze	18 (38.30%)	7 (14.9%)	0.013
Leaks when you are asleep	11 (23.4%)	3 (6.4%)	0.008
Leaks when you are physically active/exercising	16 (34.04%)	7 (14.9%)	0.035
Leaks when you have finished urinating	9 (19.15%)	2 (4.3%)	0.039
Leaks for no obvious reason	15 (31.91%)	2 (4.3%)	<0.001
Leaks all the time	2 (4.25%)	0 (0.0%)	NA
ICIQ-SF item 1 and 2 = 0	2	19	<0.001
ICIQ-SF item 1 or 2 > 0	45	27	
ICIQ-SF = 0	2	12	0.002
ICIQ-SF > 0	45	34	
	M (SD)	*M (SD)*	*Change (95% CI)*
Total score	13.40 (4.5)	5.13 (4.5)	−8 (−10.0; −6.5) p value 0.000*

Statistical tests: Student's t-test (variables with normal distribution) or Wilcoxon signed rank test (*variables with nonnormal distribution); **McNemar.

TABLE 3: Changes 3D from baseline in the 3 DVD tool at 12 months of treatment with OXY-TDS (naive/nonnaive patients).

3 DVD	Naive (n = 15) mean (SD)	Nonnaive (n = 32) mean (SD)	Diff (95% CI)	p value
DUF (episodes/day)*	7.07 (1.8)	6.9 (1.5)	0.4 (−0.7; 1.3)	0.341
NUF (episodes/night)*	0.87 (0.7)	0.7 (0.8)	0.0 (−3.0; 0.7)	0.411
UF/24 hours (episodes/day)*	8.0 (2.1)	7.6 (1.7)	6.3 (−0.4; 1.7)	0.298
Maximum UV (ml)*	444.6 (486.1)	302.1 (83.1)	24.1 (−41.7; 100.0)	0.461
Nocturnal UV (ml)	112.6 (84.9)	143.83 (168.9)	−31.2 (−135.9; 73.5)	0.550
Mean UV (ml)	205.5 (54.9)	191.0 (NA)	14.5 (−180.6; 209.6)	0.828
Urgency (episodes/day)	1.5 (2.1)	1.5 (1.2)	0.5 (−0.9; 1.0)	0.892
Urgency grade*	1.8 (1.3)	2.5 (1.3)	−0.7 (−1.3; 0.0)	0.071
UUI (episodes/day)*	0.2 (0.5)	0.6 (1.0)	0.0 (−0.3; 0.0)	0.328
SUI (episodes/day)*	0.0 (0.0)	0.2 (0.6)	0.0 (0.0; 0.0)	0.110
Pad/underwear changes (number/day)*	0.6 (1.0)	0.8 (1.1)	0.0 (−0.6; 0.0)	0.044
Liquid intake/24 h (ml)	1484.73 (613.5)	1439.0 (481.9)	45.7 (−326.4; 417.1)	0.805
Urine output/24 h (ml)	1609.17 (446.6)	1457.89 (347.2)	151.3 (−115.5; 418.0)	0.258
Nocturnal urine output (ml)	167.77 (138.3)	185.26 (228.2)	−17.5 (−162.6; 127.6)	0.808

3 DVD: 3-day voiding diary; DUF: daytime urinary frequency; NUF: night-time urinary frequency; SD: standard deviation; SUI: stress urinary incontinence; UF/24 h: 24-hour urinary frequency (total number of episodes/24 hours); UUI: urge urinary incontinence. p values: Student's t-test or *Wilcoxon signed rank test. Change: mean difference, or *Hodges-Lehman estimator of location shift.

were clinically significant and consequently considered severe. Dry mouth and constipation were recorded in only 6 (5.7%) and 1 (0.95%) of the patients, respectively.

4. Discussion

In this study, we examined retrospective data from the real-world management of patients with OAB treated with OXY-TDS over a 12-month period. Similarly to other studies reported in the literature [8, 9, 12, 13], we found that patients receiving OXY-TDS showed a reduction in OAB symptoms, with statistically significant changes in symptoms according to the 3 DVD, and in the grade of urgency perceived by patients, as recorded on the specific urgency VAS. The combined analysis performed by Dmochowski et al., in particular, found that OXY-TDS was more effective than placebo in the reduction of daily incontinence episodes (−3.0 versus −2.0, p = 0.0004) and daily urinary frequency (−2.0 versus −1.0, p = 0.0023) [12]. Moreover, OXY-TDS showed reductions similar to other antimuscarinic drugs. Findings from a review of randomized controlled trials with antimuscarinic drugs for OAB conducted by Novara et al. included reductions in urinary frequency (between −0.7 and −3.69), urgency episodes (between −1.0 and −3.4), or urgency urinary incontinence (between −0.3 and −2.28) [3]. It is also important to note that in our study, almost all incontinent patients (4 episodes of urgency/day) before treatment became continent after being treated with OXY-TDS.

In this study, we observed an improvement in symptoms due to OXY-TDS in the first 6 months, which was maintained until the end of the 12-month observational period. This is in line with results from clinical trials, which reported

Table 4: Changes 3D from baseline in the 3 DVD at 12 months of treatment with OXY-TDS (patients < 65 years and ≥65 years).

3 DVD	<65 years (n = 33) mean (SD)	≥65 years (n = 14) mean (SD)	Diff (95% CI)	p value
DUF (episodes/day)*	6.83 (1.5)	7.2 (1.9)	−0.3 (−1.3; 0.7)	0.615
NUF (episodes/night)*	0.6 (0.7)	1.1 (0.9)	−0.3 (−1.3; 0.0)	0.053
UF/24 h (episodes/day)*	7.4 (1.6)	8.4 (2.2)	−0.7 (−2.0; 0.3)	0.129
Maximum UV (ml)*	373.5 (328.4)	284.0 (203.7)	40.0 (−26.7; 106.7)	0.221
Nocturnal UV (ml)	107.4 (109.2)	194.6 (194.4)	−87.2 (−188.3; 14.0)	0.089
Mean UV (ml)	205.5 (54.9)	191 (n/a)	—	—
Urgency (episodes/day)	1.5 (1.6)	1.5 (1.2)	−0.1 (−1.0; 0.9)	0.876
Urgency grade*	2.3 (1.3)	2.3 (1.4)	0.0 (−0.7; 0.7)	0.805
UUI (episodes/day)*	0.3 (0.5)	0.87 (1.4)	0.0 (−0.7; 0.0)	0.232
SUI (episodes/day)*	0.1 (0.2)	0.3 (0.9)	0.0 (0.0; 0.0)	0.514
Pad/underwear changes (number/day)*	0.4 (0.6)	1.5 (1.5)	−0.7 (−2.0; 0.0)	0.024
Liquid intake/24 h (ml)	1431.2 (522.3)	1508.2 (531.3)	−77.0 (−457.8; 303.7)	0.684
Urine output/24 h (ml)	1503.4 (377.6)	1506.8 (405.3)	−3.4 (−274.9; 268.1)	0.980
Nocturnal urine output (ml)	127.0 (132.7)	309.2 (282.4)	−182.3 (−317.7; 46.8)	0.063

3 DVD: 3-day voiding diary; DUF: daytime urinary frequency; NUF: night-time urinary frequency; SD: standard deviation; SUI: stress urinary incontinence; UF/24 h: 24-hour urinary frequency (total number of episodes/24 hours); UV: urinary volume; UUI: urge urinary incontinence. p values: Student's t-test or *Wilcoxon signed rank test. Change: mean difference or *Hodges-Lehman estimator of location shift.

a response in the early weeks of treatment that was maintained during the following period [6].

Results suggest no differences in response to treatment between patients who were previously treated or treatment-naive. Similarly, no differences were found between patients younger and older than 65 years of age, but further studies are required to confirm these findings. In this study, approximately half of the patients received previous treatment and continued to present symptoms, and this observation is similar to those of the MATRIX study, despite the current availability of drugs such as solifenacin and mirabegron.

The most troublesome symptoms of OAB are urgency and urge incontinence [14], which may affect work productivity, impact negatively on quality of life, and lead to depression [15]. Similarly, alleviating OAB symptoms can have a significantly positive effect on health-related quality of life [16]. In this study, the overall improvement in 3 DVD and urgency VAS scores, along with improvements in all domains evaluated in both the ICIQ-SF questionnaire and OAB-V8 scale, affirm that our patients achieved an overall improvement in quality of life. Seventeen percent of our patients had depression, so long-term follow-up studies would be of interest to study associations between improvements in OAB symptoms and improvements in depressive syndromes.

VAS is a widely accepted research tool for measuring the impact of a disease and the effects of medical interventions on quality of life and has also been useful in urinary incontinence studies. It has been used for both evaluating the effects of urinary incontinence treatments and estimating the subjective perception of the patient with regard to their urinary incontinence [15, 17, 18]. In this study, the urgency VAS tool demonstrated its ability to measure treatment response. More completed urgency VAS scales (N = 58) than completed 3 DVDs3D (N = 47) were available in the patients' clinical records, and this might be interpreted as greater acceptance of the urgency VAS tool by patients, due to its simplicity as a measure of perceived grade of incontinence. Although 3 DVD is the reference instrument in clinical trials, in clinical practice, it is very difficult for patients to use. However, the urgency VAS may be a transparent, simple-to-use instrument that is easy for the clinician to interpret.

In our study, dry mouth occurred at a rate of 5.7%, less prevalent than expected in the Summary of Product Characteristics [19] (8.6%) and with other antimuscarinic drugs. In the review by Novara et al., the adverse event of dry mouth was between 13% and 86% depending on the study and antimuscarinic drug [3].

The MATRIX study, a 6-month phase IV trial carried out in the US in patients from urology, primary care, gynecology, and geriatrics departments, evaluated changes in health-related quality of life and work productivity in patients with OAB treated with OXY-TDS and found significant improvements in study parameters, along with good tolerability [20]. Two reviews of oxybutynin concluded that the transdermal formulation is generally well tolerated by OAB patients, with a low rate of anticholinergic-related adverse events, most of which were local, such as skin irritation at the site of application of the patch [6, 21]. The transdermal form of oxybutynin may offer a better tolerated therapeutic alternative to patients with OAB and urge incontinence in the management of their symptoms and thus may improve treatment adherence by patients [5, 20, 22].

In line with the MATRIX study [20], in which dermatitis, in the form of irritation, redness, and pruritus at the site of application of the patch, occurred in 14.0% of patients, adverse events related with site of application were also the most common in our study. Neither of the local adverse events (skin irritation) considered severe because of their clinical significance required hospital admission nor they did produce disability; in 1 case, the patient had a history of atopic dermatitis that she had not reported previously.

Treatment adherence with OXY-TDS was high in pre-approval clinical trials, in which 86–87.1% of participating patients completed the entire study treatment period [8, 9]. In our study, conducted in a standard clinical practice setting, 55.2% of the patients were continuing treatment at

12 months. Adverse events and failure to respond as expected were the most common reasons for discontinuation, in line with published reviews [23]. It is important to highlight that the persistence rate achieved in our study is high, and at least as high as that with other treatments options (23.7–66%), possibly associated with differences in efficacy and tolerability [24–27].

In general, however, adverse events were not serious, and treatment discontinuation could suggest that for many patients, the treatment benefits do not outweigh the drawbacks. Further studies are needed to gain more insight into how patients weigh up the difference between expected response and adverse events and what leads them to decide to maintain or discontinue a certain treatment.

To our knowledge, the OSCAR study is the first real-world study carried out in Europe recruiting patients exclusively from urology departments. In the MATRIX study, a 6-month phase IV trial carried out in the US including patients from different departments, the primary endpoint was changes in quality of life, but the 3 DVD was not used for evaluating effectiveness, even 3D as a secondary endpoint. The OSCAR study evaluated changes in signs and symptoms at 12 months as a primary endpoint, using a patient urinary diary and the OAB-V8 and ICI-Q questionnaires. In addition, cognitive function, adherence, and satisfaction were evaluated as secondary endpoints.

The limitations of this study are those typical of retrospective cohort studies and include among others bias in patient selection and missing data that might affect the final results. Nevertheless, in order to reduce possible bias, strict criteria were applied to the selection of patients, and data were evaluated for each variable according to the number of patients from whom those data were available. It is probable that patients who continue treatment have better results in terms of improvement of symptoms; however, this study did not evaluate symptoms in patients who discontinued. Another possible limitation is that the 3 participating sites were not randomly selected and results may not reflect the reality observed in other regions of Spain. However, that may be an advantage since all 3 centers belonged to the same health-care region that uses a standardized record system.

In conclusion, in view of the results of OSCAR study, it seems that there is currently an important place for OXY-TDS in the treatment of OAB, although further real-life studies should be carried out to extend knowledge of the use and effects of the drug in real practice.

Acknowledgments

This work was funded by the study sponsor (Asociación Gaditana de Investigación Urológica). The authors would like to thank GOC Networking for their advice on statistics, methodology, and manuscript preparation.

References

[1] P. Abrams, L. Cardozo, M. Fall et al., "The standardisation of terminology of lower urinary tract function: report from the Standardisation Sub-Committee of the International Continence Society," *American Journal of Obstetrics and Gynecology*, vol. 187, no. 1, pp. 116–126, 2002.

[2] E. Martinez Agullo, J. L. Ruiz Cerda, L. Gomez Perez et al., "Prevalence of urinary incontinence and hyperactive bladder in the Spanish population: results of the EPICC study," *Actas Urologicas Españolas*, vol. 33, no. 2, pp. 159–166, 2009.

[3] G. Novara, A. Galfano, S. Secco et al., "A systematic review and meta-analysis of randomized controlled trials with antimuscarinic drugs for overactive bladder," *European Urology*, vol. 54, no. 4, pp. 740–764, 2008.

[4] C. R. Chapple, R. Martinez-Garcia, L. Selvaggi et al., "A comparison of the efficacy and tolerability of solifenacin succinate and extended release tolterodine at treating overactive bladder syndrome: results of the STAR trial," *European Urology*, vol. 48, no. 3, pp. 464–470, 2005.

[5] G. W. Davila, J. S. Starkman, and R. R. Dmochowski, "Transdermal oxybutynin for overactive bladder," *Urologic Clinics of North America*, vol. 33, no. 4, pp. 455–463, 2006.

[6] J. Salinas-Casado, M. Esteban-Fuertes, O. Serrano, and J. Galvan, "The value of oxybutynin in transdermal patches for treating overactive bladder," *Actas Urológicas Españolas*, vol. 39, no. 10, pp. 599–604, 2015.

[7] G. W. Davila, C. A. Daugherty, S. W. Sanders, and TOS Group, "A short-term, multicenter, randomized double-blind dose titration study of the efficacy and anticholinergic side effects of transdermal compared to immediate release oral oxybutynin treatment of patients with urge urinary incontinence," *Journal of Urology*, vol. 166, no. 1, pp. 140–145, 2001.

[8] R. R. Dmochowski, G. W. Davila, N. R. Zinner et al., "Efficacy and safety of transdermal oxybutynin in patients with urge and mixed urinary incontinence," *Journal of Urology*, vol. 168, no. 2, pp. 580–586, 2002.

[9] R. R. Dmochowski, P. K. Sand, N. R. Zinner, M. C. Gittelman, G. W. Davila, and S. W. Sanders, "Comparative efficacy and safety of transdermal oxybutynin and oral tolterodine versus placebo in previously treated patients with urge and mixed urinary incontinence," *Urology*, vol. 62, no. 2, pp. 237–242, 2003.

[10] K. S. Coyne, T. Zyczynski, M. K. Margolis, V. Elinoff, and R. G. Roberts, "Validation of an overactive bladder awareness tool for use in primary care settings," *Advances in Therapy*, vol. 22, no. 4, pp. 381–394, 2005.

[11] M. Espuna Pons, P. Rebollo Alvarez, and M. Puig Clota, "Validation of the Spanish version of the international consultation on incontinence questionnaire-short form. A questionnaire for assessing the urinary incontinence," *Medicina Clínica*, vol. 122, no. 8, pp. 288–292, 2004.

[12] R. R. Dmochowski, V. Nitti, D. Staskin, K. Luber, R. Appell, and G. W. Davila, "Transdermal oxybutynin in the treatment of adults with overactive bladder: combined results of two randomized clinical trials," *World Journal of Urology*, vol. 23, no. 4, pp. 263–270, 2005.

[13] O. Yamaguchi, E. Uchida, N. Higo et al., "Efficacy and safety of once-daily oxybutynin patch versus placebo and propiverine in Japanese patients with overactive bladder: a randomized double-blind trial," *International Journal of Urology*, vol. 21, no. 6, pp. 586–593, 2014.

[14] I. Milsom, S. A. Kaplan, K. S. Coyne, C. C. Sexton, and Z. S. Kopp, "Effect of bothersome overactive bladder symptoms on health-related quality of life, anxiety, depression, and treatment seeking in the United States: results from EpiLUTS," *Urology*, vol. 80, no. 1, pp. 90–96, 2012.
[15] C. C. Sexton, K. S. Coyne, C. Thompson, T. Bavendam, C. I. Chen, and A. Markland, "Prevalence and effect on health-related quality of life of overactive bladder in older Americans: results from the epidemiology of lower urinary tract symptoms study," *Journal of the American Geriatrics Society*, vol. 59, no. 8, pp. 1465–1470, 2011.
[16] C. J. Kelleher, L. Cardozo, C. R. Chapple, F. Haab, and A. M. Ridder, "Improved quality of life in patients with overactive bladder symptoms treated with solifenacin," *BJU International*, vol. 95, no. 1, pp. 81–85, 2005.
[17] B. Stach-Lempinen, E. Kujansuu, P. Laippala, and R. Metsanoja, "Visual analogue scale, urinary incontinence severity score and 15 D–psychometric testing of three different health-related quality-of-life instruments for urinary incontinent women," *Scandinavian Journal of Urology and Nephrology*, vol. 35, no. 6, pp. 476–483, 2001.
[18] T. Shamliyan, J. F. Wyman, R. Ramakrishnan, F. Sainfort, and R. L. Kane, "Benefits and harms of pharmacologic treatment for urinary incontinence in women: a systematic review," *Annals of Internal Medicine*, vol. 156, no. 12, pp. 861–874, W301-10, 2012.
[19] European Medicines Agency, *Summary of Product Characteristic of Transdermal Oxybutynin*, European Medicines Agency, London, UK, 2009, http://www.ema.europa.eu/docs/es_ES/document_library/EPAR_-_Product_Information/human/000532/WC500040171.pdf.
[20] P. Sand, N. Zinner, D. Newman et al., "Oxybutynin transdermal system improves the quality of life in adults with overactive bladder: a multicentre, community-based, randomized study," *BJU International*, vol. 99, no. 4, pp. 836–844, 2007.
[21] S. A. Macdiarmid, "The evolution of transdermal/topical overactive bladder therapy and its benefits over oral therapy," *Reviews in Urology*, vol. 11, no. 1, pp. 1–6, 2009.
[22] G. W. Davila, "Transdermal oxybutynin in the treatment of overactive bladder," *Clinical Interventions in Aging*, vol. 1, no. 2, pp. 99–105, 2006.
[23] J. S. Benner, M. B. Nichol, E. S. Rovner et al., "Patient-reported reasons for discontinuing overactive bladder medication," *BJU International*, vol. 105, no. 9, pp. 1276–1282, 2010.
[24] C. R. Chapple, J. Nazir, Z. Hakimi et al., "Persistence and adherence with mirabegron versus antimuscarinic agents in patients with overactive bladder: a retrospective observational study in UK clinical practice," *European Urology*, vol. 72, no. 3, pp. 389–399, 2017.
[25] D. Kato, H. Tabuchi, and S. Uno, "Safety, efficacy, and persistence of long-term mirabegron treatment for overactive bladder in the daily clinical setting: interim (1-year) report from a Japanese post-marketing surveillance study," *LUTS: Lower Urinary Tract Symptoms*, 2017, In press.
[26] A. S. Wagg, S. Foley, J. Peters, J. Nazir, L. Kool-Houweling, and L. Scrine, "Persistence and adherence with mirabegron vs antimuscarinics in overactive bladder: retrospective analysis of a UK general practice prescription database," *International Journal of Clinical Practice*, vol. 71, no. 10, article e12996, 2017.
[27] D. Sussman, A. Yehoshua, J. Kowalski et al., "Adherence and persistence of mirabegron and anticholinergic therapies in patients with overactive bladder: a real-world claims data analysis," *International Journal of Clinical Practice*, vol. 71, no. 3-4, article e12824, 2017.

10

High-Intensity Focused Ultrasound (HIFU) Focal Therapy for Localized Prostate Cancer with MRI-US Fusion Platform

Chi-Hang Yee, Peter Ka-Fung Chiu, Jeremy Yuen-Chun Teoh, Chi-Fai Ng, Chi-Kwok Chan, and See-Ming Hou

S. H. Ho Urology Centre, Department of Surgery, Prince of Wales Hospital, The Chinese University of Hong Kong, Hong Kong

Correspondence should be addressed to Chi-Hang Yee; yeechihang@surgery.cuhk.edu.hk

Academic Editor: Jason M. Hafron

Objective. The study aimed at investigating the outcome of prostate HIFU focal therapy using the MRI-US fusion platform for treatment localization and delivery. *Methods.* It is a prospectively designed case series of HIFU focal therapy for localized prostate cancer. The inclusion criteria include clinical tumor stage ≤T2, visible index lesion on multiparametric MRI less than 20 mm in diameter, absence of Gleason 5 pattern on prostate biopsy, and PSA ≤ 20 ng/ml. HIFU focal therapy was performed in the conventional manner in the beginning 50% of the series, whereas the subsequent cases were performed with MRI-US fusion platform. The primary outcome was treatment failure rate which is defined by the need of salvage therapy. Secondary outcomes included tumor recurrence in follow-up biopsy, PSA change, perioperative complications, and postoperative functional outcomes. *Results.* Twenty patients underwent HIFU focal ablation. HIFU on an MRI-US fusion platform had a trend of a longer total operative time than the conventional counterpart (124.2 min vs. 107.1 min, $p = 0.066$). There was no difference in the mean ablation volume to lesion volume ratio between the two. The mean PSA percentage change from baseline to 6-month is more significant in the conventional group (63.3% vs. 44.6%, $p = 0.035$). No suspicious lesion was seen at 6-month mpMRI in all 20 patients. Two patients, one from each group, eventually underwent radical treatment because of the presence of clinically significant prostate cancer in the form of out-of-field recurrences during follow-up biopsy. No significant difference was observed before and after HIFU concerning uroflowmetry, SF-12 score, and EPIC-26 score. It was observed that energy used per volume was positively correlated with PSA density of the patient ($r = 0.6364$, $p = 0.014$). *Conclusion.* In conclusion, HIFU with conventional or MRI-US fusion platform provided similar oncological and functional outcomes.

1. Introduction

High-intensity focused ultrasound (HIFU) has been evaluated for the treatment of several benign and malignant conditions, such as uterine fibroids, thyroid nodules, and breast cancers. The first experience with the use of HIFU for prostate cancer management was reported in 1996 [1], and the initial role of HIFU was for whole-gland ablation when patients refused or were not eligible for radical prostatectomy [2, 3]. The use of HIFU for focal treatment represents a more recent concept aiming to provide the best balance between oncological control and minimizing the side effect profile. Such focal treatment extends from the initial report as a salvage therapy for focal recurrence after radiotherapy [4] to being the primary treatment for nonmetastatic prostate cancer [5, 6].

The diagnostic pathway of prostate cancer has been revolutionized by the use of mpMRI. MRI-ultrasound (US) guided prostate biopsy has been validated for its ability to increase the detection rate of clinically significant cancers with a reduction in the overdiagnosis of clinically insignificant cancers [7, 8]. While precision of prostate biopsy has been improved by the MRI-US fusion platform, such precision in lesion localization has not been incorporated in the conventional focal therapy delivery. Conventional HIFU focal therapy has been performed relying on transrectal ultrasound only. Recently, the MRI-US fusion software has been introduced to HIFU focal therapy platform in an attempt to enhance treatment precision. Our study aimed to describe the results and change in prostate parameters after MRI-US fusion HIFU focal therapy.

2. Materials and Methods

This was a prospective observational study on consecutive patients with localized prostate cancer who underwent HIFU focal therapy between April 2019 and September 2020. Men aged between 40 and 80 years old who were diagnosed of prostate cancer with the following criteria were considered potential candidate for HIFU focal therapy: clinically tumor stage ≤T2, visible index lesion(s) on multiparametric MRI less than 20 mm in diameter, position of tumor less than 40 mm from rectum on MRI, absence of Gleason 5 pattern on prostate biopsy, and PSA ≤ 20 ng/ml. Patients were excluded from the study if they had active urinary tract infection, if they were on anticoagulation, and if they were unfit for contrast multiparametric MRI exam. The study protocol was approved by the local institutional ethics review board (CREC 2018.556-T) and was conducted in accordance with the ethical standards of the Helsinki Declaration of 1975 and its later versions. Written informed consent was obtained from all patients for study enrolment.

All patients who entered the study had prior mpMRI of the prostate. Diagnosis of prostate cancer was either by template systematic biopsy or MRI-guided ultrasound fusion biopsy. Once the patient was identified to fulfil the aforementioned inclusion and exclusion criteria after recruitment, he would have the following assessments: TRUS (transrectal ultrasound) to assess if there is any calcification in close proximity to the lesion that would hinder HIFU energy delivery, PSA, International Prostate Symptom Score (IPSS), overactive bladder symptom score (OABSS), International Index of Erectile Function (IIEF-5), 12-item short form survey (SF-12), expanded prostate cancer index composite (EPIC-25), and uroflowmetry.

2.1. HIFU Treatment. HIFU therapy was performed using the Sonablate® 500 device (Sonacare Inc., USA), and treatments were delivered in a focal lesion ablation or quadrant fashion depending on the gland volume, tumor volume, and its location. Administration of HIFU focal therapy was based on the strategy of index lesion ablation, i.e., only index lesion was ablated in patients with multifocal disease when untreated areas did not exhibit any Gleason 6 lesion more than 3 mm in diameter. While conventional HIFU ablation was performed with cognitive recognition of lesion location, fusion of MRI and ultrasound images for the localization of lesion during HIFU treatments was performed with the Sonafuse™-MIM Symphony™ platform in the later 50% of the case series. The Sonafuse™-MIM Symphony™ platform adopted a similar fusion process as in bkFusion™ for prostate biopsy, with prior installation of MRI images and subsequent contouring of the gland and index lesions. Limitation of the fusion platform could be attributed to its rigid fusion instead of elastic fusion mode of operation. Ablation margin of 7 mm was adopted in the treatment. The whole treatment procedure was performed under general anaesthesia with real-time ultrasound monitoring (supplementary video). A urethral catheter was inserted during or after the procedure depending on the location of the lesion.

mpMRI was performed on postoperative day 7 and postoperative 6 months for evaluation. Routine follow-up biopsy was arranged after 6-month MRI. Prostate volume, lesion volume, and ablation zone volume were reconstructed and evaluated by OsiriX MD 12.0. Functional assessment and PSA were checked at 3 months and 6 months. The primary outcome was treatment failure rate which is defined by the need of salvage therapy. Secondary outcomes included tumor recurrence in follow-up biopsy, PSA change, perioperative complications, and postoperative functional outcomes.

Statistical analysis was performed using SPSS 26.0 (IBM Corp., Armonk, NY, USA). Postoperative changes in continuous variables were compared by the *t*-test. Comparison of more than 2 variables was performed by the one-way repeated measures ANOVA test, and linear regression was performed by the Pearson correlation test. A p value of <0.05 was regarded as significant.

3. Results

A total of 20 patients with 22 index lesions underwent HIFU focal therapy for prostate cancer over the study period (Table 1). Mean PSA level of the patients was 8.70 ± 3.5 ng/ml. Six patients had their cancer diagnosed by transrectal biopsy and 14 patients had transperineal prostate biopsy under local anaesthesia. All lesions were visible on preoperative mpMRI. The two patients with ISUP grade group 4 disease had isolated target biopsy of Gleason 4 + 4 prostate cancer at the target in an 18–24-core template. Twelve patients had lesions belonging to ISUP grade group 1, of which 10 of them had tumor volume $>0.5\ cm^3$ on MRI images. The other two patients with tumor volume $<0.5\ cm^3$ refused the option of active surveillance and agreed to HIFU focal treatment. Most lesions were located at the peripheral zone.

All patients underwent focal or quadrant ablation. No hemiablation or whole-gland ablation was performed. The decision of having urethral catheter in situ during HIFU therapy depended on the proximity of the lesion to the urethra. The first 10 patients underwent conventional HIFU focal therapy, and the later 10 patients had MRI-US fusion-guided treatment. Perioperative data of HIFU focal therapy are given in Table 2. A trend of a longer total operative time was observed for patients with fusion platform than without fusion platform (124.2 min vs. 107.1 min, $p = 0.066$). No statistically significant difference was observed between the two modalities with respect to ablation volume to lesion volume ratio. In the first six cases of the series, urethral catheter was removed on postoperative day 1. Four patients failed to initiate self-void on day 1 or were readmitted soon after discharge for retention of urine, requiring reinsertion of catheter. As a result, we subsequently kept the catheter for 1 week for the rest of the patients. Among the remaining 14

Table 1: Baseline characteristics of the patients.

Characteristics	
Mean age (years) ± SD	68.4 ± 5.9
Mean BMI (kg/m^2) ± SD	23.8 ± 3.0
PSA	
<4 ng/mL (*n*)	1 (5%)
4–10 ng/mL (*n*)	13 (65%)
>10–20 ng/mL (*n*)	6 (30%)
Mode of diagnosis	
MRI-USG fusion target + systematic biopsy (*n*)	14 (70%)
Mapping transperineal systematic biopsy (*n*)	6 (30%)
Number of index lesions per HIFU surgery	
1 (*n*)	18 (90%)
2 (*n*)	2 (10%)
Characteristics of index lesions under treatment on MRI	
Visible on MRI (*n*)	22 (100%)
PI-RADS 3 (*n*)	1 (5%)
PI-RADS 4 (*n*)	14 (70%)
PI-RADS 5 (*n*)	5 (25%)
ISUP grade group of index lesions under treatment	
Grade group 1 (*n*)	12 (54.5%)
Grade group 2 (*n*)	5 (22.7%)
Grade group 3 (*n*)	3 (13.6%)
Grade group 4 (*n*)	2 (9.1%)
Grade group 5 (*n*)	0
Index lesion location	
Peripheral zone (*n*)	18 (81.8%)
Transitional zone (*n*)	4 (18.2%)
Apex (*n*)	5 (22.7%)
Middle (*n*)	9 (40.9%)
Base (*n*)	8 (36.4%)
Mean distance between the lesion from rectum (mm)	15.7 ± 8.3
Mean index lesion size (cm^3) ± SD	0.89 ± 0.95

SD, standard deviation; BMI, body mass index; PSA, prostatic specific antigen.

patients, 3 patients failed to void on day 7, requiring another attempt to wean off catheter later. For the three patients with Clavien-Dindo grade 1 complications, 3 were retention of urine requiring readmission and 1 was haematuria managed conservatively.

mpMRI at post-HIFU 1 week revealed that ablation zone had covered region of interest in all patients. Mean percentage drop of PSA at 6-month was 44.6% in the fusion group and 63.3% in the conventional group ($p = 0.035$). At 6-month mpMRI, no suspicious lesion was observed in all 20 patients. Twelve patients went on to have a follow-up biopsy. Two patients (one from fusion HIFU on a peripheral zone lesion and one from conventional HIFU on a transitional zone lesion) were found to have clinically significant prostate cancer and both of them were out-of-field recurrence (GS 4 + 4 1 mm focus and GS 4 + 5 2 mm focus). These two patients eventually received radical treatment (one with robotic radical prostatectomy and the other one with radiotherapy). The radical prostatectomy specimen yielded a pT2aN0 prostate cancer, with a GS 4 + 5 tumor focus occupying 5% of the prostate volume. Another 2 patients with nonclinically significant prostate cancer (ISUP grade group 1) out-of-field recurrence was found on follow-up biopsy. The mean 6-month PSA of those in the cohort without recurrence and those with recurrence was 4.3 ± 3.2 and 3.4 ± 1.4, respectively ($p = 0.348$). The mean PSA nadir of these 2 groups was 3.6 ± 2.4 and 3.4 ± 1.4, respectively ($p = 0.096$).

Significant increase in prostate volume was observed at postoperative 7 days compared with baseline (54.5 ± 20.1 cm^3 vs. 39.5 ± 14.9 cm^3, $p = 0.004$). However, the mean prostate volume at 6 months (38.5 ± 21.8 cm^3) was similar to baseline (Figure 1). PSA showed a significant drop after the surgery, with mean PSA <4 ng/ml at 6 months (Table 3). Comparison between baseline mean IPSS and post-HIFU 3-month mean IPSS showed a significant improvement (11.2 ± 5.8 vs. 8.4 ± 5.1, $p = 0.034$). Preoperatively 13 patients were on alpha blocker for lower urinary tract symptoms (LUTS). Among these 13 patients, 8 patients were taken off alpha blockers at 6 months. No significant difference was observed before and after HIFU concerning uroflowmetry, SF-12 score, and EPIC-26 score. With respect to erectile function, at 3 months, a significant difference in the mean IIEF-5 score was found compared with baseline (11.7 ± 8.5 vs. 15.1 ± 6.5, $p = 0.001$), yet not the same was observed with respect to the 6-month mean IIEF (13.7 ± 7.6 vs. 15.1 ± 6.5, $p = 0.314$). The number of patients on phosphodiesterase type 5 inhibitor (PDE5-I) at baseline, 3 months, and 6 months was 0, 3, and 6, respectively.

Concerning the technical aspect of HIFU application, the relationship between the following factors were investigated: total energy applied, ablation zone volume, and PSA change. It was observed that energy used per volume was positively correlated with PSA density of the patient (Figure 2). However, total energy used was not correlated with PSA change ($p = 0.2431$) and percentage change in PSA ($p = 0.374$). Comparing the cases of HIFU focal therapy with or without fusion assistance, no difference was observed with respect to mean ablation zone volume to lesion volume ratio (62.8 and 66.4, $p = 0.473$). However, the mean PSA percentage change from baseline to 6-month was more significant in the conventional group than in the fusion group (44.6 vs. 63.3, $p = 0.035$).

4. Discussion

Focal therapy with HIFU ablation has proven to be an effective treatment option for prostate cancer with short-to-medium term results [9]. Besides oncological criteria, the size of the prostate gland also determines the outcome of treatment. The transrectal route of energy delivery by the HIFU probe may hinder access to anterior lesion [10], and the tissue swelling after HIFU treatment renders the placement of a urethral or suprapubic catheter, a common practice after the procedure [11]. Such change in prostate size has led to some centres performing transurethral resection of prostate (TURP) before or simultaneously with the HIFU procedure [12]. Previously, Shoji et al. reported the result of prostate swelling and shift after partial gland and whole-gland HIFU ablation [13]. Our study also investigated the perioperative change in prostate dimensions in focal HIFU ablation for prostate cancer by using the OsiriX MD

Table 2: HIFU surgery and perioperative details.

Parameters	With fusion	Without fusion	Overall	*P* value
Mean total operative time (mins) ± SD	124.2 ± 16.9	107.1 ± 28.3	115.2 ± 24.6	0.066
Mean actual HIFU time (s) ± SD	37.4 ± 10.9	42.9 ± 13.2	40.3 ± 12.2	0.172
HIFU with urethral catheter in situ (*n*)	4	3	7 (35%)	0.639
Lesion visible on ultrasound during HIFU (*n*)	5	6	11 (55%)	0.653
Number of ablation zones used during HIFU				
1 (*n*)	0	0	0 (0%)	
2 (*n*)	0	5	5 (25%)	
3 (*n*)	10	5	15 (75%)	
Mean ablation volume to lesion volume ratio	62.8	66.4	65.1	0.473
Mean urethral catheter in situ days ± SD	8.7 ± 7.2	9.8 ± 5.7	9.3 ± 6.4	0.355
Same day discharge from the hospital (*n*)	8	3	11	0.025
90-day complication (Clavien-Dindo grade) (*n*)				
Grade 1	1	3	4	0.264
Grades 2–5	0	0	0	
Mean PSA percentage change from baseline to 6-month (%) ± SD	44.6 ± 21.0	63.3 ± 22.4	53.9 ± 23.2	0.035

PSA, prostate-specific antigen; SD, standard deviation.

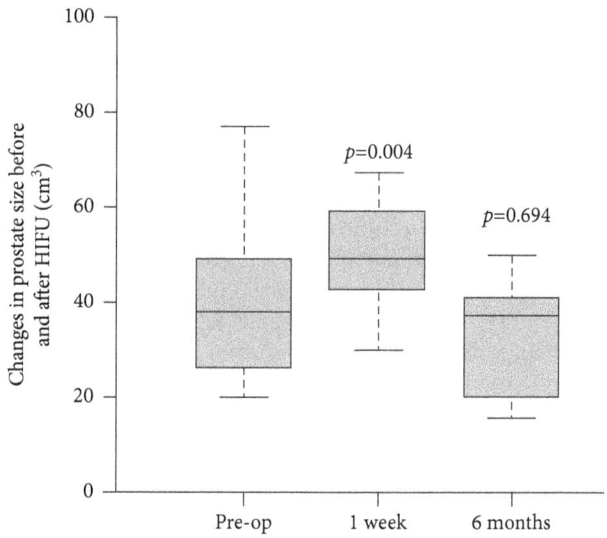

Figure 1: Boxplot of the change in prostate size before and after HIFU treatment. *P* value reflects the *t*-test comparison against the preoperative baseline value.

software. A statistically significant increase in prostate volume was observed on postoperative day 7, which eventually returned to baseline at 6 months (Figure 1). This accounts for the static results at 3 months and 6 months with respect to IPSS, OABSS, EPIC-26 LUTS score, and uroflowmetry parameters (Table 3).

The availability of MRI-US-targeted prostate biopsy has made localization of prostate tumor more precise. This has encouraged focal HIFU therapy to be an alternative to the whole-gland or hemiablation treatment in the past. As a result, there is a call for a more accurate localization of the lesion during HIFU surgery. The MRI-US fusion platform for HIFU application allows the operator to plan the treatment zone with a reference location of the target tumor in sight, minimizing the potential error from cognitive fusion for the index lesion location. In the current HIFU series, a rigid MRI-US fusion platform was adopted. Taking from the experience of prostate fusion biopsy, in a systematic review by Venderink et al., the authors did not find any difference in clinically significant cancer detection between rigid and elastic registration for MRI-TRUS fusion-guided biopsy [14]. Similarly, Hale et al. [15] found no difference in registration errors between rigid and elastic registration overall, but rigid registration decreased the registration error of targets near the prostate edge, which would be a common location of tumor for HIFU ablation. Thus, a rigid MRI-US fusion platform was incorporated into our present study.

Our series have observed that with the fusion platform, there was a trend of a longer operative time without an increase in ablation time. It could be explained by the extra time consumed during mapping, fusion, and planning during treatment. By evaluating the ratio between tumor volume and eventual ablation volume, we would like to assess if the use of MRI-US fusion platform during HIFU treatment would bring about a more focal ablation. We found that the PSA drop was more significant in the conventional group, with a higher mean ablation volume to lesion volume ratio, eventhough it has not yet reached a statistically significant difference. It could be accounted by the tendency that without a clear tumor location in sight, operators tend to ablate a larger area to minimize the chance of missing any lesion. It thus results in a larger ablation volume and a bigger PSA drop after HIFU treatment. Sivaraman et al. retrospectively reviewed their cohort of HIFU patients with Ablatherm® (no fusion platform) and Focal-One® (with fusion platform) [16]. No significant difference was found with respect to perioperative complications, but the group with fusion platform had significantly lower urine leak at 3 months. In our series, no patient experienced any incontinence in both modalities. Further evaluation is needed to confirm the benefits of MRI-US fusion HIFU treatment.

Some authors have advocated the use of contrast-enhanced ultrasound to define the ablation zone after HIFU [17]. Early postoperative MRI can be another option for the same purpose. An area of hypointensity surrounded by a peripheral rim of enhancement could be observed in patients

Table 3: Overall changes in parameters after HIFU focal therapy.

Parameters	Baseline	3 months	*P* value[#]	6 months	*P* value*
Mean PSA (ng/ml) ± SD	8.4 ± 3.3	4.2 ± 3.1	<0.001	3.7 ± 2.4	<0.001
Mean IPSS ± SD	11.2 ± 5.8	8.4 ± 5.1	0.034	8.8 ± 5.8	0.122
Mean QoL ± SD	2.4 ± 1.3	2.1 ± 1.2	0.281	2.5 ± 1.0	0.377
Mean OABSS ± SD	4.5 ± 2.6	4.2 ± 1.9	0.325	4.6 ± 2.2	0.500
Mean IIEF-5 ± SD	15.1 ± 6.5	11.7 ± 8.5	0.001	13.7 ± 7.6	0.314
Mean SF-12 ± SD					
Physical score	48.4 ± 5.9	49.7 ± 7.4	0.304	49.3 ± 6.5	0.346
Mental score	47.6 ± 10.8	49.0 ± 7.7	0.339	48.3 ± 7.0	0.422
Mean EPIC-26 score ± SD					
Incontinence	91.3 ± 13.7	90.0 ± 18.6	0.426	90.5 ± 15.1	0.449
LUTS	81.7 ± 15.2	86.7 ± 12.2	0.165	85.8 ± 11.7	0.204
Bowel function	87.8 ± 14.6	88.4 ± 13.3	0.456	85.1 ± 17.1	0.330
Sexual function	49.6 ± 30.5	43.3 ± 30.5	0.301	40.8 ± 31.0	0.237
Hormonal function	97.5 ± 6.6	97.2 ± 5.8	0.444	97.2 ± 4.8	0.440
Uroflowmetry					
Qmax (ml/s) ± SD	14.9 ± 6.3	14.6 ± 5.2	0.451	14.4 ± 6.9	0.428
PVRU (ml)	68.6 ± 41.1	53.2 ± 48.1	0.194	47.5 ± 42.2	0.104

SD, standard deviation; PSA, prostatic specific antigen; PHI, prostate health index; IPSS, International Prostate Symptom Score; QoL, quality of life; OABSS, overactive bladder symptom score; IIEF-5, International Index of Erectile Function; SF-12, 12-item short form survey; EPIC-25, expanded prostate cancer index composite; LUTS, lower urinary tract symptoms; Qmax, maximal voiding velocity; PVRU, postvoid residual urine. [#]Comparison of 3-month data against the baseline value. *Comparison of 6-month data against the baseline value.

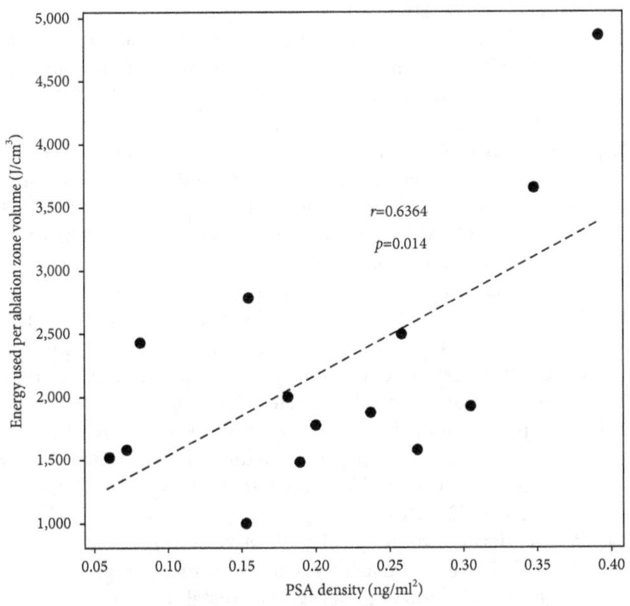

Figure 2: Scatter plot of the energy used per ablation zone volume in correlation to PSA density of the respective prostate gland.

after HIFU as early as postoperative day 2 [18] to day 14 [19]. Thus, our study used MRI on day 7 for assessment of ablation zone. PSA has been commonly used for follow-up after focal therapy. Some series have adopted the Phoenix ASTRO definition as a way to document biochemical recurrence [20, 21]. On the other hand, Huber et al. found that PSA criteria have significant variability in performance characteristics to rule out or detect failure after focal HIFU therapy. Furthermore, the diagnostic performance of PSA demonstrates a wide range of accuracy metrics at different time points [22]. Our series made use of a trimodality assessment which includes PSA, MRI, and biopsy for follow-up after HIFU focal therapy. In contrast to von Hardenberg et al. who found that out of the 20 patients that had biopsies at 12 months, 8 patients had a positive biopsy within the ablation zone, and our series did not reveal any in-field recurrence [23] which was similar to Shoji et al. [21]. The two significant prostate cancers picked up by follow-up biopsy in the series could not be identified with PSA and MRI alone early in the follow-up period. The series by Ganzer et al. also demonstrated limited sensitivity of posttreatment MRI for clinically significant prostate cancer [24]. Dellabella et al. identified 38.4% of their patients having prostate cancer on 1-year biopsy, of whom 61.8% of patients went on for another line of treatment [25]. Further study is warranted to investigate the role of routine biopsy in evaluating recurrence after focal therapy for prostate cancer.

HIFU leads to tissue destruction by means of thermal and mechanical effects. Pressure fluctuations inside tissue induce hyperthermia and the mechanical effects of ultrasound results in tissue damage by cavitation and radiation force [11]. The deposition of HIFU energy brings about coagulative necrosis known as biological focal region (BFR), of which its dimension depends on the acoustic pressure, exposure time, and tissue characteristics [26]. Our series demonstrated the positive correlation between total energy used for sonication and the eventual volume of coagulative necrosis shown on MRI. Furthermore, the energy consumption per volume of coagulative necrosis is found to be correlated to the preoperative PSA density of the patient. Such observation may be explained by the differential tissue response to HIFU energy in different cases. During HIFU focal therapy session, there is continuous real-time monitoring of the thermal effects by ultrasound visualization of the intraprostatic acoustic pattern changes which include any "popcorn effect" as caused by collapse of gas bubbles. Because, in our experience, the degree of the popcorn effect was different in every case, and not every tumor ablation would result in popcorn acoustic appearance on ultrasound; there might be a difference in HIFU energy requirement between normal tissue and tumor lesions and between different tumors. Energy delivery level is adjusted by the surgeon in real-time along the whole course of HIFU treatment in order to ensure an adequate tissue response. Difference in PSA density between different prostate cancer cases can represent a difference in architecture of the tumors. Prostate cancer cells do not make more PSA [27], and the elevated serum PSA levels are a product of disruption of cellular structure within the prostate gland [28]. Taking reference from the investigation of bioimpedance of prostate tissue, bioimpedance increases with increasing distortion of gland architecture [29]. The difference in PSA density can entail a difference in tissue characteristics, implying a difference in HIFU energy requirement to deliver the same acoustic visual feedback on ultrasound.

There are limitations of our study. In our series, only 60% of the patients underwent the 12-month follow-up biopsy after HIFU treatment. While our results with respect to PSA, PHI, and MRI provided the early outcome profile of HIFU treatment, a more complete histological assessment of the cohort at 12 months would be desired. However, patient resistance to compliance with follow-up biopsy was common in the absence of rising PSA or an indication of residual disease on MRI. In the major focal HIFU therapy series in the literature, it was reported that only 37.1–52.4% patients complied to a follow-up biopsy after HIFU therapy [5, 30]. Another limitation of our study is the lack of randomization in the comparison of the results between conventional HIFU platform and MRI-US fusion HIFU platform. The results from our prospectively designed case series can be used as the basis for future randomized controlled trial to investigate the treatment outcome of the fusion HIFU platform.

5. Conclusion

HIFU focal therapy for prostate cancer resulted in an early tumor clearance on MRI assessment, with a significant drop in PSA and PHI after treatment. Energy consumption during HIFU therapy is positively correlated with ablation volume and tissue characteristic as reflected by PSA density. While MRI-US fusion platform for HIFU focal therapy could allow visualization of the lesion during planning and ablation, further evaluation is needed to confirm the benefits of MRI/US-fusion HIFU treatment.

References

[1] A. Gelet, J. Y. Chapelon, R. Bouvier et al., "Treatment of prostate cancer with transrectal focused ultrasound: early clinical experience," *European Urology*, vol. 29, no. 2, pp. 174–183, 1996.

[2] L. Poissonnier, J.-Y. Chapelon, O. Rouvière et al., "Control of prostate cancer by transrectal HIFU in 227 patients," *European Urology*, vol. 51, no. 2, pp. 381–387, 2007.

[3] A. Blana, B. Walter, S. Rogenhofer, and W. F. Wieland, "High-intensity focused ultrasound for the treatment of localized prostate cancer: 5-year experience," *Urology*, vol. 63, no. 2, pp. 297–300, 2004.

[4] H. U. Ahmed, P. Cathcart, N. McCartan et al., "Focal salvage therapy for localized prostate cancer recurrence after external beam radiotherapy: a pilot study," *Cancer*, vol. 118, no. 17, pp. 4148–4155, 2012.

[5] S. Guillaumier, M. Peters, M. Arya et al., "A multicentre study of 5-year outcomes following focal therapy in treating clinically significant nonmetastatic prostate cancer," *European Urology*, vol. 74, no. 4, pp. 422–429, 2018.

[6] H. U. Ahmed, R. G. Hindley, L. Dickinson et al., "Focal therapy for localised unifocal and multifocal prostate cancer: a prospective development study," *The Lancet Oncology*, vol. 13, no. 6, pp. 622–632, 2012.

[7] H. U. Ahmed, A. El-Shater Bosaily, L. C. Brown et al., "Diagnostic accuracy of multi-parametric MRI and TRUS biopsy in prostate cancer (PROMIS): a paired validating confirmatory study," *The Lancet*, vol. 389, no. 10071, pp. 815–822, 2017.

[8] V. Kasivisvanathan, A. S. Rannikko, M. Borghi et al., "MRI-targeted or standard biopsy for prostate-cancer diagnosis," *New England Journal of Medicine*, vol. 378, no. 19, pp. 1767–1777, 2018.

[9] Y. He, P. Tan, M. He et al., "The primary treatment of prostate cancer with high-intensity focused ultrasound: a systematic review and meta-analysis," *Medicine*, vol. 99, no. 41, Article ID e22610, 2020.

[10] P. M. Huber, N. Afzal, M. Arya et al., "Focal HIFU therapy for anterior compared to posterior prostate cancer lesions," *World Journal of Urology*, vol. 39, no. 4, pp. 1115–1119, 2021.

[11] A. Napoli, G. Alfieri, R. Scipione et al., "High-intensity focused ultrasound for prostate cancer," *Expert Review of Medical Devices*, vol. 17, no. 5, pp. 427–433, 2020.

[12] Y.-T. Wu and P. H. Chiang, "Cohort study of high-intensity focused ultrasound in the treatment of localised prostate cancer treatment: medium-term results from a single centre," *PLoS One*, vol. 15, no. 7, Article ID e0236026, 2020.

[13] S. Shoji, T. Uchida, M. Nakamoto et al., "Prostate swelling and shift during high intensity focused ultrasound: implication for targeted focal therapy," *The Journal of Urology*, vol. 190, no. 4, pp. 1224–1232, 2013.

[14] W. Venderink, M. de Rooij, J. P. M. Sedelaar, H. J. Huisman, and J. J. Fütterer, "Elastic versus rigid image registration in magnetic resonance imaging-transrectal ultrasound fusion prostate biopsy: a systematic review and meta-analysis," *European Urology Focus*, vol. 4, no. 2, pp. 219–227, 2018.

[15] G. R. Hale, M. Czarniecki, A. Cheng et al., "Comparison of elastic and rigid registration during magnetic resonance imaging/ultrasound fusion-guided prostate biopsy: a multi-operator phantom study," *The Journal of Urology*, vol. 200, no. 5, pp. 1114–1121, 2018.

[16] A. Sivaraman, G. Marra, A. Stabile et al., "Does mpMRI guidance improve HIFU partial gland ablation compared to conventional ultrasound guidance? Early functional outcomes and complications from a single center," *International Brazilian Journal of Urology*, vol. 46, no. 6, pp. 984–992, 2020.

[17] A. N. Ashrafi, N. Nassiri, I. S. Gill, M. Gulati, D. Park, and A. L. de Castro Abreu, "Contrast-enhanced transrectal ul-

trasound in focal therapy for prostate cancer," *Current Urology Reports*, vol. 19, no. 10, p. 87, 2018.

[18] O. Rouvière, D. Lyonnet, A. Raudrant et al., "MRI appearance of prostate following transrectal HIFU ablation of localized cancer," *European Urology*, vol. 40, no. 3, pp. 265–274, 2001.

[19] S. Shoji, A. Tonooka, A. Hashimoto et al., "Time-dependent change of blood flow in the prostate treated with high-intensity focused ultrasound," *International Journal of Urology*, vol. 21, no. 9, pp. 942–945, 2014.

[20] M. Roach, G. Hanks, H. Thames Jr. et al., "Defining biochemical failure following radiotherapy with or without hormonal therapy in men with clinically localized prostate cancer: recommendations of the RTOG-ASTRO phoenix consensus conference," *International Journal of Radiation Oncology, Biology, Physics*, vol. 65, no. 4, pp. 965–974, 2006.

[21] S. Shoji, S. Hiraiwa, K. Uemura et al., "Focal therapy with high-intensity focused ultrasound for the localized prostate cancer for Asian based on the localization with MRI-TRUS fusion image-guided transperineal biopsy and 12-cores transperineal systematic biopsy: prospective analysis of oncological and functional outcomes," *International Journal of Clinical Oncology*, vol. 25, no. 10, pp. 1844–1853, 2020.

[22] P. M. Huber, N. Afzal, M. Arya et al., "Prostate specific antigen criteria to diagnose failure of cancer control following focal therapy of nonmetastatic prostate cancer using high intensity focused ultrasound," *The Journal of Urology*, vol. 203, no. 4, pp. 734–742, 2020.

[23] J. von Hardenberg, N. Westhoff, D. Baumunk et al., "Prostate cancer treatment by the latest focal HIFU device with MRI/TRUS-fusion control biopsies: a prospective evaluation," *Urologic Oncology*, vol. 36, no. 9, p. 401, 2018.

[24] R. Ganzer, B. Hadaschik, S. Pahernik et al., "Prospective multicenter phase II study on focal therapy (hemiablation) of the prostate with high intensity focused ultrasound," *The Journal of Urology*, vol. 199, no. 4, pp. 983–989, 2018.

[25] M. Dellabella, A. Branchi, M. Di Rosa et al., "Oncological and functional outcome after partial prostate HIFU ablation with focal-one®: a prospective single-center study," *Prostate Cancer and Prostatic Diseases*, vol. 24, no. 4, pp. 1189–1197, 2021.

[26] I. A. Shehata, "Treatment with high intensity focused ultrasound: secrets revealed," *European Journal of Radiology*, vol. 81, no. 3, pp. 534–541, 2012.

[27] F. J. Meng, A. Shan, L. Jin, and C. Y. Young, "The expression of a variant prostate-specific antigen in human prostate," *Cancer Epidemiology, Biomarkers & Prevention*, vol. 11, no. 3, pp. 305–309, 2002.

[28] T. A. Stamey, N. Yang, A. R. Hay, J. E. McNeal, F. S. Freiha, and E. Redwine, "Prostate-specific antigen as a serum marker for adenocarcinoma of the prostate," *New England Journal of Medicine*, vol. 317, no. 15, pp. 909–916, 1987.

[29] B. R. Lee, W. W. Roberts, D. G. Smith et al., "Bioimpedance: novel use of a minimally invasive technique for cancer localization in the intact prostate," *The Prostate*, vol. 39, no. 3, pp. 213–218, 1999.

[30] R. Bass, N. Fleshner, A. Finelli, J. Barkin, L. Zhang, and L. Klotz, "Oncologic and functional outcomes of partial gland ablation with high intensity focused ultrasound for localized prostate cancer," *The Journal of Urology*, vol. 201, no. 1, pp. 113–119, 2019.

11

The Benefits of Using a Small Caliber Ureteroscope in Evaluation and Management of Urethral Stricture

Walid Shahrour,[1] **Pankaj Joshi,**[2] **Craig B. Hunter,**[2] **Vikram S. Batra,**[2] **Hazem Elmansy,**[1] **Sandesh Surana,**[2] **and Sanjay Kulkarni**[2]

[1]*Thunder Bay Regional Health Sciences Center, Northern Ontario School of Medicine, Division of Clinical Sciences, Thunder Bay, Canada*
[2]*Kulkarni Reconstructive Urology Center, Pune, India*

Correspondence should be addressed to Walid Shahrour; walid.shahrour@gmail.com

Academic Editor: Miroslav Djordjevic

Introduction and Objective. The proper evaluation of urethral strictures is an essential part of the surgical planning in urethral reconstruction. The proper evaluation of the stricture can be challenging in certain situations, especially when the meatus is involved. We propose that the use of a small caliber ureteroscope (4.5 Fr and 6.5 Fr) can offer additional help and use for the surgical planning in urethroplasty. *Methods.* We prospectively collected data on 76 patients who underwent urethroplasties in Kulkarni Reconstructive Urology Center, Pune, India and Thunder Bay Regional Health Sciences Center, Thunder Bay, Canada. Patients had retrograde and micturition urethrograms performed preoperatively. The stricture was assessed visually using a 6.5 Fr ureteroscope. If the stricture was smaller than 6.5 Fr, we attempted using the 4.5 Fr ureteroscope. In nonobliterated strictures, we attempted bypassing the stricture making sure not to dilate the stricture. A glide wire would be passed to the bladder under vision. Stricture length, tissue quality, presence of other proximal strictures, false passages, and bladder tumors or stones would be assessed visually. If the penile stricture was near obliterative (smaller than 4.5 Fr caliber), a two-staged procedure is elected to be performed. For proximal bulbar strictures, if the urethral caliber is less than 4.5 Fr and the stricture length is less than 1 cm, we perform a nontransecting anastomotic urethroplasty (NTAU). If the stricture length is >1 cm, we perform a double-face augmented urethroplasty (DFAU). If the urethral caliber is >4.5 Fr and particularly those who are sexually active, ventral inlay with buccal mucosal grafts (BMGs) is performed. In mid to distal bulbar strictures, if the urethral caliber is >4.5 Fr, our procedure of choice is dorsal onlay with BMG. For those with urethral caliber <4.5 Fr and a stricture less than 1 cm, we perform a NTAU. For strictures longer than 1 cm, we perform a DFAU. With the exception of trauma, we very rarely transect the urethra. For panurethral strictures, we almost exclusively perform Kulkarni one-sided dissection. *Results.* Urethroscopy was performed in 76 patients who presented for urethroplasty from July 2014 to September 2014 (in Pune) and between April 2016 and September 2017 (in Thunder Bay). Bypassing the stricture was achieved in 68 patients (89%) while it was unsuccessful in 8 patients (11%). In all unsuccessful urethroscopies, the stricture was near obliterative <4.5 Fr. Our surgical planning changed in (13) 17% of the cases. Out of 43 bulbar strictures, the decision was changed in (9) 21% where we performed 4 DFAU, 3 AAU (augmented anastomotic urethroplasty), and 2 EAU (end anastomotic urethroplasty). In 13 penile strictures, we opted for staged urethroplasty including 3 Johansons and 1 first-stage Asopa in 30.7%. In 20 panurethral urethroplasties, 1 patient (5%) had a urethral stone found in a proximal portion of the bulbar urethra distal to a stricture ring that was removed using an endoscopic grasper. *Conclusion.* The use of the small caliber ureteroscope can help in evaluation of the stricture caliber, length, and tissue quality. The scope can also aid in placing a guide wire, evaluating the posterior urethra, and screening for urethral or bladder stones. It can also improve the preoperative patient counselling and avoid unwanted surprises.

1. Introduction

Urethroplasty with its different techniques has evolved significantly over the last three decades. Many reconstructive urologists perform formal urethrography (retrograde and antegrade) as a part of their surgical planning either preoperatively or perioperatively. Apart from the usual uses of urethroscopy in dilation, direct visual internal urethrotomy, and primary endoscopic realignment in pelvic fracture urethral injury, the use of urethroscopy is important for planning and performance of urethroplasty [1–4].

Historically, the endoscopes used have been rigid scopes of sizes ranging from 17 Fr to 22 Fr. Later, flexible cystoscopes were introduced with sizes ranging between 15 and 17 Fr. The average ureteroscope has a size of 7.5–9 Fr. The development of smaller caliber scopes (6.5 Fr and 4.5 Fr) can be of benefit to the reconstructive surgeon in their assessment of the urethral stricture without dilation or disruption of the stricture. We propose that the use of small caliber ureteroscopes (6 Fr and 4.5 Fr) can offer additional help and use for the surgical planning and technique in urethroplasty.

2. Materials and Methods

We prospectively collected data on 76 patients who underwent urethroplasties in two centers: Kulkarni Reconstructive Urology Center, Pune, India, and Thunder Bay Regional Health Sciences Center, Thunder Bay, Canada. These patients were undergoing various types of urethroplasties for anterior urethral strictures. We excluded patients with posterior urethral stricture. All patients had urethroscopy other than those who were excluded. Patients were consented appropriately and had retrograde urethrogram (RGU) performed preoperatively. Some of the patients had micturition cystourethrogram (MCU) done as well depending on the RGU results, feasibility, and the pathology of the disease. If the RGU was not conclusive, the stricture was obliterated, or the urethra proximal to the stricture was not properly visualized, MCU would be performed. All patients received appropriate preoperative antibiotics.

6.5 Fr ureteroscope is introduced into the meatus. The scope was passed slowly through the urethra till the stricture site. The stricture caliber and length were evaluated under vision. Assessment of the stricture was done visually to differentiate obliterative (no lumen) from near-obliterative (<4.5 Fr) and nonobliterative (>4.5 Fr) stricture. If the 6.5 Fr scope can easily bypass the stricture without dilating it, the 4.5 Fr ureteroscope was not used. If the stricture was smaller than 6.5 Fr, the 4.5 Fr ureteroscope would be used instead. After assessment of the stricture, a glide wire (0.365 mm) would be passed to the bladder under vision. Length, tissue quality, presence of other proximal stricture, false passages, and bladder for tumors or stones would be assessed visually. Occasionally, the wire passes first to guide the passage of the small caliber endoscope. In cases of near obliteration less than 4.5 Fr, the wire would be passed under vision without bypassing the stricture. If the stricture was completely obliterated and the patient had suprapubic catheter, an antegrade cystoscopy was done to evaluate the bladder, bladder neck, and posterior urethra till the verumontanum.

2.1. Management. We usually perform one-stage procedure for all different strictures. Our algorithm is presented in Figure 1. If the urethroscopy findings were different than our initial RGU, we changed our initial operative plan. If the penile stricture was near obliterative (smaller than 4.5 Fr caliber), a two-staged procedure is elected to be performed. For proximal bulbar strictures, if the urethral caliber is less than 4.5 Fr and the stricture length is less than 1 cm, we perform a nontransecting anastomotic urethroplasty (NTAU). If the stricture length is >1 cm, we perform a double-face augmented urethroplasty (DFAU). If the urethral caliber is >4.5 Fr and particularly those who are sexually active, ventral inlay with buccal mucosal grafts (BMGs) is performed. In mid to distal bulbar strictures, if the urethral caliber is >4.5 Fr, our procedure of choice is dorsal onlay with BMG. For those with urethral caliber <4.5 Fr and a stricture less than 1 cm, we perform a NTAU. For strictures longer than 1 cm, we perform a DFAU. With the exception of trauma, we very rarely transect the urethra. For panurethral strictures, we almost exclusively perform Kulkarni one-sided dissection with BMG.

3. Results

Urethroscopy using a small caliber endoscope was performed in 76 patients who were presenting with obstructive urinary symptoms from July 2014 to September 2014 in Pune, India, and between April 2016 and September 2017 in Thunder Bay, Canada. Patient data are presented in Table 1. Mean age was 49 years (range 22–78 years). The assumed etiologies of the strictures were instrumentation 17.1% (13 patients), lichen sclerosis 19.7% (15 patients), catheter-induced 10.5% (8 patients), failed hypospadias 11.8% (9 patients), infectious 2.6% (2 patients), and idiopathic 38.1% (29 patients). Mean stricture length was 6.3 cm (range 2–16). Stricture sites were found to be bulbar urethra in 57% (43 patients), panurethral in 26% (20 patients), and penile in 17% (13 patients). 71% (54 patients) had a previous visual internal urethrotomy with a mean of 1.6 (range 0–5). 26.3% (20 patients) had a previous urethroplasty. 35.5% (27 patients) were on self-dilation and CIC prior to referral. Successful urethroscopy was achieved in 91% (69 patients), while it was unsuccessful in 9% (7 patients). In all the 7 patients who had failed urethroscopy, they had near-obliterative strictures that were smaller than 4.5 Fr. 16 patients (21%) had strictures <6.5 Fr but >4.5 Fr.

Among those with penile strictures, 30.7% (4 patients) the operative procedure was changed from single-stage approach to 2-staged approach. Of those, 3 patients underwent first-stage Johansons and 1 patient had first-stage Asopa.

In bulbar strictures, the decision to go from ventral inlay or dorsal onlay to DFAU, NTAU, and end anastomotic urethroplasty (EAU) was observed in 21% (9 patients; 4 DFAU, 3 NTAU, and 2 EAU). In one patient (5%) with panurethral stricture, a urethral stone was encountered. The stone was found in a proximal portion of the bulbar urethra distal to one of the strictured rings. After the urethra was opened during the urethroplasty, a scope was passed and the stone was removed with a grasper. Out of the 13 patients in whom the decision was changed after urethroscopy, 8 (62%) had a near-obliterative stricture that was less than 4.5 Fr. The other 5 (38%) patients had strictures that were slightly larger than 4.5 Fr.

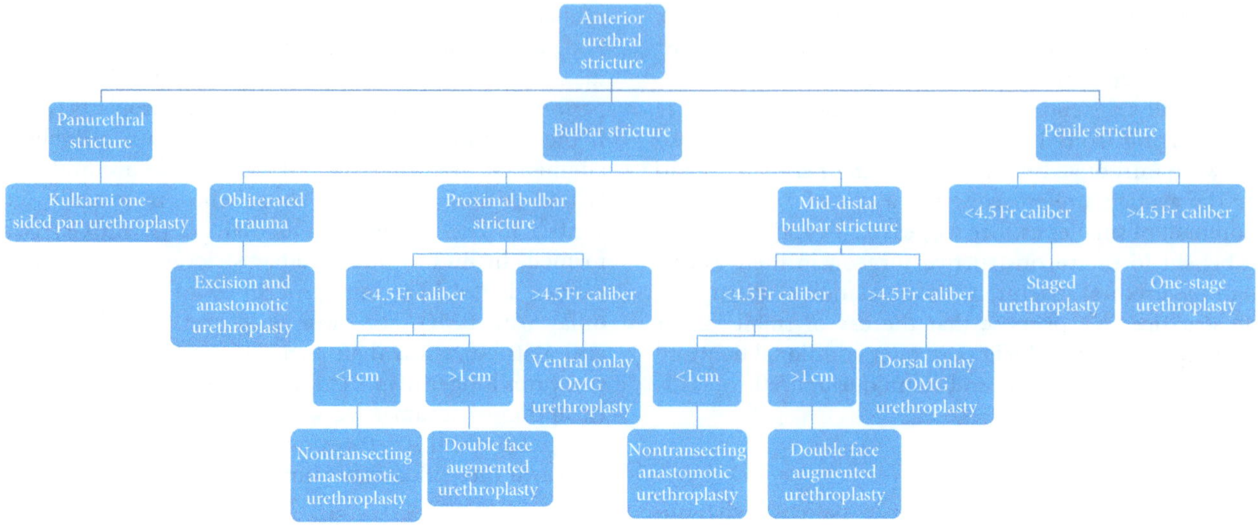

FIGURE 1: Anterior urethral stricture management algorithm (Postpost urethroscopy). BMG: Buccal Mucosal Graft.

TABLE 1: Patient demographics.

Mean age	49 (22–78)
Etiology	
Instrumentation	17% (13)
1. catheter	10.5% (8)
2. lichen scleroses	20% (15)
3. Failed hypospadias	12% (9)
4. infectious	2.5% (2)
5. idiopathic	38% (29)
6. mean stricture length	6.3 cm (1–16)
Stricture location	
1. bulbar	57% (43)
2. penile	17% (13)
3. pan-urethral	26% (20)
Previous direct visual urethrotomy (DVIU)	71% (54)
Mean DVIU	1.6 (0–5)
Previous urethroplasty	26.3% (20)
Patients on self-dilation	35.5% (27)
Decision changed after urethroscopy	17% (13)
Successful urethroplasty	89% (68)
Percentage of near obliterative stricture <4.5 Fr	11% (8)
Percentage of stricture >4.5 Fr and <6.5 Fr	26% (20)

4. Discussion

The choice of the surgical technique of urethroplasty can vary among different reconstructive surgeons. While the evaluation techniques are almost universal, the complete evaluation of the clinical situation can be of crucial importance. The use of retrograde urethrogram has been the cornerstone of the evaluation of stricture disease [2, 5]. The value of the RGU is limited by the experience of the urologist and the radiologists' ability to interpret the results. The RGU usually underestimates the stricture length [5, 6]. Some reports favor sonourethrography for determining the stricture length and extent of spongiofibrosis which can help in operative planning [7–9]. Most reconstructive surgeons would concur with the use of urethroscopy for evaluation of the urethral stricture [1–4, 10]; there is no consensus on size of the scope. The use of a smaller caliber 4.5 Fr ureteroscope can provide several benefits. These benefits include the following:

(1) The proper assessment of the length of the stricture even beyond the distal narrowed ring/strictured areas: the small caliber can navigate easily through a 5–6 Fr narrowed urethra without affecting the stricture or causing an unwanted dilation effect of the larger scopes. Hence, the number of proximal strictures that can be properly assessed would be increased given the smaller caliber endoscopes.

(2) The proper assessment of the posterior urethra, bladder, and bladder neck contracture: as demonstrated by Hosseini et al. [1], the assessment of the posterior urethra and the bladder is very important. Identification of bladder tumour can greatly alter the disposition of the patient. In addition to that, the possible presence of urethral tumors, false passages, or diverticulae proximal to the stricture can be identified visually. These can easily be missed on RGU for either technical or clinical difficulties while performing the study. In our study, we had a patient who had a stone in the proximal portion of his long stricture. If the usual male sound was passed blindly during the procedure to assess proximal patency, this stone might have been pushed into the bladder or into the urethral mucosa creating another stricture in the future.

(3) Passing the ureteroscope beyond the narrowed/strictured areas to pass a guide wire the bladder: when there is a difficulty in passing the guide wire into the bladder, the small caliber scope can help in passing the guide wire under vision. This avoids false passage placement of the wire and increased confidence of proper placement into the bladder.

(4) Reinsertion of displaced Foley catheter in the early postoperative period: the small caliber scope can aid in the passage of a new catheter over a guide wire.

The reinsertion of the catheter can be tricky with the aim not to cause any false passage, disruption of sutures, or damage to the graft by blind insertion of catheter or guide wire.

(5) In cases of patients with combined urethral stricture and benign prostatic hyperplasia: the use of small caliber ureteroscope can help in assessing the prostate and deciding if there is a possible need for prostate surgery prior to urethroplasty.

(6) Scoping the bladder and the posterior urethra is important in cases with complete urethral obliteration, or pelvic fracture urethral injury patients to rule out stones, or tumors, and to assess bladder neck and posterior urethra. While the usual size of the suprapubic catheter is around 14 Fr, the use of a small caliber scope would avoid the need to dilate the suprapubic canal since the flexible cystoscope is around 15-16 Fr.

(7) Resection of postanastomotic polyp: this polyp is an outgrowth of mucosa at the site of anastomosis that could cause future obstruction of the urethra. These polyps can be assessed and resected with a small ureteroscope and laser.

(8) Flexible cystoscopy is not yet available in many developing countries where stricture incidence is higher.

(9) The availability of a small caliber ureteroscope could benefit in the pediatric population as well as the adult population with stricture disease.

(10) The evaluation of the posterior urethra that cannot be properly assessed using the RGU and needs MCU to be assessed: MCU can be painful and difficult to perform on the patient in addition to time consumption in filling the bladder in a retrograde fashion and with increased radiation exposure. Despite repeated attempts at proper MCU, the resulting images are sometimes inadequate.

In the cases where the urethroscopy was successful, there were 16 patients (21%) who had nonobliterative (Figure 2) stricture (>4.5 Fr and <6.5 Fr) that were yet successfully evaluated because of the small caliber of the scope used. While definition of near-obliterative stricture can be loose, we aim to define it as a tight stricture that is less than 4.5 Fr in which we can see a lumen. Having the ability to properly assess the stricture and pass the guide wire safely into the bladder under vision helped in the evaluation and the surgical planning.

In cases of panurethral stricture, the urethroscopy was successful and aided in determining the length of grafts needed. The added information increased the efficiency of the operative time by providing data for the second team harvesting BMG although this has not been addressed in this study.

Urethroscopy was not successful in 8 patients (11%). The strictures were near obliterative in all of them (Figures 3-4), becoming almost like pin point strictures. In those cases, the

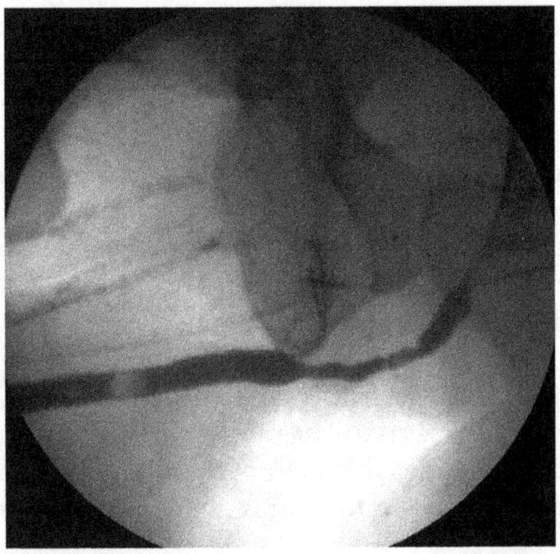

Figure 2: RGU demonstration of a bulbar stricture (>4.5 Fr and <6.5 Fr).

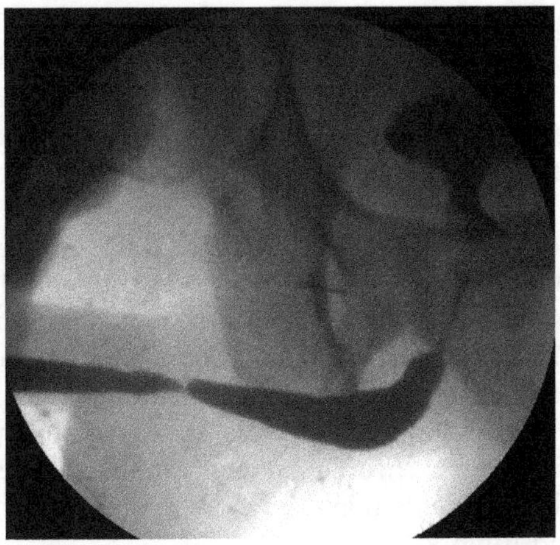

Figure 3: RGU of a peno-bulbar stricture that is nearly obliterative <4.5 Fr.

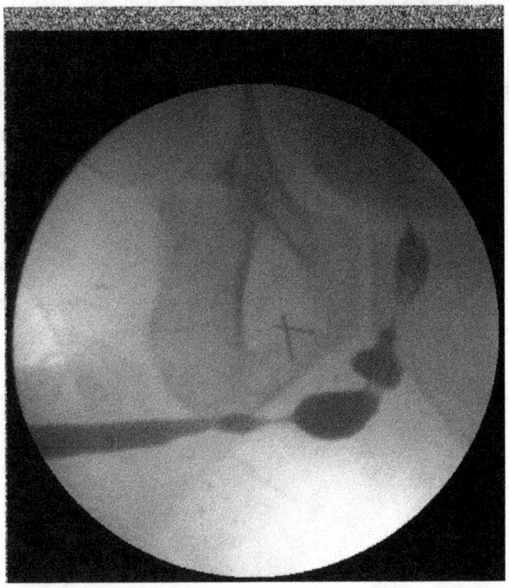

Figure 4: RGU of a peno-bulbar stricture that is nearly obliterative <4.5 Fr.

guide wire was passed through the pin point stricture under vision but the urethra proximal to that stricture was not assessed. After the urethra was opened, the scope was passed proximally into the bladder. The change in the planned procedure was decided after the assessment of the stricture type, length, caliber, and quality of the urethra proximally and distally. Initially, the procedure was planned based on the findings on the RGU and MCU. We observed a change in the planned procedure in 13 patients (17%) after the urethroscopy. We consider this to be significant yet the impact can vary depending on the surgical technique and the algorithm used for surgical planning. We did not perform a statistical analysis as this was not the aim of our study. This would be addressed in the future with another prospective study.

RGU has limitations. An RGU for nearly obliterated urethral stricture will underestimate the caliber of the urethra proximal to the nearly obliterated portion. A proximal narrow urethra on RGU can either be secondary to a tight distal ring or a long strip of narrow urethra. Using the small caliber endoscope would allow the surgeon to go through the stricture and formulate the surgical plan. It is also not always possible to perform a voiding urethrogram in those very tight strictures unless they have a suprapubic catheter.

26% of the cases had a urethra that is smaller than 6.5 Fr that required the use of a 4.5 Fr scope. Putting the glide wire under vision in the 8 patients (11%) who had a stricture less than 4.5 Fr was important. Blind guide wire insertion might lead to false passages and worsening spongiofibrosis.

Patient population of urethral strictures might suffer from urine stasis, chronic catheterization, and retention. Hence, these patients might be at increased risk of bladder stones and tumors.

The possible criticism of urethroscopy in general is that it might cause dilation. This would be negated with the use of a very small caliber as the one we used in this study. Other possible criticisms would be the increased operative time from that extrastep. In our opinion, these extrafew minutes spent for the proper evaluation would be compensated with the proper evaluation and decision-making. The time can also be saved by deciding to harvest the graft early on or going for EAU as compared to waiting till the urethra is formally opened and the stricture is evaluated. The cost factor should always be considered. Given that the scope is always an added value to the armamentarium of reconstructive surgeons, this should not be a limiting factor.

Depending on the urology clinic setup, urethroscopy could be performed preoperatively. This would help in counselling and involving the patient in the decision-making process.

5. Conclusion

The use of a small caliber ureteroscope in the operative setting of urethroplasty can add value to the initial evaluation. It can also help in properly evaluating the stricture, planning the surgery appropriately, and avoiding unwanted surprises during the surgery without damaging the urethra.

References

[1] S. J. Hosseini, A. Kaviani, M. Jabbari, M. M. Hosseini, A. Haji-Mohammadmehdi-Arbab, and N. R. Simaei, "Diagnostic application of flexible cystoscope in pelvic fracture urethral distraction defects," *Urology Journal*, vol. 3, no. 4, pp. 204–207, 2006.

[2] K. Rourke and K. Rourke, "Imaging of urethra stricture disease," *Translational Andrology and Urology*, vol. 4, no. 1, pp. 2–9, 2015.

[3] S. K. Goonesinghe, C. J. Hillary, T. R. Nicholson, N. I. Osman, and C. R. Chapple, "Flexible cystourethroscopy in the follow-up of posturethroplasty patients and characterisation of recurrences," *European Urology*, vol. 68, no. 3, pp. 523–529, 2015.

[4] M. L. Gallentine and A. F. Morey, "Imaging of the male urethra for stricture disease," *Urologic Clinics of North America*, vol. 29, no. 2, pp. 361–372, 2002.

[5] A. F. Morey and J. W. McAninch, "Role of preoperative sonourethrography in bulbar urethral reconstruction," *Journal of Urology*, vol. 158, no. 4, pp. 1376–1379, 1997.

[6] S. Gupta, B. Majumdar, A. Tiwari, R. K. Gupta, A. Kumar, and R. B. Gujral, "Sonourethrography in the evaluation of anterior urethral strictures: correlation with radiographic urethrography," *Journal of Clinical Ultrasound*, vol. 21, no. 4, pp. 231–239, 1993.

[7] A. F. Morey and J. W. McAninch, "Ultrasound evaluation of the male urethra for assessment of urethral stricture," *Journal of Clinical Ultrasound*, vol. 24, no. 8, pp. 473–479, 1996.

[8] J. W. McAninch, F. C. Laing, and R. B. Jeffrey Jr., "Sonourethrography in the evaluation of urethral strictures: a preliminary report," *Journal of Urology*, vol. 139, no. 2, pp. 294–297, 1988.

[9] S. Choudhary, P. Singh, E. Sundar, S. Kumar, and A. Sahai, "A comparison of sonourethrography and retrograde urethrography in evaluation of anterior urethral strictures," *Clinical Radiology*, vol. 59, no. 8, pp. 736–742, 2004.

[10] T. L. C. Kuo, S. Venugopal, R. D. Inman, and C. R. Chapple, "Surgical tips and tricks during urethroplasty for bulbar urethral strictures focusing on accurate localisation of the stricture: results from a tertiary centre," *European Urology*, vol. 67, no. 4, pp. 764–770, 2015.

12

Dual-Tracer Positron-Emission Tomography Using Prostate-Specific Membrane Antigen and Fluorodeoxyglucose for Staging of Prostate Cancer

Stephen McGeorge,[1,2,3] Michael Kwok,[2,3] Andrew Jiang,[3] Louise Emmett,[4,5] David A. Pattison,[3,6] Paul A. Thomas,[3,6] John W. Yaxley,[1,3,7] and Matthew J. Roberts[1,2,3,8]

[1]*Department of Urology, Royal Brisbane and Women's Hospital, Butterfield St, Herston 4029, Queensland, Australia*
[2]*Department of Urology, Redcliffe Hospital, Anzac Avenue, Redcliffe 4020, Queensland, Australia*
[3]*Faculty of Medicine, The University of Queensland, Herston 4006, Queensland, Australia*
[4]*Department of Theranostics and Nuclear Medicine, St. Vincent's Hospital Sydney, 390 Victoria St, Darlinghurst 2010, New South Wales, Australia*
[5]*Garvan Institute of Medical Research, 384 Victoria St, Darlinghurst 2010, New South Wales, Australia*
[6]*Department of Nuclear Medicine & Specialised PET Services, Royal Brisbane and Women's Hospital, Butterfield St, Herston 4029, Queensland, Australia*
[7]*Wesley Urology Clinic, Wesley Hospital, 451 Coronation Dr, Auchenflower 4066, Queensland, Australia*
[8]*University of Queensland Centre for Clinical Research, Faculty of Medicine, Building 71/918 RBWH, Butterfield St, Herston 4029, Queensland, Australia*

Correspondence should be addressed to Matthew J. Roberts; m.roberts2@uq.edu.au

Academic Editor: Mohammad H. Ather

PSMA PET is more accurate than conventional imaging (CT/bone scan) for staging of intermediate- or high-risk prostate cancer (PCa), but 5–10% of primary tumours have low PSMA ligand uptake. FDG PET has been used to further define disease extent in end-stage castrate-resistant PCa and may be beneficial earlier in the disease course for more accurate staging. The objective of this study was to review the available evidence for patients undergoing both FDG and PSMA PET for PCa staging at initial diagnosis and in recurrent disease. A systematic literature review was performed for studies with direct, intraindividual comparison of PSMA and FDG PET for staging of PCa. Assessment for radioligand therapy eligibility was not considered. Risk of bias was assessed. 543 citations were screened and assessed. 13 case reports, three retrospective studies, and one prospective study were included. FDG after PSMA PET improved the detection of metastases from 65% to 73% in high-risk early castration-resistant PCa with negative conventional imaging (M0). Positive FDG PET was found in 17% of men with negative PSMA PET for postprostatectomy biochemical recurrence. Gleason score ≥8 and higher PSA levels predicted FDG-avid metastases in BCR and primary staging. Variant histology (ductal and neuroendocrine) was common in case reports, resulting in PSMA-negative FDG-positive imaging for 3 patients. Dual-tracer PET for PCa may assist in characterising high-risk disease during primary staging and restaging. Further studies are required to determine the additive benefit of FDG PET and if the FDG-positive phenotype may indicate a poorer prognosis.

1. Introduction

Prostate cancer (PCa) is the most commonly diagnosed internal malignancy and high-ranking cause of mortality in men worldwide [1, 2]. An increased incidence of *de novo* metastatic PCa has been observed since 2004, most significantly in men aged 55 to 69 years, potentially contributing to higher mortality [3, 4]. Modern approaches to metastatic PCa treatment incorporate aggressive systemic therapy, such as taxane-based chemotherapy, androgen receptor inhibitors, and radioligand therapy (RLT) [5, 6]. Additionally, earlier use of systemic therapy prior to treatment of high-risk, locally advanced disease has been reported and is the subject of ongoing clinical trials [7–10]. However, accurate patient selection for systemic therapy remains one of the key challenges in urologic oncology.

Despite limitations, conventional imaging with computed tomography (CT) and technetium-based bone scan are widely used for staging [11]. However, cumulative evidence indicates that prostate-specific membrane antigen (PSMA) positron-emission tomography (PET) should be a centrepiece of staging for intermediate- to high-risk patients [11–16]. A prospective, randomised trial by Hofman and colleagues determined that PSMA PET/CT was 27% (95% CI: 23–31) more accurate than conventional imaging [12]. However, 5–10% of primary PCa tumours have low PSMA activity which evade detection by PSMA PET, mostly in high-grade and variant tumour types [14–18].

18-F-Fluorodeoxyglucose (FDG) PET use in PCa has previously been of limited benefit in primary staging and biochemical recurrence (BCR) [19, 20]. In a study of 41 men with Gleason score ≥8 PCa who had FDG PET/CT for primary staging, 11 men had nodal metastasis from histopathology, and only 3 of these men (27%) had corresponding lymph node FDG uptake [21]. Increasing use of FDG PET to aid patient selection for RLT and other therapies in mCRPCa has provided insight into tumour heterogeneity and benefits of dual-tracer PET imaging [22, 23]. Discordant findings have been attributed to the increased anaerobic glycolysis detected by FDG PET in patients with more aggressive histological types [24]. Whilst the use of PSMA and FDG PET imaging in PCa has been examined individually, the potential diagnostic impact for individual patients to undergo dual-tracer PET imaging remains unclear. Additional use of FDG PET may improve disease characterisation in patients with high-risk localised and metastatic PCa, with inconclusive conventional imaging and negative PSMA PET.

We sought to summarise the available evidence for the use of dual-tracer PET, being 18-F-fluorodeoxyglucose (FDG) PET in addition to PSMA PET, for PCa staging at initial diagnosis and in recurrent disease.

2. Methods

2.1. Search Strategy. A systematic literature search was performed in April 2021 (Table S1) in accordance with the preferred reporting items for systematic reviews and meta-analysis (PRISMA) and the Cochrane Handbook guidelines [25, 26]. The review protocol was registered (CRD42020201307) and published in the International Prospective Register of Systematic Reviews (PROSPERO). Citation searches were conducted from included reports to ensure all relevant studies were captured. All included studies received ethical approval, and the source data were publicly available, so ethical approval was not sought [27].

2.2. Study Selection. All original research reports that directly compared PSMA and FDG PET in the setting of histologically diagnosed or clinically suspected PCa were considered. Editorials, review articles, and animal studies were excluded, as were studies comparing PSMA and FDG PET for the purpose of RLT, as this topic was felt to be beyond the scope of the current review. Furthermore, records were excluded if they assessed other primary malignancies or active systemic disease accounting for tracer uptake, PCa was not specifically diagnosed, or they compared alternative tracers that were not FDG or PSMA.

2.3. Quality Assessment. Methodological quality was appraised using checklists recommended by the Cochrane Guidelines [28, 29]. Each article was assessed for bias by two independent authors, with a third reviewer used to resolve disagreements (Tables S2 and S3).

2.4. Data Management. The data from case reports included, where available, patient age, PSA at the time of imaging, indication for dual-tracer use, sites of metastatic lesions, ligand uptake patterns for FDG and PSMA, previous PCa treatments, histological PCa type, and Gleason score. Cases were considered to be positive if ligand uptake (according to criteria used in each case) was reported in either the prostate or at sites of metastatic disease. Discordant ligand uptake was reported when both FDG and PSMA PET were positive, but there were different sites of the disease. If multiple PSA values were reported, the PSA at the time of PET imaging was used for this comparison. For articles concerning a population, these data were collected as a range, where applicable, as well as the inclusion and exclusion criteria.

Included studies displayed significant heterogeneity and small overall population, so a quantitative assessment was not possible (Table S4).

3. Results

The database search yielded 543 citations. Following screening and assessment (Figure 1), one single-arm prospective trial, three retrospective observational studies, and 13 case reports were included in the final analysis (Tables 1 and 2).

3.1. Castration-Resistant Disease. A prospective single-arm trial investigated the prevalence of PSMA-negative FDG-positive lesions in 37 men with negative conventional imaging (M0) in the setting of high-risk early castration resistance (defined as PSA progression with PSA ≤2 ng/ml and PSA doubling time ≤10 months) who were restaged using PSMA and then FDG PET [33]. 65% of men had metastatic disease on initial PSMA PET, while an additional 5% had localised PSMA avidity within the prostate, which was concordant with FDG PET. Among 30% of men with no PSMA avidity, 27% (8% overall) showed metastatic disease according to FDG PET, increasing the detection of metastases from 65% to 73%.

High-grade disease, defined as Gleason grade group of four or higher, correlated with nodal or distant metastases on FDG PET (OR = 13.09, $p = 0.02$). A PSA doubling time less

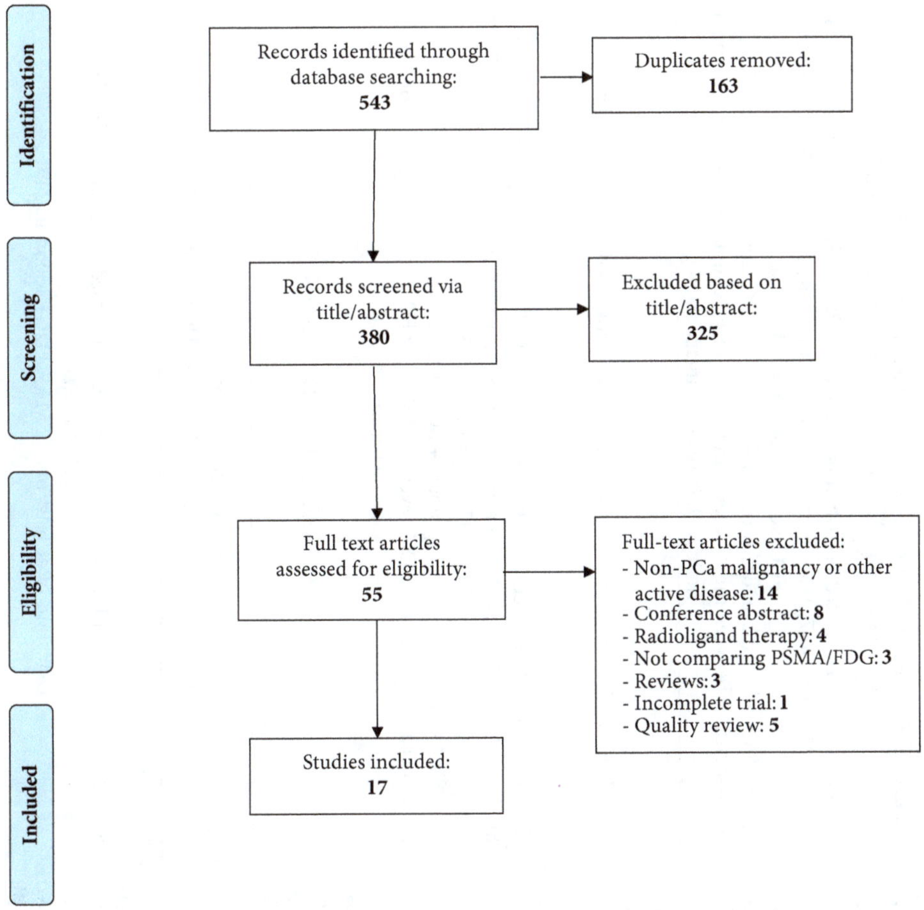

FIGURE 1: PRISMA 2009 flow diagram.

than six months was associated with the presence of PSMA-positive metastatic disease (OR = 8.00, $p = 0.009$), but not for FDG-positive metastases ($p = 0.29$). Discordant lesions (PSMA-negative FDG-positive) were more common for axial bone lesions compared to concordant PSMA-FDG-positive patients ($p = 0.02$). Metastatic disease burden was according to CHAARTED criteria and was unchanged in the use of FDG PET [47]. However, use of FDG PET was estimated to enable an additional six men (19 in total) precise lesion targeting for oligometastatic-directed therapy according to SABR-COMET trial criteria [48].

Within the same manuscript, an additional analysis of a retrospective cohort of 41 men was reported. The cohort included 14 men with BCR, 18 men with hormone-sensitive PCa (HSPCa), and 9 men with mCRPCa. Metastatic disease according to PSMA PET was detected in 29%, 39%, and 100% of men (with FDG concordant disease for 100%, 86%, and 67%) with BCR, HSPCa, and mCRPCa, respectively. PSMA-negative FDG-positive disease was rare in HSPCa (6%) and more commonly observed for CRPCa (33%).

3.2. Biochemically Recurrent Hormone-Sensitive Disease. Predictive factors for FDG-positive PET in men with BCR (PSA >0.2 ng/ml) after radical prostatectomy and a negative PSMA PET were determined in a retrospective case-control study ($n = 72$) [32]. The median PSA was 3.4 ng/ml, and 53% had prior adjuvant therapy. FDG PET was positive in 17% of men, where serum PSA (16.7 versus 0.8 ng/ml) and Gleason scores (34.4% with Gleason score ≥8 vs. 2.5% with Gleason score <8; $p < 0.001$) were higher than the FDG-negative group. There were no differences in age, PSA doubling time, interval between PSMA and FDG PET, or adjuvant therapies. A PSA cutoff of 2.3 ng/ml was 91.7% accurate for FDG PET positivity (area under the curve of 0.872, $p < 0.001$). The group was divided into three groups for the prediction of positive FDG in the setting of negative PSMA, being low potential (PSA <2.3 ng/ml and Gleason score <8), moderate potential (PSA ≥2.3 ng/ml or Gleason score ≥8, but not both), and high potential (PSA ≥2.3 ng/ml and Gleason score ≥8). These groups showed 0% (36/36), 11.5% (3/26), and 90% (9/10) positive FDG PET results, respectively.

A retrospective evaluation of 138 men who underwent ^{68}Ga-PSMA-11 and FDG PET for differentiating lymph node metastases from peripheral ganglia was examined for oncological outcomes [31]. Imaging was for primary staging in 47% ($n = 65$) and BCR in 53% ($n = 73$). 47% of men had Gleason ≥8 disease, and mean PSA was 56.4 ng/mL (IQR: 18.5–99.7) and 1.1 ng/mL (IQR: 0.4–4.1) in the primary staging and BCR cohorts, respectively. 42% of patients demonstrated PSMA-avid lymph node metastases, totalling 83 metastases, with FDG concordance in 63% ($n = 52$).

Table 1: Summary of included cohort studies, comprising prospective trials and retrospective analyses, across the spectrum of prostate cancer (PCa) including primary staging, biochemical recurrence (BCR), hormone-sensitive PCa (HSPCa), and castrate-resistant PCa (CRPCa).

Category	*N*	Study	*N*	Criteria	Characteristics	Findings
Primary staging	86	Zhou et al. [30]	21	(i) No prior treatment	Median PSA: 41.2 ng/mL 53% ISUP ≥4	PSMA PET/CT identified more bone (50 vs. 32) and lymph node (25 vs. 22) metastases, with less benign lesions (21% vs. 49%) than FDG PET
		Shi et al. [31]	65	(i) No treatment between PSMA and FDG PET/CT (ii) <2 weeks of interval in imaging	Median PSA: 56.4 ng/ml	PSMA/FDG PET detected N+ when both are avid (PSMA SUV_{max} >2.05 and FDG SUV_{max} >4.1; $n = 43/47$, 92%) compared to low or no avidity (PSMA SUV_{max} <2.05 and FDG SUV_{max} <4.1; $n = 3/334$, 1%) 83 PSMA-avid lymph nodes (primary + BCR) with FDG uptake in 53% ($n = 52/83$) No association between the PSA level and PSMA or FDG uptake in ganglia or lymph node metastases in primary staging
BCR	159	Chen et al. [32]	72	(i) PSA >0.2 ng/ml after RP (ii) Not on androgen deprivation (iii) N0M0 on Ga68 PSMA PET/CT	Median PSA: 0.5 ng/mL 44% ISUP ≥4 38% prior adjuvant ADT	FDG-avid disease found in 17% of patients with negative PSMA PET/CT
		Shi et al. [31]	73	(i) No treatment between PSMA and FDG PET/CT (ii) <2 weeks of interval in imaging	Median PSA: 1.1 ng/mL	PSMA/FDG PET detected N+ when both are avid (PSMA SUV_{max} >2.05 and FDG SUV_{max} >4.1; $n = 43/47$, 92%) compared to low or no avidity (PSMA SUV_{max} <2.05 and FDG SUV_{max} <4.1; $n = 3/334$, 1%) 83 PSMA-avid lymph nodes (primary + BCR) with FDG uptake in 53% ($n = 52/83$) No association between the PSA level and PSMA or FDG uptake in ganglia or lymph node metastases in BCR
		Wang et al. [33] (retrospective)	14	(i) Not defined	Median PSA: 0.35 ng/mL 50% ISUP ≥4 100% after RP	0% with PSMA− FDG+ lesions
HSPCa	18	Wang et al. [33] (retrospective)	18	(i) Not defined	Median PSA: 14.5 ng/mL 33% on ADT	29% of patients N+/M+ on PSMA PET/CT Detection of at least one PSMA− FDG+ lesion in 6%
CRPCa	46	Wang et al. [33] (trial group)	37	(i) Rising PSA ≤2 ng/ml (ii) Testosterone <50 ng/dL (iii) PSA doubling time ≤10 months (iv) N0M0 on CT and bone scan	Median PSA: 0.57 ng/mL 73% ISUP ≥4 100% after RP 19% postop EBRT	Subsequent addition of FDG after PSMA PET/CT increased detection of N+/M+ from 65% to 73% Detection of at least one PSMA− FDG+ lesion in 24%
		Wang et al. [33] (retrospective)	9	(i) Not defined	Median PSA: 2.26 ng/mL 89% ISUP ≥4	Detection of at least one PSMA− FDG+ lesion in 33%

TABLE 2: Summary of case report data, considering use at different stages of prostate cancer (PCa) including primary staging, recurrent disease, and castrate-resistant PCa.

Ref.	Reason for dual-tracer PET	Avidity pattern	Metastatic/localised	Histology	PSMA+ lesions	FDG+ lesions	PSA	Gleason score
A-primary staging								
[34]	Staging for ductal variant	PSMA+ FDG+ discordant	L	Ductal	Prostate, mild bilaterally	Prostate, extensively in the left lobe	0.2	4 + 5 = 9
[35]	Synchronous rectal cancer and PCa	PSMA+ FDG+ discordant	L	Adenocarcinoma	Prostate	Rectum, presacral lymph node	37	Not documented
[36]	High-grade histology, low PSMA avidity of the prostate, equivocal staging	PSMA+ FDG+ discordant	M	Adenocarcinoma	Pelvic lymph nodes, T8 vertebrae	Prostate, pelvic lymph nodes, T8 vertebrae, right acetabulum	16.3	5 + 5 = 10
[37]	Infection vs. locally advanced disease in frail elderly patient	PSMA+ FDG−	M	Neuroendocrine (presumed)	Prostate, bladder	None	49	No histology
[38]	Staging for neuroendocrine PCa	PSMA− FDG+	M	Neuroendocrine	None	Prostate, bladder, rectum, lymph nodes, bone	163	5 + 4 = 9
B-restaging of the recurrent disease								
[34]	BCR in ductal variant with lung nodules	PSMA− FDG+	M	Ductal	None	Lung	5.9	4 + 5 = 9
[39]	BCR with lung nodules	PSMA− FDG+	M	Ductal	None	Lung	0.59	Not documented
[40]	Neuroendocrine transformation	PSMA+ FDG+ discordant	M	Neuroendocrine	Bone	Bone, left pelvic soft tissue, penis	8	4 + 3 = 7
[41]	BCR with lung nodules	PSMA+ FDG+ discordant	M	Adenocarcinoma	Two lung nodules	One lung nodule	0.275	Not documented
[42]	BCR with lung nodules	PSMA+ FDG+ discordant	M	Adenocarcinoma Sarcomatoid metastasis	Pelvic lymph node, lung	Lung	4.63	4 + 4 = 8
[43]	BCR with lung nodules	PSMA+ FDG−	M	Adenocarcinoma Mucinous metastasis	Lung	None	0.2	4 + 3 = 7
[44]	BCR with negative FDG PET	PSMA+ FDG−	M	Adenocarcinoma	Mediastinal lymph nodes	None	7.1	4 + 4 = 8
C-castrate-resistant prostate cancer								
[45]	Onset of castration resistance with unclear FDG PET	PSMA+ FDG+ discordant	M	Not documented	Prostate, bone, pelvic lymph nodes	Prostate, mild bone avidity	10	Not documented
[46]	Onset of castration resistance with adrenal mass	PSMA+ FDG+ concordant	M	Adenocarcinoma	Right adrenal mass	Right adrenal mass	1.9	4 + 5 = 9

Significantly less ganglia showed FDG uptake ($p < 0.001$), so the PSMA/FDG PET combination was shown to detect lymph node metastases when both were avid (PSMA SUV_{max} >2.05 and FDG SUV_{max} >4.1; 43/47, 92%) compared to low or no avidity (PSMA SUV_{max} <2.05 and FDG SUV_{max} <4.1; 3/334, 1%). No correlation was found for PSMA or FDG uptake (according to SUV_{max}) with Gleason scores or PSA level (binary grouping, not defined, $p > 0.05$) in both primary staging and BCR cohorts.

3.3. Primary Staging. Staging with dual-tracer PSMA/FDG PET/CT prior to treatment was examined in one retrospective study of 21 men [30]. 68.7% ($n = 11/16$) of men had Gleason scores ≥8, and median PSA at diagnosis was 41.2 ng/mL (range: 5–200). All patients had ^{18}F-PSMA-1007 uptake within the prostate; however, 66.7% had local FDG uptake. PSMA PET/CT identified more bone (50 vs. 32) and lymph node (25 vs. 22) metastases, with less benign lesions (21% vs. 49%) than FDG PET. Most patients with metastases on FDG PET had Gleason scores ≥8. SUV_{max} (median: 10.72 vs. 4.42), SUV_{mean} (median: 6.67 vs. 2.59), and tumour-to-background ratio (13.3 vs. 7.91) of identified metastases were all higher for ^{18}F-PSMA-1007 than FDG PET ($p < 0.001$).

3.4. Case Reports. Case report data are summarised in Table 2 (Ref. A–C) according to indication for dual-tracer use with subgrouping according to the ligand uptake pattern. The most common indication was for men with BCR requiring characterisation of lung nodules seen on conventional imaging (5/14 patients) [34, 39, 41–43]. Variant histology was also common, with three cases of ductal variant and three cases of neuroendocrine differentiation, although one of these was presumed on the basis of a raised serum chromogranin A level in combination with DOTATOC PET avidity [34, 37–40].

PSMA and FDG ligand uptake patterns were discordant in the majority of cases, although this was not consistently reported for each individual lesion in every patient (Table 2). Three cases reported a negative PSMA PET with positive FDG PET, all of which had either ductal or neuroendocrine histology. Serum PSA levels were highly variable for all patterns of ligand uptake according to the tracer, being 0.2–37 ng/ml for discordant PSMA-positive FDG-positive, 0.2–49 ng/ml for PSMA-positive FDG-negative, and 0.59–163 ng/ml in PSMA-negative FDG-positive.

4. Discussion

The role of dual-tracer PET for localised or recurrent PCa is unclear, and available data are limited. Despite significant heterogeneity in patient populations, indications, and performance which limit meta-analysis, discordant imaging and altered staging classification were observed. Imaging discordance was more likely to be observed in more advanced disease, presumably due to greater tumour clone heterogeneity.

An important application of dual-tracer PET/CT may be in the identification of additional sites of disease amenable to oligometastatic directed therapy. In the early castrate-resistant population discussed by Wang et al., 24% of patients had at least one PSMA− FDG+ lesion which would have been otherwise missed [33]. The SABR-COMET trial found an overall survival benefit with stereotactic ablative radiotherapy, and results from the ORIOLE trial showed that the total consolidation of all PSMA-avid diseases gave significant progression-free survival and distant metastasis-free survival advantages [48, 49]. Therefore, dual PSMA/FDG PET/CT may improve oncological outcomes by identifying additional sites of the disease amenable to oligometastatic directed therapy.

Furthermore, the PSMA-negative FDG-positive phenotype may represent a population at a greater risk of rapid disease progression. These poor oncological outcomes have been reported in the context of RLT, with Suman and colleagues reporting that, among 40 patients who underwent ^{177}Lu-PSMA-617 RLT, high FDG uptake (SUV_{max} >15) was reported to correlate with worse 12-month progression-free survival (PFS; $p = 0.05$) and poor response to RLT (disease progression in 12/15 patients) [50]. Furthermore, a study of 16 men with poor PSMA avidity or significantly discordant FDG avidity ineligible for ^{177}Lu-PSMA-617 RLT reported a median overall survival of 2.3 months when FDG avidity was high [51]. While PSMA-negative imaging may suggest aggressive disease, a lower ratio of PSMA SUV_{max} to FDG SUV_{max} may better predict PSA reduction ≥30% following RLT ($p < 0.02$) [23]. However, FDG findings alone were not predictive of response, and no imaging factors correlated with PSA response ≥50%. Conversely, 59% of men with low FDG uptake (SUV_{max} <15) reported improved or stable disease with RLT in one study, while absent PSMA and FDG avidity following RLT was indicative of favourable treatment response [50].

We observed low PSMA avidity in FDG-positive disease to be a common finding among papers included in this review. Low PSMA avidity in advanced PCa is hypothesised to be due to dedifferentiation or neuroendocrine transformation. Biomarker-focused research supports this hypothesis, with a retrospective analysis in 66 patients referred for RLT, of which 41 patients (62%) had at least one PSMA-negative FDG-positive lesion and demonstrated higher levels of neuron-specific enolase, a neuroendocrine marker [52]. Furthermore, neuroendocrine PCa has a more aggressive course and thereby an expectation of increased anaerobic glycolysis with consequent FDG avidity [24]. This is in keeping with existing evidence on divergent clonal evolution of CRPCa and the "genomic overlap" between conventional adenocarcinoma and neuroendocrine PCa in the development of castration resistance [53]. There is also support in the correlation between levels of glucose uptake-associated genes with neuroendocrine gene signatures and low PSMA expression [54]. Given the poor prognosis in these patients, further research on dual-tracer PET may help streamline earlier diagnosis of this PCa phenotype and thereby prompt earlier escalation to more aggressive treatment to improve oncological outcomes.

PSMA PET has been shown to be superior to conventional imaging for the initial staging of intermediate- and high-risk PCa [12]. However, approximately 5–10% of primary PCa has insufficient PSMA avidity for PET detection due to contributions of both low- (usually of lower volume) and high-grade disease [14]. In the latter population, the available data suggest that FDG may detect primary and metastatic disease that would otherwise not be observed on PSMA PET or conventional imaging. Thus, the potential for FDG PET use in the primary staging of high-grade PCa, especially with neuroendocrine or ductal variation, may be an early independent identifier of aggressive disease and poorer oncological outcomes with conventional therapies.

The limitations of this review include limited available studies and details of data included in these studies, including their mostly retrospective nature and limited coverage of each disease state. Furthermore, we were unable to adjust for selection and publication bias in the included studies. Conversely, to our knowledge, this review represents the first summary of the available literature of the intra-individual assessment of PSMA and FDG PET.

In conclusion, the diagnostic utility of dual-tracer FDG/PSMA PET/CT for PCa may assist in characterising high-risk disease during primary staging and restaging. Addition of FDG PET can identify additional sites of the disease amenable to oligometastatic directed therapy. Patients with FDG-positive disease in advanced PCa states have a poor prognosis, especially with concurrently negative PSMA PET. When applied to high-risk (high-grade or variant histology), hormone-sensitive disease in the localised or recurrent stage, detection of the FDG-positive phenotype may signal a poorer prognosis to prompt more aggressive intervention earlier in the disease course. Further studies are required to validate the prognostic insights outlined here and selective incorporation into therapeutic clinical trials.

Acknowledgments

MJR was supported by a Clinician Research Fellowship from the Metro North Office of Research, Queensland Health, and a Doctor in Training Research Scholarship from Avant Mutual Group Pty Ltd.

References

[1] C. H. Pernar, E. M. Ebot, K. M. Wilson, and L. A. Mucci, "The epidemiology of prostate cancer," *Cold Spring Harbor Perspectives in Medicine*, vol. 8, no. 12, 2018.

[2] Global Burden of Disease Cancer Collaboration, C. Fitzmaurice, C. Allen et al., "Global, regional, and national cancer incidence, mortality, years of life lost, years lived with disability, and disability-adjusted life-years for 32 cancer groups, 1990 to 2015: a systematic analysis for the global burden of disease study," *JAMA Oncology*, vol. 3, no. 4, pp. 524–548, 2017.

[3] S. Smith and P. Wolanski, "Metastatic prostate cancer incidence in Australia after amendment to prostate-specific antigen screening guidelines," *ANZ Journal of Surgery*, vol. 88, no. 7-8, pp. E589–E593, 2018.

[4] A. B. Weiner, R. S. Matulewicz, S. E. Eggener, and E. M. Schaeffer, "Increasing incidence of metastatic prostate cancer in the United States (2004–2013)," *Prostate Cancer and Prostatic Diseases*, vol. 19, no. 4, pp. 395–397, 2016.

[5] M. Perera, M. J. Roberts, L. Klotz et al., "Intermittent versus continuous androgen deprivation therapy for advanced prostate cancer," *Nature Reviews Urology*, vol. 17, no. 8, pp. 469–481, 2020.

[6] P. Cornford, R. C. N. Van den Bergh, E. Briers et al., "EAU-EANM-ESTRO-ESUR-SIOG guidelines on prostate cancer. Part II-2020 update: treatment of relapsing and metastatic prostate cancer," *European Urology*, vol. 79, no. 2, pp. 263–282, 2021.

[7] J. A. Eastham, G. Heller, S. Halabi et al., "Cancer and leukemia group B 90203 (alliance): radical prostatectomy with or without neoadjuvant chemohormonal therapy in localized, high-risk prostate cancer," *Journal of Clinical Oncology*, vol. 38, no. 26, pp. 3042–3050, 2020.

[8] B. Montgomery, M. S. Tretiakova, A. M. Joshua et al., "Neoadjuvant enzalutamide prior to prostatectomy," *Clinical Cancer Research*, vol. 23, no. 9, pp. 2169–2176, 2017.

[9] T. R. McClintock, N. Von Landenberg, A. P. Cole et al., "Neoadjuvant androgen deprivation therapy prior to radical prostatectomy: recent trends in utilization and association with postoperative surgical margin status," *Annals of Surgical Oncology*, vol. 26, no. 1, pp. 297–305, 2019.

[10] N. Dhiantravan, J. Violet, R. Eapen et al., "Clinical trial protocol for LuTectomy: a single-arm study of the dosimetry, safety, and potential benefit of (177)Lu-PSMA-617 prior to prostatectomy," *European Urology Focus*, vol. 7, no. 2, pp. 234–237, 2021.

[11] M. S. Litwin and H.-J. Tan, "The diagnosis and treatment of prostate cancer," *Journal of the American Medical Association*, vol. 317, no. 24, pp. 2532–2542, 2017.

[12] M. S. Hofman, N. Lawrentschuk, R. J. Francis et al., "Prostate-specific membrane antigen PET-CT in patients with high-risk prostate cancer before curative-intent surgery or radiotherapy (proPSMA): a prospective, randomised, multicentre study," *The Lancet*, vol. 395, no. 10231, pp. 1208–1216, 2020.

[13] P. Donato, M. J. Roberts, A. Morton et al., "Improved specificity with 68Ga PSMA PET/CT to detect clinically significant lesions "invisible" on multiparametric MRI of the prostate: a single institution comparative analysis with radical prostatectomy histology," *European Journal of Nuclear Medicine and Molecular Imaging*, vol. 46, no. 1, pp. 20–30, 2019.

[14] T. Maurer, M. Eiber, M. Schwaiger, and J. E. Gschwend, "Current use of PSMA-PET in prostate cancer management," *Nature Reviews Urology*, vol. 13, no. 4, pp. 226–235, 2016.

[15] M. J. Roberts, A. Morton, P. Donato et al., "68Ga-PSMA PET/CT tumour intensity pre-operatively predicts adverse pathological outcomes and progression-free survival in localised prostate cancer," *European Journal of Nuclear Medicine and Molecular Imaging*, vol. 48, no. 2, pp. 477–482, 2021.

[16] T. Lengana, I. O. Lawal, T. G. Boshomane et al., "68Ga-PSMA PET/CT replacing bone scan in the initial staging of skeletal metastasis in prostate cancer: a fait accompli?" *Clinical Genitourinary Cancer*, vol. 16, no. 5, pp. 392–401, 2018.

[17] A. Ghosh and W. D. W. Heston, "Tumor target prostate specific membrane antigen (PSMA) and its regulation in prostate cancer," *Journal of Cellular Biochemistry*, vol. 91, no. 3, pp. 528–539, 2004.

[18] P. S. Chakraborty, M. Tripathi, K. K. Agarwal, R. Kumar, M. K. Vijay, and C. Bal, "Metastatic poorly differentiated prostatic carcinoma with neuroendocrine differentiation," *Clinical Nuclear Medicine*, vol. 40, no. 2, pp. e163–e166, 2015.

[19] K. L. Wallitt, S. R. Khan, S. Dubash, H. H. Tam, S. Khan, and T. D. Barwick, "Clinical PET imaging in prostate cancer," *RadioGraphics*, vol. 37, no. 5, pp. 1512–1536, 2017.

[20] H. Jadvar, "Imaging evaluation of prostate cancer with 18F-fluorodeoxyglucose PET/CT: utility and limitations," *European Journal of Nuclear Medicine and Molecular Imaging*, vol. 40, no. Suppl 1, pp. S5–S10, 2013.

[21] J.-M. Beauregard, A.-C. Blouin, V. Fradet et al., "FDG-PET/CT for pre-operative staging and prognostic stratification of patients with high-grade prostate cancer at biopsy," *Cancer Imaging*, vol. 15, no. 1, p. 2, 2015.

[22] M. S. Hofman, J. Violet, R. J. Hicks et al., "[177 Lu]-PSMA-617 radionuclide treatment in patients with metastatic castration-resistant prostate cancer (LuPSMA trial): a single-centre, single-arm, phase 2 study," *The Lancet Oncology*, vol. 19, no. 6, pp. 825–833, 2018.

[23] L. Emmett, M. Crumbaker, B. Ho et al., "Results of a prospective phase 2 pilot trial of 177Lu-PSMA-617 therapy for metastatic castration-resistant prostate cancer including imaging predictors of treatment response and patterns of progression," *Clinical Genitourinary Cancer*, vol. 17, no. 1, pp. 15–22, 2019.

[24] M. P. Mannas, T. Lee, M. Pourghiasian, D. C. Wilson, and P. C. Black, "Incidentalomas of the prostate detected by 18-fluoro-2-deoxy-D-glucose positron emission tomography/computed tomography," *Canadian Urological Association Journal = Journal de l'Association des urologues du Canada*, vol. 14, no. 5, pp. E180–E184, 2020.

[25] J. P. T. Higgins and Cochrane Collaboration, *Cochrane Handbook for Systematic Reviews of Interventions*, Wiley-Blackwell, Hoboken, NJ, USA, Second edition, 2020.

[26] D. Moher, A. Liberati, J. Tetzlaff, D. G. Altman, and P. Group, "Preferred reporting items for systematic reviews and meta-analyses: the PRISMA statement," *PLoS Medicine*, vol. 6, no. 7, Article ID e1000097, 2009.

[27] H. Suri, "Ethical considerations of conducting systematic reviews in educational research," in *Systematic Reviews in Educational Research: Methodology, Perspectives and Application*, O. Zawacki-Richter, M. Kerres, S. Bedenlier, M. Bond, and K. Buntins, Eds., Springer Fachmedien Wiesbaden, Wiesbaden, Germany, pp. 41–54, 2020.

[28] Joanna Briggs Institute, *Checklist for Case Reports [The Joanna Briggs Institute Critical Appraisal Tools for Use in JBI Systematic Reviews]*, http://joannabriggs.org/assets/docs/critical-appraisal-tools/JBI_Critical_Appraisal-Checklist_for_Case_Reports.pdf, Joanna Briggs Institute, Adelaide, Australia, 2016, http://joannabriggs.org/assets/docs/critical-appraisal-tools/JBI_Critical_Appraisal-Checklist_for_Case_Reports.pdf.

[29] P. F. Whiting, A. W. Rutjes, M. E. Westwood et al., "QUADAS-2: a revised tool for the quality assessment of diagnostic accuracy studies," *Annals of Internal Medicine*, vol. 155, no. 8, pp. 529–536, 2011.

[30] X. Zhou, Y. Li, X. Jiang et al., "Intra-individual comparison of 18F-PSMA-1007 and 18F-FDG PET/CT in the evaluation of patients with prostate cancer," *Frontiers in oncology*, vol. 10, Article ID 585213, 2020.

[31] Y. Shi, L. Xu, Y. Zhu, Y. Wang, R. Chen, and J. Liu, "Use of 68Ga-PSMA-11 and 18F-FDG PET-CT dual-tracer to differentiate between lymph node metastases and ganglia," *Frontiers in Oncology*, vol. 11, Article ID 646110, 2021.

[32] R. Chen, Y. Wang, Y. Shi et al., "Diagnostic value of (18)F-FDG PET/CT in patients with biochemical recurrent prostate cancer and negative (68)Ga-PSMA PET/CT," *European Journal of Nuclear Medicine and Molecular Imaging*, vol. 48, no. 9, pp. 2970–2977, 2021.

[33] B. Wang, C. Liu, Y. Wei et al., "A prospective trial of 68Ga-PSMA and 18F-FDG PET/CT in nonmetastatic prostate cancer patients with an early PSA progression during castration," *Clinical Cancer Research*, vol. 26, no. 17, pp. 4551–4558, 2020.

[34] L. M. McEwan, D. Wong, and J. Yaxley, "Flourodeoxyglucose positron emission tomography scan may be helpful in the case of ductal variant prostate cancer when prostate specific membrane antigen ligand positron emission tomography scan is negative," *Journal of Medical Imaging and Radiation Oncology*, vol. 61, no. 4, pp. 503–505, 2017.

[35] A. Kichloo, R. Amir, M. Aljadah et al., "FDG-PET versus PSMA-PET: a patient with prostate cancer," *Journal of investigative medicine high impact case reports*, vol. 8, 2020.

[36] T. Cakir, S. Guven, B. Muezzinoglu, C. Erol, M. Y. Boz, and T. Atasever, "Intense fluoro-2-deoxyglucose uptake in high-grade prostatic adenocarcinoma with negligible prostate-specific membrane antigen expression," *Urology Annals*, vol. 11, no. 4, pp. 439–442, 2019.

[37] S. Chen, S. K. Cheung, K.-N. Wong, K. K. Wong, and C.-L. Ho, "68Ga-DOTATOC and 68Ga-PSMA PET/CT unmasked a case of prostate cancer with neuroendocrine differentiation," *Clinical Nuclear Medicine*, vol. 41, no. 12, pp. 959-960, 2016.

[38] G. K. Parida, S. Tripathy, S. Datta Gupta et al., "Adenocarcinoma prostate with neuroendocrine differentiation," *Clinical Nuclear Medicine*, vol. 43, no. 4, pp. 248-249, 2018.

[39] D. Shetty, H. Loh, C. Bui, R. Mansberg, A. Hadjashrafi, and V. Do, "Non-prostate-specific membrane antigen-avid metastatic lung nodule from primary prostatic adenocarcinoma," *Clinical Nuclear Medicine*, vol. 41, no. 10, pp. 776–778, 2016.

[40] R. Parghane and S. Basu, "Small cell transformation of metastatic prostate adenocarcinoma diagnosed by dual-tracer PET/CT (68Ga-PSMA and 18F-FDG): potential clinical utility in therapeutic decision making and treatment monitoring," *Journal of Nuclear Medicine Technology*, vol. 47, no. 1, pp. 85–87, 2019.

[41] P. M. Perez, T. A. Hope, S. C. Behr, A. Van Zante, E. J. Small, and R. R. Flavell, "Intertumoral heterogeneity of 18F-FDG and 68Ga-PSMA uptake in prostate cancer pulmonary metastases," *Clinical Nuclear Medicine*, vol. 44, no. 1, pp. e28–e32, 2019.

[42] L. Geraldo, F. Ceci, C. Uprimny, D. Kendler, and I. Virgolini, "Detection of sarcomatoid lung metastasis with 68GA-PSMA PET/CT in a patient with prostate cancer," *Clinical Nuclear Medicine*, vol. 41, no. 5, pp. 421-422, 2016.

[43] G. Polverari, F. Ceci, M. Allen-Auerbach et al., "Solitary mucinous prostate adenocarcinoma lung metastasis detected

by Ga-68-PSMA-11 PET/CT," *Clinical Genitourinary Cancer*, vol. 17, no. 1, pp. E53–E55, 2019.

[44] M. A. Queiroz, P. Viana, A. Santos, D. Bastos, E. Etchebehere, and G. Cerri, "Clinical impact of Ga-68-PSMA PET/CT in a patient with biochemical recurrence of prostate cancer," *Clinical Nuclear Medicine*, vol. 41, no. 9, pp. E417–E419, 2016.

[45] I. Sarikaya, A. Elgazzar, A. Sarikaya, and M. Alfeeli, "Fluorodeoxyglucose, sodium fluoride, and prostate-specific membrane antigen positron emission tomography studies for treatment response assessment in prostate cancer," *World Journal of Nuclear Medicine*, vol. 17, no. 3, pp. 207–210, 2018.

[46] S. McGeorge, R. Phillips, N. J. Rukin, J. Reynolds, and M. J. Roberts, "Solitary castrate-resistant prostate cancer metastasis to adrenal gland with concordant intense avidity on PSMA and FDG PET," *Urology Case Reports*, vol. 38, Article ID 101696, 2021.

[47] C. J. Sweeney, Y.-H. Chen, M. Carducci et al., "Chemohormonal therapy in metastatic hormone-sensitive prostate cancer," *New England Journal of Medicine*, vol. 373, no. 8, pp. 737–746, 2015.

[48] D. A. Palma, R. Olson, S. Harrow et al., "Stereotactic ablative radiotherapy versus standard of care palliative treatment in patients with oligometastatic cancers (SABR-COMET): a randomised, phase 2, open-label trial," *The Lancet*, vol. 393, no. 10185, pp. 2051–2058, 2019.

[49] R. Phillips, W. Y. Shi, M. Deek et al., "Outcomes of observation vs stereotactic ablative radiation for oligometastatic prostate cancer," *JAMA Oncology*, vol. 6, no. 5, pp. 650–659, 2020.

[50] S. Suman, R. V. Parghane, A. Joshi et al., "Therapeutic efficacy, prognostic variables and clinical outcome of 177Lu-PSMA-617 PRLT in progressive mCRPC following multiple lines of treatment: prognostic implications of high FDG uptake on dual tracer PET-CT vis-à-vis Gleason score in such cohort," *British Journal of Radiology*, vol. 92, no. 1104, 2019.

[51] S. P. Thang, J. Violet, S. Sandhu et al., "Poor outcomes for patients with metastatic castration-resistant prostate cancer with low prostate-specific membrane antigen (PSMA) expression deemed ineligible for 177Lu-labelled PSMA radioligand therapy," *European Urology Oncology*, vol. 2, no. 6, pp. 670–676, 2019.

[52] F. Rosar, K. Ribbat, M. Ries et al., "Neuron-specific enolase has potential value as a biomarker for [18F]FDG/[68Ga]Ga-PSMA-11 PET mismatch findings in advanced mCRPC patients," *EJNMMI Research*, vol. 10, no. 1, 2020.

[53] H. Beltran, D. Prandi, J. M. Mosquera et al., "Divergent clonal evolution of castration-resistant neuroendocrine prostate cancer," *Nature Medicine*, vol. 22, no. 3, pp. 298–305, 2016.

[54] M. K. Bakht, J. M. Lovnicki, J. Tubman et al., "Differential expression of glucose transporters and hexokinases in prostate cancer with a neuroendocrine gene signature: a mechanistic perspective for 18F-FDG imaging of PSMA-suppressed tumors," *Journal of Nuclear Medicine*, vol. 61, no. 6, pp. 904–910, 2020.

[55] E. Acar and G. Ç. Kaya, "18F-FDG, 68Ga-DOTATATE and 68Ga-PSMA positive metastatic large cell neuroendocrine prostate tumor," *Clinical Nuclear Medicine*, vol. 44, no. 1, pp. 53-54, 2019.

[56] V. Prati, F. Munoz, O. Dal Canton et al., "68GA-PSMA: high sensibility, specificity and detection rate tracer even with low PSA level: case report," *Anticancer Research*, vol. 37, no. 4, pp. 2058-2059, 2017.

[57] F. H. Cornelis, J. C. Durack, M. J. Morris, H. I. Scher, and S. B. Solomon, "Effective prostate-specific membrane antigen-based 18F-DCFPyL-Guided cryoablation of a single positive site in a patient believed to be more metastatic on 11C-choline PET/CT," *Clinical Nuclear Medicine*, vol. 42, no. 12, pp. e516–e518, 2017.

[58] B. L. Liu, J. J. Hong, K. Tang, J. Lin, and X. W. Zheng, "18F-PSMA-1007 uptake in pulmonary lymphangitic carcinomatosis metastasis from prostate cancer," *Clinical Nuclear Medicine*, vol. 46, no. 7, pp. e355–e357, 2021.

[59] C. Soydal, E. Ozkan, H. Yerlikaya, G. Utkan, and O. N. Kucuk, "Widespread metastatic prostate carcinoma shown by 68Ga-PSMA PET/CT," *Clinical Nuclear Medicine*, vol. 41, no. 6, pp. e294–e295, 2016.

13

Adolescent and Young Adult Testicular Germ Cell Tumors: Special Considerations

Amanda F. Saltzman and Nicholas G. Cost

Department of Surgery, Division of Urology, University of Colorado School of Medicine and Children's Hospital Colorado, Aurora, CO, USA

Correspondence should be addressed to Nicholas G. Cost; nicholas.cost@ucdenver.edu

Academic Editor: Costantine Albany

While testicular germ cell tumors (T-GCTs) make up only 0.5% of pediatric malignancies and less than 2% of adult malignancies, they comprise 14% of adolescent malignancies, making it the most common solid tumor in this age group. The transition in incidence at this age is also accompanied by a transition in tumor histology with adolescents having mostly pure embryonal carcinoma and mixed nonseminomatous germ cell tumors. Similar to T-GCTs of all ages, surgical excision with orchiectomy is the standard initial step in treatment. Chemotherapy, retroperitoneal lymph node dissection, and targeted treatment of distant metastases make even widely disseminated disease treatable and curable. For this reason, in many ways, the future focus has expanded beyond survival alone to emphasize quality of life issues such as fertility and hypogonadism. However, adolescents remain the age group least studied or understood as they fall in between the ages included in most study designs. Also, they require the most psychosocial support because of the challenges unique to the adolescent period. In this review, we aim to highlight the known outcome data for T-GCTs in this population and also to discuss the unique aspects of treatment and support for this age group.

1. Introduction

In pediatric oncology, significant advances have been made in survival of a variety of malignancies. The OS of children with cancer as a group approaches 80%, largely due to the collaborative efforts of cooperative groups [1]. However, numerous reports have shown that this triumph has not been evenly distributed across patients of all ages—the adolescent age group has not enjoyed the same success as younger children, and this has been specifically demonstrated for T-GCTs [2]. In fact, cancer in those aged 15–29 years kills more patients than any disease except suicide [3]. This is due to a host of reasons: delayed presentation and diagnosis [4], transition between adult and pediatric providers which may limit access to care [5], the disproportionate presence of high-risk pathologic components [6], poor treatment compliance [7], and a paucity of clinical trials and research focused on adolescents specifically. Perhaps the most relevant, however, is the lack of awareness of this age group as being unique [3].

Often, we assess adolescents along with those just slightly older and consider this group as adolescents and young adults (AYAs). The AYA population with cancer is a vulnerable group [4]. Compared with older adults with testicular cancer specifically, survival patterns differ [8], there are insurance coverage issues [5], and these patients are less likely to participate in clinical trials, are more likely to experience delays in diagnosis or treatment [9], and are more likely to suffer psychosocial problems and decreased quality of life related to their diagnosis [10, 11]. Because of these disparities, in 2006, the American Cancer Society and National Cancer Institute with help from the LIVESTRONG Young Adult Alliance called for future research to focus on cancer outcomes in AYA patients and established the AYA Oncology Progress Review Group [12]. Similarly, COG and SWOG have established dedicated AYA committees, and recently, the Society for Adolescent and Young Adult Oncology was funded. It is very important to understand that this term is used differently between studies and between large study groups: SEER 15–29 yr, NCI's AYA Oncology

Progress Review Group 15–39 yr, and NCCN guideline 15–39 yr [13].

To properly develop a focus on AYA testicular cancer, there needs to be focus beyond just diagnosis and treatment—and must include a focus on fertility preservation, emotional support for patients and families, socioeconomic support, educational encouragement, palliative care, and survivorship specialists to meet the needs of this unique population [5]. There also must be collaboration and cooperation of providers who care for children and adults and fluid transition between the two.

2. Disease-Specific Aspects Unique to the AYA Population

2.1. Ethnicity. Testicular cancer is the most common urologic cancer in the AYA males [4, 13, 14]. Worldwide, it disproportionately affects men living in developed nations (USA, Canada, Denmark, Switzerland, Norway, Australia, New Zealand, etc.), where its incidence is attenuating over recent generations. In contrast, the incidence is rapidly increasing in countries undergoing developmental transition (Croatia, Slovenia, Singapore, the Philippines, China, Costa Rica, etc.) [15]. Testis cancer in general, disproportionately affects white men. While the incidence of testis cancer in AYAs is increasing overall, there has been a very large (58%) increase in the Hispanic population over the non-Hispanic white population (7%) [16]. Also, within the AYA group, in the adolescent population specifically, there appears to be a disproportionate population of Hispanic males affected [17]. While survival after testicular cancer is high, several large population-based studies of men with testicular cancer of all ages have shown that non-Hispanic whites have an increased OS when compared to Hispanic whites [18], African Americans [17, 19], and nonwhites [20]. This has been confirmed in the AYA population, with African Americans and Hispanics having worse OS and CSS than whites, even after adjustment for neighborhood socioeconomic status [21]. When looking at patients with pure seminoma, however, the racial disparities are less impactful for unclear reasons [21].

2.2. Neighborhood/Socioeconomic Status. A recent study using the California Cancer Registry examined the association between the patients' sociodemographic factors (race/ethnicity and neighborhood socioeconomic status) and survival of AYAs with testicular cancer from 1998 to 2000 [21]. They identified just over 14,000 patients and found that AYAs from middle and low socioeconomic neighborhoods had a much lower OS and cancer-specific survival than AYAs from high socioeconomic neighborhoods, even when controlling for race/ethnicity. This difference was seen in both patients with seminoma and those with non-seminoma [21]. This trend, worse outcomes in lower socioeconomic neighborhoods, has been well described in the oncologic literature, across various cancers and in both children and adults [17, 22, 23]. It has been suggested that neighborhood socioeconomic status is an independent risk factor for survival, not just a surrogate for individual socioeconomic status, and it mediates poorer outcomes through neighborhood level factors, such as social environment, reduced quality and availability of healthcare and support services, and chronic stress [21].

2.3. Age. Patients aged 15–24 years with T-GCTs had an improved OS, but not cancer-specific survival, than those aged 25–39 years [21]. However, when comparing patients aged 15–19 years to those <15 years, there are significant decreases in OS [1]. When examining event free survival (EFS), patients aged 13–19 years have been shown to have a 3-year EFS of 60%, significantly worse than patients aged < 13 years (87%) and patients aged >19 years (80%) [2]. The seeming contradictions of these studies are apparent; however, it is very important to identify the endpoint specified, because a disease like T-GCTs is very salvageable, even after metastasis and recurrence. Thus, differences in OS may not be appreciated despite difference in EFS and other measures. There can also be differences in histology (high incidence of embryonal component and rare seminomas) as well as more advanced disease at presentation for adolescents. Specifically, it appears that the incidence of clinical stage I disease decreases with age: 70–80% of prepubertal children with T-GCT, 50–60% of adolescents with T-GCT, and 40–50% of adults with NSGCT [24–27]. Another factor associated with age is marital status. Married AYAs with testicular cancer had improved OS and cancer-specific survival than their unmarried counterparts [17, 21].

2.4. Histology. Interestingly, T-GCTs in prepubertal males are usually pure yolk sac tumors, which rarely metastasize [28], and pure teratoma, which is benign in this age group [29]. Pure seminoma is rare in the pediatric and adolescent population. When compared to pure seminoma, non-seminoma is most common in the AYA population and generally is of mixed histology, more frequently involves metastatic disease at presentation, and has a higher rate of relapse [30]. These mixed tumors, especially with embryonal components, are the most common seen in AYAs [31].

Stokes et al. [32] recently performed an analysis of the NCDB looking at patterns of care and survival outcomes for AYAs (age ≥ 15 years) with seminoma treated with primary surgery, known histology, and known outcomes. They identified 12,880 AYAs and compared this group to both adults aged 40–55 years (8,022) and >55 years (1,459). Compared to their adult counterparts, AYAs in this cohort were more likely to be nonwhite/nonblack, be uninsured, have fewer comorbidities, have clinical stage 1 disease at presentation, receive care at a high-volume institution, forego RPLND, and undergo surveillance over adjuvant therapy. Unadjusted 5- and 10-year OS was significantly better for AYAs than their older counterparts (98% and 96.1%, resp.). Factors associated with improved OS included AYA age, private insurance, high facility volume, stage 1 disease, and receipt of radiation therapy. Even controlling for other factors, AYA status remains significantly associated with improved OS. Interestingly, race was not significantly associated with OS, unlike previous studies, while socio-economic factors (insurance status) were associated with OS. The authors suggest that the less frequent use of adjuvant therapy by AYAs than older adults highlights progress for these patients; judicious use of these therapies, all of which carry significant side effects over the long term, has still allowed an extremely high OS [32]. This study mirrors findings from a SEER database analysis and European registry data [33].

A complementary paper on NSGCT in the AYA population investigated the SEER database to evaluate the association between age and outcomes [17]. The authors identified 1,496 adolescents (13–19 years) and 12,467 adults (>19 years) with a median follow up of 71 months. 5-year OS for adolescents was 94% and adults was 92% ($p = 0.007$) with 5-year CSS of 95% and 94%, respectively ($p = 0.139$). Age was a significant predictor of both OS and CSS when controlling for other factors. They also found that, despite presenting more often with metastatic disease, adolescents had improved OS and CSS than adults.

2.5. Risk Factors for Metastatic Disease. Active surveillance is the current recommendation for both adults and children [34] with clinical stage 1 T-GCTs. However, we know that a significant proportion (20–30%) will harbor occult disease. In the adult population, the identification of high-risk features for harboring of occult metastases—lymphovascular invasion and an increasing component of embryonal carcinoma for NSGCT [35] and size > 4 cm and rete testis invasion for seminoma [36]—has allowed a risk-stratified treatment approach to be employed [34]. Cost et al. [37] reviewed 23 patients aged 7–21 years and found that about half of all patients had high-risk features (≥40% embryonal carcinoma or lymphovascular invasion), and almost 60% with high-risk features harbored occult metastatic disease. No patients without high-risk features had metastatic disease. This confirmed that these same high-risk features for NSGCT in the adult population confer a similar risk for harboring occult metastatic disease in the pediatric and AYA population. While all relapses were successfully managed with 100% survival, the validation of these same high-risk features in the AYA population may lend themselves to counseling points for families and perhaps future incorporation into treatment strategies; however, they are currently not part of any treatment guidelines.

2.6. Surgery. Traditional teaching calls for radical orchiectomy for all testicular masses concerning for malignancy. Recent data suggest that partial orchiectomy/excisional biopsy via an inguinal incision may be safe in certain highly selected patients, and this has become common practice for the management of prepubertal pediatric testis tumors, regardless of the preoperative suspicion of teratoma [38]. For postpubertal boys, the authors' current practice involves performing a partial orchiectomy if patients have a mass < 2 cm *and* normal tumor markers, regardless of suspected pathology (manuscript in submission). Intraoperative frozen section is then utilized; if there is any concern for T-GCT, a radial orchiectomy is completed at the same setting. However, if the pathology returns benign or not concerning for T-GCT, the partial orchiectomy is completed and that testis has retained fertility and hormonal function [39]. Partial orchiectomy is not being advocated for or used to treat T-GCTs, but rather it is proposed as an initial step to preserve gonadal function in patients with small testicular masses and normal tumor markers due to the associated high rate of benign pathology. Although unilateral radical orchiectomy preserves contralateral testicular function, Leydig cell dysfunction and hypogonadism may develop prematurely, making T-GCT survivors at risk for androgen deficiency into adulthood [40].

2.7. Treatment. Because of similar tumor biology, postpubertal T-GCTs are best managed using adult algorithms. Individual pubertal status needs to be determined before discussing any treatment. Traditional pediatric regimens have been thought to undertreat adolescents with T-GCTs and may contribute to worse outcomes in adolescents over adults [6]. Indeed, the staging is different for patients with T-GCTs that are prepubertal (COG staging system) compared to postpubertal (AJCC TNMS system and IGCCCG system for metastatic disease), and the emphasis on postchemotherapy surgery differs. These differences are highlighted in Table 1. Additionally, COG remains concerned about long-term effects of cisplatin exposure (ototoxicity, nephrotoxicity, peripheral neuropathy, etc.) and is investigating the role of carboplatin versus cisplatin for children with T-GCTs. While adult studies have demonstrated a superior effect of cisplatin, pediatric studies have shown that higher dose carboplatin is associated with similarly good outcomes for children with T-GCTs [41]. Many adult urologic oncologists may be hesitant to place patients onto this COG study given their belief that randomization to the carboplatin arm is substandard of care therapy. COG protocols generally target patients aged 15 years and younger, with most postpubertal patients, which would include AYAs, being treated per adult algorithms [5].

The vast majority of adolescents and AYAs with clinical stage I disease should undergo active surveillance, per NCCN guidelines. The relapse rate is 20–30%, with excellent survival after salvage therapy. Even in the presence of high-risk features and high risk of relapse, the potential for morbidity with overtreatment of 70–80% of patients without a clear survival advantage makes an aggressive upfront treatment approach less desirable [42]. This approach prevents overtreatment and associated side effects while reserving highly effective salvage therapy for those who truly need it.

2.8. Long-Term Outcomes. There have been huge advances with long-term survival of AYAs with testicular cancer, so there has been a focus shift towards quality of life and late effects of treatment. A recent review of quality of life outcomes has shown that long-term testicular cancer survivors were comparable to age-matched controls, including mental health and sexual function, and that any decreases in quality of life were not related to treatment modality [43, 44]. For

Table 1: AJCC versus COG staging for testicular tumors [5].

Stage	AJCC	COG
I	$pT_{1\text{-}4}N_0M_0S_0$ IA: $pT_1N_0M_0S_0$ IB: $pT_{2\text{-}4}N_0M_0S_0$ IS: $pT_{1\text{-}4}N_0M_0S_{1\text{-}3}$	Tumor limited to testis, completely resected by high inguinal orchiectomy; no clinical, radiographic, or histologic evidence of disease beyond the testis Normal or unknown tumor markers at diagnosis must have negative ipsilateral RPLND to confirm stage I disease if imaging shows LNs > 2 cm Scrotal orchiectomy with high ligation of the cord is also considered stage I
II	$pT_{1\text{-}4}N_{1\text{-}3}M_0S_{0\text{-}1}$ IIA: $pT_{1\text{-}4}N_1M_0S_{0\text{-}1}$ IIB: $pT_{1\text{-}4}N_2M_0S_{0\text{-}1}$ IIC: $pT_{1\text{-}4}N_3M_0S_{0\text{-}1}$	Transscrotal biopsy; microscopic disease in scrotum or high in spermatic cord (< 5 mm from proximal cord margin) Failure of tumor markers to normalize or decrease with an appropriate half-life
III	$pT_{1\text{-}4}N_{1\text{-}3}M_1S_{0\text{-}1}$ IIIA: $pT_{1\text{-}4}N_{1\text{-}3}M_{1a}S_{0\text{-}1}$ IIIB: $pT_{1\text{-}4}N_{1\text{-}3}M_{0\text{-}1b}S_2$ IIIC: $pT_{1\text{-}4}N_{1\text{-}3}M_{0\text{-}1b}S_3$	Retroperitoneal LN involvement without visceral or extraabdominal involvement LNs > 4 cm by CT or 2–4 cm if biopsy proven metastatic
IV		Distant metastasis, including liver

those treated during adolescence, however, lower rates of fertility, body image, and sexual function have been described [45].

3. Late Effects

Important to consider is that this group of patients has a longer life expectancy than older adults. Thus, the long-term sequelae of systemic treatments (radiation, chemotherapy, and surgery) should be seriously considered, and monitoring for these complications is necessary. The NCCN has published a clinical guideline for AYA oncology patients, which all providers caring for this group of patients should review and have readily available. This nicely summarizes risks specific to this patient population as well as screening guidelines for survivors [13].

3.1. Fertility. All adjunctive treatment strategies beyond radical orchiectomy (chemotherapy, RPLND, and radiation) are associated with potential fertility issues, either transient or permanent. A recent survey of cancer survivors ranked fertility questions as the second most common concern behind mortality [46]. Every effort should be made to perform nerve sparing RPLND when necessary, and some advocate for referral to high-volume centers. Sperm cryopreservation is the most effective method to maintain fertility potential, but this must be initiated prior to treatment for testicular cancer. There are a host of issues surrounding cryopreservation, including young age and collection methods, anxiety associated with cancer diagnosis, and high cost of preservation. AYA patients and their families may not immediately think of fertility to be important given a diagnosis of malignancy and the patient's current life stage, so it is the responsibility of the provider to address this issue head on, prior to treatment initiation. Early involvement of an oncofertility specialist can help patients and families work through banking [5].

3.2. Secondary Malignancy. For at least 35 years after treatment, patients who have received chemotherapy or radiation are at higher risk of developing a secondary malignancy over the general population who has not been exposed to these agents [47]. The relative risk of development of a secondary malignancy is 1.8 for radiation, 2 for chemotherapy, and 2.9 for a combination of chemotherapy and radiation [48]. Etoposide specifically carries a risk of developing a secondary leukemia that is highly resistant to available therapies. This risk is correlated with total dose received and is increased in combination with radiation exposure [49]. Smoking and excessive alcohol consumption, common behaviors in AYA cancer survivors, has been shown to increase the risk of malignancy in bladder/prostate rhabdomyosarcoma patients, who are also at increased risk of secondary malignancy due to the chemotherapeutic agents and radiation used to treat their disease [50]. Patients with T-GCTs may receive similar therapies to the rhabdomyosarcoma population, albeit with differing doses, fields, and agents. However, they too are at higher risk for secondary malignancies and probably also engage in cigarette use and excessive alcohol consumption. It is not unreasonable to infer that these patients may be further increasing their risk of malignancy with these behaviors and should be counseled to avoid these activities.

3.3. Chemotherapy. Cisplatin-related nephrotoxicity via proximal tubular dysfunction is well described. Decreases in glomerular filtration rate, hypomagnesemia, and proteinuria have all been reported with this drug that is highly effective for T-GCTs. A recent study calculated a 10% risk of stage 3 chronic kidney disease for those exposed to a median of 4 cycles of cisplatin during treatment, and rate of progression increased with more cycles of chemotherapy [51]. Another review of 63 children treated with cis- or carboplatin showed no significant change in renal function over time, measured 10 years after completion of therapy. However, 11% of patients had an eGFR < 60 mL/min/1.73 m^2, which is not insignificant. Older age at the initiation of therapy was associated with a lower GFR [52].

About 1 in 6 patients will report peripheral neuropathy, and this is due to cisplatin exposure [53]. Similarly, high-frequency hearing loss is seen in 20–40% of patients exposed to cisplatin (dose-dependent), and this is usually permanent

[54]. Other long-term effects of cisplatin exposure include cardiovascular disease, paresthesia, hypogonadism, hypercholesterolemia, and hypertension. Interestingly, studies have confirmed that platinum and platinum-based residuals remain in circulation up to 20 years, and it is thought that perhaps these contribute to long-term complications [55]. In this same study, renal function 1 year after treatment was associated with the level of platinum remaining, meaning that the relationship between renal function and drug goes both ways—the drug damages the kidneys, and because of this, there is more drug left in the system, perpetuating its effects [55]. It is postulated that there may be therapy-related vascular changes that could contribute to the increased cardiovascular disease and increased incidence (6%) of myocardial infarction in these patients, illustrating that the implication of a single agent/therapy as the cause for a specific complication has been difficult to determine thus far [56].

Bleomycin has been linked to lung disease in a dose-related fashion, with about 5% of patients developing pulmonary fibrosis. Risk factors for bleomycin toxicity include increased age, concomitant chest radiation, decreased renal function, and elevated concentrations of inspired oxygen. Unfortunately, radiographic evidence of bleomycin toxicity may be seen as pleural-based nodules, which may be mistaken for relapsed or refractory disease (these resolve over time) [54].

Metabolic syndrome has been reported to occur in about 25% of T-GCT survivors. The exact mechanism for this is unknown, but testosterone and Leydig cell function have been implicated, although not uniformly across studies [57].

Hypogonadism is estimated to occur in 10–15% of patients after unilateral orchiectomy [58, 59], resulting in the need for androgen replacement. Preserving gonadal function may also reduce the clinically underrecognized but real rates of osteopenia and osteoporosis in these patients [60].

3.4. Psychosocial Effects. Adolescence is a tumultuous time in life, where all changes and experiences are amplified. Most teenagers feel that even ordinary challenges are difficult to overcome and that they are facing these challenges alone. On top of this baseline feeling, a cancer diagnosis clearly radically changes the patient's life and their needs when confronted with cancer are greater than older patients. The AYA population has a significant need for psychosocial support; cancer and subsequent therapy will create significant change in their social lives and interactions, which are central to being a teenager. There are obvious changes that will occur; self-image will be affected by hair loss, weight changes, mood alterations, nausea, febrile illness and hospitalizations, isolation due to infectious risk, etc. Impaired sexual function due to infertility, impotence, and an inability to feel that the patient was having any type of intimate relationship are major issues during this life stage. While these issues are common for an adult urologist to discuss with their patients, regardless of whether the patient has cancer, pediatric patients and providers are often uncomfortable discussing these personal details. Conversely, adult providers rarely acknowledge the impact of adolescence and puberty on a patient's everyday health, attitudes, and compliance [32].

Patients in the AYA age group are often at a cross roads with respect to education and career decisions. Cancer obviously detracts from the attention that is usually paid to these decisions, which seriously impact a person's identity. Pursuing treatment may affect a patient's ability to work and earn an income, which may lead to financial challenges that are then augmented by the cost of cancer treatment and insurance issues that are already prevalent in this age group. In addition to the obvious financial implications, this may be associated with guilt about not being able to meet basic expectations. After therapy, in the survivorship stage, resuming normal work or school life activities can be difficult. More than half of cancer survivors have problems continuing work or education after therapy cessation [61]. Expectation for both the patient and employer/school is one of the biggest factors in the success of transitioning back to normal life. Additionally, maintaining some type of involvement in work/school life during therapy, even if minimal, is associated with increased success with reentry long term [61].

Relationships, both with friends and partners, are central to AYA lives and can be severely impacted by cancer diagnosis and treatment. Partners may be lost or have feelings of fear of relapse, guilt, or sympathy. A father or brother with testicular cancer increases a male's risk of testicular cancer four times over the general population (2 or more relatives, 10x increased risk), and the development of testicular cancer tends to be at a similar age, but not necessarily the same histology [62]. Thus, there are unknown genetics and predisposition for existing children and when considering expanding families, which may result in tension between partners and thus a strained relationship [5]. Additionally, care of young children during cancer treatment can be unpredictable and yet another source of strain on a relationship [13].

These challenges are more than those experienced in either the adult or pediatric population and thus providers are usually unprepared to handle them. Providers generally provide a narrow, focused, technical view of diagnosis and treatment, which may further isolate the patient and his family, marginalizing their concerns. To fix this, early involvement of a multidisciplinary team, including mental health providers, is necessary. Not only will this improve mental health, stress levels, and quality of life, but it will increase compliance and hopefully survival, a central issue with the AYA population. Being aware of the issues, creating a team, and being prepared is the first step to face these issues head on [5].

4. Conclusions and Future Directions

For all the above reasons, the AYA population truly is unique with its own particular set of challenges. While the end goal is to improve outcomes, namely survivorship, there are a host of other issues that need to be addressed. These issues will not be able to be tackled without a multilayered approach to both clinical and translational research. AYA oncology education and awareness need to be increased, areas of research that will most directly lead to improved survivorship or quality of life for need to be prioritized, and there needs to be increased funding for researchers committed to studying this population. Increased awareness on the national level with various new societies and groups is occurring, but urologists need to be advocates at the institutional level to raise awareness and education about this unique population [5].

Recently, novel biomarkers such as microRNA clusters have been identified that are uniformly overexpressed in all malignant GCTs, regardless of patient age, subtype, or site. While these remain a research tool and are not yet prevalent in everyday practice, they remain an exciting possibility for diagnosis (new staging criteria?) and surveillance (instead of CT scans?) of patients with T-GCTs [63].

Patient care collaboration through the development of and referral to highly experienced treatment teams have been shown to improve outcome for patients with T-GCTs. With increasing technology available to share information between centers, expertise can reach farther than a single institution into smaller community practices for advice and allows for improved coordinated referrals to these large volume centers [64]. A huge area in need of improvement for this group is clinical trial participation. More than 90% of children participate in clinical trials, while about 10% of teenagers and even fewer young adults do participate [28]. Providers need to educate patients and families about study trial opportunities that exist and need to create trials that specifically target this population [5].

Abbreviations

OS: Overall survival
AYA: Adolescent and young adult
NCCN: National Comprehensive Cancer Network
NCI: National Cancer Institute
CSS: Cancer-specific survival
T-GCT: Testicular germ cell tumor
NSGCT: Nonseminomatous germ cell tumor
EFS: Event free survival
NCDB: National Cancer Database
RPLND: Retroperitoneal lymph node dissection
SEER: Surveillance, Epidemiology and End Results Program
COG: Children's Oncology Group
SWOG: Southwest Oncology Group
AJCC: American Joint Committee on Cancer
TNMS: Tumor, node, metastasis, serum
IGCCCG: International Germ Cell Cancer Collaborative Group
eGFR: Estimated glomerular filtration rate.

Acknowledgments

The study was supported by the Etkin Family Fund of the Aspen Community Foundation.

References

[1] A. Bleyer, "Adolescent and young adult (AYA) oncology: the first A," *Pediatric Hematology and Oncology*, vol. 24, no. 5, pp. 325–336, 2007.

[2] N. G. Cost, J. D. Lubahn, M. Adibi et al., "A comparison of pediatric, adolescent, and adult testicular germ cell malignancy: pediatric, adolescent, and adult testicular GCTs," *Pediatric Blood and Cancer*, vol. 61, no. 3, pp. 446–451, 2014.

[3] V. Subbiah, "Adolescent oncology: who cares?—the new KID on the block," *Supportive Care in Cancer*, vol. 18, no. 6, pp. 771–773, 2010.

[4] A. Bleyer, R. Barr, B. Hayes-Lattin, D. Thomas, C. Ellis, and B. Anderson, "The distinctive biology of cancer in adolescents and young adults," *Nature Reviews Cancer*, vol. 8, no. 4, pp. 288–298, 2008.

[5] N. G. Cost, C. R. Cost, J. I. Geller, and W. R. DeFoor, "Adolescent urologic oncology: current issues and future directions," *Urologic Oncology: Seminars and Original Investigations*, vol. 32, no. 2, pp. 59–69, 2014.

[6] E. C. Grantham, B. T. Caldwell, and N. G. Cost, "Current urologic care for testicular germ cell tumors in pediatric and adolescent patients," *Urologic Oncology: Seminars and Original Investigations*, vol. 34, no. 2, pp. 65–75, 2016.

[7] G. Pentheroudakis and N. Pavlidis, "Juvenile cancer: improving care for adolescents and young adults within the frame of medical oncology," *Annals of Oncology*, vol. 16, no. 2, pp. 181–188, 2005.

[8] M. C. DeRouen, S. L. Gomez, D. J. Press, L. Tao, A. W. Kurian, and T. H. M. Keegan, "A population-based observational study of first-course treatment and survival for adolescent and young adult females with breast cancer," *Journal of Adolescent and Young Adult Oncology*, vol. 2, no. 3, pp. 95–103, 2013.

[9] H. M. Parsons, L. C. Harlan, N. L. Seibel, J. L. Stevens, and T. H. M. Keegan, "Clinical trial participation and time to treatment among adolescents and young adults with cancer: does age at diagnosis or insurance make a difference?," *Journal of Clinical Oncology*, vol. 29, no. 30, pp. 4045–4053, 2011.

[10] K. M. Bellizzi, A. Smith, S. Schmidt et al., "Positive and negative psychosocial impact of being diagnosed with cancer as an adolescent or young adult: impact of cancer," *Cancer*, vol. 118, no. 20, pp. 5155–5162, 2012.

[11] A. W. Smith, K. M. Bellizzi, T. H. M. Keegan et al., "Health-related quality of life of adolescent and young adult patients with cancer in the United States: the Adolescent and Young Adult Health Outcomes and Patient Experience study," *Journal of Clinical Oncology*, vol. 31, no. 17, pp. 2136–2145, 2013.

[12] C. Schmidt, "Lack of progress in teen and young adult cancers concerns researchers, prompts study," *Journal of the National Cancer Institute*, vol. 98, no. 24, pp. 1760–1763, 2006.

[13] NCCN Guidelines® and Clinical Resources, *NCCN Clinical Practice Guidelines in Oncology-Adolescent and Young Adult (AYA) Oncology*, National Comprehensive Cancer Network, Fort Washington, PA, USA, 2017.

[14] J. S. Townsend, L. C. Richardson, and R. R. German, "Incidence of testicular cancer in the United States, 1999–2004," *American Journal of Men's Health*, vol. 4, no. 4, pp. 353–360, 2010.

[15] A. Znaor, J. Lortet-Tieulent, M. Laversanne, A. Jemal, and F. Bray, "International testicular cancer incidence trends: generational transitions in 38 countries 1900–1990," *Cancer Causes and Control*, vol. 26, no. 1, pp. 151–158, 2015.

[16] F. L. Chien, S. M. Schwartz, and R. H. Johnson, "Increase in testicular germ cell tumor incidence among Hispanic adolescents and young adults in the United States: increasing TGCT Among Hispanic AYAs," *Cancer*, vol. 120, no. 17, pp. 2728–2734, 2014.

[17] A. Amini, T. V. Waxweiler, P. D. Maroni et al., "Survival outcomes of adolescent and adult patients with non-seminomatous testicular germ-cell tumors: a population-based study," *Journal of Pediatric Urology*, vol. 12, no. 6, pp. 405.e1–405.e9, 2016.

[18] T. V. Johnson, W. Hsiao, A. Jani, and V. A. Master, "Increased mortality among Hispanic testis cancer patients independent of neighborhood socioeconomic status: a SEER study," *Journal of Immigrant and Minority Health*, vol. 13, no. 5, pp. 818–824, 2011.

[19] M. Sun, F. Abdollah, D. Liberman et al., "Racial disparities and socioeconomic status in men diagnosed with testicular germ cell tumors: a survival analysis," *Cancer*, vol. 117, no. 18, pp. 4277–4285, 2011.

[20] S. D. Fosså, M. Cvancarova, L. Chen et al., "Adverse prognostic factors for testicular cancer–specific survival: a population-based study of 27,948 patients," *Journal of Clinical Oncology*, vol. 29, pp. 963–970, 2011.

[21] M. C. DeRouen, M. Mujahid, S. Srinivas, and T. H. M. Keegan, "Disparities in adolescent and young adult survival after testicular cancer vary by histologic subtype: a population-based study in California 1988–2010," *Journal of Adolescent and Young Adult Oncology*, vol. 5, no. 1, pp. 31–40, 2016.

[22] T. E. Byers, H. J. Wolf, K. R. Bauer et al., "The impact of socioeconomic status on survival after cancer in the United States: findings from the National Program of Cancer Registries Patterns of Care Study," *Cancer*, vol. 113, no. 3, pp. 582–591, 2008.

[23] E. E. Kent, R. A. Morris, J. A. Largent, A. Ziogas, L. S. Sender, and H. Anton-Culver, "Socioeconomic impacts on survival differ by race/ethnicity among adolescents and young adults with Non-Hodgkin's lymphoma," *Journal of Cancer Epidemiology*, vol. 2010, Article ID 824691, 10 pages, 2010.

[24] M. Schlatter, F. Rescorla, R. Giller et al., "Excellent outcome in patients with stage I germ cell tumors of the testes: a study of the Children's Cancer Group/Pediatric Oncology Group," *Journal of Pediatric Surgery*, vol. 38, no. 3, pp. 319–324, 2003.

[25] M. L. Curto, F. Lumia, R. Alaggio et al., "Malignant germ cell tumors in childhood: results of the first Italian cooperative study ?TCG 91?," *Medical and Pediatric Oncology*, vol. 41, pp. 417–425, 2003.

[26] R. G. Feltbower, C. Siller, E. Woodward et al., "Treatment and survival patterns for germ cell tumors among 13- to 24-year olds in Yorkshire, UK," *Pediatric Blood and Cancer*, vol. 56, no. 2, pp. 282–288, 2011.

[27] T. B. Powles, J. Bhardwa, J. Shamash, S. Mandalia, and T. Oliver, "The changing presentation of germ cell tumours of the testis between 1983 and 2002," *BJU International*, vol. 95, no. 9, pp. 1197–1200, 2005.

[28] R. Haas, P. Schmidt, U. Göbel, and H. Deiter, "Testicular germ cell tumors, an update. Results of the German cooperative studies 1982–1997," *Klinische Pädiatrie*, vol. 211, no. 4, pp. 300–304, 1999.

[29] U. Gobel, D. T. Schneider, G. Calaminus, R. J. Haas, P. Schmidt, and D. Harms, "Germ cell tumors in childhood and adolescence," *Annals of Oncology*, vol. 11, no. 3, pp. 263–271, 2000.

[30] D. R. Feldman, G. J. Bosl, J. Sheinfeld, and R. J. Motzer, "Medical treatment of advanced testicular cancer," *JAMA*, vol. 299, no. 6, pp. 672–684, 2008.

[31] S. Taskinen, R. Fagerholm, J. Aronniemi, R. Rintala, and M. Taskinen, "Testicular tumors in children and adolescents," *Journal of Pediatric Urology*, vol. 4, no. 2, pp. 134–137, 2008.

[32] W. Stokes, A. Amini, P. D. Maroni et al., "Patterns of care and survival outcomes for adolescent and young adult patients with testicular seminoma in the United States: a National Cancer Database analysis," *Journal of Pediatric Urology*, vol. 13, no. 4, pp. 386.e1–386.e7, 2017.

[33] R. H. A. Verhoeven, A. Gondos, M. L. G. Janssen-Heijnen et al., "Testicular cancer in Europe and the USA: survival still rising among older patients," *Annals of Oncology*, vol. 24, no. 2, pp. 508–513, 2013.

[34] F. J. Rescorla, J. H. Ross, D. F. Billmire et al., "Surveillance after initial surgery for Stage I pediatric and adolescent boys with malignant testicular germ cell tumors: report from the Children's Oncology Group," *Journal of Pediatric Surgery*, vol. 50, no. 6, pp. 1000–1003, 2015.

[35] Y. Vergouwe, E. W. Steyerberg, M. J. C. Eijkemans, P. Albers, and J. D. F. Habbema, "Predictors of occult metastasis in clinical stage I nonseminoma: a systematic review," *Journal of Clinical Oncology*, vol. 21, no. 22, pp. 4092–4099, 2003.

[36] J. L. Boormans, J. Mayor de Castro, L. Marconi et al., "Testicular tumour size and rete testis invasion as prognostic factors for the risk of relapse of clinical stage I seminoma testis patients under surveillance: a systematic review by the testicular cancer guidelines panel," *European Urology*, 2017.

[37] N. G. Cost, J. D. Lubahn, M. Adibi et al., "Risk stratification of pubertal children and postpubertal adolescents with clinical stage I testicular nonseminomatous germ cell tumors," *Journal of Urology*, vol. 191, no. 5, pp. 1485–1490, 2014.

[38] A. R. Shukla, C. Woodard, M. C. Carr et al., "Experience with testis sparing surgery for testicular teratoma," *Journal of Urology*, vol. 171, no. 1, pp. 161–163, 2004.

[39] B. T. Caldwell, D. T. Wilcox, and N. G. Cost, "Current Management for Pediatric Urologic Oncology," *Advances in Pediatrics*, vol. 64, no. 1, pp. 191–223, 2017.

[40] C. Nord, T. Bjøro, D. Ellingsen et al., "Gonadal hormones in long-term survivors 10 years after treatment for unilateral testicular cancer," *European Urology*, vol. 44, no. 3, pp. 322–328, 2003.

[41] F. Shaikh, P. C. Nathan, J. Hale, E. Uleryk, and L. Frazier, "Is there a role for carboplatin in the treatment of malignant germ cell tumors? A systematic review of adult and pediatric trials," *Pediatric Blood and Cancer*, vol. 60, no. 4, pp. 587–592, 2013.

[42] C. R. Nichols, B. Roth, P. Albers et al., "Active surveillance is the preferred approach to clinical stage I testicular cancer," *Journal of Clinical Oncology*, vol. 31, no. 28, pp. 3490–3493, 2013.

[43] A. A. Dahl, A. Mykletun, and S. D. Fosså, "Quality of life in survivors of testicular cancer," *Urologic Oncology: Seminars and Original Investigations*, vol. 23, no. 3, pp. 193–200, 2005.

[44] A. Mykletun, A. A. Dahl, C. F. Haaland et al., "Side effects and cancer-related stress determine quality of life in long-term survivors of testicular cancer," *Journal of Clinical Oncology*, vol. 23, no. 13, pp. 3061–3068, 2005.

[45] M. Y. Carpentier, and J. D. Fortenberry, "Romantic and sexual relationships, body image, and fertility in adolescent and young adult testicular cancer survivors: a review of the literature," *Journal of Adolescent Health*, vol. 47, no. 2, pp. 115–125, 2010.

[46] M. J. Loscalzo, and K. L. Clark, "The psychosocial context of cancer-related infertility," *Cancer Treatment and Research*, vol. 138, pp. 180–190, 2007.

[47] L. B. Travis, S. D. Fosså, S. J. Schonfeld et al., "Second cancers among 40576 testicular cancer patients: focus on long-term survivors," *JNCI: Journal of the National Cancer Institute*, vol. 97, no. 18, pp. 1354–1365, 2005.

[48] R. Abouassaly, S. D. Fossa, A. Giwercman et al., "Sequelae of treatment in long-term survivors of testis cancer," *European Urology*, vol. 60, no. 3, pp. 516–526, 2011.
[49] U. B. Chaudhary and J. R. Haldas, "Long-term complications of chemotherapy for germ cell tumours," *Drugs*, vol. 63, no. 15, pp. 1565–1577, 2003.
[50] J. A. Punyko, A. C. Mertens, J. G. Gurney et al., "Long-term medical effects of childhood and adolescent rhabdomyosarcoma: a report from the childhood cancer survivor study," *Pediatric Blood and Cancer*, vol. 44, no. 7, pp. 643–653, 2005.
[51] N. G. Cost, M. Adibi, J. D. Lubahn et al., "Effect of testicular germ cell tumor therapy on renal function," *Urology*, vol. 80, no. 3, pp. 641–648, 2012.
[52] R. Skinner, A. Parry, L. Price, M. Cole, A. W. Craft, and A. D. J. Pearson, "Persistent nephrotoxicity during 10-year follow-up after cisplatin or carboplatin treatment in childhood: relevance of age and dose as risk factors," *European Journal of Cancer*, vol. 45, no. 18, pp. 3213–3219, 2009.
[53] C. Fung et al., "Multi-institutional assessment of adverse health outcomes among North American testicular cancer survivors after modern cisplatin-based chemotherapy," *Journal of Clinical Oncology*, vol. 35, no. 11, pp. 1211–1222, 2017.
[54] B. Hayes-Lattin and C. R. Nichols, "Testicular cancer: a prototypic tumor of young adults," *Seminars in Oncology*, vol. 36, no. 5, pp. 432–438, 2009.
[55] H. Boer, J. H. Proost, J. Nuver et al., "Long-term exposure to circulating platinum is associated with late effects of treatment in testicular cancer survivors," *Annals of Oncology*, vol. 26, no. 11, pp. 2305–2310, 2015.
[56] L. B. Travis, C. Beard, J. M. Allan et al., "Testicular cancer survivorship: research strategies and recommendations," *JNCI: Journal of the National Cancer Institute*, vol. 102, no. 15, pp. 1114–1130, 2010.
[57] M. Bandak, N. Jørgensen, A. Juul et al., "Leydig cell dysfunction, systemic inflammation and metabolic syndrome in long-term testicular cancer survivors," *European Journal of Cancer*, vol. 84, pp. 9–17, 2017.
[58] L. Jacobs, and D. Vaughn, "Hypogonadism and infertility in testicular cancer survivors," *Journal of the National Comprehensive Cancer Network*, vol. 10, no. 4, pp. 558–563, 2012.
[59] M. Sprauten, M. Brydoy, H. Haugnes et al., "Longitudinal serum testosterone, luteinizing hormone, and follicle-stimulating hormone levels in a population-based sample of long-term testicular cancer survivors," *Journal of Clinical Oncology*, vol. 32, no. 6, pp. 571–578, 2014.
[60] M. Ondrusova, D. Ondrus, L. Dusek, and B. Spanikova, "Damage of hormonal function and bone metabolism in long-term survivors of testicular cancer," *Neoplasma*, vol. 56, no. 6, pp. 473–479, 2009.
[61] H. M. Parsons, L. C. Harlan, C. F. Lynch et al., "Impact of cancer on work and education among adolescent and young adult cancer survivors," *Journal of Clinical Oncology*, vol. 30, no. 19, pp. 2393–2400, 2012.
[62] E. Kharazmi, K. Hemminki, E. Pukkala et al., "Cancer risk in relatives of testicular cancer patients by histology type and age at diagnosis: a joint study from five Nordic countries," *European Urology*, vol. 68, no. 2, pp. 283–289, 2015.
[63] M. J. Murray, R. A. Huddart, and N. Coleman, "The present and future of serum diagnostic tests for testicular germ cell tumours," *Nature Reviews Urology*, vol. 13, no. 12, pp. 715–725, 2016.
[64] T. Tandstad, C. K. Kollmannsberger, B. J. Roth et al., "Practice makes perfect:the rest of the story in testicular cancer as a model curable neoplasm," *Journal of Clinical Oncology*, vol. 35, no. 31, pp. 3525–3528, 2017.

14

Initial Evaluation of Computer-Assisted Radiologic Assessment for Renal Mass Edge Detection as an Indication of Tumor Roughness to Predict Renal Cancer Subtypes

Rahul Rajendran,[1] Kevan Iffrig,[2] Deepak K Pruthi,[2] Allison Wheeler,[2] Brian Neuman,[2] Dharam Kaushik,[2] Ahmed M Mansour,[2] Karen Panetta,[3] Sos Agaian,[4] and Michael A. Liss[2,5]

[1]*University of Texas San Antonio, Department of Electrical and Computer Engineering, San Antonio, TX, USA*
[2]*University of Texas Health San Antonio, Department of Urology, San Antonio, TX, USA*
[3]*Tufts University, School of Engineering, Medford, MA, USA*
[4]*College of Staten Island, The City University of New York (CSI-CUNY), New York City, NY, USA*
[5]*University of Texas San Antonio, Department of Biology, San Antonio, TX, USA*

Correspondence should be addressed to Michael A. Liss; mliss008@gmail.com

Guest Editor: Xuanyu Chen

Objective. To develop software to assess the potential aggressiveness of an incidentally detected renal mass using images. *Methods.* Thirty randomly selected patients who underwent nephrectomy for renal cell carcinoma (RCC) had their images independently reviewed by engineers. Tumor "Roughness" was based on image algorithm of tumor topographic features visualized on computed tomography (CT) scans. Univariant and multivariant statistical analyses are utilized for analysis. *Results.* We investigated 30 subjects that underwent partial or radical nephrectomy. After excluding poor image-rendered images, 27 patients remained (benign cyst = 1, oncocytoma = 2, clear cell RCC = 15, papillary RCC = 7, and chromophobe RCC = 2). The mean roughness score for each mass is 1.18, 1.16, 1.27, 1.52, and 1.56 units, respectively ($p < 0.004$). Renal masses were correlated with tumor roughness (Pearson's, $p = 0.02$). However, tumor size itself was larger in benign tumors ($p = 0.1$). Linear regression analysis noted that the roughness score is the most influential on the model with all other demographics being equal including tumor size ($p = 0.003$). *Conclusion.* Using basic CT imaging software, tumor topography ("roughness") can be quantified and correlated with histologies such as RCC subtype and could lead to determining aggressiveness of small renal masses.

1. Introduction

Kidney cancer (renal cell carcinoma; RCC) is expected to account for 3.8% of all new cancers diagnosed in 2017 and will be responsible for an estimated 14,400 deaths [1]. The widespread use of radiologic imaging likely accounts for the increased incidence of new cancer cases diagnosed in the United States since the 1970s. Up to 40% of these incidental masses are localized, and approximately 15–20% of these small renal masses are ultimately benign. [2–7].

Small renal masses are typically not aggressive and are slow growing with low malignant potential; therefore, urologists have adapted a monitoring program to follow these masses over time called active surveillance [8]. Active surveillance heavily relies on growth of tumors in size and lacks uniform standardization usually citing every 6-month imaging [9]. While size is an important factor in renal tumors, it does not solely predict the malignant potential of a small renal mass. In a study by Daugherty et al., proposed the need for different size cutoffs for the various renal cancer subtypes indicating the clear cell cancer has the most malignant potential and should be smaller than 4 cm and chromophobe has the lowest malignant potential and could wait until 7 cm size [10]. While active surveillance in appropriately selected patients is a viable alternative to surgical intervention, it still carries the burden of uncertainty, patient anxiety, risk of disease progression, and the associated financial cost to the patient [11]. As the diagnosis of small renal masses remains primarily radiographic, the development of software to assess the potential aggressiveness of a mass would be a useful aid in the clinicians' armamentarium for shared decision-making. Previous studies have attempted to discern tumor histology through the use of current imaging techniques and automated image analysis with varying degrees of success [12–16].

In order to provide additional information on malignant potential of small renal masses without needing a biopsy, we utilize computed tomographic (CT) scans with image enhancement techniques and edge detection to calculate the surface irregularities of renal masses scheduled for partial nephrectomy. Using this technology, we create an overall "Tumor Roughness Score" (TRS) to determine the distinction of renal tumor subtype and potential aggressiveness. The initial assessment of this technique is to determine its utility in active surveillance clinical follow-up and potential research trials.

2. Methods

2.1. Patient Population. Thirty patients who underwent nephrectomy for RCC from our institution represent cases of clear cell RCC ($n = 10$), papillary RCC ($n = 10$), and chromophobe RCC ($n = 10$). Limited demographic and follow-up data were available. We excluded patients with known hereditary disorders and those deemed to have poor quality CT images.

2.2. Tumor Roughness Measure by Using Multilevel Voxel Box Counting. The "roughness" measure of a kidney tumor requires contrast-enhanced CT scans, which automatically detect, quantitatively measure, and distinguish lymph node involvement and local tumor invasion based on the tumor's topography [17]. The extensive computer simulation validates the proposed roughness measure acquisition that requires a three-stage algorithm.

2.2.1. Improving the Image Quality and Contrast. In general, the quality of images is affected by factors such as restricted image dimension and pixel resolution along with the compulsive effects caused due to noise and poor contrast. To overcome these problems, we utilize well-described enhancement methods such as guided filtering, edge enhancement, and image fusion to improve the contrast and quality of the image [18, 19].

2.2.2. Enhanced Image Multilevel Segmentation Using Its Alpha-Trimmed Mean and Variance. Multiple-level segmentation aims to obtain more than one threshold for a given image and segment the image into specific regions of interest (tumor) overlying one background [20]. The method assumes that the image contains only foreground and background information. Traditional multilevel segmentation techniques are usually susceptible to Gaussian and impulse noise. The algorithm is a modification of the multilevel thresholding technique for image segmentation that eliminates noise and performs a comprehensive search for a threshold that minimizes the intraclass (foreground and background) alpha-trimmed variance [21]. The critical component of this method is the selection of a threshold such that it separates the pixels into multiple classes by maximizing the between-class variance. The between-class variance is defined as

$$\sigma^2 = \sum_{i=1}^{M} P_i (\mu_i - \mu_T), \tag{1}$$

where σ^2 is the between-class variance, P_i is the probability of class i, μ_i is the mean value of class i, and μ_T is the total mean of the histogram.

2.2.3. Computation of the Average of Hausdorff's Measure of the Regions of Interest (Tumor). The Hausdorff measure is a scale of closeness of two groups of points that are subclasses of a metric space [22]. The measure assigns a scalar score to the similarity between two paths, data clouds, or any group of points. It is defined by equations (2) and (3). Let (A, d) be a metric space. For any subset $M \subset A$, $\operatorname{diam}(M)$ will denote the diameter of M. For any $M \subset A$, any $\delta \in [0, \infty]$, and any $\alpha \in [0, \infty]$, the outer measure is given by

$$H_\delta^\alpha(M) = \inf\left\{\sum_{i=1}^{\infty} \operatorname{diam}(M_i)^\alpha : M \subset \bigcup_i E_i \text{ and } \operatorname{diam}(M_i) < \delta\right\}. \tag{2}$$

Hence, the Hausdorff α-dimensional measure of M is

$$H^\alpha(M) = \lim_{\delta \longrightarrow 0} H_\delta^\alpha(M). \tag{3}$$

The system uses the box counting method to generate feature points based on the presence of edges in the image. Based on these feature points, the Hausdorff dimension is estimated and the slope of the best fit line generates a roughness score. In our case, Hausdorff's measure is an outer measure that calculates the roughness of each level and a combined score is generated. This score is referred to as the Tumor Roughness Score.

3. Statistical Analysis

Continuous variables were analyzed with either T-tests or ANOVA for comparisons of the five renal mass subtype groups. ANOVA post hoc analysis used least significant difference (LSD). All p values are two-tailed with a significance of $p < 0.05$, unless otherwise specified. The Pearson correlation coefficient is used to determine correlation analysis specifically between renal mass size and tumor roughness because larger tumors are more likely to be aggressive. We utilized a linear regression model to identify the factors that are most influential on predicting tumor subtype.

4. Results

Of the thirty patients selected, we excluded three patients due to poor quality CT images. We selected the data from 27 patients for analysis composed of the following subtypes: benign cyst ($n = 1$), oncocytoma ($n = 2$), clear cell RCC ($n = 15$), papillary RCC ($n = 7$), and chromophobe RCC ($n = 2$). Overall demographics include median age of 56 (IQR 48–63), median body mass index of 30.4 (27.6–32.0), median tumor size of 2.5 cm (IQR 1.8–4 cm), and four positive margins (14.8%, 4/27) and consisted of 93% men (25/27). Only one tumor was upgraded to pT3a and a total of three to pT1b, with all other tumors being pT1a. Race/ethnicity includes 59% of European descent and 41% of non-European descent. We display the demographics of each subtype and comparisons in Table 1. At a median follow-up of 3.9 years (interquartile range (IQR) 2.2, 5.4 years), there were no patient deaths. None of the patients had a documented recurrence. The majority of the cases were stage 1 disease; two cases did not have a recorded stage, and none of the subjects had documented metastasis or received neoadjuvant therapy before surgical resection (Table 1). We display an example of the adaptive segmentation technique for image processing for the calculation of the tumor roughness score in Figure 1. We obtain standard clinical CT scans and segment the kidney and tumor for surface enhancement separately. To investigate tumor irregularity, we take the tumor slice by slice using edge detection and other techniques described in Methods to obtain a 3-dimensional surface irregularity. These slices are calculated into a composite score of tumor roughness.

Of the 27 patients, tumor size associated with benign renal masses (Figure 2, $p = 0.01$). The mean roughness score for each mass is 1.18, 1.16, 1.27, 1.52, and 1.56 units, respectively (Figure 3(a), $p < 0.004$). The mean TRS did trend along the renal cancer subtype associated with tumor aggressiveness. The lowest quartile is 1.32 and would indicate the lowest risk based on this dataset and is visually displayed in the waterfall plot of TRS and colored by the corresponding tumor subtype. The stage T3a-upgraded tumor has a TRS of 1.46. The mean scores of positive and negative margins were identical ($p = 0.9$), but both above the lowest quartile. We investigated those tumors with Furman score ($n = 23$) and did not show significant differences between high grade tumors vs. low grade tumors ($p = 0.7$); however, 83% (19/23) were documented as Furman Grade 2 (low grade) and therefore, there was not an acceptable range of tumor cellular aggressiveness based on histopathology. Renal masses size correlates with tumor roughness (Pearson's, $p = 0.02$, Figure 4). However, tumor size itself was larger in benign tumors rather than malignant tumors ($p = 0.01$) giving the indication that size would not be a significant factor for aggressiveness. Linear regression analysis noted that the roughness score is the most influential on the model with all other demographics being equal including tumor size ($p = 0.003$) (Table 2).

5. Discussion

Herein, we describe a data image processing technique to provide a tumor roughness score that can have additional information beyond tumor size. Currently, physicians use tumor size and growth rate in active monitoring strategies. However, this strategy has not shown to be accurate regarding tumor subtype or tumor aggressiveness. We show that the TRS can be a useful adjunct to image assessment and has the potential for automation using artificial intelligence and machine learning. TRS provides additional information regarding tumor subtype which correlates with the traditional RCC aggressiveness without a renal mass biopsy. This information is already available to physicians; however, computer-assisted techniques remain limited for evaluation. The roughness scoring could provide information regarding those tumors that may be less aggressive from the clear cell and papillary cancers. We plan on using these techniques in future clinical trials and to potentially implement machine learning protocols, which would enhance its predictive ability with more comprehensive datasets.

We distinguish our analysis from previous manuscripts describing the surface contact area, which has also been shown to predict postoperative outcomes but was not investigated regarding tumor subtype [23, 24]. Tumor surface contact areas only represent how much tumor is touching the kidney parenchyma, and essentially, the test is an indicator of how exophytic a renal tumor is to its surrounding tissue. Our technique enhances and outlines the entire tumor surface for irregularity not based on exophytic or endophytic which is usually reserved for surgical resection planning. Another utilization of CT imaging is the texture analysis performed by Khene and colleagues noting the texture on CT could predict malignant or benign tumors as well as adherent perinephric fat during surgical intervention [25, 26]. Closure to our analysis is the work performed by Linguraru et al. who developed semiautomated quantification and classification of renal tumors to classify benign or malignant tumors especially those patients with genetic abnormalities prone for forming multiple kidney tumors [27]. Considerable effort has been placed to detect papillary renal cancer from clear cell including subtypes based on contrast enhancement largely because papillary renal neoplasms have a poor or delayed enhancement that can be difficult to discern from hyperdense renal cysts [28, 29]. In addition, papillary subtype tumors are less likely to have a thick pseudocapsule around the tumor which would coincide with having more irregular edges to the tumor [30]. Our technique could assist with this particular question in more extensive studies.

Data science with the use of deep learning based-automated methods is ever increasing and merging with clinical care [31]. Other authors have utilized similar techniques for image analysis. Pattern recognition is essential in radiology; however, utilization of quantitative image analysis will provide objective additional data on

TABLE 1: Demographics by tumor subtype.

Renal cancer subtype	Benign cyst	Oncocytoma	Chromophobe	Clear cell	Papillary	p value
Number of patients (N)	1	2	2	15	7	
Age	60	45 (42–45)	54 (51–54)	56 (42–66)	57 (51–63)	0.9
Body mass index	24.9	26.3 (24.1–26.3)	31.8 (31.3–31.8)	30.1 (27.3–31.6)	32.01 (29.9–40.7)	0.05
Race/ethnicity (white %)	1/1 (100%)	1/2 (50%)	0/2 (0%)	9/15 (60%)	5/7 (71%)	0.4
Biologic gender (male %)	0/1 (0%)	1/2 (50%)	2/2(100%)	15/15 (100%)	7/7 (100%)	0.001
Tumor size (cm)	1.8	5.3 (4.0–5.3)	4.45 (4.4–4.45)	2.3 (1.5–3.8)	2.5 (2.0–2.7)	0.01
Tumor stage (stage 3)	0/1 (0%)	0/2 (0%)	0/2 (0%)	1/15 (7%)	0/7 (0%)	0.3
Tumor surface roughness	1.18	1.16 (1.12–1.16)	1.27 (1.21–1.27)	1.52 (1.38–1.55)	1.56 (1.43–1.66)	0.004

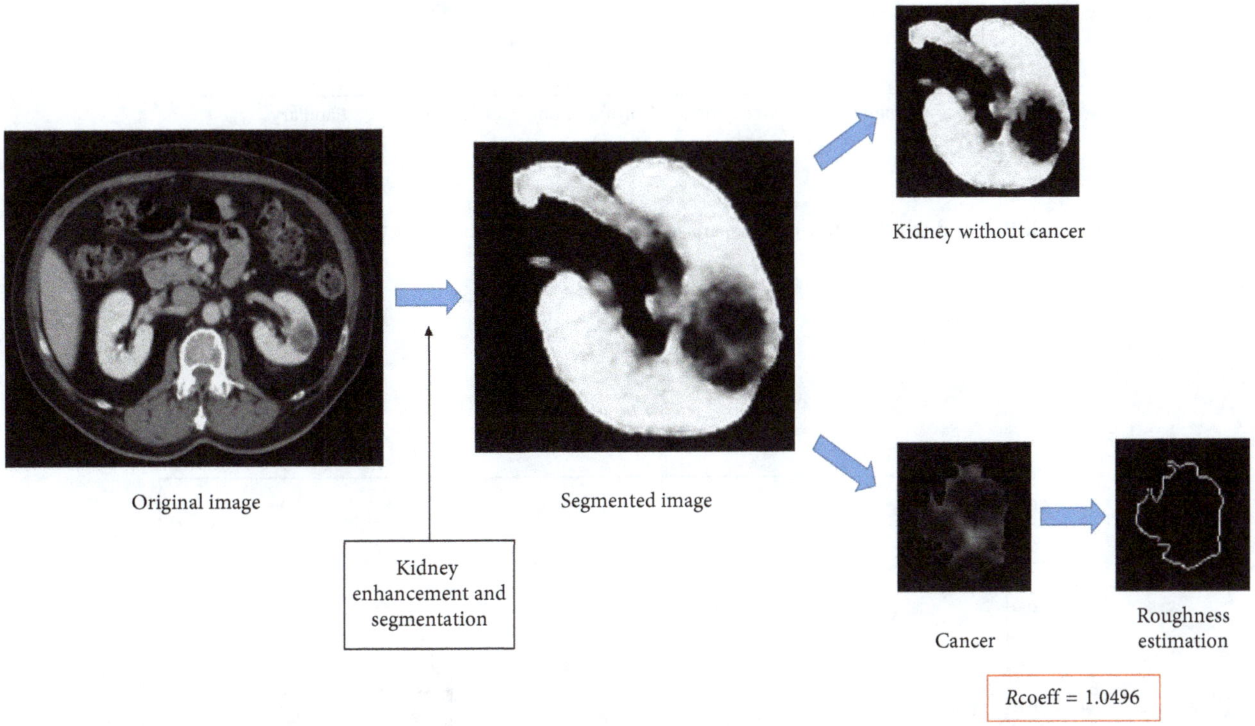

(a)

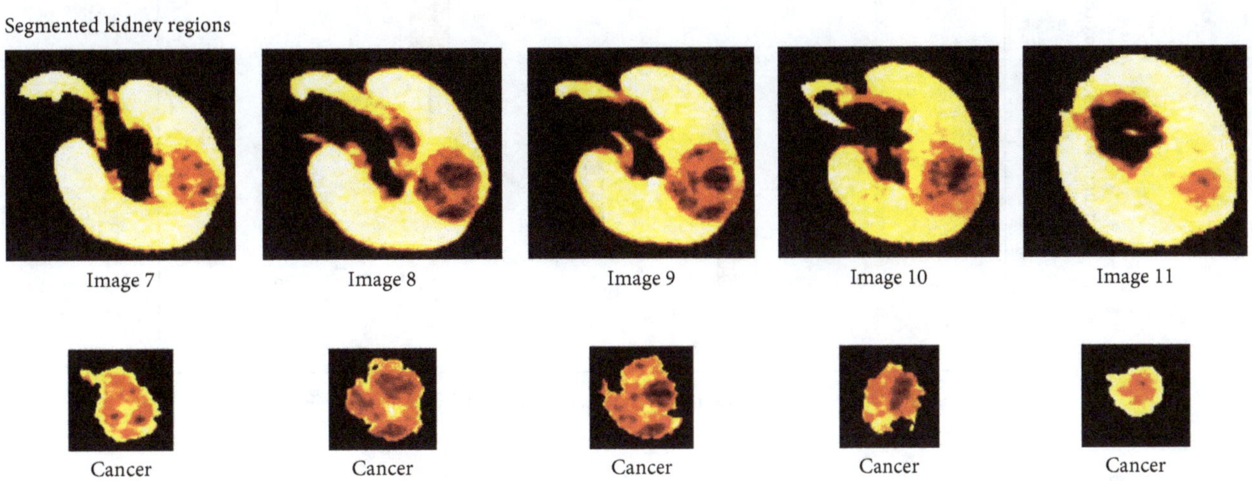

(b)

FIGURE 1: Tumor roughness score image analysis. Adaptive segmentation technique developed to segment the kidney and tumor for surface enhancement and investigate tumor irregularity. The summary irregularity score ($R_{avg} = 1.0413$) is averaged across all segments of the tumor.

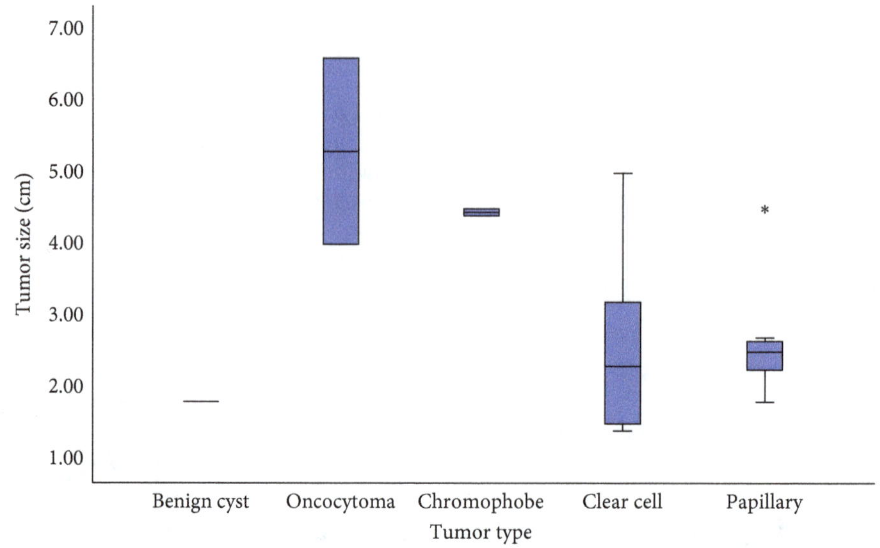

FIGURE 2: Box and whisker plot of renal mass size compared to the renal tumor subtype for trend.

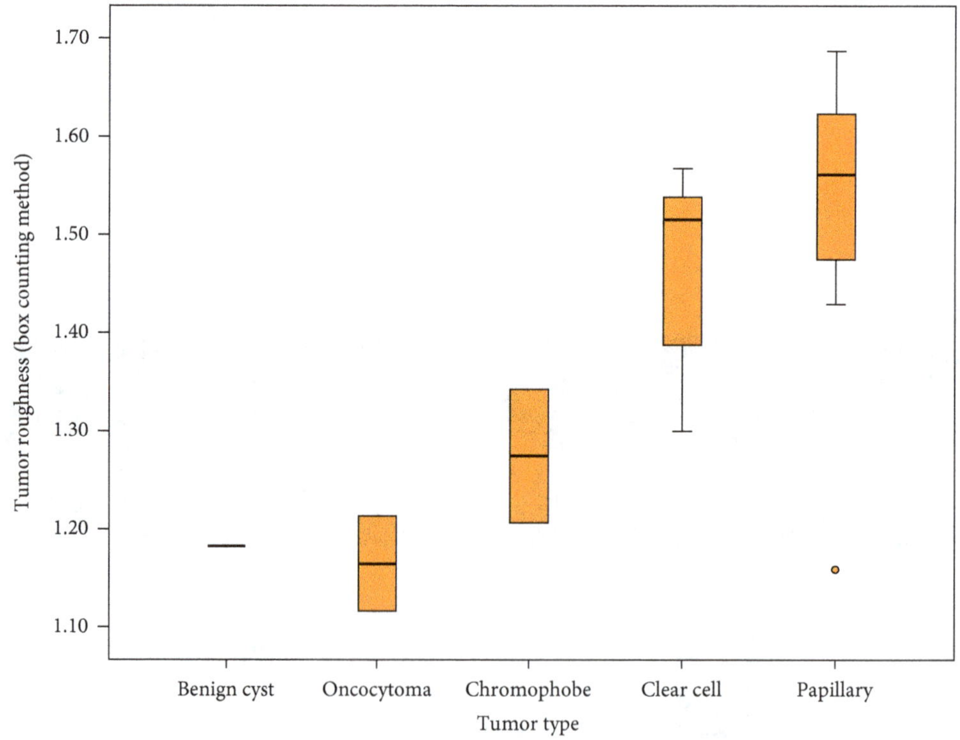

(a)

FIGURE 3: Continued.

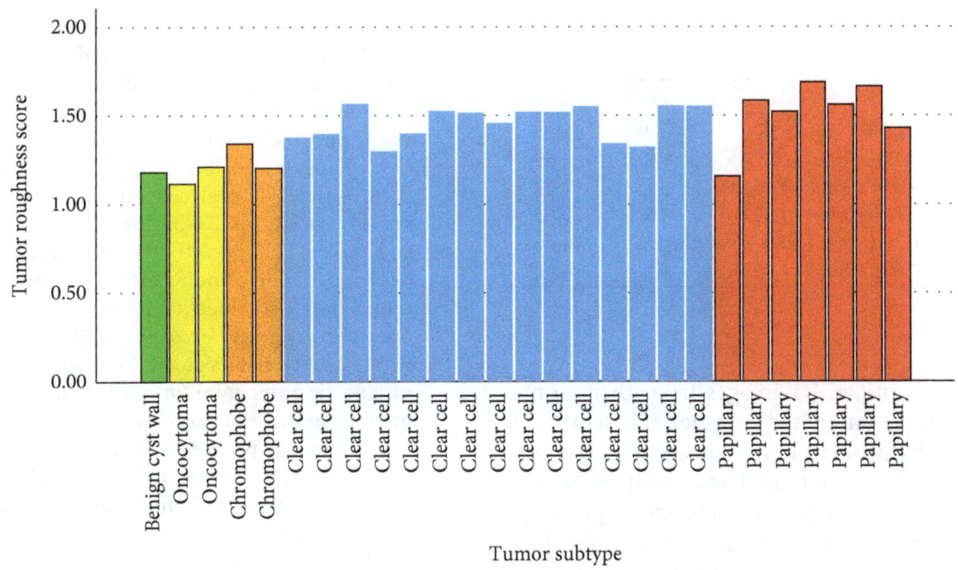

(b)

FIGURE 3: (a) Box and whisker plot displaying the tumor surface roughness score compared to each renal mass subtype for trend. (b) Waterfall plot for tumor roughness score with each renal tumor subtype listing less aggressive tumors to the left and more aggressive tumors to the right.

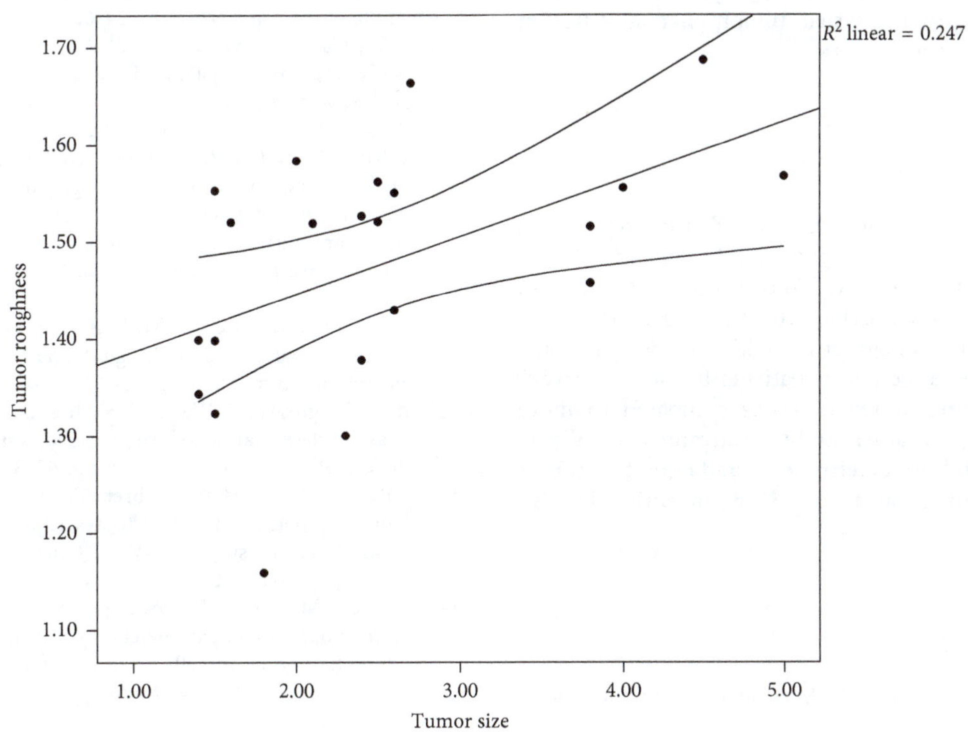

FIGURE 4: Scatter plot noting the correlation between renal mass size and tumor roughness score (Pearson's $p = 0.02$).

tumor aggressiveness. These techniques have been applied in lung cancer and others [32–34]. A review on other techniques for small renal mass characterization will be utilized in further evaluation and improvements [35, 36]. We seek to add to the expanding literature using image analysis techniques to utilize data science to implement actionable data to physicians and patients.

There are some limitations to this study. First, while we identified some potentially significant associations, this is a pilot study in a small cohort of patients without validated findings. Secondly, our cohort included CT scans performed at different institutions using different CT scanners, which could insert variability into the quality of the roughness score. However, in practical use, this would be the norm as

Table 2: Multivariable linear regression model or the outcome of kidney cancer subtype.

Demographic	Coefficient (95% CI)	t score	p value
Constant	2.59 (−5.8–0.58)	−1.709	0.1
Age	0.004 (0.17–0.025)	0.9	0.69
Body mass index	0.049 (0.008–0.107)	2.7	0.09
White (yes vs. no)	0.114 (0.364–0.592)	0.5	0.62
Tumor size	1.71 (−0.351–0.009)	−1.2	0.06
Roughness score	2.601 (0.977–4.225)	4.2	0.003

other clinicians would utilize CT images from their home institutions. We assume that the tumor roughness score will have more applicability in small renal masses to have more influence on future decision making. Unfortunately, we are unable to compare our method with methods of previous authors because specific algorithms have not been published [37]. We acknowledge the fast moving field of image analysis and new techniques to separate target lesions in imaging with new techniques such as topographical assessments [38]. We included all renal mass types because until surgical removal, the subtype is completely unknown, giving us impetus for this study. We are currently developing validation profiles of our work and development of AI technology that can provide visual tumor characteristics in quantitative form as a biomarker.

6. Conclusion

Using existing CT imaging in this proof of concept study, renal mass tumoral topography can be quantified and correlated with histology and biological aggressiveness in small renal masses. We provide preliminary data to suggest the use of imaging topography could provide additional information in the selection of patients for active surveillance or monitoring of renal masses compared to more aggressive therapy. A larger study is warranted to validate these findings and to determine if radiographic tumor surface analysis can obviate the need for conventional serum or urine biomarkers.

Acknowledgments

This work was supported by the SA Cancer Council Circle of Hope.

References

[1] R. L. Siegel, K. D. Miller, and A. Jemal, "Cancer statistics, 2019," *CA: A Cancer Journal for Clinicians*, vol. 69, no. 1, pp. 7–34, 2019.

[2] D. C. Johnson, J. Vukina, A. B. Smith et al., "Preoperatively misclassified, surgically removed benign renal masses: a systematic review of surgical series and United States population level burden estimate," *Journal of Urology*, vol. 193, no. 1, pp. 30–35, 2015.

[3] C. J. Kane, K. Mallin, J. Ritchey, M. R. Cooperberg, and P. R. Carroll, "Renal cell cancer stage migration," *Cancer*, vol. 113, no. 1, pp. 78–83, 2008.

[4] A. Kutikov, L. K. Fossett, P. Ramchandani et al., "Incidence of benign pathologic findings at partial nephrectomy for solitary renal mass presumed to be renal cell carcinoma on preoperative imaging," *Urology*, vol. 68, no. 4, pp. 737–740, 2006.

[5] B. R. Lane, D. Babineau, M. W. Kattan et al., "A preoperative prognostic nomogram for solid enhancing renal tumors 7 cm or less amenable to partial nephrectomy," *Journal of Urology*, vol. 178, no. 2, pp. 429–434, 2007.

[6] A. Mathew, S. S. Devesa, J. F. Fraumeni Jr., and W.-H. Chow, "Global increases in kidney cancer incidence, 1973–1992," *European Journal of Cancer Prevention*, vol. 11, no. 2, pp. 171–178, 2002.

[7] M. M. Nguyen, I. S. Gill, and L. M. Ellison, "The evolving presentation of renal carcinoma in the United States: trends from the surveillance, epidemiology, and end results program," *Journal of Urology*, vol. 176, no. 6, pp. 2397–2400, 2006.

[8] I. S. Gill, M. Aron, D. A. Gervais, and M. A. S. Jewett, "Clinical practice. Small renal mass," *New England Journal of Medicine*, vol. 362, no. 7, pp. 624–634, 2010.

[9] C. W. Liaw, J. S. Winoker, and R. Mehrazin, "Imaging protocols for active surveillance in renal cell carcinoma," *Current Urology Reports*, vol. 19, no. 10, p. 81, 2018.

[10] M. Daugherty, D. Sedaghatpour, O. Shapiro, S. Vourganti, A. Kutikov, and G. Bratslavsky, "The metastatic potential of renal tumors: influence of histologic subtypes on definition of small renal masses, risk stratification, and future active surveillance protocols," *Urologic Oncology: Seminars and Original Investigations*, vol. 35, no. 4, pp. 153 e115–153 e120, 2017.

[11] S. Campbell, R. G. Uzzo, M. E. Allaf et al., "Renal mass and localized renal cancer: AUA guideline," *Journal of Urology*, vol. 198, no. 3, pp. 520–529, 2017.

[12] M. G. Linguraru, S. Wang, F. Shah et al., "Automated noninvasive classification of renal cancer on multiphase CT," *Medical Physics*, vol. 38, no. 10, pp. 5738–5746, 2011.

[13] R. Papalia, A. L. De Castro Abreu, V. Panebianco et al., "Novel kidney segmentation system to describe tumour location for nephron-sparing surgery," *World Journal of Urology*, vol. 33, no. 6, pp. 865–871, 2015.

[14] F. Chen, M. Gulati, D. Hwang et al., "Voxel-based whole-lesion enhancement parameters: a study of its clinical value in differentiating clear cell renal cell carcinoma from renal oncocytoma," *Abdominal Radiology*, vol. 42, no. 2, pp. 552–560, 2017.

[15] H. Coy, J. R. Young, M. L. Douek, M. S. Brown, J. Sayre, and S. S. Raman, "Quantitative computer-aided diagnostic algorithm for automated detection of peak lesion attenuation in differentiating clear cell from papillary and chromophobe renal cell carcinoma, oncocytoma, and fat-poor angiomyolipoma on multiphasic multidetector computed tomography," *Abdominal Radiology*, vol. 42, no. 7, pp. 1919–1928, 2017.

[16] N. J. Farber, Y. Wu, L. Zou, P. Belani, and E. A. Singer, "Challenges in RCC imaging: renal insufficiency, post-operative surveillance, and the role of radiomics," *Kidney Cancer Journal*, vol. 13, no. 4, pp. 84–90, 2015.

[17] J. W. Cho, S. C. Choi, J. Y. Jang et al., "Lymph node metastases in esophageal carcinoma: an endoscopist's view," *Clinical Endoscopy*, vol. 47, no. 6, pp. 523–429, 2014.
[18] K. He, J. Sun, and X. Tang, "Guided image filtering," *IEEE Transactions on Pattern Analysis and Machine Intelligence*, vol. 35, no. 6, pp. 1397–1409, 2013.
[19] K. Panetta, Y. Yicong Zhou, S. Agaian, and H. Hongwei Jia, "Nonlinear unsharp masking for mammogram enhancement," *IEEE Transactions on Information Technology in Biomedicine*, vol. 15, no. 6, pp. 918–928, 2011.
[20] S. Arora, J. Acharya, A. Verma, and P. K. Panigrahi, "Multilevel thresholding for image segmentation through a fast statistical recursive algorithm," *Pattern Recognition Letters*, vol. 29, no. 2, pp. 119–125, 2008.
[21] K. M. Kamath, R. Rajendran, K. Panetta, and S. Agaian, "A human visual based binarization technique for histological images," in *Proceedings of the Mobile Multimedia/Image Processing, Security, and Applications*, Anaheim, CA, USA, April 2017.
[22] I. Banič and A. Taranenko, "Measuring closeness of graphs—the Hausdorff distance," *Bulletin of the Malaysian Mathematical Sciences Society*, vol. 40, no. 1, pp. 75–95, 2017.
[23] V. Ficarra, A. Crestani, R. Bertolo et al., "Tumour contact surface area as a predictor of postoperative complications and renal function in patients undergoing partial nephrectomy for renal tumours," *BJU International*, vol. 123, no. 4, pp. 639–645, 2019.
[24] S. Leslie, I. S. Gill, A. L. de Castro Abreu et al., "Renal tumor contact surface area: a novel parameter for predicting complexity and outcomes of partial nephrectomy," *European Urology*, vol. 66, no. 5, pp. 884–893, 2014.
[25] Z. E. Khene, K. Bensalah, A. Largent et al., "Role of quantitative computed tomography texture analysis in the prediction of adherent perinephric fat," *World Journal of Urology*, vol. 36, no. 10, pp. 1635–1642, 2018.
[26] B. A. Varghese, F. Chen, D. H. Hwang et al., "Differentiation of predominantly solid enhancing lipid-poor renal cell masses by use of contrast-enhanced CT: evaluating the role of texture in tumor subtyping," *American Journal of Roentgenology*, vol. 211, no. 6, pp. W288–W296, 2018.
[27] M. G. Linguraru, S. Wang, F. Shah et al., "Computer-aided renal cancer quantification and classification from contrast-enhanced CT via histograms of curvature-related features," in *Proceedings of the 2009 Annual International Conference of the IEEE Engineering in Medicine and Biology Society*, pp. 6679–6682, Minneapolis, MN, USA, September 2009.
[28] N. D. Egbert, E. M. Caoili, R. H. Cohan et al., "Differentiation of papillary renal cell carcinoma subtypes on CT and MRI," *American Journal of Roentgenology*, vol. 201, no. 2, pp. 347–355, 2013.
[29] R. P. Kopp, L. Aganovic, K. L. Palazzi, F. H. Cassidy, K. Sakamoto, and I. H. Derweesh, "Differentiation of clear from non-clear cell renal cell carcinoma using CT washout formula," *Canadian Journal of Urology*, vol. 20, no. 3, pp. 6790–6797, 2013.
[30] J. M. Jacob, S. R. Williamson, D. D. Gondim et al., "Characteristics of the peritumoral pseudocapsule vary predictably with histologic subtype of T1 renal neoplasms," *Urology*, vol. 86, no. 5, pp. 956–961, 2015.
[31] L. Carin and M. J. Pencina, "On deep learning for medical image analysis," *Journal of the American Medical Association*, vol. 320, no. 11, pp. 1192-1193, 2018.
[32] G. Buizza, I. Toma-Dasu, M. Lazzeroni et al., "Early tumor response prediction for lung cancer patients using novel longitudinal pattern features from sequential PET/CT image scans," *Physica Medica*, vol. 54, pp. 21–29, 2018.
[33] W. Sun, M. Jiang, J. Dang, P. Chang, and F. F. Yin, "Effect of machine learning methods on predicting NSCLC overall survival time based on radiomics analysis," *Radiation Oncology*, vol. 13, no. 1, p. 197, 2018.
[34] F. L. Bayisa, X. Liu, A. Garpebring, and J. Yu, "Statistical learning in computed tomography image estimation," *Medical Physics*, vol. 45, no. 12, pp. 5450–5460, 2018.
[35] K. Sasaguri and N. Takahashi, "CT and MR imaging for solid renal mass characterization," *European Journal of Radiology*, vol. 99, pp. 40–54, 2018.
[36] S. Hemachander, A. Verma, S. Arora, and P. K. Panigrahi, "Locally adaptive block thresholding method with continuity constraint," *Pattern Recognition Letters*, vol. 28, no. 1, pp. 119–124, 2007.
[37] M. Srivastava, S. K. Singh, and P. K. Panigrahi, "A semi-automated statistical algorithm for object separation," *Circuits, Systems, and Signal Processing*, vol. 32, no. 6, pp. 3059–3078, 2013.
[38] H. Cui, X. Wang, J. Zhou et al., "A topo-graph model for indistinct target boundary definition from anatomical images," *Computer Methods and Programs in Biomedicine*, vol. 159, pp. 211–222, 2018.

15

Understanding the Impact of Urinary Incontinence in Persons with Dementia: Development of an Interdisciplinary Service Model

Patrick Juliebø-Jones,[1,2,3] **Elizabeth Coulthard**,[1,3] **Elizabeth Mallam**,[1] **Hilary Archer**,[1] **and Marcus J. Drake**[2,3]

[1]*Bristol Brain Centre, Southmead Hospital, Bristol, UK*
[2]*Bristol Urological Institute, Southmead Hospital, Bristol, UK*
[3]*University of Bristol, Bristol, UK*

Correspondence should be addressed to Patrick Juliebø-Jones; patrick.jones1@nhs.net

Academic Editor: Jason M. Hafron

Introduction. Prevalence of urinary symptoms such as incontinence (UI) in patients with dementia is estimated to exceed 50%. The resultant psychological and socio-economic burden can be substantial. Our aim was to develop a dedicated urology service within a cognitive impairment clinic in order to treat and better understand the bothersome urinary symptoms suffered by persons with dementia. *Methods.* Patients attending this clinic were invited to be assessed and interviewed by urologist, together with their family and/or carer. In addition, formal history, examination and relevant investigations, themes of importance such as quality of life, and select question items were drawn from validated questionnaires. Multidisciplinary team (MDT) meeting was carried out on the same day. Outcomes of the first 75 patients with UI and dementia have been reported. *Results.* Average age was 70 years (range 58–98). Majority of persons had a diagnosis of Alzheimer's disease ($n = 43$, 57%). Average score for how much urine leakage interferes with everyday life was 7.7/10 (range 2–10). 58.7% ($n = 44$) revealed some degree of sleep disturbance due to UI. 83% ($n = 62$) stated daily activities were limited due to UI. Two-thirds of persons with dementia ($n = 50$) stated their bladder problem makes them feel anxious. 88% ($n = 67$) felt the topic was socially embarrassing. All carers stated that the person's continence issues affect the care they provide. Less than one-third of carers (30.7%, $n = 23$) were aware of or had been in contact with any bladder and bowel community service. More than half of the carers ($n = 46$, 65%) were concerned incontinence may be a principal reason for future nursing home admission. *Conclusion.* UI can be distressing for persons with dementia. Care partners were concerned about loss of independence and early nursing home admission. Awareness of bladder and bowel services should be increased.

1. Introduction

The psychological and socio-economic impact of urinary incontinence (UI) can be very burdensome for patients, families, and carers. These effects are magnified when dementia is also present. Dementia will affect over 1 million people in the UK by 2021 and the prevalence of concomitant urinary symptoms such as incontinence is estimated to exceed 50% [1]. The prevalence is likely underestimated given that many are believed to not report it. Urinary incontinence (UI), defined as the complaint of involuntary loss of urine, negatively affects quality of life [2]. It is now widely recognised as a key risk factor and precipitant for premature admission to nursing home (NH) residency [3]. Independent of any physical comorbidities, dementia is also a risk factor for hospital admission [4]. However, despite the reality that bothersome urinary symptoms in this population represent a pressing research priority, as recognised by the World Health Organisation (WHO), such activity is lacking and available evidence to direct treatment pathways remains under-reported [5, 6].

Our aim was to develop and pilot a dedicated urology service within a cognitive impairment clinic led by neurologists. The principal objective of this was to improve understanding and treatment of bothersome urinary symptoms suffered by these patients, with a principal focus on patients with dementia and UI. To our knowledge, this has not been described previously. The findings of the first 75 persons with dementia and UI have been reported as well as the views of their carer.

1.1. Action Plan for Implementing the Intervention. The setting was a dedicated cognitive impairment outpatient clinic at the Bristol Brain Centre. This established service already implemented a multidisciplinary approach with involvement of psychologist, psychiatrist, specialist nursing team, and academic researchers in dementia.

Such as the range of complex needs in patients with dementia, there is now increasing recognition regarding the merits of such an approach in their healthcare [7]. It also allows the clinician to focus more on their area of expertise [8]. Chase et al. recently published findings from their study, which incorporated semistructured interviews, focus group discussions, and shadowing of caregivers. The conclusions revealed lack of existing integrated frameworks and the significant day-to-day challenges faced by practitioners in this regard [8].

The first step in the development of such an approach was for the urologist to adopt an observer role in all parts of this existing clinic over a three-month period. Collett et al. outlined recommendations for setting up a multidisciplinary clinic and how can it be built over time with new specialities becoming involved. The authors highlighted the importance of team members understanding the roles of their colleagues in different specialities [9]. This period of familiarisation allowed learning of the typical clinical cases attending for assessment and review as well as the organisation of the clinic.

Later, persons attending this clinic, together with their carer(s), were invited to be assessed and interviewed by a urologist. In addition, formal history, exam and relevant investigations, themes of importance such as impact on quality of life, and select question items were drawn from validated questionnaires such as the King's Health Questionnaire (KHQ) and relevant International Consultation on Incontinence Questionnaire (ICIQ) modules such as ICIQ-short form (SF) [10–14]. A round table discussion with relevant continence experts (from disciplines of urology, nursing, dementia, and elderly medicine) had taken place at start of the project to determine the themes and areas of importance. These were determined to be the interruption to activities of daily life (physical, social, and sleep), unmet care needs, stigma, and carer burden. This was led and coordinated by a research fellow in dementia. Care partners were also involved. The items generated were consistent with a scoping review carried out by Kalánková et al. and a previous European cross-sectional survey [15, 16]. This study was carried out as part of an audit of service provision and therefore no specific ethical approval was deemed to be required. The Standard for QUality Improvement Reporting Excellence (SQUIRE) checklist was adhered to [17]. Clinician funding was supplied in select cases by National Institute Health Research (NIHR).

1.2. Services Offered. For persons with dementia attending the clinic, the urologist routinely carried out history, physical exam, and basic tests including assessment to rule out any reversible causes of UI such as infection, constipation, restricted mobility, pharmacotherapy, and excess fluid [18]. Medication advice could be given and summarised for the persons, their carer(s), and primary care team. In persons where special tests, e.g., uroflowmetry, were required, these were referred internally. Bladder diaries are a validated tool to aid the quantitative measurement of micturition and temporal micturition patterns [19]. Persons with sufficient cognitive function were issued with such a diary to complete and return. Each person was kept on a prospective database and followed up as required. Also, recorded were the responses given to the predetermined question items drawn from the aforementioned validated questionnaires. For patients with severe cognitive impairment (MoCA < 12), the questionnaire responses for the persons were gathered by carer proxy. All persons with dementia attended the clinic with a carer and they were also present during the consultation. Carers were also asked select question items, such as whether continence care affects care they provide (and if so, to what degree), contact with community support, and any concerns regarding whether UI may be the principal reason for future NH admission.

Referrals and liaison with bladder and bowel team were made if needed. All the cases were routinely discussed in a multidisciplinary team (MDT) format at the end of the clinic. Figure 1 provides overview of the clinic pathway.

1.3. Evolution of Service and Challenges. In order to help recruitment and support identification of persons more suitable for assessment, electronic case notes were screened in advance, for example, if previous referrals from primary care or inpatient care summaries had mentioned urinary problems, but no formal evaluation had taken place. These were then highlighted to other team members as part of the clinic briefing. In addition, being asked by neurologists, persons were also asked at the end of Montreal Cognitive Assessment (MoCA) by the psychologist and given a large print card as a kind of "passport" reminder. A checklist sheet was later developed and held at reception to ensure the person was seen by the urology if required. The urologist later goes to spend time with the bladder and bowel team to learn their perspective on this issue as it emerged how valuable this resource was.

2. Results

The overall sample size was 150 (75 persons with dementia and 75 carers. Average age of persons with dementia was 72 years (range 56–98). The majority of persons with dementia

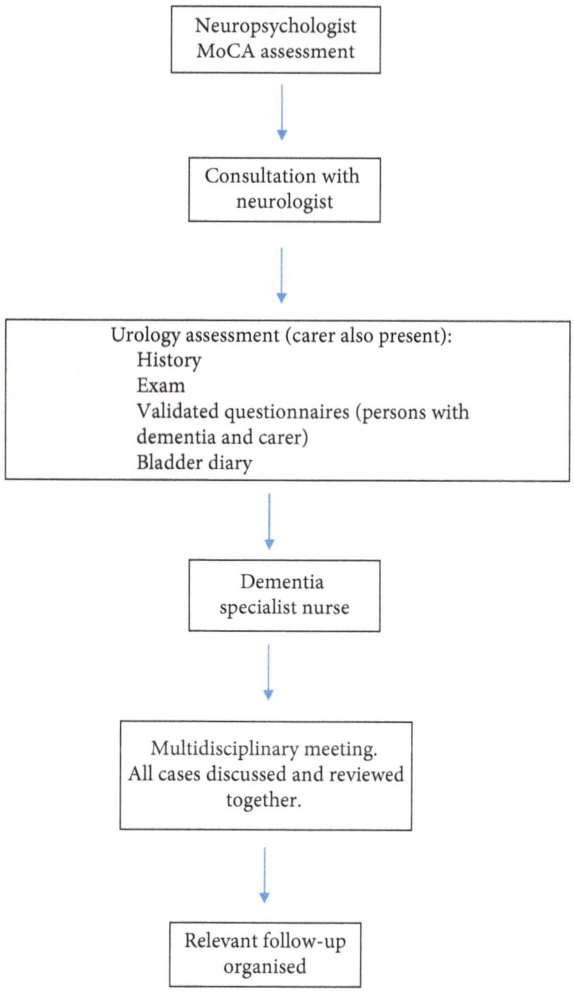

FIGURE 1: Flow diagram of the clinic set-up.

(94.7%, $n = 71$) lived in the community with carer support. Table 1 outlines baseline information. Tables 2 and 3 show responses to question items from persons with dementia and their carers, respectively. In addition to these results, 88% ($n = 67$) of persons with dementia felt the topic was socially embarrassing for them to discuss, both among their families, and with health professionals. Interestingly, those patients who responded that UI was not embarrassing had lived with the condition for a long time and stated that, in the beginning, it had indeed been very embarrassing. More than half of the patients (60%, $n = 45$) reported that they had not disclosed their struggles with incontinence previously. 34% had concurrent faecal incontinence.

Family caregivers were able to describe in great detail the first-time leakage had occurred in a public place. While all respondents stated that continence issues affected the care they provided; this was heightened in those who could not afford additional (self-funded) assistance compared to those who could (6.9/10 versus 8.3/10). Those from more socio-economically privileged backgrounds appeared to manage better as extra care and supplies could supplement standard resources.

3. Discussion

3.1. Key Findings. This coordinated approach to the management of dementia and bothersome urinary tract symptoms has revealed how much persons with dementia can struggle with UI. The disruption to daily life includes sleep, normal daily outings, and relationships with their community. This affects not only the person with dementia but also the care, which family and carers provide which was confirmed by everyone. Bladder and bowel continence teams appear to be an under-recognised resource, and therefore, it is key that awareness is raised accordingly.

3.2. How Do These Findings Compare with Relevant Literature? Our findings were consistent with previous research by Engberg et al. with regard to the range of self-care behaviours persons with dementia adopt such as strict fluid restriction in an attempt to remedy UI [20]. The burden of UI appeared under-reported due to the common misconception that it is an inevitable part of the disease and ageing process and that no treatment strategies are available.

Samuelsson et al. reported how heavy a toll the financial elements of continence care can have [21]. We also found that worries regarding access to continence products and the associated financial burden weighed heavily in the minds of many family caregivers. One of the basic tests we performed included measurement of postvoid residual bladder volumes with a mobile scanner to rule out chronic urinary retention. While the latter is not generally clinically significant, sometimes it can be. Parson et al. evaluated feasibility of intermittent self-catheterisation (ISC) in elderly patients and reported the overall success rate was 82% in patients over 65 years of age [22]. In carefully selected cases, ISC can also be performed by a carer. While ISC may not be an option in patients with severe cognitive impairment, we found that patients with earlier/milder disease appear to still be suitable candidates. Research on continence in patients with cognitive impairment reveals that for disclosure of issues surrounding UI, the self-referral rate for UI among the elderly is lower [23]. Drennan et al. recorded that carers would try to preserve patient dignity and therefore tended to under-report the extent of the problem(s) [5]. We also found that time and active listening were required for patients to reveal continence problems. Cole et al. added to this by finding that patients often prefer not to complain as they do not want to burden the carer [23]. Of the many stigmas held by individuals and society, the shame associated with lack of self-control of urine and faeces can be very powerful [24], such as the human response to such a matter that powerful emotions and tensions can be triggered [25]. The impact of shame and embarrassment highlighted in these studies was consistent with our findings in this clinic.

3.3. Limitations and Future Research. Our study does not provide any estimate of prevalence of bothersome urinary symptoms among dementia patients. Questions asked during the assessment were drawn from validated

Table 1: Summary of demographics and baseline information.

Overall sample size	150
Persons with dementia	75
Carer	75
Mean age	72 years (range 56–98)
Male-to-female ratio	1.6 : 1
Nursing home residency/community dwelling	4 (5.3%)/71 (94.7%)
Dementia type	
(i) Alzheimer's	57% ($n = 43$)
(ii) FTD	16% ($n = 12$)
(iii) Lewy body	10.7% ($n = 8$)
(iv) Vascular	9.3% ($n = 7$)
(v) Others, e.g., dementia associated with multiple sclerosis (MS) or progressive supranuclear palsy (PSP).	5.3% ($n = 4$)
Mean MoCA score	18/30 (range 9–25)
Distibution of MoCA scores	
Mild (20–24)	40% ($n = 30$)
Moderate (13–20)	55% ($n = 41$)
Severe (<12)	5%. ($n = 4$)
Concurrent faecal incontinence and urinary incontinence	34% ($n = 18$)
Transient causes	
Urinary tract infection	11% ($n = 8$)
Constipation	35% ($n = 26$)
Urinary retention	4% ($n = 3$)
Patients requiring changes to medication	39% ($n = 29$)
Referrals to bladder and bowel services	44% ($n = 33$)

Table 2: Responses of persons with dementia to question items.

Question	Response
How often do you leak urine?	
(i) About once a week	12% ($n = 9$)
(ii) Two or three times a week	21.3% ($n = 16$)
(iii) About once a day	18.7 ($n = 14$)
(iv) Several times a day	30.7% ($n = 23$)
(v) All the time	17.3% ($n = 13$)
How much urine do you leak?	
(i) Small amount	54.7% ($n = 41$)
(ii) Moderate amount	27% ($n = 21$)
(iii) Large amount	17.3% ($n = 13$)
How much does leaking of urine interferes with everyday life? (on a scale of 1–10)	Mean score 7.7/10 (range 2–10)
Does urine leakage interfere with your sleep?	
(i) Slightly	14.7% ($n = 11$)
(ii) Moderately	18.7% ($n = 14$)
(iii) A lot	25.3% ($n = 19$)
(iv) Not at all	31.3% ($n = 31$)
Are your daily activities limited due to incontinence?	
(i) Slightly	17.3% ($n = 13$)
(ii) Moderately	24% ($n = 18$)
(iii) A lot	41.3% ($n = 31$)
(iv) Not at all	17.3% ($n = 13$)
How much does your bladder problem make you feel more anxious?	
(i) Slightly	14.7% ($n = 11$)
(ii) Moderately	30.7% ($n = 23$)
(iii) A lot	21.3% ($n = 16$)
(iv) Not at all	33.3% ($n = 25$)
Is continence a socially embarrassing topic to discuss?	Yes = 88% ($n = 67$)

Table 3: Responses of carers to question items.

Question	Response
Does continence care affect the care you provide?	Yes = 100% (n = 75)
How much does incontinence affect the care you provide? (on a scale of 1 to 10)	7.7/10 (range 5–10)
Are you concerned that UI may be a principal reason for future nursing home admission?	Yes = 65% (n = 46)
Are you aware of or have you been in contact with community bladder and bowel services?	Yes = 30.7% (n = 23)
Would more awareness and teaching on continence care be beneficial?	Yes = 100% (n = 75)

questionnaires, which is a strength. However, in four persons with severe cognitive impairment (MoCA score <12), questions were answered by carer proxy. While this was only required in a few cases, this can introduce bias. This is a recognised difficulty in assessments related to quality of life in persons with dementia. Boyer et al. reported the potential discrepancies between persons and their carer proxy [26]. A novel solution for this to improve assessment of continence issues in persons with dementia is the "ICIQ Cog." This is a patient-reported outcome measure (PROM) specifically designed for the assessment of urinary tract symptoms in patients with cognitive impairment, which is currently under development. While its properties have been finalised, it has yet to be formally validated for clinical use [13]. The final version will serve as useful outcome measure in future studies, particularly when assessing continence interventions. Given how valuable the use of a formal bladder diary is in the assessment of patients with bothersome urinary symptoms, development of a modified version for application in cognitively impaired patients, which can be completed by care giver, would be of benefit [19]. A validated pad diary would also be a valuable resource. While there is still value in using the current version available, our experience highlighted it is more suited to those with milder cognitive impairment.

Given the important role of community bladder and bowel services and the financial pressures faced by the National Health Service (NHS), it is imperative that such services are appreciated and supported through this.

This project, while limited by small numbers of persons with dementia, shows the potential benefits of a coordinated approach between specialities. In financially pressured healthcare systems, the next step in our hospital is for the development of a tailored referral pathway between neurologists and urologists to identify those persons with dementia who would benefit most from urology input. In addition to this, establishment of a referral pathway between neurology services and the bladder and bowel community services is also considered to be a valuable initiative to pursue.

4. Conclusion

In persons with dementia who develop UI, it can be distressing and disrupt many facets of daily life. Moreover, it can serve as the precursor to loss of independence and even early nursing home admission. Bladder and bowel services are invaluable and awareness of the benefits of such resources should be increased across primary and secondary care. Development and expansion of models like this one and improved interspeciality referral pathways are important steps improving care.

Acknowledgments

Patrick Juliebø-Jones had his salary funded by the National Institute of Health Research (NIHR).

References

[1] I. Milsom, D. Altman, R. Cartwright et al., "Epidemiology of urinary incontinence (UI) and other lower urinary tract symptoms (LUTS), pelvic organ prolapse (POP) and anal incontinence (AI)," in *Incontinence: 5th International Consultation on Incontinence, Paris, February 2012*, pp. 15–107, ICUD-EAU, Paris, France, 2013.

[2] D. Bedretdinova, X. Fritel, M. Zins, and V. Ringa, "The effect of urinary incontinence on health-related quality of life: is it similar in men and women?" *Urology*, vol. 91, pp. 83–89, 2016.

[3] R. Andel, K. Hyer, and A. Slack, "Risk factors for nursing home placement in older adults with and without dementia," *Journal of Aging and Health*, vol. 19, no. 2, pp. 213–228, 2007.

[4] A. Sommerlad, G. Perera, C. Mueller et al., "Hospitalisation of people with dementia: evidence from English electronic health records from 2008 to 2016," *European Journal of Epidemiology*, vol. 34, no. 6, pp. 567–577, 2019.

[5] V. M. Drennan, L. Cole, and S. Iliffe, "A taboo within a stigma? a qualitative study of managing incontinence with people with dementia living at home," *BMC Geriatrics*, vol. 11, no. 1, p. 75, 2011.

[6] D. Gove, A. Scerri, J. Georges et al., "Continence care for people with dementia living at home in Europe: a review of literature with a focus on problems and challenges," *Journal of Clinical Nursing*, vol. 26, no. 3-4, pp. 356–365, 2017.

[7] J. H. Grand, S. Grand, and S. W. Macdonald, "Clinical features and multidisciplinary approaches to dementia care," *Journal of Multidisciplinary Healthcare*, vol. 4, pp. 125–147, 2011.

[8] E. A. Crooks and D. S. Geldmacher, "Interdisciplinary approaches to Alzheimer's disease management," *Clinics in Geriatric Medicine*, vol. 20, no. 1, pp. 121–139, 2004.

[9] B.-J. Collett, C. Cordle, and C. Stewart, "Setting up a multidisciplinary clinic," *Best Practice & Research Clinical Obstetrics & Gynaecology*, vol. 14, no. 3, pp. 541–556, 2000.

[10] R. Luz, I. Pereira, A. Henriques, A. L. Ribeirinho, and A. Valentim-Lourenço, "King's health questionnaire to assess subjective outcomes after surgical treatment for urinary incontinence: can it be useful?" *International Urogynecology Journal*, vol. 28, no. 1, pp. 139–145, 2017.

[11] K. N. L. Avery, J. L. H. R. Bosch, M. Gotoh et al., "Questionnaires to assess urinary and anal incontinence: review and recommendations," *Journal of Urology*, vol. 177, no. 1, pp. 39–49, 2007.

[12] P. Abrams, K. Avery, N. Gardener, J. Donovan, and I. A. Board, "The international consultation on incontinence modular questionnaire: www.iciq.net," *Journal of Urology*, vol. 175, no. 3, pp. 1063–1066, 2006.
[13] E. Volz-Sidiropoulou, T. Rings, A. S. Wagg et al., "Development and initial psychometric properties of the "ICIQ-Cog": a new assessment tool to measure the disease-related impact and care effort associated with incontinence in cognitively impaired adults," *BJU International*, vol. 122, no. 2, pp. 309–316, 2018.
[14] A. Dowling-Castronovo and J. K. Specht, "How to try this," *AJN American Journal of Nursing*, vol. 109, no. 2, pp. 62–71, 2009.
[15] D. Kalánková, M. Stolt, P. A. Scott, E. Papastavrou, and R. Suhonen, "Unmet care needs of older people: a scoping review," *Nursing Ethics*, vol. 28, no. 2, pp. 149–178, 2020.
[16] M. Herr, J.-J. Arvieu, P. Aegerter, J.-M. Robine, and J. Ankri, "Unmet health care needs of older people: prevalence and predictors in a French cross-sectional survey," *The European Journal of Public Health*, vol. 24, no. 5, pp. 808–813, 2014.
[17] G. Ogrinc, S. E. Mooney, C. Estrada et al., "The SQUIRE (standards for quality improvement reporting excellence) guidelines for quality improvement reporting: explanation and elaboration," *Quality and Safety in Health Care*, vol. 17, no. Suppl 1, pp. i13–i32, 2008.
[18] P. Yap and D. Tan, "Urinary incontinence in dementia-a practical approach," *Australian Family Physician*, vol. 35, no. 4, pp. 237–241, 2006.
[19] E. Bright, M. J. Drake, and P. Abrams, "Urinary diaries: evidence for the development and validation of diary content, format, and duration," *Neurourology and Urodynamics*, vol. 30, no. 3, pp. 348–352, 2011.
[20] S. Engberg, J. Kincade, and D. Thompson, "Future directions for incontinence research with frail elders," *Nursing Research*, vol. 53, no. Supplement, pp. S22–S29, 2004.
[21] E. Samuelsson, L. Månsson, and I. Milsom, "Incontinence aids in Sweden: users and costs," *BJU International*, vol. 88, no. 9, pp. 893–898, 2001.
[22] B. A. Parsons, A. Narshi, and M. J. Drake, "Success rates for learning intermittent self-catheterisation according to age and gender," *International Urology and Nephrology*, vol. 44, no. 4, pp. 1127–1131, 2012.
[23] L. Cole and V. M. Drennan, "Living with incontinence: the experience of people with dementia," *Dementia*, vol. 18, no. 5, pp. 1826–1839, 2019.
[24] F. Olsson and C. Berterö, "Living with faecal incontinence: trying to control the daily life that is out of control," *Journal of Clinical Nursing*, vol. 24, no. 1-2, pp. 141–150, 2015.
[25] A. Milne, "The "D" word: reflections on the relationship between stigma, discrimination and dementia," *Journal of Mental Health*, vol. 19, no. 3, pp. 227–233, 2010.
[26] F. Boyer, J.-L. Novella, I. Morrone, D. Jolly, and F. Blanchard, "Agreement between dementia patient report and proxy reports using the Nottingham health profile," *International Journal of Geriatric Psychiatry*, vol. 19, no. 11, pp. 1026–1034, 2004.

16

Pediatric Germ Cell Tumors: A Developmental Perspective

Joshua L. Pierce,[1,2] **A. Lindsay Frazier,**[3] **and James F. Amatruda**[1,2,4]

[1]*Department of Pediatrics, University of Texas Southwestern Medical Center, Dallas, TX 75390, USA*
[2]*Department of Molecular Biology, University of Texas Southwestern Medical Center, Dallas, TX 75390, USA*
[3]*Department of Pediatric Oncology, Children's Hospital Dana-Farber Cancer Care, Boston, MA 02115, USA*
[4]*Department of Internal Medicine, University of Texas Southwestern Medical Center, Dallas, TX 75390, USA*

Correspondence should be addressed to James F. Amatruda; james.amatruda@utsouthwestern.edu

Academic Editor: Costantine Albany

Germ cell tumors (GCTs) arising in infants, children, and adolescents present a set of special challenges. GCTs make up about 3% of malignancies in children aged 0–18 and nearly 15% of cancers in adolescents. Epidemiologic and molecular evidence suggests that GCTs in young children likely represent a distinct biologic group as compared to GCTs of older adolescents and adults. Despite this difference, pediatric GCTs are typically treated with cisplatin-based multiagent regimens similar to those used in adults. There is evidence that children are particularly vulnerable to late effects of conventional therapy, including ototoxicity, pulmonary abnormalities, and secondary malignancies, motivating the search for molecular targets for novel therapies. Evidence is accumulating that the genes and mechanisms controlling normal germ cell development are particularly relevant to the understanding of germ cell tumorigenesis. Perturbations in the epigenetic program of germ cell differentiation, with resulting effects on the regulation of pluripotency, may contribute to the marked histologic variability of GCTs. Perturbations in the KIT receptor signaling pathway have been identified via next-generation sequencing studies and in genome-wide association studies of testicular cancer susceptibility. Here, we review these and other biological insights that may fuel further translational and clinical research in childhood GCTs.

1. Introduction

"Pediatric germ cell tumor" is the term used to describe malignant cancers of germline cells in patients aged 0–18 years. These cancers may arise in the testis, the ovary, or the extragonadal sites including the sacrococcygeal area and the mediastinum. Germ cell tumors (GCTs) also occur in the brain in children and young adults. Though intracranial GCTs (iGCTs) are histologically similar to extracranial GCTs, it is unclear if tumors in the different sites arise by similar or different mechanisms, and the treatment approaches used are somewhat different; for these reasons, iGCTs are not further considered here.

Though the biology and clinical presentation of pediatric GCTs share significant overlap with that of adult testicular (T) GCTs, there are important differences that should be kept in mind. First, epidemiologic data reveal two distinct peaks in GCT incidence, one in young children (aged approximately 0–4 years) and a second peak beginning in puberty [1]. While the histologic presentation and molecular biology of GCTs arising in adolescents appear similar to those in adult TGCTs, germ cell tumors in very young children have important differences (reviewed below), suggesting that they may represent a distinct disease. Altogether GCTs make up about 3% of malignancies in children aged 0–18 and incidence rises with onset of puberty, GCTs account for 15% of the malignancies diagnosed during adolescence. As with adult TGCTs, the mainstay of treatment for pediatric GCTs is cisplatin-based multiagent regimens that have proved to be highly effective even in the setting of advanced disease. However, increasing evidence has emerged of adverse late effects in adult male survivors of TGCT, including a doubling of the risk of early-onset cardiovascular disease [2] and second malignancies [3, 4]. It is worth noting that GCTs were not included in the malignancies studied in the landmark Children's Cancer Survival Study, and thus, the potential long-term toxicities of

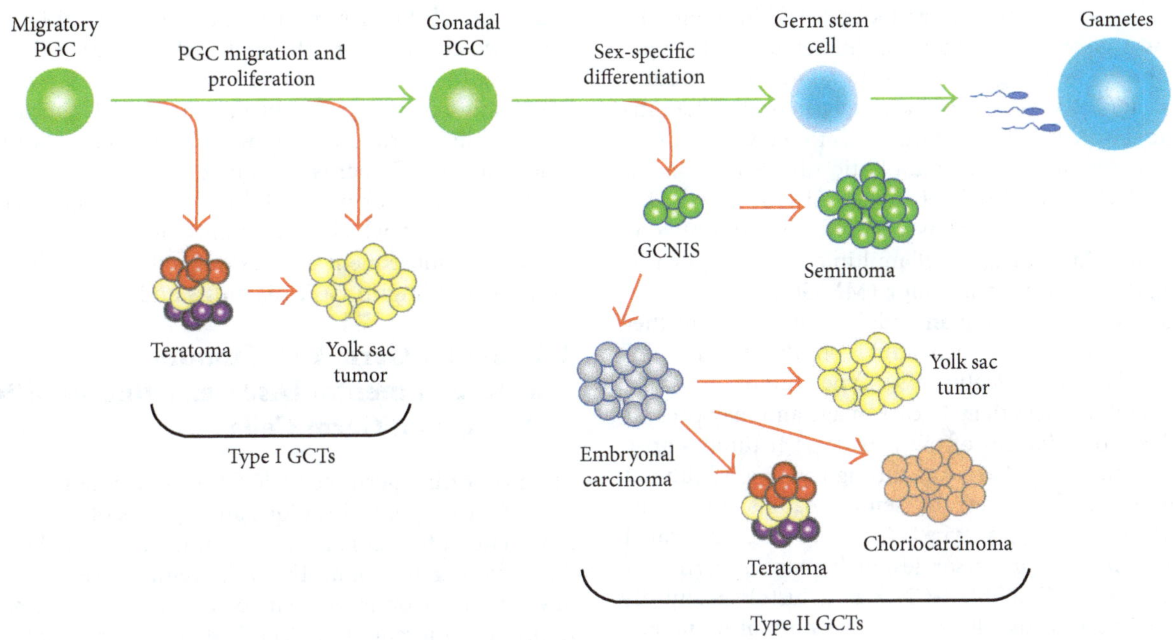

FIGURE 1: Germline development and histologic subtypes of GCTs. Primordial germ cells (PGCs) are specified early in embryogenesis and migrate through the embryo to the developing gonad. Type I GCTs exhibit a limited histologic spectrum, a partial erasure of genomic imprinting, and a propensity for development at extragonadal sites, all suggesting a derivation from early stages of germ cell development. Type II GCTs frequently contain foci of germ cell neoplasia in situ (GCNIS) and exhibit the full range of seminoma and nonseminoma histologies. Together with a more complete erasure of imprinting, these features suggest that the Type II tumors arise at a later stage of germline development.

conventional chemotherapy in pediatric GCT patients are still largely unknown. There is evidence that children are particularly vulnerable to late effects of therapy, especially ototoxicity and pulmonary abnormalities [5]. In a large cohort study, the cumulative risk of secondary malignancy also increased with decreasing age at diagnosis [4].

Finally, treatment regimens for pediatric GCT have largely been based on clinical trial results from adult men with TGCT, who represent the largest patient population. Whether these results apply equally to children with gonadal or extragonadal GCT remains to be established. In recent years, investigators in the Children's Oncology Group (USA) and the Children's Cancer and Leukaemia Group (UK) have joined forces to form the Malignant Germ Cell Tumor International Collaborative (MaGIC) Consortium to improve outcomes for patients with germ cell tumors (GCTs) by generating new insights into etiology, prognosis, toxicity reduction, and optimal treatment. MaGIC investigators have produced a revised evidence-based risk stratification for pediatric and adolescent GCTs based on amalgamation of 25 years of clinical trial data from the US and the UK [6] that separated patients into low-, standard-, and poor-risk groups. This risk stratification has in turn informed the development of the clinical trial AGCT1531 recently opened by the Children's Oncology Group (https://clinicaltrials.gov/show/NCT03067181), which aims to eliminate unnecessary chemotherapy in patients with Stage I disease at all sites (testicular, ovarian, and extragonadal) likely cured with surgery alone who will undergo active surveillance. AGCT1531 will also test whether the less-toxic carboplatin can be substituted for cisplatin in standard-risk patients. The COG will also be opening in the near future a trial for poor-risk patients, testing the efficacy of standard BEP chemotherapy versus accelerated BEP given every 2 weeks instead of every 3 weeks. This trial is conducted by the Australian and New Zealand Urogenital and Prostate Cancer Trials Group (ANZUP). The clinical management of pediatric GCTs was recently comprehensively reviewed [7].

2. Histologic Presentation of Germ Cell Tumors

Several lines of evidence suggest that GCTs do not arise from a mature gonadal cell (e.g., a spermatogonial stem cell) but rather from a germ cell in early stages of development. This was discovered through an interesting set of observations that linked etiological phenomena to characteristics of the developing germline [8]. GCTs can be classified into two major types based on histology, known as seminomatous GCTs and nonseminomatous GCTs (Figure 1). Seminomatous GCTs are tumors which are made of undifferentiated germ cells which can histologically resemble early spermatogonia, oogonia, or even germ cells from developmental lineages. These tumors are called seminoma when present in the testis, dysgerminoma when present in the ovary, and germinoma when found in an extragonadal site. Nonseminomatous GCTs can be further subdivided into the distinct histologies of embryonal carcinoma (EC), yolk sac tumor (YST), teratoma (TER), and choriocarcinoma (CC). EC comprised undifferentiated cells that histologically resemble embryonic cells from the blastocyst. YST is the most common malignant GCT of young children. These tumors have a very complex endodermal morphology with components of both embryonic and extraembryonic endoderm. TER histologically presents as a disordered mixture of differentiated cell types from all three somatic germ layers. In some cases, a component of a TER may acquire a unique neural differentiation state, known as an immature teratoma. CC is a rare histology and represents trophoblastic differentiation. In general, NSGCTs are more likely to be resistant to standard therapies. GCTs may present as a pure form with only one histology or as an amalgam of multiple types, known as mixed malignant germ cell tumor (MMGCT).

GCTs arising in children and adolescents can be further classified into two types depending on the age at presentation and histologic features [9]. Type I tumors generally present in children less than 4 years of age and may present as TER, YST, or mixtures of the two. Type II tumors arise around the time of puberty up through young adulthood and exhibit the full range of seminomatous and nonseminomatous histologies. Type II GCTs are often associated with a presumptive precursor lesion known as germ cell neoplasia in situ (GCNIS). GCNIS is a histologically diagnosed cell pattern usually seen in the normal tissue adjacent to the tumor [10] and is composed of undifferentiated germ cells that have proliferated within a seminiferous tubule [11]. GCNIS is not observed adjacent to Type I tumors, which are thus designated as non GCNIS-associated GCTs. These differences, along with molecular features discussed below, suggest that Type I and Type II GCTs may develop from germ cells at different stages of development.

3. Molecular Genetics of Pediatric GCTs

The most frequent chromosomal aberrations in Type II GCTs are amplification of chromosome 12p, usually through creation of isochromosome 12p, and amplification of the X chromosome. However, X amplification is an uncommon event in pediatric germ cell tumors, and 12p gain, while present, is infrequent [12]. Instead, pure YST, the most common malignant Type I GCT, has been shown to most commonly possess gain of 1q, 11q, 20q, and 22 and loss of 1p, 6q, and 16q [13]. Germ cell tumors also exhibit loss of genomic imprinting, which is partial in Type I GCTs and more complete in Type II GCTs. Since primordial germ cells undergo erasure of imprinting during germline development, this difference further suggests that Type I GCTs may arise from an earlier stage of development compared to Type II GCTs [14].

While the spectrum of somatic mutations in TGCTs is beginning to be defined (reviewed in this issue by Woldu et al.), little is known about the mutational status of pediatric GCTs. Addeo et al. found that *BAX* mutations in pediatric GCTs correlated with outcome [15]. At the transcriptional level, Palmer and coworkers found that Type I and Type II GCTs exhibit distinct gene expression profiles, even when controlling for histologic subtype [16]. Another important finding within GCTs is that the landscape of microRNAs (miRNAs) is changed relative to the normal gonad [17]. Palmer and coworkers demonstrated that the eight main miRNAs from the miR-371–373 and miR-302/367 clusters were overexpressed in all malignant GCT tissues [18]. Murray et al. further showed that levels of miRNAs from these two clusters were elevated in the serum at the time of diagnosis of an extragonadal malignant GCT, with levels falling and remaining low during uneventful clinical follow-up [19]. These serum findings were confirmed in extracranial malignant GCTs across a range of representative ages (pediatric/adult), anatomical sites, and histological subtypes, the majority of which were tumor marker negative [17]. These and subsequent studies suggest a possible role for miRNA profiling in GCT diagnosis and risk stratification.

4. Pediatric Germ Cell Tumors as a Developmental Disease: Vulnerabilities in Primordial Germ Cells

The primordial germ cell (PGC), responsible for specification of the germline, is unique among cells of the body in its requirement to maintain the pluripotent potential necessary for gamete generation. This requirement creates a unique developmental cycle which involves stages of vulnerability to improper differentiation. The PGC must be specified from the rest of the developing embryo through genetic and epigenetic events; it subsequently migrates throughout the body to the site of the gonad, and it must then undergo sex specific differentiation. Each of these stages reflects both a developmental feature and a clue related to the phenotypes and characteristics of germ cell tumors.

5. PGC Specification and Pluripotency

The first event in the development of the germline is the specification of PGCs in the early embryo. This specification event endows the PGCs with pluripotency as marked by a unique histological and genetic signature. PGC specification in humans occurs at ~2 weeks after fertilization when BMP signals target to the mesendoderm of the preprimitive streak embryo, which leads to the induction of SOX17 which, with BLIMP1, suppresses endodermal differentiation and activates PGC differentiation [20]. These cells express the pluripotency-associated markers OCT3/4, LIN28A, and NANOG histologically and begin a process of global DNA demethylation necessary for the later establishment of sex-specific gametic imprinting [21–23]. This genetic and epigenetic state creates the platform for development of the gamete, which leads to formation of the totipotent zygote after fertilization.

This unique developmental licensing of pluripotency is likely partially responsible for the extremely heterogeneous histological variation amongst germ cell tumors. Unlike most other tumor types, germ cell tumors may present with cells from each of the three germ layers as well as undifferentiated germline and extraembryonic cells [24]. In addition to GCTs exhibiting histological heterogeneity, it has been shown that both seminomas and nonseminomas retain pluripotency-associated protein expression (SALL4, OCT3/4, and LIN28A), which indicates the pluripotent growth potential even amongst the different differentiation states [24]. Furthermore, it has been shown that LIN28A expression in malignant GCTs is responsible for maintaining an undifferentiated state through repression of the tumor suppressive let-7 miRNA family [25]. Additionally, the protein EPCAM, which is expressed in undifferentiated embryonic stem cells (ESCs), is associated with malignant nonseminomatous GCTs and has been suggested as a serum diagnostic marker in the treatment of GCTs [26, 27].

The second step of PGC specification, global demethylation, is another hallmark of GCTs and may be related to GCT susceptibility [20]. GWAS studies have revealed a GCT-associated SNP near the gene *PRDM14*, a key PGC pluripotency marker in mice [28, 29]. Though the function of PRDM14 is still being elucidated in humans, it is possible that it is involved in maintenance of the pluripotent state through the initiation of global demethylation, as it is in mice [30]. DNA demethylation at this stage allows for biallelic expression of genes [31]. Research on methylation states of the gene *SNRPN* revealed that most GCTs possess hypomethylation which lends credence to the idea that GCTs were derived from PGCs [32]. In addition to connecting GCTs to PGCs, this loss of transcriptional control likely provides a vulnerability in GCT development as loss of imprinting is a common event in many cancers [33]. This open epigenetic environment is thought to be protected by activation of the repressive chromatin modifications H3K27me3 and H3K9me3 concurrent with global demethylation. However, another testis cancer GWAS SNP near *ATF7IP*, a gene related to chromatin dynamics, may play a role in disrupting this repressive mark [34, 35]. Disregulation of ATF7IP with its cofactor SETDB1 may interfere with proper repressive chromatin marks, as it is known to be involved in creation of H3K9me3 marks, though further work is needed to establish this connection [36, 37]. It is likely that the pluripotent specification of PGCs as well as the physiological loss of imprinting naturally provides two pro-oncogenic conditions that may be coopted by improper differentiation cues.

This creation and maintenance of the pluripotent state prior to and during migration may explain the histologies specific to Type I GCTs, namely teratoma (TER) and yolk sac tumor (YST) [24]. As mentioned previously, TER frequently presents in a mature form with fully differentiated cell types. It is likely that these tumors are the result of improper regulation of pluripotency in which reacquisition of epiblast-like pluripotency during improper PGC specification results in cells that attempt to recapitulate embryonic development, including creation of the three germ layers. Cells in teratomas may not, however, receive the very specific spatial and temporal differentiation cues needed for proper embryogenesis, resulting in disorganized development. Type I teratomas are likely benign because the improper differentiation is the result of a failure of development rather than the acquisition of an oncogenic mutation.

In contrast to teratomas, YSTs are highly malignant. Old and new insights into PGC development may reveal why this tumor, which is composed of one germ layer, that is, endoderm (or two if one considers embryonic and extraembryonic endoderms separately), takes on a much more traditional tumorigenic phenotype. These tumors histologically resemble many differentiated endodermal structures, possess regions of primitive endoderm histology, and grow rapidly requiring treatment through surgical resection and adjuvant chemotherapy [24, 38]. As mentioned previously, PGC specification is controlled by a concerted effort between SOX17 and BLIMP1, the second of which is responsible for preventing endodermal differentiation [39]. This is required because SOX17 in the absence of BLIMP1 or even in excess of BLIMP1 is responsible for specification of the definitive endoderm, an endodermal structure responsible, through complex differentiation programs, for the development of most adult endodermal structures [40]. Kobayashi et al. recently showed in porcine, monkey, and human systems that even after PGC priming of mesendoderm cells, overexpression of SOX17 or loss of BLIMP1 resulted in differentiation to definitive endoderm [41]. Interestingly, almost 3 decades ago, it was shown in rats that externalization of fetal yolk sac primitive endoderm after fetectomy was capable of formation of malignant YSTs which could be transplanted to syngeneic rats [42]. This provides evidence that primitive endoderm cells have the capacity to grow rapidly and acquire oncogenic lesions which enhance growth when removed from their normal developmental location. Rather than terminally differentiating like their teratoma counterparts, they grow rapidly and act as the source of their own growth regulatory signals, as do many endodermal compartments [43]. This proliferative licensing of primitive endoderm may serve as the explanation for the GWAS SNP associated with HNF1β, which is an important transcription factor related to endoderm differentiation and maintenance [44]. Aberrations in HNF1β signaling in the context of a PGC may favor primitive endoderm misdifferentiation and subsequent YST formation.

6. PGC Migration and Proliferation

After the PGCs have been specified as the independent germ lineage, they must make their way to the gonadal ridge, proliferating en route, where they will receive subsequent differentiation cues for sex-specific development. However, this journey serves as a source of developmental vulnerabilities that may explain the frequent extragonadal localization of pediatric GCTs. After specification of the PGCs in the early mesendoderm ~2 weeks after conception, they make their way to the wall of the yolk sac endoderm [45]. Subsequently, PGCs migrate along the hindgut and midgut endoderm until near the gonadal ridge (GR) [46]. At this point, they migrate through the dorsal mesentery to the dorsal body wall where they migrate laterally to the GR. This migration generally results in the specific localization of viable PGCs to the GR; however, multiple sections of this tightly controlled migratory pathway present developmental vulnerabilities.

Pediatric germ cell tumors frequently present in extragonadal locations in pediatric patients. These locations are limited to midline structures such as the sacrococcygeal, retroperitoneal, mediastinal, cervical, and intracranial regions. The migratory route coupled with the molecular mechanisms governing PGC migration is likely the causal factor in GCT localization. Though the exact mechanism by which PGC migration is controlled is not fully understood, multiple cytokine mechanisms have been implicated. Interruptions of these pathways have revealed ectopic germ cell localization. The GWAS SNP most strongly correlated to GCT risk resides in the *KITLG* locus. KITLG is the ligand of the KIT tyrosine kinase receptor, which is thought to regulate migration from the midgut to the GR, among other roles [47, 48]. Knockdown of CXCR4 and its ligand CXCL12 results in PGC mismigration and failure to reach the gonadal ridge after PGCs reach the dorsal wall [49]. β-integrin and E-cadherin cell surface proteins as well as surface lipids have been implicated in migration along the midgut endoderm [50]. Finally, a study by Runyan et al. revealed that PGCs that fail to exit the midline to enter the gonadal ridge are cleared through a BAX-dependent apoptotic program [51]. Intriguingly, GWAS studies found that an SNP near the *BAK1* locus, which is an important member of the BCL2-BAX-BAK1 antiapoptotic axis, was associated with GCT risk [52]. These observations together reveal the developmental vulnerabilities of PGC migration.

If perturbations of these migratory mechanisms result in failure to appropriately reach the GR, we might expect to find extragonadal GCTs (EGGCTs) in body regions that develop from the tissues along which PGCs migrate. The germ cells must migrate past the dorsal aorta from the dorsal mesentery on the way to the GR. Migration failure at this point would result in PGCs residing along and near the aorta which eventually reside in the mediastinum and the retroperitoneum, two frequent sites of EGGCTs [46]. Anterior-posterior, rather than lateral, mismigration along the body wall may be the mechanism for EGGCTs occurring in the sacrococcygeal and cervical regions. Aberrant migration from the hindgut could explain sacrococcygeal GCT prevalence as this structure is caudal and adjacent to the region which will form the tailbone. Intriguingly, another mechanism based on nerve fibers may explain the distal localization of some EGGCTs. Mollgard et al. found that PGCs migrate along nerve fibers from the midgut along the dorsal mesentery and into the GR. These PGCs associated intimately with the peripheral Schwann cells [53]. These data suggest that cells of the autonomic nervous system (ANS) may be responsible for secreting cytokines which PGCs recognize as migration and proliferative cues. This idea is further corroborated by studies involving the secreted neural signaling molecules PACAP and GDNF, both of which have migratory and proliferative effects on germ cells in vitro [53–55]. These proteins are both secreted by the ANS and could explain the cranial, cervical, and sacrococcygeal localization of ectopic PGCs and EGGCTs as these regions are thoroughly enervated by the ANS. Based on this evidence, further investigation of the link between PGC migration and ANS signaling is warranted.

During the migratory phase of PGC development, their numbers expand rapidly in order to properly colonize the GR. This proliferative step may be a key in the initiation of pediatric GCTs. The primary determinant of this proliferative step is KIT signaling. As PGCs migrate from the midgut to the GR, somatic KIT ligand (KITLG) secretion induces rapid PGC proliferation and suppresses apoptotic pathways used to clear ectopic cells [56]. The signaling axis relating to KIT-controlled proliferation has proven especially interesting due to the fact that two primary interactors have been discovered to have associated SNPs linked to GCT risk. SNP variants near the KITLG have revealed a GCT-associated odds ratio of approximately 2.5 which represents the strongest GCT SNP association to date and one of the highest general cancer associations described [47, 48, 57]. Mahakali et al. showed through a series of mutations to the KITL (murine KITLG homolog) that interruption of KITLG signaling resulted in diminished PGC proliferation [56]. In vitro assays have shown that excess KITLG can induce rapid proliferation of PGCs [58]. The KITLG association with GCTs may thus be due to a variation that causes some increase in KIT signaling, resulting in more robust PGC proliferation. This expansion of the pool would create two independent vulnerabilities to GCT development. Firstly, the rapidly dividing pool of cells is vulnerable to acquisition of mutations that may drive oncogenesis and becomes doubly so when proliferation is increased through excess KITLG secretion. Secondly, KIT signaling activates prosurvival pathways that would allow for expansion of cells that have acquired genetic lesions as well as survival of ectopic PGCs if the range of KITLG secretion was increased by the SNP variants. Further evidence strengthening the relationship of the KIT axis to GCTs is the discovery that an SNP near the gene SPRY4 is associated with GCT risk [47]. SPRY4 is an inhibitor of RTK signaling and has been shown to abrogate KIT signaling [59, 60]. An SNP at this locus resulting in reduced SPRY4 expression could serve a function similar to KITLG increase by failing to reduce KIT signaling. It has also been found that KIT is frequently mutated in intracranial germinomas; however, this finding may be an independent mechanism that helps to drive RAS signaling in Type II GCTs rather than an aberration of normal developmental pathways as would be the case in KITLG-mediated PGC proliferation [61]. This might explain why KITLG is associated with GCT risk for all histologies, while KIT mutations are limited to germinomas. These results suggest that pediatric GCTs are the result of specific aberrations in normal developmental pathways.

7. Germline Differentiation

Upon arrival to the nascent gonad, the PGCs must begin the transition from migratory pluripotent cells to either sperm or egg progenitors. This process is controlled through induction of sex-specific gene expression mediated by ligand secretion from the somatic cells of the gonad as well as circulating hormones. The set of developmental processes responsible for sex determination is tightly controlled, and interruption of these differentiation mechanisms represents the final set of vulnerabilities to pediatric GCT development. Work from Looijenga and colleagues has carefully laid out the case that failure of sexual development in the context of disorders of sex development (DSDs) is the proximate cause of the additional GCT risk observed in these patients [62].

As described above, Type II GCTs frequently exhibit a precursor lesion known as germ cell neoplasia in situ

(GCNIS) in otherwise normal gonadal tissue adjacent to tumor tissue [9]. These lesions exhibit histological markers, methylation status, and gene expression profiles that are remarkably similar to PGCs, which should normally be absent at the developmental stages at which GCNIS is observed [63]. The molecular mechanisms leading to the development of GCNIS and the transition of GCNIS to invasive cancer, including the possible role of oncogenic mutations, are active areas of investigation. In vitro, PGCs can dedifferentiate to a state resembling a pluripotent embryonic germ cell (EGC), under the control of Akt/PI3 kinase signaling [64]. EGCs exhibit epiblast pluripotency marks such as OCT3/4 and SOX2 and are capable of teratoma formation [65]. Additionally, newly discovered SNP variants of the embryonic pluripotency-related genes ZFP42 and TFCP2L1 have been associated with GCT risk [66, 67]. Taken together, these experimental results emphasize the importance of the OCT3/4-SOX2-SOX17-BLIMP1 network in controlling the fate of developing germ cells. If primitive germ precursors indeed exist in a metastable state between pluripotency and differentiation, perturbations in this network could explain how GCTs can present with such varied histologies.

The unique susceptibility of PGCs to aberrant differentiation may explain the variety of genes implicated in GCT GWAS studies. Rather than traditional SNPs involved in pro-oncogenic or tumor suppressive activities, such as MYC or CDKN1A in colorectal cancer [68, 69], GCT SNPs may cause slight perturbations in PGC development that lead to differentiation failure, mismigration, or aberrant proliferation. This hypothesis is evidenced by multiple mouse models in which the loss of genes responsible for PGC maintenance and eventual sexual differentiation occurs, and testicular teratomas resembling Type I pediatric GCTs result [70, 71]. Two sentinel GWAS loci near the genes DAZL and DMRT1, which are responsible for specification of the germline during sexual development, have also been implicated in teratoma susceptibility [28, 47]. Loss of any of these three genes releases suppression of proliferation and pluripotency in PGCs [72, 73].

8. Conclusions

As the only nonsomatic tumor lineage in the body, GCTs exhibit a unique combination of varied histology, wide range of sites of presentation, and apparent lack of traditional oncogenic drivers, suggesting a prominent role for aberrant developmental pathways in the etiology of these cancers. A perspective that focuses on these mechanisms could be key to the development of differentiation-based therapies using either exogenous signaling ligands or small molecule activators or inhibitors of the relevant pathways, which might one day supplement or substitute for conventional cytotoxic therapies. The challenges of long-term adverse effects that arise in the treatment of malignant tumors in young children and adolescents create a powerful incentive for pursuing such approaches.

References

[1] A. L. Frazier and J. F. Amatruda, "Germ cell tumors," in *Nathan and Oski's Textbook of Pediatric Hematology-Oncology*, D. E. Fisher, D. Nathan, and A. T. Look, Eds., Elsevier, London, UK, 2009.

[2] R. A. Huddart, A. Norman, M. Shahidi et al., "Cardiovascular disease as a long-term complication of treatment for testicular cancer," *Journal of Clinical Oncology*, vol. 21, no. 8, pp. 1513–1523, 2003.

[3] L. B. Travis, R. E. Curtis, H. Storm et al., "Risk of second malignant neoplasms among long-term survivors of testicular cancer," *Journal of the National Cancer Institute*, vol. 89, no. 19, pp. 1429–1439, 1997.

[4] L. B. Travis, S. D. Fossa, S. J. Schonfeld et al., "Second cancers among 40,576 testicular cancer patients: focus on long-term survivors," *Journal of the National Cancer Institute*, vol. 97, no. 18, pp. 1354–1365, 2005.

[5] G. A. Hale, N. M. Marina, D. Jones-Wallace et al., "Late effects of treatment for germ cell tumors during childhood and adolescence," *Journal of Pediatric Hematology/Oncology*, vol. 21, no. 2, pp. 115–122, 1999.

[6] A. L. Frazier, J. P. Hale, C. Rodriguez-Galindo et al., "Revised risk classification for pediatric extracranial germ cell tumors based on 25 years of clinical trial data from the United Kingdom and United States," *Journal of Clinical Oncology*, vol. 33, no. 2, pp. 195–201, 2015.

[7] F. Shaikh, M. J. Murray, J. F. Amatruda et al., "Paediatric extracranial germ-cell tumours," *The Lancet Oncology*, vol. 17, no. 4, pp. e149–e162, 2016.

[8] J. W. Oosterhuis and L. H. Looijenga, "Testicular germ-cell tumours in a broader perspective," *Nature Reviews Cancer*, vol. 5, no. 3, pp. 210–222, 2005.

[9] D. M. Berney, L. H. Looijenga, M. Idrees et al., "Germ cell neoplasia in situ (GCNIS): evolution of the current nomenclature for testicular pre-invasive germ cell malignancy," *Histopathology*, vol. 69, no. 1, pp. 7–10, 2016.

[10] N. E. Skakkebaek, "Carcinoma in situ of the testis: frequency and relationship to invasive germ cell tumours in infertile men," *Histopathology*, vol. 2, no. 3, pp. 157–170, 1978.

[11] E. Rajpert-De Meyts, "Developmental model for the pathogenesis of testicular carcinoma in situ: genetic and environmental aspects," *Human Reproduction Update*, vol. 12, no. 3, pp. 303–323, 2006.

[12] R. D. Palmer, N. A. Foster, S. L. Vowler et al., "Malignant germ cell tumours of childhood: new associations of genomic imbalance," *British Journal of Cancer*, vol. 96, no. 4, pp. 667–676, 2007.

[13] B. Summersgill, H. Goker, S. Weber-Hall, R. Huddart, A. Horwich, and J. Shipley, "Molecular cytogenetic analysis of adult testicular germ cell tumours and identification of regions of consensus copy number change," *British Journal of Cancer*, vol. 77, no. 2, pp. 305–313, 1998.

[14] J. A. Ross, P. T. Schmidt, J. P. Perentesis, and S. M. Davies, "Genomic imprinting of H19 and insulin-like growth factor-2 in pediatric germ cell tumors," *Cancer*, vol. 85, no. 6, pp. 1389–1394, 1999.

[15] R. Addeo, S. Crisci, V. D'Angelo et al., "Bax mutation and overexpression inversely correlate with immature phenotype and prognosis of childhood germ cell tumors," *Oncology Reports*, vol. 17, no. 5, pp. 1155–1161, 2007.

[16] R. D. Palmer, N. L. Barbosa-Morais, E. L. Gooding et al., "Pediatric malignant germ cell tumors show characteristic transcriptome profiles," *Cancer Research*, vol. 68, no. 11, pp. 4239–4247, 2008.

[17] M. J. Murray and N. Coleman, "Testicular cancer: a new generation of biomarkers for malignant germ cell tumours," *Nature Reviews Urology*, vol. 9, no. 6, pp. 298–300, 2012.

[18] R. D. Palmer, M. J. Murray, H. K. Saini et al., "Malignant germ cell tumors display common microRNA profiles resulting in global changes in expression of messenger RNA targets," *Cancer Research*, vol. 70, no. 7, pp. 2911–2923, 2010.

[19] M. J. Murray, D. J. Halsall, C. E. Hook, D. M. Williams, J. C. Nicholson, and N. Coleman, "Identification of microRNAs from the miR-371~373 and miR-302 clusters as potential serum biomarkers of malignant germ cell tumors," *American Journal of Clinical Pathology*, vol. 135, no. 1, pp. 119–125, 2011.

[20] W. W. Tang, T. Kobayashi, N. Irie, S. Dietmann, and M. A. Surani, "Specification and epigenetic programming of the human germ line," *Nature Reviews Genetics*, vol. 17, no. 10, pp. 585–600, 2016.

[21] H. G. Leitch, K. Blair, W. Mansfield et al., "Embryonic germ cells from mice and rats exhibit properties consistent with a generic pluripotent ground state," *Development*, vol. 137, no. 14, pp. 2279–2287, 2010.

[22] J. A. West, S. R. Viswanathan, A. Yabuuchi et al., "A role for Lin28 in primordial germ-cell development and germ-cell malignancy," *Nature*, vol. 460, no. 7257, pp. 909–913, 2009.

[23] M. De Felici, "Nuclear reprogramming in mouse primordial germ cells: epigenetic contribution," *Stem Cells International*, vol. 2011, Article ID 425863, 15 pages, 2011.

[24] D. Rakheja and L. Teot, "Pathology of germ cell tumors," in *Pediatric Germ Cell Tumors*, A. L. F. Amatruda, Ed., Springer, Berlin, Germany, 2014.

[25] M. J. Murray, H. K. Saini, C. A. Siegler et al., "LIN28 expression in malignant germ cell tumors downregulates let-7 and increases oncogene levels," *Cancer Research*, vol. 73, no. 15, pp. 4872–4884, 2013.

[26] S. Schonberger, V. Okpanyi, G. Calaminus et al., "EPCAM-A novel molecular target for the treatment of pediatric and adult germ cell tumors," *Genes Chromosomes and Cancer*, vol. 52, no. 1, pp. 24–32, 2013.

[27] V. Y. Ng, S. N. Ang, J. X. Chan, and A. B. Choo, "Characterization of epithelial cell adhesion molecule as a surface marker on undifferentiated human embryonic stem cells," *Stem Cells*, vol. 28, no. 1, pp. 29–35, 2010.

[28] E. Ruark, S. Seal, H. McDonald et al., "Identification of nine new susceptibility loci for testicular cancer, including variants near DAZL and PRDM14," *Nature Genetics*, vol. 45, no. 6, pp. 686–689, 2013.

[29] Y. Ohinata, B. Payer, D. O'Carroll et al., "Blimp1 is a critical determinant of the germ cell lineage in mice," *Nature*, vol. 436, no. 7048, pp. 207–213, 2005.

[30] N. Okashita, Y. Suwa, O. Nishimura et al., "PRDM14 drives OCT3/4 recruitment via active demethylation in the transition from primed to naive pluripotency," *Stem Cell Reports*, vol. 7, no. 6, pp. 1072–1086, 2016.

[31] J. Lee, K. Inoue, R. Ono et al., "Erasing genomic imprinting memory in mouse clone embryos produced from day 11.5 primordial germ cells," *Development*, vol. 129, no. 8, pp. 1807–1817, 2002.

[32] K. J. Bussey, H. J. Lawce, E. Himoe et al., "SNRPN methylation patterns in germ cell tumors as a reflection of primordial germ cell development," *Genes Chromosomes and Cancer*, vol. 32, no. 4, pp. 342–352, 2001.

[33] P. Jelinic and P. Shaw, "Loss of imprinting and cancer," *Journal of Pathology*, vol. 211, no. 3, pp. 261–268, 2007.

[34] J. A. Hackett, J. P. Reddington, C. E. Nestor et al., "Promoter DNA methylation couples genome-defence mechanisms to epigenetic reprogramming in the mouse germline," *Development*, vol. 139, no. 19, pp. 3623–3632, 2012.

[35] C. Turnbull, E. A. Rapley, S. Seal et al., "Variants near DMRT1, TERT and ATF7IP are associated with testicular germ cell cancer," *Nature Genetics*, vol. 42, no. 7, pp. 604–607, 2010.

[36] A. Basavapathruni, J. Gureasko, M. Porter Scott et al., "Characterization of the enzymatic activity of SETDB1 and its 1:1 complex with ATF7IP," *Biochemistry*, vol. 55, no. 11, pp. 1645–1651, 2016.

[37] T. Ichimura, S. Watanabe, Y. Sakamoto, T. Aoto, N. Fujita, and M. Nakao, "Transcriptional repression and heterochromatin formation by MBD1 and MCAF/AM family proteins," *Journal of Biological Chemistry*, vol. 280, no. 14, pp. 13928–13935, 2005.

[38] F. F. Nogales, O. Preda, and A. Nicolae, "Yolk sac tumours revisited. A review of their many faces and names," *Histopathology*, vol. 60, no. 7, pp. 1023–1033, 2012.

[39] N. Irie, L. Weinberger, W. W. Tang et al., "SOX17 is a critical specifier of human primordial germ cell fate," *Cell*, vol. 160, no. 1-2, pp. 253–268, 2015.

[40] L. Ying, J. A. Mills, D. L. French, and P. Gadue, "OCT4 coordinates with WNT signaling to pre-pattern chromatin at the SOX17 locus during human ES cell differentiation into definitive endoderm," *Stem Cell Reports*, vol. 5, no. 4, pp. 490–498, 2015.

[41] T. Kobayashi, H. Zhang, W. W. C. Tang et al., "Principles of early human development and germ cell program from conserved model systems," *Nature*, vol. 546, no. 7658, pp. 416–420, 2017.

[42] H. Sobis, A. Verstuyf, and M. Vandeputte, "Visceral yolk sac-derived tumors," *International Journal of Developmental Biology*, vol. 37, no. 1, pp. 155–168, 1993.

[43] M. L. Stevens, P. Chaturvedi, S. A. Rankin et al., "Genomic integration of Wnt/β-catenin and BMP/Smad1 signaling coordinates foregut and hindgut transcriptional programs," *Development*, vol. 144, no. 7, pp. 1283–1295, 2017.

[44] W. Kristiansen, R. Karlsson, T. B. Rounge et al., "Two new loci and gene sets related to sex determination and cancer progression are associated with susceptibility to testicular germ cell tumor," *Human Molecular Genetics*, vol. 24, no. 14, pp. 4138–4146, 2015.

[45] N. Aeckerle, C. Drummer, K. Debowski, C. Viebahn, and R. Behr, "Primordial germ cell development in the marmoset monkey as revealed by pluripotency factor expression: suggestion of a novel model of embryonic germ cell translocation," *Molecular Human Reproduction*, vol. 21, no. 1, pp. 66–80, 2015.

[46] L. S. Mamsen, C. B. Brochner, A. G. Byskov, and K. Mollgard, "The migration and loss of human primordial germ stem cells from the hind gut epithelium towards the gonadal ridge," *International Journal of Developmental Biology*, vol. 56, no. 10–12, pp. 771–778, 2012.

[47] J. N. Poynter, A. J. Hooten, A. L. Frazier, and J. A. Ross, "Associations between variants in KITLG, SPRY4, BAK1, and DMRT1 and pediatric germ cell tumors," *Genes Chromosomes and Cancer*, vol. 51, no. 3, pp. 266–271, 2012.

[48] S. Chanock, "High marks for GWAS," *Nature Genetics*, vol. 41, no. 7, pp. 765-766, 2009.

[49] M. Doitsidou, M. Reichman-Fried, J. Stebler et al., "Guidance of primordial germ cell migration by the chemokine SDF-1," *Cell*, vol. 111, no. 5, pp. 647–659, 2002.

[50] M. De Felici, M. L. Scaldaferri, and D. Farini, "Adhesion molecules for mouse primordial germ cells," *Frontiers in Bioscience*, vol. 10, no. 1–3, pp. 542–551, 2005.

[51] C. Runyan, Y. Gu, A. Shoemaker, L. Looijenga, and C. Wylie, "The distribution and behavior of extragonadal primordial germ cells in Bax mutant mice suggest a novel origin for sacrococcygeal germ cell tumors," *International Journal of Developmental Biology*, vol. 52, no. 4, pp. 333–344, 2008.

[52] L. M. Lindqvist and D. L. Vaux, "BCL2 and related prosurvival proteins require BAK1 and BAX to affect autophagy," *Autophagy*, vol. 10, no. 8, pp. 1474-1475, 2014.

[53] K. Mollgard, A. Jespersen, M. C. Lutterodt, C. Yding Andersen, P. E. Hoyer, and A. G. Byskov, "Human primordial germ cells migrate along nerve fibers and Schwann cells from the dorsal hind gut mesentery to the gonadal ridge," *Molecular Human Reproduction*, vol. 16, no. 9, pp. 621–631, 2010.

[54] L. Dovere, S. Fera, M. Grasso et al., "The niche-derived glial cell line-derived neurotrophic factor (GDNF) induces migration of mouse spermatogonial stem/progenitor cells," *PLoS One*, vol. 8, no. 4, article e59431, 2013.

[55] M. Pesce, R. Canipari, G. L. Ferri, G. Siracusa, and M. De Felici, "Pituitary adenylate cyclase-activating polypeptide (PACAP) stimulates adenylate cyclase and promotes proliferation of mouse primordial germ cells," *Development*, vol. 122, no. 1, pp. 215–221, 1996.

[56] A. M. Zama, F. P. Hudson, and M. A. Bedell, "Analysis of hypomorphic KitlSl mutants suggests different requirements for KITL in proliferation and migration of mouse primordial germ cells," *Biology of Reproduction*, vol. 73, no. 4, pp. 639–647, 2005.

[57] R. Hersmus, H. Stoop, G. J. van de Geijn et al., "Prevalence of c-KIT mutations in gonadoblastoma and dysgerminomas of patients with disorders of sex development (DSD) and ovarian dysgerminomas," *PloS one*, vol. 7, no. 8, article e43952, 2012.

[58] G. H. Moe-Behrens, F. G. Klinger, W. Eskild, T. Grotmol, T. B. Haugen, and M. De Felici, "Akt/PTEN signaling mediates estrogen-dependent proliferation of primordial germ cells in vitro," *Molecular Endocrinology*, vol. 17, no. 12, pp. 2630–2638, 2003.

[59] H. Felfly and O. D. Klein, "Sprouty genes regulate proliferation and survival of human embryonic stem cells," *Scientific Reports*, vol. 3, no. 1, p. 2277, 2013.

[60] M. A. Cabrita and G. Christofori, "Sprouty proteins, masterminds of receptor tyrosine kinase signaling," *Angiogenesis*, vol. 11, no. 1, pp. 53–62, 2008.

[61] Y. Kamakura, M. Hasegawa, T. Minamoto, J. Yamashita, and H. Fujisawa, "*c-kit* gene mutation: common and widely distributed in intracranial germinomas," *Journal of Neurosurgery: Pediatrics*, vol. 104, no. 3, pp. 173–180, 2006.

[62] L. H. Looijenga, T. Van Agthoven, and K. Biermann, "Development of malignant germ cells-the genvironmental hypothesis," *International Journal of Developmental Biology*, vol. 57, no. 2–4, pp. 241–253, 2013.

[63] H. Stoop, F. Honecker, G. J. van de Geijn et al., "Stem cell factor as a novel diagnostic marker for early malignant germ cells," *Journal of Pathology*, vol. 216, no. 1, pp. 43–54, 2008.

[64] T. Kimura and T. Nakano, "Induction of pluripotency in primordial germ cells," *Histology and Histopathology*, vol. 26, no. 5, pp. 643–650, 2011.

[65] F. Attari, H. Sepehri, H. Ansari et al., "Efficient induction of pluripotency in primordial germ cells by dual inhibition of TGF-beta and ERK signaling pathways," *Stem Cells and Development*, vol. 23, no. 10, pp. 1050–1061, 2014.

[66] W. W. Tang, S. Dietmann, N. Irie et al., "A unique gene regulatory network resets the human germline epigenome for development," *Cell*, vol. 161, no. 6, pp. 1453–1467, 2015.

[67] K. B. Scotland, S. Chen, R. Sylvester, and L. J. Gudas, "Analysis of Rex1 (zfp42) function in embryonic stem cell differentiation," *Developmental Dynamics*, vol. 238, no. 8, pp. 1863–1877, 2009.

[68] B. W. Kang, H. S. Jeon, Y. S. Chae et al., "Association between GWAS-identified genetic variations and disease prognosis for patients with colorectal cancer," *PLoS One*, vol. 10, no. 3, article e0119649, 2015.

[69] J. Dai, J. Gu, M. Huang et al., "GWAS-identified colorectal cancer susceptibility loci associated with clinical outcomes," *Carcinogenesis*, vol. 33, no. 7, pp. 1327–1331, 2012.

[70] T. Noguchi and M. Noguchi, "A recessive mutation (ter) causing germ cell deficiency and a high incidence of congenital testicular teratomas in 129/Sv-ter mice," *Journal of the National Cancer Institute*, vol. 75, no. 2, pp. 385–392, 1985.

[71] K. K. Youngren, D. Coveney, X. Peng et al., "The Ter mutation in the dead end gene causes germ cell loss and testicular germ cell tumours," *Nature*, vol. 435, no. 7040, pp. 360–364, 2005.

[72] H. H. Chen, M. Welling, D. B. Bloch et al., "DAZL limits pluripotency, differentiation, and apoptosis in developing primordial germ cells," *Stem Cell Reports*, vol. 3, no. 5, pp. 892–904, 2014.

[73] A. D. Krentz, M. W. Murphy, S. Kim et al., "The DM domain protein DMRT1 is a dose-sensitive regulator of fetal germ cell proliferation and pluripotency," *Proceedings of the National Academy of Sciences*, vol. 106, no. 52, pp. 22323–22328, 2009.

17

Penile Hemodynamic Response to Phosphodiesterase Type V Inhibitors after Cavernosal Sparing Inflatable Penile Prosthesis Implantation: A Prospective Randomized Open-Blinded End-Point (PROBE) Study

Adham Zaazaa,[1] Michaela Bayerle-Eder,[2] Ramzy Elnabarawy,[1] Mahmoud Elbitar,[1] and Taymour Mostafa[1]

[1]*Department of Andrology, Sexology & STIs, Faculty of Medicine, Cairo University, Cairo 11562, Egypt*
[2]*Department of Endocrinology & Metabolism, Medical University of Vienna, Währinger Gürtel 18–20, Vienna 1090, Austria*

Correspondence should be addressed to Adham Zaazaa; adhamzaazaa@gmail.com

Academic Editor: Mohammad H. Ather

Forceful corporal dilatation amidst penile prosthesis implantation may injure cavernosal arteries compromising penile vasculature. In this study, we aimed to compare the conventional and cavernosal sparing techniques regarding cavernosal artery preservation. Overall, 33 patients underwent inflatable penile prosthesis implantation with Coloplast Titan Touch® three-piece inflatable penile implants. 16 patients had conventional implantations with serial vigorous dilatations, while 17 patients were implanted with the cavernosal sparing technique, consisting of a single minimal corporal dilatation after an intraoperative intracavernosal injection (ICI) of Alprostadil. Postoperatively, a penile duplex Doppler ultrasound study was performed. Whenever a cavernosal artery was spared and thus successfully probed, its hemodynamics were studied before and after an oral administration of a phosphodiesterase type 5 inhibitor (PDE5i). A cavernosal artery was successfully probed in 16/17 (94%) of patients in the cavernosal sparing group compared to 5/16 (31%) of patients in the conventional group with a significant statistical difference ($P = 0.001$). This demonstrated that the cavernosal sparing technique was superior to the conventional approach in preserving the cavernosal artery (odds ratio 35.2, 95% IC 3.5–344.2; $P = 0.0022$). Whenever a cavernosal artery could be probed, its hemodynamic responsiveness was also preserved. This trial is registered with NCT03733860.

1. Background

Since the advent of the inflatable penile prosthesis (IPP) in 1973, it has become the surgical gold standard in treating patients with refractory erectile dysfunction (ED) [1, 2]. Three-piece inflatable implants have shown greater satisfaction among patients compared to the semi-rigid rods, due to their better concealability and more natural erections [3]. Patients' satisfaction rates after three-piece inflatable implants have been estimated to be up to 98% and up to 96% among their partners [4].

Corporal dilatation during penile prosthesis implantation procedures can injure the cavernosal arteries. This would compromise the blood supply of the corpora and make them solely dependent on the dorsal and bulbourethral arteries. The postoperative application of tight dressings could then potentially compress these arteries against the underlying cylinders resulting in distal ischemia [5].

Cavernosal arteries also play an indirect role in glandular tumescence. The glans penis is mainly supplied by the dorsal arteries and the terminal branches of the spongiosal arteries. Glandular tumescence is partly caused by compression of the deep dorsal and circumflex veins between the engorged corpora cavernosa, supplied by the cavernosal arteries, and the surrounding tissues [6]. Thus, a lack of glans engorgement might be one of the indirect sequelae of cavernosal artery injury during penile prosthesis implantation. Additionally, postoperative loss of subjective penile tumescence and decreased penile girth often occur due to corporal tissue damage [6]. The erection obtained by means of a penile implant may therefore be perceived as "artificial" when it is uncoupled from physiological tumescence.

Efforts have been made to preserve some postoperative residual erectile function in the form of spontaneous tumescence and increased penile girth during sexual activity, which may play an important role in inciting female arousal [7, 8]. Therefore, PDE5i were prescribed after penile prosthesis implantations to increase patients' and partners' satisfaction by enhancing glans engorgement [9, 10]. In that context, Mulhall et al. [11] pointed out that patient satisfaction was indeed significantly increased with the implant-PDE5i combination compared to the implant alone. Grasso et al. [12] also noted an improvement in PSV in response to PDE5i, up to 6 years postimplantation. Lastly, Zaazaa and Mostafa [13] were able to detect pulsating cavernosal arteries by penile duplex Doppler ultrasound (PDDU), after malleable penile prostheses were implanted using the cavernosal sparing technique. In the present study, we adapted that technique to three-piece inflatable penile implantations in an attempt to spare the cavernosal arteries.

2. Materials and Methods

The study protocol was approved by the Institutional Ethical Committee and Review Board and informed consent was taken from all patients before the start of the study. The study took place from March 2019 to December 2020. Eligibility criteria included males over 18 years of age with ED of more than one year, unsatisfied with all types of medical treatment. All patients underwent a preoperative PDDU study, in which penile hemodynamics, peak systolic velocity (PSV), end-diastolic velocities (EDV), and resistivity index (RI) were recorded at baseline and 20 minutes after an ICI of 20 μg Alprostadil. Erection was assessed with the erection hardness grading scale. Only patients with adequate cavernosal artery arterial perfusion (PSV >30 cm/sec), obvious veno-occlusive mechanism disorder (EDV ≥6 cm/sec), and an erectile response ranging from 2 to 3 on the erection hardness grading scale were included [14–19].

Patients excluded from the study were patients who had previously undergone penile surgeries (e.g., hypospadias repair, correction of curvature, previous penile prosthesis implantation, and removal), patients with history of priapism or Peyronie's disease (whether causing a palpable mass and/or curvature or deformity on examination), and patients on organic nitrates and unwilling to retake PDE5i postoperatively.

Forty-two patients met the eligibility criteria. Nine patients were excluded from the study, four patients for choosing a different treatment modality, and five patients for declining to participate. Patients meeting the inclusion criteria were randomized to cavernosal sparing and conventional implantation groups using sealed envelopes. All patients were implanted with Coloplast Titan Touch® three-piece inflatable penile implants (Titan Touch, Coloplast, Minneapolis, MN, USA).

2.1. General Operative Considerations. Trichotomy was performed on the table and the skin was cleansed twice with Sterillium® disinfectant (HARTMANN International, Heidenheim Germany) before the application of povidone-iodine 10% (Betadine® Solution, Avrio Health LP, USA). The patient was placed in a supine position under spinal anesthesia and was catheterized with an indwelling foley urinary catheter. A purely scrotal longitudinal incision was chosen over the traditional penoscrotal incision due to its more esthetic healing. Two longitudinal corporotomies were performed, each between two sets of double stay sutures of 2/0 Monocryl. Double suturing (two sutures on each side of the corporotomy) ensured the stay sutures were less liable to tear during dilatation and implantation. Dilatation was deemed adequate when each dilator proximally reached a bone stopping point and distally extended well beyond the coronal sulcus. The lengths of the cylinders were deemed suitable when neither buckling nor a dropped glans were encountered intraoperatively after cylinder inflation. The same stay sutures were used to close the corporotomies.

2.2. Hemostatic Considerations. To decrease the occurrence of a postoperative scrotal hematoma, we adopted a 3-step approach to ensure better hemostasis. Before closing the scrotal incision, a 2 ml solution of ephedrine HCl was instilled into the scrotal cavity. A fairly tight wrap was applied to the scrotum to which the patients were advised to continuously apply ice packs for 3 days postoperatively. To avoid any urine soiling the wrap, the foley catheter was left in place until all bandages were removed.

2.3. Conventional Implantation. In the conventional surgery group, serial dilations of the corpora were carried out with Hegar dilators ranging from a size 8 up to a size 13 whenever possible. Dilatations were carried out with no prior intraoperative intracavernosal injection. Each dilator was passed twice proximally and twice distally, once in the dorsomedial plane and once in the ventrolateral plane, to ensure maximal dilatation.

2.4. Cavernosal Sparing Implantation. Unlike what we did in the group undergoing conventional surgery, patients that underwent cavernosal sparing implantation were intraoperatively injected with 40 μg Alprostadil intracorporeally to achieve intraoperative tumescence. Dilation was carried out with a size 7 Hegar dilator only, aiming at minimally disrupting the cavernous tissue and to avoid severing the cavernosal artery during implantation. It is worth noting that dilating tumescent corpora with engorged cavernous sinusoids was remarkably smoother than dilating through a detumescent penis with contracted cavernous tissue.

2.5. Postoperative PDDU Study. PDDU study was performed by a blinded operator, 4 to 6 weeks after implantation. A 7.5 MHz linear ultrasound transducer in superficial mode was used (Shenzhen Mindray Bio-Medical Electronics, Shenzhen, China). The presence of a pulsating cavernosal artery, around the inflated cylinders in the shaft of the penis, was probed. Care was taken not to confuse the dorsal artery pulsations with the cavernosal artery which should typically appear adjacent to the cylinders. If the cavernosal artery was not detected in both corpora, or segments of it detected with no pulsatile blood flow, it was deemed severed during dilatation or implantation. In case a pulsatile cavernosal artery was detected in either corpus, its hemodynamics were recorded both at baseline and after combined pharmacological and manual stimulation.

With the implants inflated (Figure 1), PSV, EDV, and RI were recorded at baseline (Figure 2). The patients were then administered a 10 mg orodispersible tablet of Vardenafil hydrochloride (Vivanza, Bayer). After 10 minutes, they were instructed to manually stimulate their penis for about 10 more minutes. PSV, ESV, and RI were recorded once more after sexual stimulation (Figure 3).

2.6. Statistical Analysis. Statistical analysis was performed using SPSS version 23 (SPSS Inc, Chicago, IL, USA). Paired *t*-test, ANOVA, and Fisher Exact test were used as statistical tools. P value <0.05 was set as statistically significant.

3. Results

Overall, 33 patients were randomized into 2 arms (16 patients received conventional implantations and 17 patients received cavernosal sparing implantations). The mean baseline PSV in both the cavernosal sparing and conventional groups at baseline as well as after ICI showed nonsignificant differences ($P = 0.553$; $P = 0.314$, respectively). Patients in both groups showed veno-occlusive dysfunction with no significant differences between their EDV ($P = 0.561$) (Table 1).

3.1. Postoperative Measurements. The postoperative detection of at least one pulsating cavernosal artery was achieved in 16/17 (94%) of patients in the cavernosal sparing group compared to 5/16 (31%) of patients in the conventional group ($P < 0.001$). The cavernosal sparing technique was thus superior to the conventional approach in preserving the cavernosal artery (odds ratio 35.2, 95% IC 3.5–344.2; $P = 0.0022$). In the cavernosal sparing group, both PSV and EDV increased in response to PDE5i administration ($P < 0.001$; $P = 0.001$, respectively). In the conventional group, PSV increased significantly in response to PDE5i administration ($P < 0.001$), while EDV showed nonsignificant change ($P = 0.720$) (Table 2). Hence, whenever an artery was spared, its PSV hemodynamic response to PDE5i was similarly preserved, whether it was spared by means of the cavernosal sparing technique or during a conventional implantation.

3.2. Surgical Complications. One patient in the conventional group exhibited posterior perforation and surgery was resumed with sling sutures applied to the rear tip extender [20]. No perforations were encountered in the cavernosal sparing group. Two patients in the cavernosal sparing group developed a postoperative scrotal hematoma that was treated conservatively. All of these aforementioned complications were of grade I of the Clavien–Dindo classification [21].

4. Discussion

One of the key steps of conventional penile prosthesis implantations is serially dilating the corpora with dilators of incrementally increasing sizes. This step might inevitably cause cavernous tissue damage evident by the ubiquitous scarring in redo cases. Therefore, many attempts have been made to minimize corporal tissue injury during this step.

In their randomized controlled trial on 100 patients, Moncada et al. [22] suggested omitting the dilatation step altogether in virgin cases. This not only lessened postoperative pain due to less tissue damage but also preserved some residual erectile function, enabling patients to score higher on questions 1 to 3 of the International Index of Erectile Function (IIEF) questionnaire.

Zaazaa and Mostafa [13] proposed an additional cavernous tissue-sparing technique consisting of minimal dilatation after pharmacologically induced tumescence. In that randomized controlled trial on 92 patients, the cavernous tissue-sparing technique yielded a higher incidence of postoperative subjectively reported tumescence. Postoperative ultrasound imaging showed superior radial cavernous tissue thickness translating into a significantly higher postoperative penile girth.

In this context, tumescence, with its subsequent increased penile girth, not only is important for subjective arousal but also enhances the partner's excitement in terms of the perception of "being desired" [7, 8, 23]. Another advantage of preserving cavernous tissue would be the preservation of postoperative tumescence hence decreasing the likelihood of a "floppy glans" thus enabling easier vaginal penetration [24].

In the current study, we applied the cavernosal sparing technique to inflatable penile prosthesis implantation. We then studied residual erectile function in the form of cavernosal artery responsiveness to PDE5i. The preservation of a cavernosal artery and hence its PDE5i responsiveness was noted in 16/17 (94%) of patients in the cavernosal sparing group versus 5/16 (31%) of patients in the conventional group with significant difference.

Intraoperative tumescence and minimal dilatation are the two principal steps in the cavernosal sparing technique. In the current series, the cavernosal artery was spared in 5/16 (31%) of patients in the conventional group despite serial dilatations. It could be postulated that this might be due to suboptimal dilatations and/or accidental intraoperative tumescence. Welti and Brodsky [25] as well as Baltogiannis et al. [26] have reported intraoperative erections with an incidence of up to 2.4%, suggesting that intraoperative tumescence, not full erection, might be of even higher

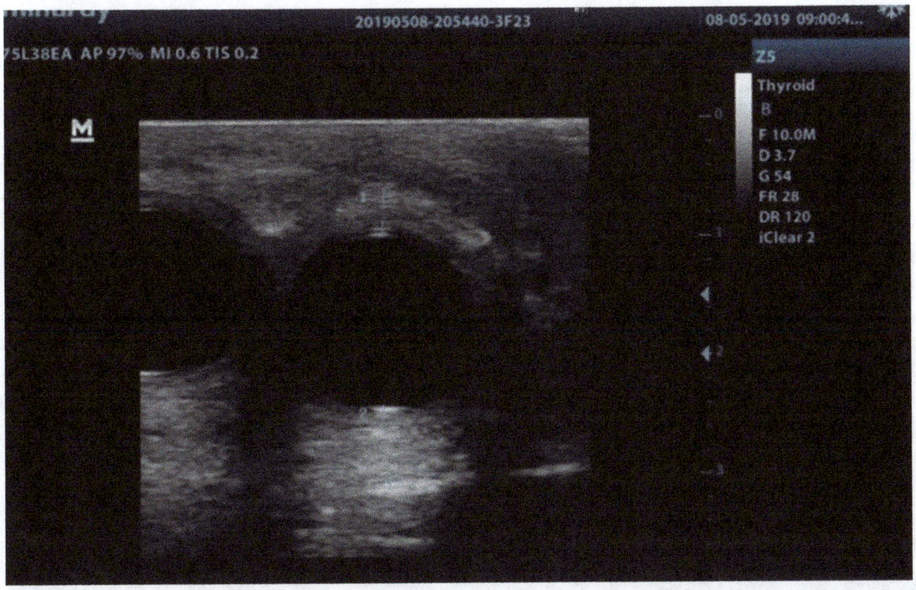

FIGURE 1: Inflated cylinders. 2D ultrasound image showing the inflated cylinders before penile hemodynamic measurement.

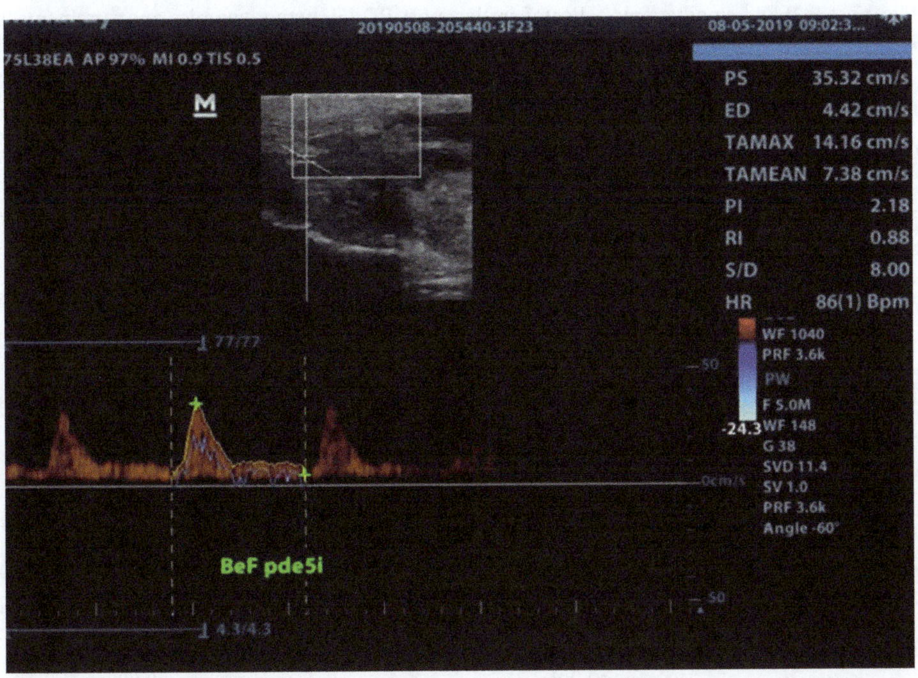

FIGURE 2: Postoperative baseline hemodynamics. PDDU showing postoperative baseline hemodynamics before administration of PDE5i. Note that Figures 2 and 3 are for the same patient.

incidence, but would pass unnoticed or unreported. Inline, Manning et al. [27] reported spontaneous tumescence after 3-piece prosthesis implantation in 53% of their cases. Another case report by Yildirim et al. [28] reported the occurrence of a complete rigid erection without inflating the implant cylinders.

Other than spontaneous tumescence, PDE5i-induced tumescence was also noted after penile prosthesis implantation. In their study, Mulhall et al. [11] endorsed prescribing up to 100 mg sildenafil citrate after penile prosthesis implantations to enhance glans engorgement, with a significantly better IIEF score achieved in those patients compared to patients not receiving PDE5i. In the current study, penile hemodynamic responsiveness to PDE5i was used as our outcome measure instead of the IIEF score.

In another series of 12 patients with Peyronie's disease undergoing malleable penile implantations for correction of acquired penile curvatures, Grasso et al. [12] demonstrated improved cavernous tissue thickness from 5 mm to 9 mm and increased PSV from 7.5 cm/s to 16.5 cm/s both at

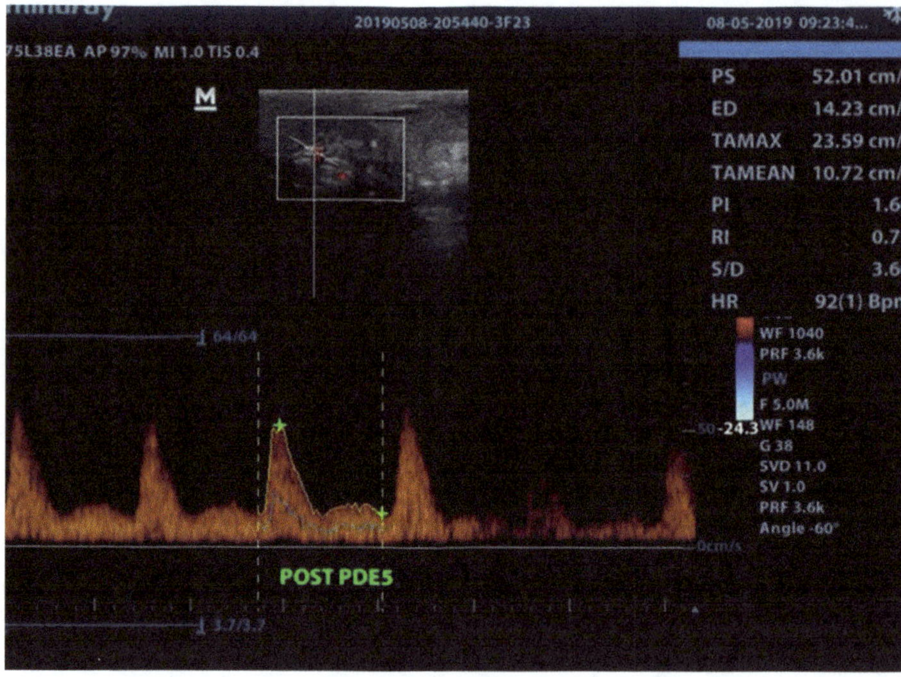

Figure 3: Postoperative post-PDE5i hemodynamics. Postoperative post-PDE5i hemodynamics measurements showing pronounced cavernosal artery waves, recorded 20 minutes after PDE5i administration and manual stimulation. Please note that Figures 2 and 3 are for the same patient.

Table 1: Patients' characteristics and preoperative baseline measurements (mean ± SD, range).

	Cavernosal sparing group ($n = 17$)	Conventional group ($n = 16$)	P
Age (years)	47.4 ± 12.3 (30.0–69.0)	54.3 ± 11.8 (36.0–71.0)	0.1106
BMI (kg/m^2)	27.2 ± 1.3 (25.0–29.7)	26.8 ± 1.1 (25.2–29.1)	0.3489
ED duration (years)	4.7 ± 2.1 (2.0–8.0)	5.1 ± 2.4 (2.0–9.0)	0.6134
Basal PSV (cm/s)	17.7 ± 5.8 (10–30)	19.1 ± 4.1 (11.3–27.7)	0.4321
PSV (cm/s) after ICI	49.9 ± 13.2 (30.9–80.0)	45.6 ± 10.9 (32.23–71.7)	0.3516
Basal EDV (cm/s)	0.1 ± 0.4 (0.0–1.4)	0 (0)	—
EDV (cm/s) after ICI	12.6 ± 4.0 (6.1–20.9)	11.8 ± 3.6 (6.1–20.1)	0.5512

BMI: body mass index; PSV: peak systolic velocity; EDV: end-diastolic velocity; ICI: intracavernosal injection.

Table 2: Postoperative measurements of spared cavernosal artery (mean ± SD, range).

	Cavernosal sparing group ($n = 16$)	Conventional group ($n = 5$)	P
PSV baseline (cm/s)	33.5 ± 7.6 (17.7–43.2)	28.4 ± 7.8 (18.1–40.1)	0.0708
PSV (cm/s) after PDE5i	56.4 ± 11.5 (36.8–83.4)	51.2 ± 5.7 (45.5–60.2)	0.1156
P	<0.001	<0.001	
EDV baseline (cm/s)	5.7 ± 4.7 (0.0–13.7)	11.6 ± 7.4 (0.0–26.9)	0.1708
EDV (cm/s) after PDE5i	8.4 ± 5.5 (2.3–15.2)	9.4 ± 2.3 (7.3–13.1)	0.7173
P	0.001	0.720	

Paired t-test. PSV: peak systolic velocity; EDV: end-diastolic velocity; PDE5i: phosphodiesterase type 5 inhibitor.

baseline and then after administration of 50 mg sildenafil citrate, up to 6 years postimplantation. This postoperative increase in PSV was reproduced in our study whenever a cavernosal artery could be probed.

In our experience, corporal dilatation was found to be smoother with intraoperative tumescence, as the dilator would glide in a path of least resistance, through blood-filled sinusoidal spaces, as opposed to being pushed through the contracted cavernous tissue of a flaccid penis [29]. Additionally, intraoperative tumescence enhanced the assessment of penile size and shape, allowed for a better grip during surgical manipulations, and enabled easier installations of the paracorporotomy stay sutures.

In response to the omnipresent question among implant surgeons: to dilate or not to dilate? It could be assumed from the current series that minimal dilatation should suffice in virgin cases. Serial dilatations can be reserved for cases with corporal fibrosis and scarring, such as Peyronie's disease, neglected priapism, or redo cases.

Previously reported advantages of the cavernosal sparing technique include preserving subjectively reported tumescence [13], optimizing postimplantation penile dimensions [30], and theoretically nonetheless, enhancing postoperative antibiotics reach to the plane around the implants [31]. This study proposes the cavernosal sparing implantation technique as a means of further enhancing postoperative PDE5i hemodynamic responsiveness, after inflatable penile prosthesis implantations.

Still, the current study's main limitations are the lack of placebo control and validated questionnaires such as the Erectile Dysfunction Inventory of Treatment Satisfaction (EDITS) questionnaire [32] or IIEF score [33]. Further studies are also needed to correlate between the sonographic hemodynamic responsiveness and clinical manifestations such as glans engorgement and penile tumescence.

5. Conclusions

The present study gives an ultrasonographic rationale for the use of PDE5i after inflatable penile prosthesis implantations. Given the observed results, we recommend the use of the cavernosal sparing technique in virgin inflatable penile prosthesis implantations to potentially enhance the postoperative response to pharmacological adjuvant therapies.

Abbreviations

ED: Erectile dysfunction
EDITS: Erectile dysfunction inventory of treatment satisfaction
EDV: End-diastolic velocity
ICI: Intracavernosal injection
IIEF: International index of erectile function
IPP: Inflatable penile prosthesis
PDDU: Penile duplex Doppler ultrasound
PDE5i: Phosphodiesterase type 5 inhibitors
PROBE: Prospective randomized open-blinded end-point
PSV: Peak systolic velocity
RI: Resistivity index.

Consent

Informed consent was taken from all the patients before the start of the study.

Authors' Contributions

A. Zaazaa and T. Mostafa contributed to conception and design; A. Zaazaa, T. Mostafa, R. Elnabarawy, and M. Elbitar contributed to administrative support; A. Zaazaa contributed to provision of patients; all authors contributed to collection and assembly of data, data analysis and interpretation, manuscript writing, and final approval of manuscript. The authors are accountable for all aspects of the work in ensuring that questions related to the accuracy or integrity of any part of the work are appropriately investigated and resolved.

References

[1] F. Brantley Scott, W. E. Bradley, G. W. Timm, and G. W. Timm, "Management of erectile impotence Use of implantable inflatable prosthesis," *Urology*, vol. 2, no. 1, pp. 80–82, 1973.
[2] L. Trost and W. J. G. Hellstrom, "History, contemporary outcomes, and future of penile prostheses: a review of the literature," *Sexual Medicine Reviews*, vol. 1, no. 3, pp. 150–163, 2013.
[3] L. A. Levine, E. Becher, A. Bella et al., "Penile prosthesis surgery: current recommendations from the international consultation on sexual medicine," *The Journal of Sexual Medicine*, vol. 13, no. 4, pp. 489–518, 2016.
[4] F. Montorsi, P. Rigatti, G. Carmignani et al., "AMS three-piece inflatable implants for erectile dysfunction: a long-term multi-institutional study in 200 consecutive patients," *European Urology*, vol. 37, no. 1, pp. 50–55, 2000.
[5] S. K. Wilson, C. Mora-Estaves, P. Egydio et al., "Glans necrosis following penile prosthesis implantation: prevention and treatment suggestions," *Urology*, vol. 107, pp. 144–148, 2017.
[6] U. B. Zaid, X. Zhang, and T. F. Lue, "Physiology of penile erection," *Male Sexual Dysfunction*, vol. 14–21, 2016.
[7] B. P. Jiann, C. C. Su, and J. Y. Tsai, "Is female sexual function related to the male partners' erectile function?" *The Journal of Sexual Medicine*, vol. 10, no. 2, pp. 420–429, 2013.
[8] R. Basson, "Human sexual response," *Neurology of Sexual and Bladder Disorders*, vol. 130, pp. 11–18, 2015.
[9] A. O. Mireku-Boateng, M. Dennery, and J. Littlejohn, "Use of sildenafil in penile implant patients," *Urologia Internationalis*, vol. 66, no. 3, pp. 149–151, 2001.
[10] E. Lledó garcia, I. Moncada iribarren, J. Jara rascón et al., "Tratamiento con sildenafilo del síndrome de glande frio tras implante de prótesis hidráulica de pene," *Actas Urológicas Españolas*, vol. 28, no. 6, pp. 443–446, 2004.
[11] J. P. Mulhall, A. Jahoda, N. Aviv, R. Valenzuela, and M. Parker, "The impact of sildenafil citrate on sexual satisfaction profiles in men with a penile prosthesis in situ," *BJU International*, vol. 93, no. 1, pp. 97–99, 2004.
[12] M. Grasso, C. Lania, F. Fortuna, S. Blanco, and I. Piacentini, "Preservation of cavernosal erectile function after soft penile prosthesis implant in Peyronie's disease: long-term followup," *Advances in Urology*, vol. 2008, Article ID 646052, 2008.
[13] A. Zaazaa and T. Mostafa, "Spontaneous penile tumescence by sparing cavernous tissue in the course of malleable penile prosthesis implantation," *The Journal of Sexual Medicine*, vol. 16, no. 3, pp. 474–478, 2019.
[14] S. C. Sikka, W. J. G. Hellstrom, G. Brock, and A. M. Morales, "Standardization of vascular assessment of erectile dysfunction," *The Journal of Sexual Medicine*, vol. 10, no. 1, pp. 120–129, 2013.
[15] E. Chung, L. De Young, and G. B. Brock, "Penile duplex ultrasonography in men with peyronie's disease: is it veno-occlusive dysfunction or poor cavernosal arterial inflow that

contributes to erectile dysfunction?" *The Journal of Sexual Medicine*, vol. 8, no. 12, pp. 3446–3451, 2011.

[16] M. Mancini, M. Bartolini, and V. Maggi, "Duplex ultrasound evaluation of cavernosal peak systolic velocity and waveform acceleration in the penile flaccid state: clinical significance in the assessment of the arterial supply in patients with erectile dysfunction," *International Journal of Andrology*, vol. 23, no. 4, pp. 199–204, 2000.

[17] Y.-C. Kuo, S.-P. Liu, J.-H. Chen, H.-C. Chang, V. F. S. Tsai, and J.-T. Hsieh, "Feasability of a novel audio-video sexual stimulation system: an adjunct to the use of penile duplex Doppler ultrasonography for the investigation of erectile dysfunction," *The Journal of Sexual Medicine*, vol. 7, no. 12, pp. 3979–3983, 2010.

[18] W. Hsiao, A. B. Shrewsberry, K. A. Moses, D. Pham, and C. W. M. Ritenour, "Longer time to peak flow predicts better arterial flow parameters on penile Doppler ultrasound," *Urology*, vol. 75, no. 1, pp. 112–116, 2010.

[19] J. P. Mulhall, L. A. Levine, and K.-P. Jünemann, "Erection hardness: a unifying factor for defining response in the treatment of erectile dysfunction," *Urology*, vol. 68, no. 3, pp. 17–25, 2006.

[20] S. K. Wilson, "Surgical techniques: rear tip extender sling: a quick and easy repair for crural perforation," *The Journal of Sexual Medicine*, vol. 7, no. 3, pp. 1052–1055, 2010.

[21] D. Dindo, N. Demartines, and P.-A. Clavien, "Classification of surgical complications," *Annals of Surgery*, vol. 240, no. 2, pp. 205–213, 2004.

[22] I. Moncada, J. I. Martínez-Salamanca, J. Jara, R. Cabello, M. Moralejo, and C. Hernández, "Inflatable penile prosthesis implantation without corporeal dilation: a cavernous tissue sparing technique," *Journal of Urology*, vol. 183, no. 3, pp. 1123–1126, 2010.

[23] M. L. Chivers, M. C. Seto, M. L. Lalumière, E. Laan, and T. Grimbos, "Agreement of self-reported and genital measures of sexual arousal in men and women: a meta-analysis," *Archives of Sexual Behavior*, vol. 39, no. 1, pp. 5–56, 2010.

[24] M. Bickell, N. Manimala, J. Parker, B. Steixner, L. Wiegand, and R. Carrion, "Floppy glans syndrome: pathogenesis and treatment," *Sexual Medicine Reviews*, vol. 4, no. 2, pp. 149–156, 2016.

[25] R. S. Welti and J. B. Brodsky, "Treatment of intraoperative penile tumescence," *Journal of Urology*, vol. 124, no. 6, pp. 925-926, 1980.

[26] D. M. Baltogiannis, A. K. Charalabopoulos, X. K. Giannakopoulos, D. J. Giannakis, N. V. Sofikitis, and K. A. Charalabopoulos, "Penile erection during transurethral surgery," *Journal of Andrology*, vol. 27, no. 3, pp. 376–380, 2006.

[27] M. Manning, F. J. Martínez, P. Alken, and K.-P. Jünemann, "Spontaneous tumescence after implantation of three-piece hydraulic penile prostheses: a short-term experience," *International Journal of Impotence Research*, vol. 15, no. 3, pp. 152–155, 2003.

[28] I. Yildirim, E. Aydur, L. Tahmaz, H. C. Irkilata, B. Seçkin, and A. F. Peker, "Spontaneous and prolonged drug-induced erection in a patient with inflatable penile implant," *Andrologia*, vol. 39, no. 2, pp. 71-72, 2007.

[29] C. Costa and P. Vendeira, "Does erectile tissue angioarchitecture modify with aging? An immunohistological and morphometric approach," *The Journal of Sexual Medicine*, vol. 5, no. 4, pp. 833–840, 2008.

[30] B. B. Shah, M. Kent, and R. Valenzuela, "Advanced penile length restoration techniques to optimize penile prosthesis placement outcomes," *Sexual Medicine Reviews*, vol. 9, 2020.

[31] R. E. Fernandez-Crespo, K. Buscaino, J. Parker, and R. Carrion, "Current status for semirigid penile prosthetic devices," *Current Urology Reports*, vol. 22, no. 2, p. 7, 2021.

[32] S. E. Althof, E. W. Corty, S. B. Levine et al., "EDITS: development of questionnaires for evaluating satisfaction with treatments for erectile dysfunction," *Urology*, vol. 53, no. 4, pp. 793–799, 1999.

[33] R. Rosen, J. Cappelleri, M. Smith, J. Lipsky, and B. Peña, "Development and evaluation of an abridged, 5-item version of the international index of erectile function (IIEF-5) as a diagnostic tool for erectile dysfunction," *International Journal of Impotence Research*, vol. 11, no. 6, pp. 319–326, 1999.

18

Novel Bioceramic Urethral Bulking Agents Elicit Improved Host Tissue Responses in a Rat Model

**Travis K. Mann-Gow,[1] Benjamin J. King,[1]
Ahmed El-Ghannam,[2] Christine Knabe-Ducheyne,[3] Masatoshi Kida,[4]
Ole M. Dall,[5] Jan Krhut,[6] and Peter Zvara[1,6,7]**

[1] *Department of Surgery, University of Vermont, Burlington, VT 05405, USA*
[2] *Department of Mechanical Engineering and Engineering Science, University of North Carolina at Charlotte, Charlotte, NC 28223, USA*
[3] *Department of Medicine, Philipps University of Marburg, 35039 Marburg, Germany*
[4] *Department of Pathology and Laboratory Medicine, University of Vermont, Burlington, VT 05405, USA*
[5] *TAK Biopharma, 2000 Frederiksberg, Denmark*
[6] *Department of Surgical Sciences, Ostrava University, 703 00 Ostrava, Czech Republic*
[7] *Department of Urology and Biomedical Laboratory, Clinical Institute, University of Southern Denmark, 5000 Odense, Denmark*

Correspondence should be addressed to Peter Zvara; peter.zvara@uvm.edu

Academic Editor: Matthew Rutman

Objectives. To test the physical properties and host response to the bioceramic particles, silica-calcium phosphate (SCPC10) and Cristobalite, in a rat animal model and compare their biocompatibility to the current clinically utilized urethral bulking materials. *Material and Methods.* The novel bulking materials, SCPC10 and Cristobalite, were suspended in hyaluronic acid sodium salt and injected into the mid urethra of a rat. Additional animals were injected with bulking materials currently in clinical use. Physiological response was assessed using voiding trials, and host tissue response was evaluated using hard tissue histology and immunohistochemical analysis. Distant organs were evaluated for the presence of particles or their components. *Results.* Histological analysis of the urethral tissue five months after injection showed that both SCPC10 and Cristobalite induced a more robust fibroblastic and histiocytic reaction, promoting integration and encapsulation of the particle aggregates, leading to a larger bulking effect. Concentrations of Ca, Na, Si, and P ions in the experimental groups were comparable to control animals. *Conclusions.* This side-by-side examination of urethral bulking agents using a rat animal model and hard tissue histology techniques compared two newly developed bioactive ceramic particles to three of the currently used bulking agents. The local host tissue response and bulking effects of bioceramic particles were superior while also possessing a comparable safety profile.

1. Introduction

Approximately 130,000 surgical procedures are performed annually to treat stress urinary incontinence (SUI) in the US [1]. Urethral bulking therapy (UBT) was used frequently in the 1990s but lost popularity due to three main reasons: first, disappointing long-term efficacy; second, complications related to local host tissue response and distant tissue migration; and third, a dramatic increase in the use of polypropylene mesh. SUI treatment using mesh has, in some cases, led to severe and sometimes irreversible complications resulting in an FDA warning first released in 2008 and then again in 2011 [2, 3]. Subsequent to the warnings, there was a resurgence of interest in other forms of treatment for SUI [4]. Provided its limitations are resolved, UBT represents an ideal treatment for poor surgical candidates, patients with comorbidities, placing them in a high-risk category for anesthesia, as well as patients who opt against a more complex surgical procedure [5].

Complications related to the use of synthetic material in the treatment of SUI highlight a need for preclinical studies. Experimental animal models could be used to help assess and solve the fundamental problem associated with UBT, the absence of an ideal bulking material. The urethral bulking agent should be stable, easy to inject, nonimmunogenic, permanent, nonmigratory, nonerosive, and easily stored and handled and should possess a high safety profile [6]. All these properties can be tested on laboratory animals; however only a few such preclinical studies have been performed to date [7, 8]. We recently described a rat model for preclinical testing of urethral bulking agents, including hard microparticle bulking therapy [9]. In this study, we present a preclinical experiment comparing two new bioactive ceramic bulking materials to the three bulking agents most commonly used in treatment of SUI.

The two new bulking materials we tested were silica-calcium phosphate (SCPC10) and Cristobalite. Both of these bioactive ceramic particles have been studied extensively in bone regeneration [10]. Previous studies documented that bioceramics stimulate tissue attachment to the porous surface through serum protein adsorption, tissue formation, and cell attachment [11]. The chemical stability of bioceramics depends on the chemical composition and crystalline phases, which can be controlled by thermal treatment and compact pressure during the manufacturing process [12]. In addition, we used a new formulation of hyaluronic acid sodium salt, sodium hyaluronate, Hyaluronan (HA), with optimized viscosity, which gets absorbed by the body, leaving only the particles at the injection site where they can interact directly with the tissue. We suspended the two different experimental, bioceramic particles in HA and injected them into the proximal urethra of a rat. As a control, we used bulking materials that are currently in clinical use: silicon particles (Macroplastique, Uroplasty Inc, Minneapolis, MN, USA), calcium-hydroxyapatite particles (Copatite, Boston Scientific, Natic, MA, USA), and polyacrylamide hydrogel (Bulkamid, Contura International, Soeborg, Denmark). We used hard tissue histology techniques to evaluate particle integrity, incorporation, and host tissue reaction. In addition, we harvested the distal organs and tested them for the presence of particle and/or trace levels of their components.

2. Material and Methods

An individual bulking agent was injected into the proximal urethra of 21 female Wistar rats. Six animals per experimental group were injected with either SCPC10 or Cristobalite and three animals per control group were injected with Coaptite, Bulkamid, or Macroplastique. Organs from three healthy animals were harvested as normal controls.

2.1. Preparation of Bioceramic Particles, HA Suspension. HA, prepared in double-distilled water (ddH_2O), was used as the suspension media for the two experimental bulking agents. According to our previous research, we used HA (molecular weight of 900 kDa) at a 2.5% concentration with a bioceramic particle to HA ratio of 1 : 4 [9]. The suspension mixture was sterilized in an autoclave for 20 minutes at 121°C. Viscosity of the 2.5% HA solution was approximately 80,000 cP prior to sterilization and decreased to approximately 30,000 cP following sterilization due to a slightly lower molecular weight, which is caused by heat-induced depolymerization of the HA molecule. pH of the material was 7.2 and remained within the physiological range after dissolving in water. Once sterilized, the solution was mixed on a mixing plate for 12 hours, or until the bioceramic particles were evenly distributed throughout the suspension media.

2.2. Injection. Female Wistar rats, 6-7 months old (Charles River Laboratories, Saint-Constant, Quebec, Canada), were maintained under standard laboratory conditions with free access to food and water. The University of Vermont Institutional Animal Care and Use Committee approved all animal procedures, and appropriate measures were taken to minimize pain and discomfort to the animals. Under inhalation anesthesia, through a lower midline abdominal incision, the mid urethra was bluntly dissected to expose the injection site. Using direct visualization with an operating microscope, the urethral bulking agent was injected into the wall of the mid urethra. This injection technique was previously described in depth [9]. Microphotographs were taken to record any gross abnormalities.

2.3. Tissue Harvesting. Five months after injection, under general inhalation anesthesia, a midline abdominal incision was made and the urethra was exposed. Following removal of the urethra, the lungs, kidneys, liver, and spleen were harvested to test for levels of particle ions. All tissues were immediately fixed in an ethanol-based fixative, HistoChoice (Amresco, Solon, OH), for 7 days at room temperature.

2.4. Histological Analysis. Urethral specimens were processed using a novel technique, which facilitates immunohistochemical analysis on tissues containing hard particles [13–15]. It involves embedding the specimen in resin and cutting the sections using a sawing microtome (Leitz 1600, Wetzlar, Germany). This method was previously described in detail [9]. Immunohistochemical staining was performed using a primary mouse monoclonal antibody specific to tumor necrosis factor-alpha (TNF-α, Abcam Ltd., Cambridge, UK). Additional sections were stained using Giemsa surface stain [16]. A pathologist evaluated the urethral cross-sections to determine bead morphology and host tissue reaction.

2.5. Scanning Electron Microscopy (SEM). Bioceramic particles were analyzed with SEM prior to suspension and injection. The size, shape, and integrity of the bulking material were evaluated.

2.6. Evaluation of Distant Organs for the Presence of Particles and Their Components. Following tissue digestion, filtration, and centrifugation, the liver, kidneys, spleen, and lungs were examined microscopically for the presence of whole particles. Subsequently, organs were digested in 70% HNO_3 and the concentration of Si, P, Ca, and Na was measured using

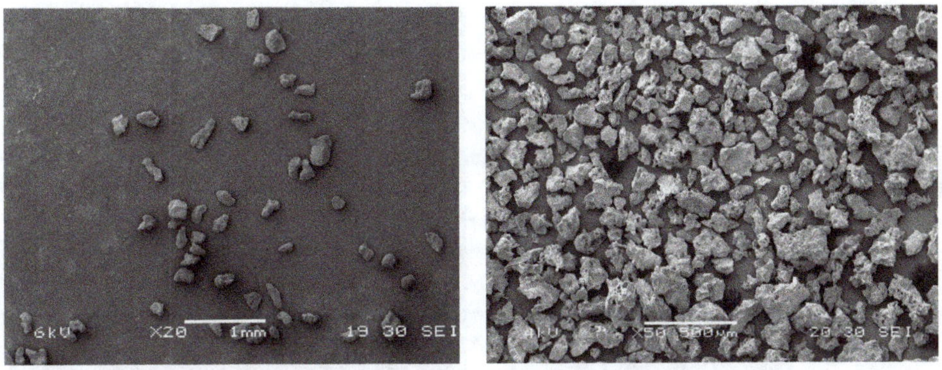

(a) (b)

FIGURE 1: Scanning electron microscopy depicting the surface of (a) Cristobalite and (b) SCPC10 particles.

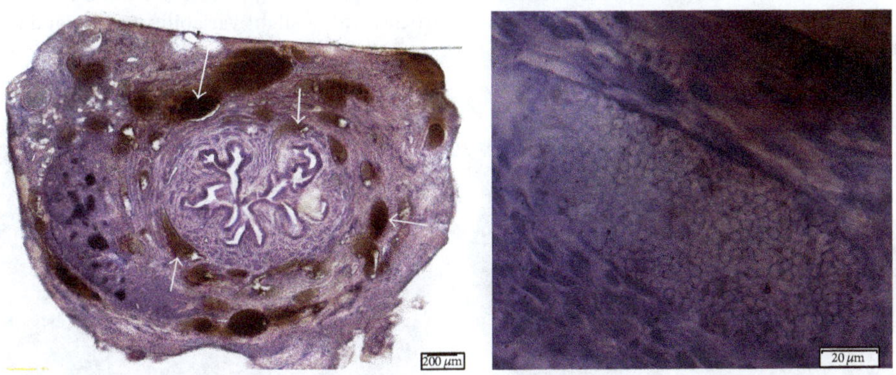

(a) (b)

FIGURE 2: Cross-sections of urethra 5 months after injection of SCPC10 particles. (a) Cross-sectional view of entire urethra with nodular particle packets in the submucosa and adventitia (10x magnification). Arrows indicate particle masses. (b) Particle packet in a well circumscribed nodule showing some surface irregularities and size variability of the individual particles (20x magnification).

inductively coupled plasma optical emission spectroscopy. A control experiment was run in parallel using organs from normal, noninjected animals.

2.7. Statistical Analysis. Quantitative values were presented as means ± standard error of the mean. All statistical calculations were performed using GraphPad PRISM (San Diego, CA, USA). Paired data were evaluated using a two-tailed Student's t-test. A one-way analysis of variance was used for comparisons of multiple groups. P values ≤ 0.05 were considered statistically significant.

3. Results

3.1. SEM Evaluation of Bioceramic Particles. Cristobalite particles were cuboidal in shape, with a cross-section size of 75–200 micrometers. Significant variation in the shape and size was noted among the SCPC10 particles, which displayed a coral-like appearance with multiple pores (Figure 1).

3.2. Intraoperative Examination. In vivo examination under the operating microscope of Cristobalite and SCPC10 particles 5 month after injection did not reveal any gross abnormalities. No signs of abscess formation, acute inflammatory changes, or florid scarring of the host tissue were noted. These observations were comparable to those obtained immediately following injection.

3.3. Histological Examination

3.3.1. SCPC10. Cross-sections of the injection site showed coaptation of the urethral mucosa, with the particles located in the submucosa and urethral smooth muscle. Surface irregularities of individual particles were noted on high-power light microscopy. Collagen fibers were densely packed around the particle mass. Immunostaining did not reveal active macrophages, signs of a robust foreign body response, or scarring. Fibroblastic proliferation around individual particles resulted in a 1.5–2 times larger volume than the injected particle mass alone (Figure 2).

3.3.2. Cristobalite. Particle aggregates were seen scattered throughout the urethral cross-sections. The aggregates were polyhedral in shape and were integrated into the tissue

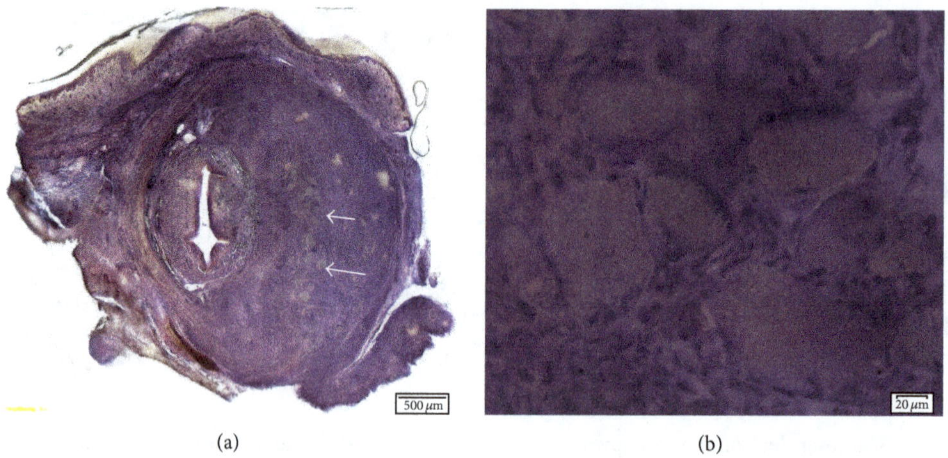

FIGURE 3: Cross-sections of rat urethra 5 months after injection of Cristobalite particles. (a) Cross-sectional view of the entire urethra (10x magnification). Arrows indicating particle mass. (b) Image showing particles with a slight variability in size and surrounding fibroblastic proliferation (20x magnification).

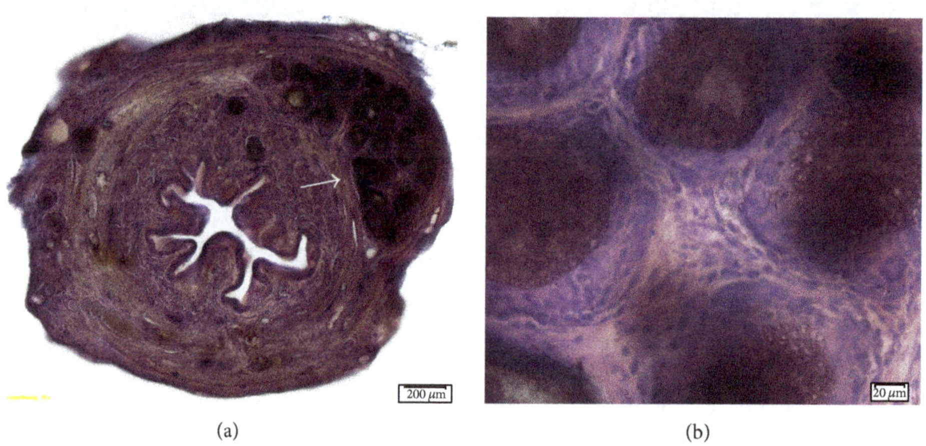

FIGURE 4: (a) Cross-sections of urethra 5 months after injection of Coaptite (10x magnification). Arrow pointing to particle mass. (b) Image showing particles surrounded by fibroblasts and giant cells. Relatively uniform size of the injected particles.

due to the surrounding mild host reaction. Fibroblastic proliferation around the particle masses and between the individual particles was noted. This proliferation resulted in a volume 2-3 times larger than the injected particle mass alone, which was noted on the urethral lumen. Some histiocytes were interspersed among the fibroblasts, indicating a mild histiocytic reaction. The particles were seen as a mass in the adventitia as well as the submucosa of the urethra (Figure 3). Overall, for both SCPC10 and Cristobalite, a minor host tissue response without florid scarring was visualized using light microscopy. The presence of macrophages and a host tissue inflammatory response was ruled out with negative TNF alpha staining.

3.3.3. Coaptite. Compared to the bioceramic particles, there were less fibroblastic changes with less mass effect. The increase in volume was approximately twofold. Fibroblastic proliferation was more localized and nodular and was surrounded by giant cells. The injected material was primarily seen in aggregates, with each aggregate containing a variable amount of material. There were also aggregates of histiocytes with giant cells interspersed. The contour of each individual calcium hydroxylapatite particle was relatively uniform. Coaptite showed calcium-hydroxyapatite particles uniform in size (70–125 microns) surrounded by fibroblasts and collagen (Figure 4).

3.3.4. Bulkamid. There were two distinct types of host tissue reaction: diffuse fibroblastic changes and nodular aggregates with mild fibroblastic proliferation. The diffuse changes were surrounded by fibroblasts, resulting in an increased volume of approximately 3-fold. The nodular type of reaction resulted in a volume increase of approximately 2-fold. The volume effect and fibroblastic reaction seen in the nodular tissue changes were similar to those seen with Coaptite. There was a large variation in size of the nodular aggregates spread throughout the tissue. Distribution of the bulking agent was seen in the

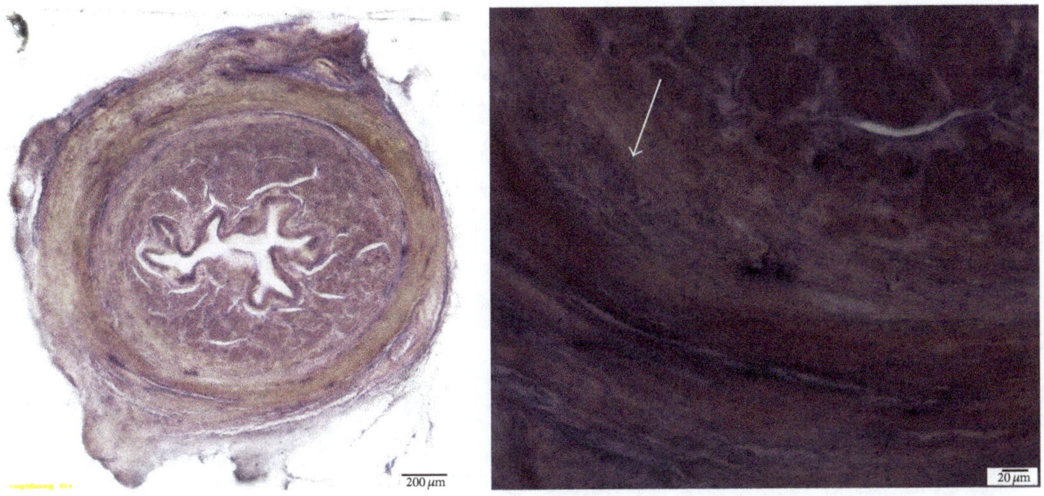

(a) (b)

FIGURE 5: Cross-sections of urethra 5 months after injection of Bulkamid. (a) Cross-section of urethra without large injection mass (10x magnification). (b) Image showing small injection aggregates in a nodular type of reaction with mild surrounding fibroblastic changes (20x magnification). Arrow indicates bulking agent mass.

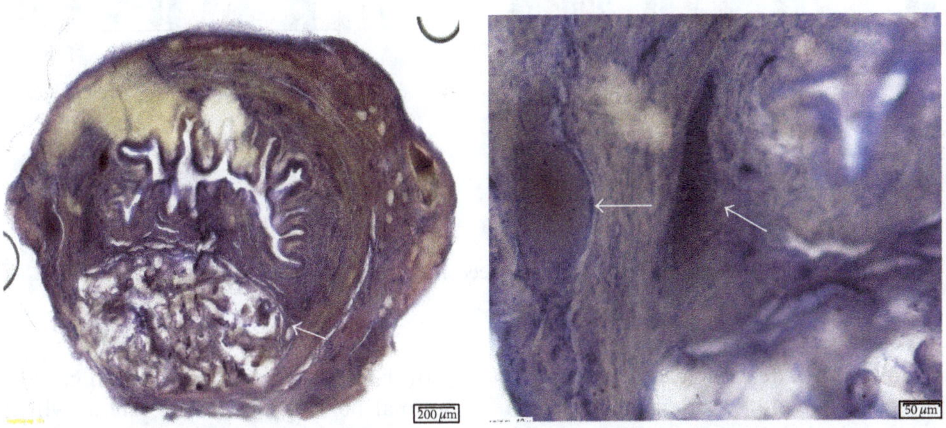

(a) (b)

FIGURE 6: Cross-sections of urethra 5 months after injection of Macroplastique. (a) Cross-section of entire urethra (10x magnification). Arrows indicate bulking material mass in the adventitia and suburothelium. (b) Injected bulking material with some surrounding fibroblastic proliferation (20x magnification).

adventitia and submucosa. The only tissue change noted with Bulkamid was mild fibroblastic proliferation (Figure 5).

3.3.5. Macroplastique. This bulking agent also displayed two distinct reaction types to the injected material: nodular aggregates and a more diffuse fibroblastic type of reaction. The nodular aggregates of material appeared to be somewhat band-like, partially folded onto itself, and surrounded predominantly by histiocytes. This resulted in an increase in volume of approximately 1.5-fold. The more diffuse reaction is primarily a fibroblastic reaction with mild, thin proliferation surrounding the injected bead masses. The injected material aggregates varied significantly in size and shape. Individual silicone beads varied in size by a factor of 8. Particles were organized in collagen-encapsulated clusters with evidence of mild fibroblast in-growth (Figure 6).

3.4. Evaluation of Distant Organs. There were no particles detected in the distant organs. Animals injected with Cristobalite and Macroplastique appeared to have higher Si concentrations in the lungs; nevertheless, the ion concentrations in all of the organs were within the biological range. Trace components (Si, P, Ca, and Na elements) from SCPC10 and Cristobalite showed comparable concentrations to the other injected bulking agents and the healthy, intact controls (Figure 7).

4. Discussion

The use of urethral bulking therapy declined significantly over the course of the last two decades, in part, due to an increase in the use of anti-incontinence procedures using polypropylene mesh. It has been well documented that this

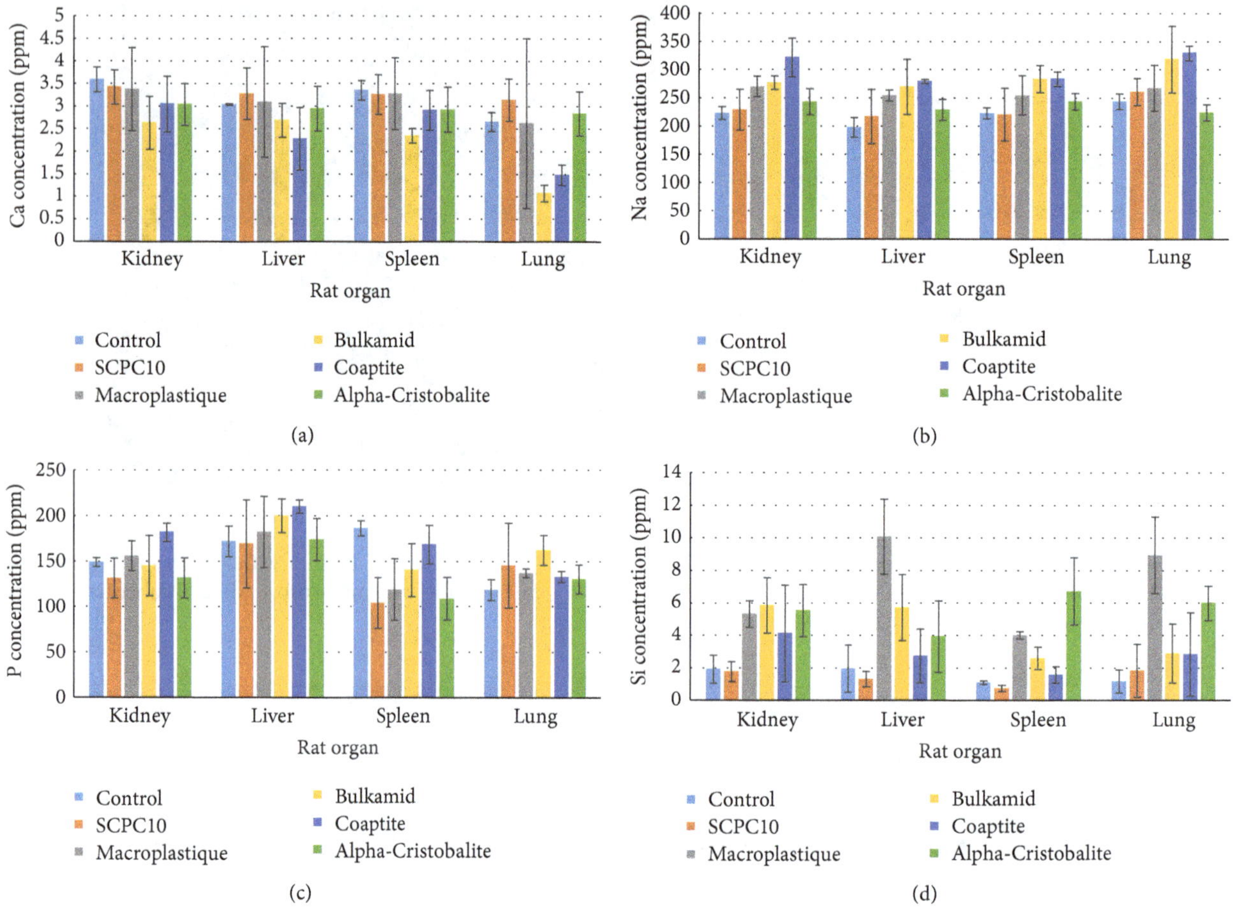

FIGURE 7: Bar graphs summarizing the ion levels of particle components in the distant organs.

therapy is not suitable for every patient and can be associated with serious complications [17, 18]. Complications from UBT are linked to the degradation of synthetic material, causing local inflammatory changes, or distant migration of the material or its components [19, 20]. UBT-induced complications were most pronounced with the use of polytetrafluoroethylene (Telfon), popularized in the 1970s [21]. Teflon is not a biologically inert substance, which leads to significant scarring as well as a foreign body granulomatous reaction locally and distantly from migration of the particles [22, 23].

We compared two types of bioactive ceramic particles, suspended in sodium hyaluronate, to bulking materials currently being used clinically, and assessed the propensity of these materials to cause complications due to local host tissue reaction and distant migration. Sodium hyaluronate is the sodium salt of hyaluronic acid. It is a natural, linear, unbranched polysaccharide belonging to the class of nonsulphated glycosaminoglycans. It occurs naturally in the human body, especially in the vitreous humor and synovial fluid, and as a major component in the extracellular matrix in the skin. It proved to be the optimal suspension media. Its high viscosity prevents plugging of the needle and facilitates uniform particle suspension. The propensity for absorption allows the surface of the bioceramic particles to better interact with the host tissue, preventing migration and providing an optimal bulking mass. The rate at which Hyaluronan gets absorbed by the body is tissue specific and depends on the flow of body fluids in the specific tissue as well as the viscosity. An additional advantage is that it does not significantly change its properties during the sterilization process [24].

Injections of SCPC10 particles showed fibroblastic proliferation, which is needed to hold the particle mass in place. Significant variation in particle size raises the concern that they may migrate to distant organs, which was previously documented on particles smaller than 80 microns [25]. However, no evidence of migration of particles or their components was documented in this study. When compared to the commonly used bulking agents, both SCPC10 and Cristobalite produced a more robust fibroblastic and histiocytic reaction, which in turn helped to integrate and encapsulate the particle aggregates. In vivo, this property effectively anchors the particles in the target tissue and generates a larger bulking effect. Cristobalite, which has the same inherent properties as SCPC10 but shows more regularity in shape and size, induced stronger fibroblastic proliferation, which in turn resulted in a larger bulking effect. Microscopic examination of tissue injected with Cristobalite was most similar to the response seen with Macroplastique but displayed some important differences. Macroplastique particle aggregates were encapsulated by a thin fibroblastic and histiocytic reaction causing less of a mass effect. When comparing all particle types, it appears that round particles elicit less of a fibroblastic tissue reaction.

Comparable levels of Ca, Na, and P ions were noted in the distant organs of all experimental animals. Animals injected with SCPC10 had comparable Si levels to healthy, noninjected controls and animals injected with Cristobalite and Macroplastique appeared to have higher concentrations of Si than controls. Nevertheless, the concentration in all organs was within the biological range [26]. The particle migration seen with previously introduced bulking agents represents a major complication, which has serious and even fatal consequences [27]. For some substances (Teflon, Durasphere, and autologous fat), migration was detected only after broader clinical use. Testing for the presence of particle ions is a novel method that provides additional evidence on the safety of these new materials. The absence of particles and their components in distant organs, shown in our study, provides initial safety data. However, experiments conducted using a rodent model do not provide a final guarantee of clinical safety. We plan to repeat these preclinical trials using larger animals.

In this study, we performed a comprehensive, side-by-side comparison of urethral bulking agents utilizing a previously established rat animal model in combination with hard tissue histologic and immunohistochemical analysis. On this basis, two newly developed bioactive ceramic particles, suspended in sodium hyaluronate, were compared to three currently used urethral bulking agents. The local host tissue response and bulking effects of both SCPC10 and Cristobalite were superior while also possessing a comparable safety profile. Although further studies are necessary, this research suggests that Cristobalite, suspended in sodium hyaluronate, produces a superior bulking effect and can provide the improved, durable long-term response needed for successful urethral bulking therapy.

Acknowledgments

This study was funded by Department of Surgery, University of Vermont, and Grant LH 13068 from the Ministry of Education, Czech Republic.

References

[1] A. D. Shah, N. Kohli, S. S. Rajan, and L. Hoyte, "The age distribution, rates, and types of surgery for stress urinary incontinence in the USA," *International Urogynecology Journal and Pelvic Floor Dysfunction*, vol. 19, no. 1, pp. 89–96, 2008.

[2] "FDA public health notification: serious complications associated with transvaginal placement of surgical mesh in repair of pelvic organ prolapse and stress urinary incontinence," 2008, http://www.fda.gov/MedicalDevices/Safety/AlertsandNotices/PublicHealthNotifications/ucm061976.htm.

[3] US Food and Drug Administration, *FDA Public Health Notification: Serious Complications Associated with Transvaginal Placement of Surgical Mesh in Repair of Pelvic Organ Prolapse and Stress Urinary Incontinence. For Updated Information about Surgical Mesh for Pelvic Organ Prolapse: Update on Serious Complications Associated with Transvaginal Placement of Surgical Mesh for Pelvic Organ Prolapse*, US Food and Drug Administration, Silver Spring, Md, USA, 2011, http://www.fda.gov/medicaldevices/safety/alertsandnotices/ucm262435.htm.

[4] C. R. Chapple, S. Raz, L. Brubaker, and P. E. Zimmern, "Mesh sling in an era of uncertainty: lessons learned and the way forward," *European Urology*, vol. 64, no. 4, pp. 525–529, 2013.

[5] W. S. Reynolds and R. R. Dmochowski, "Urethral bulking: a urology perspective," *Urologic Clinics of North America*, vol. 39, no. 3, pp. 279–287, 2012.

[6] N. Itano, S. Sweat, and D. Lightner, "The use of bulking agents for stress incontinence," *American Urological Association Update Series*, vol. 21, pp. 34–39, 2002.

[7] G. Lemperle, P. B. Lappin, C. Stone, and S. M. Lemperle, "Urethral bulking with polymethylmethacrylate microspheres for stress urinary incontinence: tissue persistence and safety studies in miniswine," *Urology*, vol. 77, no. 4, pp. 1005.e1–1005.e7, 2011.

[8] S. C. Radley, C. R. Chapple, and J. A. Lee, "Transurethral implantation of silicone polymer for stress incontinence: evaluation of a porcine model and mechanism of action in vivo," *BJU International*, vol. 85, no. 6, pp. 646–650, 2000.

[9] T. K. Mann-Gow, J. G. Blaivas, B. J. King et al., "Rat animal model for preclinical testing of microparticle urethral bulking agents," *International Journal of Urology*, vol. 22, no. 4, pp. 416–420, 2015.

[10] S. F. Hulbert, F. A. Young, R. S. Mathews, J. J. Klawitter, C. D. Talbert, and F. H. Stelling, "Potential of ceramic materials as permanently implantable skeletal prostheses," *Journal of Biomedical Materials Research*, vol. 4, no. 3, pp. 433–456, 1970.

[11] A. A. Hofmann, R. D. Bloebaum, and K. N. Bachus, "Progression of human bone ingrowth into porous-coated implants. Rate of bone growth in humans," *Acta Orthopaedica Scandinavica*, vol. 68, no. 2, pp. 161–166, 1997.

[12] A. El-Ghannam, A. Hart, D. White, and L. Cunningham, "Mechanical properties and cytotoxicity of a resorbable bioactive implant prepared by rapid prototyping technique," *Journal of Biomedical Materials Research Part A*, vol. 101, no. 10, pp. 2851–2861, 2013.

[13] C. Knabe, B. Kraska, C. Koch, U. Gross, H. Zreiqat, and M. Stiller, "A method for immunohistochemical detection of osteogenic markers in undecalcified bone sections," *Biotechnic & Histochemistry*, vol. 81, no. 1, pp. 31–39, 2006.

[14] C. Knabe, C. Koch, A. Rack, and M. Stiller, "Effect of β-tricalcium phosphate particles with varying porosity on osteogenesis after sinus floor augmentation in humans," *Biomaterials*, vol. 29, no. 14, pp. 2249–2258, 2008.

[15] M. Stiller, E. Kluk, M. Bohner, M. A. Lopez-Heredia, C. Müller-Mai, and C. Knabe, "Performance of β-tricalcium phosphate granules and putty, bone grafting materials after bilateral sinus floor augmentation in humans," *Biomaterials*, vol. 35, no. 10, pp. 3154–3163, 2014.

[16] U. M. Gross and V. Strunz, "Surface staining of sawed sections of undecalcified bone containing alloplastic implants," *Stain Technology*, vol. 52, no. 4, pp. 217–219, 1977.

[17] A. Imel, T. Malmgren, M. Dadmun, S. Gido, and J. Mays, "In vivo oxidative degradation of polypropylene pelvic mesh," *Biomaterials*, vol. 73, pp. 131–141, 2015.

[18] D. R. Ostergard, "Degradation, infection and heat effects on polypropylene mesh for pelvic implantation: what was known and when it was known," *International Urogynecology Journal and Pelvic Floor Dysfunction*, vol. 22, no. 7, pp. 771–774, 2011.

[19] D. R. Henly, D. M. Barrett, T. L. Weiland, M. K. O'Connor, A. A. Malizia, and A. J. Wein, "Particulate silicone for use in periurethral injections: local tissue effects and search for migration," *The Journal of Urology*, vol. 153, no. 6, pp. 2039–2043, 1995.

[20] C.-C. Tsai, V. Lin, and L. Tang, "Injectable biomaterials for incontinence and vesico-ureteral reflux: current status and future promise," *Journal of Biomedical Materials Research Part B: Applied Biomaterials*, vol. 77, no. 1, pp. 171–178, 2006.

[21] S. Berg, "Polytef augmentation urethroplasty: correlation of surgically incurable urinary incontinence by injection technique," *Archives of Surgery*, vol. 107, no. 3, pp. 379–381, 1973.

[22] W. Boykin, F. R. Rodriguez, J. P. Brizzolara, I. M. Thompson, and E. J. Zeidman, "Complete urinary obstruction following periurethral polytetrafluoroethylene injection for urinary incontinence," *The Journal of Urology*, vol. 141, no. 5, pp. 1199–1200, 1989.

[23] A. A. Malizia Jr., H. M. Reiman, R. P. Myers et al., "Migration and granulomatous reaction after periurethral injection of polytef (Teflon)," *The Journal of the American Medical Association*, vol. 251, no. 24, pp. 3277–3281, 1984.

[24] T. C. Laurent, U. B. G. Laurent, and J. R. E. Fraser, "The structure and function of hyaluronan: an overview," *Immunology and Cell Biology*, vol. 74, no. 2, pp. A1–A7, 1996.

[25] J. Pannek, F. H. Brands, and T. Senge, "Particle migration after transurethral injection of carbon coated beads for stress urinary incontinence," *Journal of Urology*, vol. 166, no. 4, pp. 1350–1353, 2001.

[26] "Silicon levels in human tissues," in *Biochemistry of Silicon and Related Problems*, J. H. Austin, Ed., pp. 255–268, Springer, 1978.

[27] P. E. Lee, R. C. Kung, and H. P. Drutz, "Periurethral autologous fat injection as treatment for female stress urinary incontinence: a randomized double-blind controlled trial," *The Journal of Urology*, vol. 165, no. 1, pp. 153–158, 2001.

Immune-Related Concepts in Biology and Treatment of Germ-Cell Tumors

Michal Chovanec,[1,2] Ugo De Giorgi,[3] and Michal Mego[1]

[1]*2nd Department of Oncology, Faculty of Medicine, Comenius University, National Cancer Institute, Bratislava, Slovakia*
[2]*Divison of Hematologya and Oncology, Indiana University Melvin and Bren Simon Cancer Center, Indianapolis, IN, USA*
[3]*Medical Oncology Department, Istituto Scientifico Romagnolo per lo Studio e la Cura dei Tumori (IRST), IRCCS, Via Piero Maroncelli 40, 47014 Meldola, Italy*

Correspondence should be addressed to Michal Chovanec; michal.chovanec1@gmail.com

Academic Editor: Aditya Bagrodia

Germ-cell tumors (GCTs) are highly curable with chemotherapy. Salvage chemotherapy or surgery can cure a proportion of patients, but the ones failing these treatments will die of their disease in the young age. Immune checkpoint pathways are emerging as powerful targetable biomarkers, and a significant preclinical and clinical research is underway to widen our knowledge and expand the treatment possibilities with immune therapy. The concept of immune modulation that was currently adopted in many solid tumors is understudied in GCTs. Herein, we summarize the current knowledge of published literature discussing the immune mechanisms and immune therapy in GCTs.

1. Introduction

The success story of curing germ-cell tumors (GCTs) established a cisplatin-based chemotherapy as a mainstay for achieving >95% relative overall survival rate [1]. Unfortunately, chemotherapy is not a universal cure for all patients with metastatic disease. About 40–80% of patients with relapse after initial chemotherapy will fail the salvage treatment, and their prognosis is dismal [2–4]. Researchers have spent limitless effort to further advance the anticancer treatment with the most recent substantial achievement being the discovery of modern immune therapy in numerous solid cancers. GCTs are traditionally referred to as "a model for cure" with chemotherapy; however, a scientific inquiry has risen, whether the immune mechanisms may be as important in GCTs as it is in melanoma, lung cancer, kidney cancer, or others. The failure of chemotherapy in substantial proportion of GCT patients creates a therapeutic dilemma for many decades with no major advancement since the introduction of the salvage chemotherapy. Therefore, the question whether immunity plays a significant role in the pathogenesis of GCTs is critical to answer, allowing to derive implications for future development in the treatment of this unique solid malignancy. Herein, we summarize the current knowledge of the literature to provide the insights into the immune biology of GCTs.

2. Literature Search

We performed a literature search of the PubMed/Medline database and meeting libraries of American Society of Clinical Oncology (ASCO) and ASCO Genitourinary Cancers Symposium for publications with the terms "testicular germ cell tumors," "immunity," "immune," "immunotherapy," "tumor infiltrating lymphocytes," "TIL," "inflammation," "cytokines," "check-point." Combinations of these key words were used for comprehensive search as outlined in Figure 1. The search of literature was performed on September 1, 2017. Original full-text articles published in English were reviewed, and the reference lists of key articles were further evaluated. We did not limit our search by the years of publication. Our search was conducted according to the Preferred Reporting Items for

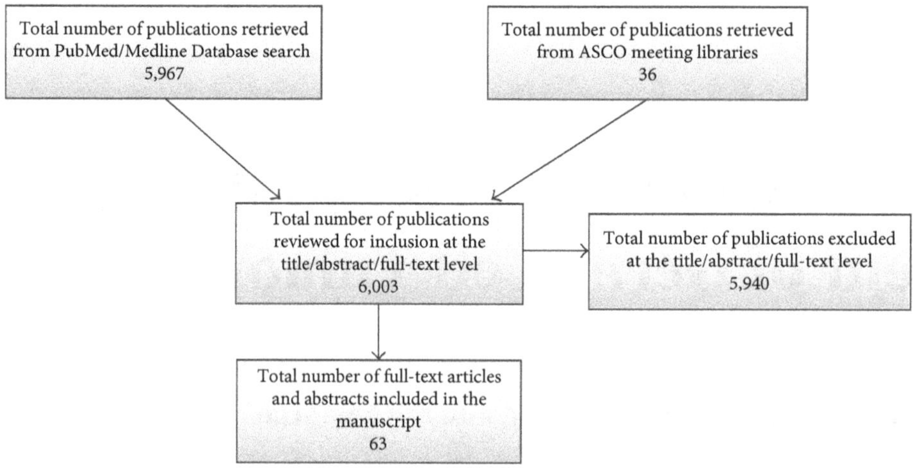

FIGURE 1

Systematic Review and Meta-Analysis (PRISMA) statement. Identified reports were reviewed according to the Consolidated Standards of Reporting Trials (CONSORT) criteria. The search resulted in overall 6003 publications. Sixty-three publications were selected for inclusion in our review article. The outline of the literature search is summarized in Figure 1.

3. Immune-Cell Infiltration, Cytokine Signaling, and Genomic Underpinnings

The observation of immune reaction induced by GCTs evidenced by lymphocytic and granulomatous intratumoral infiltrates dates as early as 1964 and was published by Marshal and Dayan from Bernhard Baron Institute of Pathology in London [5]. Rich infiltration with immune cells in testicular GCTs, particularly in seminomas, was observed by number of other earlier studies [6–11], suggesting an involvement of the immune system in GCT biology. The immune-cell characterization of seminoma by Bols et al. has shown tumor infiltrating lymphocytes (TILs) that included CD3+ and T-memory cell populations, while B-cells and plasma cells were present less frequently. Seminoma in situ (germ-cell neoplasia in situ adjacent to seminoma) was infiltrated mainly by CD4+ and CD8+ TILs and then followed by B-cells, dendritic cells, NKcells, and macrophages. This study was also among the first ones to provide data about prognostic significance of TILs, where authors showed that lower TIL count was associated with the risk of relapse [9]. Hvarness et al. provided similar observation of immune microenvironment in germ-cell neoplasia in situ describing macrophages, CD8+T-cells, CD450R0+ T-cells, and B-cells present in the GCNIS tissue [12]. T-lymphocytes and macrophages were also documented in an embryonal carcinoma [8]. Further observations presented data of characteristic cytokine signaling encompassing tumor tissue with immune-cell infiltrates. Klein and colleagues observed a presence of B-cells and dendritic cells in GCNIS, accompanied by high level of transcripts of several proinflammatory (IL6, IL-1β, and TNF-α), anti-inflammatory (TGF-β1), Th1-driven (IL-2 and IFN-γ) cytokines, and chemokines (CXCL-13, CXCL-10, and CCL-5) [13]. In vitro experiments were conducted on seminoma-derived T-cam2 and peripheral blood mononuclear cell (PBMC) coculture. PBMC exhibited a robust increase in the production of IL1β, TNF-α, TGF-β, and CCL5 transcript levels after direct, but not after indirect, contact with T-cam2 cells. PBMC previously stimulated with the mitogen phytohemaglutinin also exhibited significantly higher expression of IL-1β, IL-6, and IFN-γ. Moreover, authors provided surprising observation of the natural production of IL-6 by T-cam2 cell lines [14]. A specific cytokine signature was also observed as a response to murine testicular teratoma. Two cytokines, IL-6 and IL-10, were the most abundant allowing for subsequent promotion of humoral immune response [15]. Cytokine signatures observed to date position IL-6 signalling as one of the proposed central proinflammatory mechanisms in GCTs. Furthermore, a study by Purdue et al. that evaluated single nucleotide polymorphisms (SNPs) in immune function genes uncovered that SNPs in *TGFB*1, *LTA/TNF*, and others (*IL*2, *IFNGR*2, and *IL*10) may be responsible for an increase in the susceptibility for GCTs [16]. Recent study described distinct molecular signatures of immune cells specifically for seminoma showing elevation of expression signatures for B-cells, cytotoxic T-cells, Th17 cells, and T-regulatory cells (T-reg). This increase was associated with an increase in specific cytokines and immune checkpoints (CTLA4, LAG3, and PD-L1). Interestingly, there was no correlation between immune cells and load of mutations, neoantigens, or detected viruses, which confirms observations obtained from TCGA (The Cancer Genome Atlas) datasets [17–19]. The strongest association of growth in immune-cell populations was observed with activating mutations in *KIT* together with increased expression profiles of *KIT* and *MHC class I* and *II* genes [17]. Another in vitro study tried to address IFN-γ produced by GCT cells (NTERA and NCCIT cell lines) as a potential treatment target by a specific blocking antibody but found that autocrine production of IFN-γ was insufficient to utilize the signaling blockade in favor of the cell inhibition [20].

However, the question of the specific role of immune surveillance in GCT development remains open. Authors from Denmark assessed the immune-cell infiltrate phenotype in GCNIS versus normal tissue and infertile testicular tissue and did not find differences in immune infiltrating cells in this region. Authors, thus, speculated that immune surveillance is not the critical factor for germ-cell development [12]. According to another study evaluating canine seminomas, T-reg TILs did not prove the critical role in the immune response in canine seminoma [21]. Androgen receptor mutation specific to Sertoli cells was discovered to result in loss of testicular immune privilege, a physiological barrier to prevent an immune response against germ-cell antigens. The experiment was performed on Sertoli cell-specific androgen receptor mutant mice, who exhibited higher intratesticular levels of IgG as compared with nonmutant mice, subsequently resulting into infertility [22]. It is not clear how this observation may fit into pathogenesis of GCTs. However, assessing the androgen-receptor associated signaling in patients with GCTs may shed more light into immune surveillance and its errors in patients with metastatic disease. Interesting observations were done in several studies showing that the incidence of GCTs significantly increases in the population of acquired immunodeficiency syndrome (AIDS) patients [23–25]. The number of events from these studies prevents from the conclusion whether acquired immunodeficiency alters GCT-specific survival in this patient population. Nevertheless, the raise in incidence of GCTs may provide indirect indications of the role of overall immune health in this disease development.

4. Immune-Related Biomarkers in GCTs

Despite the fact that we are not able to clearly assess the role of the immune surveillance in the development of GCTs, the prognostic role of TILs is clear. Data regarding new biomarkers, such as immune checkpoints, started to emerge recently as a result of astonishing clinical achievements of immune checkpoint inhibition in various malignancies.

Kersemaekers et al. suggested that FAS/FASL apoptotic signaling in GCT TILs may be a contributing factor to GCT development [26]. Another similar study by Schmelz, however, failed to replicate these results [27]. One of the new promising targets in different types of tumors is programmed-death-1 receptor (PD-1; CD279) and its ligand (PD-L1; B7-H1; CD274), which deliver inhibitory signals that regulate the balance between T-cell activation, tolerance, and immune-mediated tissue damage [28]. PD-1 is a member of the immunoglobulin superfamily and is expressed on double-negative T cells in thymus and on activated CD4+ T-cells, CD8+ T-cells, natural killer cells, B-cells, and monocytes [29]. It is primarily involved in modulating T-cell activity in peripheral tissues through interaction with its ligands PD-L1 and PD-L2 [9]. PD-L1 is expressed in different organs, including placenta, heart, lung, and liver as well as on activated T-cells, B-cells, dendritic cells, macrophages, and mesenchymal stem cells [30].

PD-L1 is expressed also on various tumor cells [29]. Expression of PD-L1 is an important process by which tumor cells suppress antitumor immunity in the tumor microenvironment [31]. Prognostic significance of PD-L1 expression on tumor cells was described in various malignancies [32–37], and the inhibition of PD-1/PD-L1 interaction has become an important landmark in cancer treatment. PD-1 and PD-L1 blocking antibodies have demonstrated clinical activity in several types of cancer including melanoma, nonsmall-cell lung cancer, renal cell cancer, ovarian cancer, and head and neck cancers [38].

The discovery of the PD-1 receptor and its ligand inspired Fankhauser et al. to conduct the first study in GCTs, which described the abundant expression of PD-L1 in seminoma and nonseminoma [39]. Our study explored the prognostic significance of PD-1/PD-L1 pathway in 140 patients with GCTs. We observed abundant expression of PD-L1 but not PD-1 on tumor cells and TILs (expressed in reverse manner on tumor and TILs) that correlated with poor risk clinical characteristics and survival. The low versus high expression of PD-L1 in tumor was associated with better survival (HR = 0.43; 95% CI 0.15–1.23; $P = 0.04$ for OS) [40]. In contrast, high PD-L1 on TILs correlated with better survival (HR = 0.08; 95% CI 0.04–0.16; $P = 0.001$ for OS). Based on these results, we developed a prognostic tool using PD-L1 on tumors and TILs independently of International Germ Cell Cancer Collaborative Group (IGCCCG) criteria [41]. Siska et al. performed a deep exploration of immune infiltrates in GCTs by immunohistochemistry and gene expression profiling and identified that activated T-cell infiltration correlated with seminoma and good prognosis. Advanced GCTs were associated with decreased T-cell and NK-cell signatures, while T-regs, mastocytes, and macrophages proved to be activated in patients with advanced stage disease. Authors also observed increased PD-L1 signalling in seminomas compared with nonseminomas using immunohistochemistry [42]. A study conducted on 102 patients from Japan evaluated the prognostic role of tumor-infiltrating neutrophils (TIN) by assessing CD66b+ TIN and found that they correlated with nodal and distant metastases, S stage, and nonseminoma histology. CD66b+ TIN were prognostic for progression-free and overall survival ($P < 0.05$ for both) [43]. The presence of inflammation in the cancer microenvironment may be identified with a simple clinical tool, the systemic immune inflammation index (SII), calculated as platelets × neutrophils/lymphocytes from the peripheral blood smear. SII proved to predict prognosis in several malignancies [18–22]. Chovanec et al. assessed the prognostic significance of SII in 240 GCT patients and discovered statistically significant differences in PFS and OS. Patients with lower levels of systemic inflammation, represented by lower SII, had significantly better prognosis compared with patients with high SII [44]. Preclinical research initiative by Terayama et al. aimed to evaluate testicular germ-cell specific autoimmunogenic antigens (AIs) in experimental mice with autoimmune orchitis. Authors immunized the serum of these mice with germ cells (nonmalignant), observing 11 specific AIs as a result. The results led to a speculation that these testis-specific AIs may provide a substrate for future research in targeting GCT novel targets [45]. The discovery of toll-like receptors (TLRs) has contributed to the expanding knowledge about the innate immune system. TLRs were proposed to contribute to cancer development [46]. TLRs 2, 3, 4, and 9 are expressed in testicular and GCT tissues; however, the expression in cancer tissue is significantly stronger [7]. Lin et al. published findings from a preclinical therapeutic trial in a mouse model using a conjugate of toll-like receptor 7 (TLR7) and OCT4. Mice were immunized with this novel agent and were subsequently challenged with the mouse embryonal carcinoma. Treatment with the conjugate resulted in significant release of IL12 and IFN-γ in vitro, and the significant increase in CD3+/CD8+ T cells occurred in vivo. Moreover, the rate of cytotoxicity in immunized mice was significantly higher, while the tumor growth decreased by 90% compared to the controls treated with OCT4 or TLR7 alone [47]. While experiments with animal models including animal cancer are difficult to interpret in the context of human biology, this study provides a pilot data of GCT immunogenicity. Vaccination with inhibin alpha was assessed and was effective against stromal cell tumors in preclinical in vitro and autochtonous mouse models but did not exhibit efficacy in GCTs [48]. Schreck et al. published an interesting observation of the loss of activation-induced cytidine deaminase (AID) in GCNIS and GCTs compared to the normal spermatocytes [49]. AID is normally involved in class-switch recombination of immunoglobulin genes in antigen-dependent B-cell maturation, suggesting that immune escape may be a mechanism participating in GCT development. This interpretation, however, may be biased and more studies are needed for validation.

5. Patterns in Cytokine and Immune-Cell Response to GCT and Its Treatment

Our research initiative investigated the patterns of cytokine signalling in peripheral blood in 79 patients with GCTs unveiling specific patterns in seminoma versus non-seminoma, nonpulmonary visceral metastases, and cerebral metastases and administered chemotherapy corresponded with the decline in the proinflammatory signature [50, 51]. These patterns generally suggest the tumor proangiogenic activity, the inhibition of immune response by low T- and NK-cell stimulation, the inhibition of T- and B-cell maturation, and the inhibition of chemoattraction and phagocytosis. The simultaneous immune stimulation and immune inhibition observed in our study was also described previously [51–53]. Further research has shown that increased pre-chemotherapy levels of cytokines promoting angiogenesis, tumorigenesis, immune stimulation, and chemoattraction correlated with shorter PFS and OS in 92 GCT patients [54]. Investigators from the University of Birmingham also observed a spontaneous CD4+ and CD8+ T-cell responses against cancer testis antigen in peripheral blood of patients with GCTs. The frequency of these T-cells substantially declined (by 89%) following orchiectomy for stage I GCTs [55].

6. Immune Therapy Efficacy and Clinical Trials

Early immunotherapy trials date to 1970s and 1980s. Undeniable efficacy of high-dose (HD) IL2 and HD IFN-α in selected patient population led to establishment of these treatments in malignant melanoma and kidney cancer. Anecdotal evidence existing in GCT patients is included in these clinical trials. The review summarized by Rosenberg et al. mentions 1 patient treated with HD IL2 + IFN- α and 1 patient treated with HD IL2 + lymphokine activated killer cells. No response was observed in either of them [56]. The concept of immune therapy has been abandoned or has never truly arisen because the excellent sensitivity of cisplatin-based chemotherapy provided substantially more powerful treatment results compared to other solid malignancies. Recent development of new biomarkers and novel immune therapies, however, raised questions, whether refractory GCTs may be candidates for immune checkpoint inhibition. A single-arm phase II study by Adra et al. from Indiana University recruited 12 patients with refractory GCTs to be treated with anti-PD1 inhibitor pembrolizumab. Although transient declines in tumor markers were noted in few cases, none of the patients had a radiographic response or a stable disease with this treatment [57]. Contradictory data to this trial exist from several case reports with platinum refractory GCTs treated with anti-PD1 agents (pembrolizumab or nivolumab) after salvage HD chemotherapy. These case reports describe possible responses in 3 out of 7 patients [58–60]. However, the interpretation of anti-PD1 treatment efficacy in these cases may be biased, as one of the patients received concomitant etoposide and the other two had only a short-term response to nivolumab. A single case report by Chi et al. provided evidence of ongoing partial remission with marker stabilization after treatment with nivolumab [61]. Based on the data from biomarker studies mentioned earlier in the article, we hypothesize that anti-PD-L1 treatment is more promising for patients with refractory GCTs and phase II trial with anti-PD-L1 inhibitor avelumab is being currently opened in Slovakia (NCT number not assigned yet). Another mechanism may be involved in immune regulation of GCTs, as proposed by Albany et al., who assessed guadecitabine, a demethylation agent, combined with cisplatin to reestablish a platinum sensitivity. A genome-wide analysis from their preclinical findings has shown that response to treatment was accompanied by activation of p53 together with the presence of immune-related pathways [62]. A phase I/II clinical study evaluating guadecitabine plus cisplatin in refractory GCTs is currently underway (NCT02429466).

7. Conclusion

GCTs and the immunity remains an understudied area. Existing evidence suggests active participation of immune system in the response to the presence of GCT and a certain level of evidence suggests its involvement in GCT development as well. Powerful biomarkers, such as PD-L1, TILs, and TLRs, are perhaps among first key elements to provide deep insight into GCT immune regulation and may certainly serve as reasonable treatment targets for future clinical trials.

Acknowledgments

This work was supported by the Slovak Research and Development Agency under Contract no. APVV-15-0086.

References

[1] N. Hanna and L. H. Einhorn, "Testicular cancer–discoveries and updates," *New England Journal of Medicine*, vol. 371, no. 21, p. 2342, 2014.

[2] R. J. Motzer, J. Sheinfeld, M. Mazumdar et al., "Paclitaxel, ifosfamide, and cisplatin second-line therapy for patients with relapsed testicular germ cell cancer," *Journal of Clinical Oncology*, vol. 18, no. 12, pp. 2413–2418, 2000.

[3] J. Mardiak, T. Salek, Z. Sycova-Mila et al., "Paclitaxel plus ifosfamide and cisplatin in second-line treatment of germ cell tumors: a phase II study," *Neoplasma*, vol. 52, no. 6, pp. 497–501, 2005.

[4] L. H. Einhorn, S. D. Williams, A. Chamness, M. J. Brames, S. M. Perkins, and R. Abonour, "High-dose chemotherapy and stem-cell rescue for metastatic germ-cell tumors," *New England Journal of Medicine*, vol. 357, no. 4, pp. 340–348, 2007.

[5] A. H. Marshall and A. D. Dayan, "An immune reaction in man against seminomas, dysgerminomas, pinealomas, and the mediastinal tumours of similar histological appearance?," *The Lancet*, vol. 284, no. 7369, pp. 1102–1104, 1964.

[6] E. Yakirevich, O. Lefel, Y. Sova et al., "Activated status of tumour-infiltrating lymphocytes and apoptosis in testicular seminoma," *Journal of Pathology*, vol. 196, no. 1, pp. 67–75, 2002.

[7] F. Saint, X. Leroy, J. P. Graziana et al., "Dendritic cell infiltration in a patient with seminomatous germ cell tumor of the testis: is there a relationship with infertility and tumor stage?," *Journal of Urology*, vol. 167, no. 4, pp. 1643–1647, 2002.

[8] A. Torres, J. F. Casanova, M. Nistal, and J. Regadera, "Quantification of immunocompetent cells in testicular germ cell tumours," *Histopathology*, vol. 30, no. 1, pp. 23–30, 1997.

[9] B. Bols, L. Jensen, A. Jensen, and O. Braendstrup, "Immunopathology of in situ seminoma," *International Journal of Experimental Pathology*, vol. 81, no. 3, pp. 211–217, 2000.

[10] N. J. Cope, P. McCullagh, and P. T. Sarsfield, "Tumour responding accessory cells in testicular seminoma: an immunohistochemical study," *Histopathology*, vol. 34, no. 6, pp. 510–516, 1999.

[11] D. A. Bell, T. J. Flotte, and A. K. Bhan, "Immunohistochemical characterization of seminoma and its inflammatory cell infiltrate," *Human Pathology*, vol. 18, no. 5, pp. 511–520, 1987.

[12] T. Hvarness, J. E. Nielsen, K. Almstrup, N. E. Skakkebaek, E. Rajpert-De Meyts, and M. H. Claesson, "Phenotypic characterisation of immune cell infiltrates in testicular germ cell neoplasia," *Journal of Reproductive Immunology*, vol. 100, no. 2, pp. 135–145, 2013.

[13] B. Klein, T. Haggeney, D. Fietz et al., "Specific immune cell and cytokine characteristics of human testicular germ cell neoplasia," *Human Reproduction*, vol. 31, no. 10, pp. 2192–2202, 2016.

[14] B. Klein, H. C. Schuppe, M. Bergmann et al., "An in vitro model demonstrates the potential of neoplastic human germ cells to influence the tumour microenvironment," *Andrology*, vol. 5, no. 4, pp. 763–770, 2017.

[15] J. Sundstrom, E. Verajnkorva, E. Salminen, L. J. Pelliniemi, and P. Pöllänen, "Experimental testicular teratoma promotes formation of humoral immune responses in the host testis," *Journal of Reproductive Immunology*, vol. 42, no. 2, pp. 107–126, 1999.

[16] M. P. Purdue, L. C. Sakoda, B. I. Graubard et al., "A case-control investigation of immune function gene polymorphisms and risk of testicular germ cell tumors," *Cancer Epidemiology Biomarkers & Prevention*, vol. 16, no. 1, pp. 77–83, 2007.

[17] D. P. Hollern, K. Hoadley, B. Vincent, C. M. Perou, and TCGA Testicular Germ Cell Tumor Ana Group, "Abstract 3703: a genomic characterization of testicular germ cell tumor immune microenvironment," *Cancer Research*, vol. 77, no. 13, p. 3703, 2017.

[18] E. Cerami, J. Gao, U. Dogrusoz et al., "The cBio cancer genomics portal: an open platform for exploring multidimensional cancer genomics data," *Cancer Discovery*, vol. 2, no. 5, pp. 401–404, 2012.

[19] J. Gao, B. A. Aksoy, U. Dogrusoz et al., "Integrative analysis of complex cancer genomics and clinical profiles using the cBioPortal," *Science Signaling*, vol. 6, no. 269, p. pl1, 2013.

[20] S. Schweyer, A. Soruri, J. Peters, A. Wagner, H. J. Radzun, and A. Fayyazi, "Malignant germ cell tumours of the testis express interferon-gamma, but are resistant to endogenous interferon-gamma," *British Journal of Cancer*, vol. 89, no. 5, pp. 915–921, 2003.

[21] J. H. Kim, S. K. Chon, K. S. Im, N. H. Kim, K. W. Cho, and J. H. Sur, "Infiltrating Foxp3+ regulatory T cells and histopathological features in canine classical and spermatocytic seminomas," *Reproduction in Domestic Animals*, vol. 48, no. 2, pp. 218–222, 2013.

[22] J. Meng, A. R. Greenlee, C. J. Taub, and R. E. Braun, "Sertoli cell-specific deletion of the androgen receptor compromises testicular immune privilege in mice," *Biology of Reproduction*, vol. 85, no. 2, pp. 254–260, 2011.

[23] T. Powles, M. Bower, G. Daugaard et al., "Multicenter study of human immunodeficiency virus-related germ cell tumors," *Journal of Clinical Oncology*, vol. 21, no. 10, pp. 1922–1927, 2003.

[24] M. U. Hentrich, N. G. Brack, P. Schmid, T. Schuster, C. Clemm, and R. C. Hartenstein, "Testicular germ cell tumors in patients with human immunodeficiency virus infection," *Cancer*, vol. 77, no. 10, pp. 2109–2116, 1996.

[25] F. Buzelin, G. Karam, A. Moreau, O. Wetzel, and F. Gaillard, "Testicular tumor and the acquired immunodeficiency syndrome," *European Urology*, vol. 26, no. 1, pp. 71–76, 1994.

[26] A. M. Kersemaekers, P. C. van Weeren, J. W. Oosterhuis, and L. H. J. Looijenga, "Involvement of the Fas/FasL pathway in the pathogenesis of germ cell tumours of the adult testis," *Journal of Pathology*, vol. 196, no. 4, pp. 423–429, 2002.

[27] H. U. Schmelz, M. Abend, K. Kraft et al., "Fas/Fas ligand system and apoptosis induction in testicular carcinoma," *Cancer*, vol. 95, no. 1, pp. 73–81, 2002.

[28] L. M. Francisco, P. T. Sage, and A. H. Sharpe, "The PD-1 pathway in tolerance and autoimmunity," *Immunological Reviews*, vol. 236, no. 1, pp. 219–242, 2010.

[29] T. Okazaki and T. Honjo, "PD-1 and PD-1 ligands: from discovery to clinical application," *International Immunology*, vol. 19, no. 7, pp. 813–824, 2007.

[30] X. Cheng, V. Veverka, A. Radhakrishnan et al., "Structure and interactions of the human programmed cell death 1 receptor," *Journal of Biological Chemistry*, vol. 288, no. 17, pp. 11771–11785, 2013.

[31] H. Noh, J. Hu, X. Wang, X. Xia, A. Satelli, and S. Li, "Immune checkpoint regulator PD-L1 expression on tumor cells by contacting CD11b positive bone marrow derived stromal cells," *Cell Communication and Signaling*, vol. 13, no. 1, p. 14, 2015.

[32] K. Azuma, K. Ota, A. Kawahara et al., "Association of PD-L1 overexpression with activating EGFR mutations in surgically resected nonsmall-cell lung cancer," *Annals of Oncology*, vol. 25, no. 10, pp. 1935–1940, 2014.

[33] J. W. Kim and J. P. Eder, "Prospects for targeting PD-1 and PD-L1 in various tumor types," *Oncology*, vol. 28, no. 3, pp. 15–28, 2014.

[34] R. Hino, K. Kabashima, Y. Kato et al., "Tumor cell expression of programmed cell death-1 ligand 1 is a prognostic factor for malignant melanoma," *Cancer*, vol. 116, no. 7, pp. 1757–1766, 2010.

[35] R. H. Thompson, S. M. Kuntz, B. C. Leibovich et al., "Tumor B7-H1 is associated with poor prognosis in renal cell carcinoma patients with long-term follow-up," *Cancer Research*, vol. 66, no. 7, pp. 3381–3385, 2006.

[36] S. J. Shi, L. J. Wang, G. D. Wang et al., "B7-H1 expression is associated with poor prognosis in colorectal carcinoma and regulates the proliferation and invasion of HCT116 colorectal cancer cells," *PLoS One*, vol. 8, no. 10, article e76012, 2013.

[37] S. Muenst, A. R. Schaerli, F. Gao et al., "Expression of programmed death ligand 1 (PD-L1) is associated with poor prognosis in human breast cancer," *Breast Cancer Research and Treatment*, vol. 146, no. 1, pp. 15–24, 2014.

[38] M. K. Callahan, M. A. Postow, and J. D. Wolchok, "CTLA-4 and PD-1 pathway blockade: combinations in the clinic," *Frontiers in Oncology*, vol. 4, p. 385, 2014.

[39] C. D. Fankhauser, A. Curioni-Fontecedro, V. Allmann et al., "Frequent PD-L1 expression in testicular germ cell tumors," *British Journal of Cancer*, vol. 113, no. 3, pp. 411–413, 2015.

[40] Z. Cierna, M. Mego, V. Miskovska et al., "Prognostic value of programmed-death-1 receptor (PD-1) and its ligand 1 (PD-L1) in testicular germ cell tumors," *Annals of Oncology*, vol. 27, no. 2, pp. 300–305, 2016.

[41] M. Chovanec, Z. Cierna, V. Miskovska et al., "Prognostic role of programmed-death ligand 1 (PD-L1) expressing tumor infiltrating lymphocytes in testicular germ cell tumors," *Oncotarget*, vol. 8, no. 13, pp. 21794–21805, 2017.

[42] P. J. Siska, R. A. N. Johnpulle, A. Zhou et al., "Deep exploration of the immune infiltrate and outcome prediction in testicular cancer by quantitative multiplexed immunohistochemistry and gene expression profiling," *Oncoimmunology*, vol. 6, no. 4, p. e1305535, 2017.

[43] Y. Yamada, T. Nakagawa, T. Sugihara et al., "Prognostic value of CD66b positive tumor-infiltrating neutrophils in testicular germ cell tumor," *BMC Cancer*, vol. 16, no. 1, p. 898, 2016.

[44] M. Chovanec, Z. Cierna, V. Miskovska et al., "Systemic immune-inflammation index is prognostic in testicular germ cell tumors with PD-L1 expressing tumor infiltrating lymphocytes," *Journal of Clinical Oncology*, vol. 35, no. 15, p. e16042, 2017.

[45] H. Terayama, S. Hirai, M. Naito et al., "Specific autoantigens identified by sera obtained from mice that are immunized with testicular germ cells alone," *Scientific Reports*, vol. 6, no. 1, p. 35599, 2016.

[46] B. Salaun, S. Lebecque, S. Matikainen, D. Rimoldi, and P. Romero, "Toll-like receptor 3 expressed by melanoma cells as a target for therapy?," *Clinical Cancer Research*, vol. 13, no. 15, pp. 4565–4574, 2007.

[47] G. Lin, X. Wang, W. Yi et al., "A conjugate of octamer-binding transcription factor 4 and toll-like receptor 7 agonist prevents the growth and metastasis of testis embryonic carcinoma," *Journal of Translational Medicine*, vol. 13, no. 1, p. 166, 2015.

[48] R. Aguilar, J. M. Johnson, P. Barrett, and V. K. Tuohy, "Vaccination with inhibin-alpha provides effective immunotherapy against testicular stromal cell tumors," *Journal for ImmunoTherapy of Cancer*, vol. 5, no. 1, p. 37, 2017.

[49] S. Schreck, M. Buettner, E. Kremmer, M. Bogdan, H. Herbst, and G. Niedobitek, "Activation-induced cytidine deaminase (AID) is expressed in normal spermatogenesis but only infrequently in testicular germ cell tumours," *Journal of Pathology*, vol. 210, no. 1, pp. 26–31, 2006.

[50] J. Mardiak, D. Cholujova, I. Jurisica et al., "A cytokine and angiogenic factor (CAF) analysis in plasma in testicular germ cell tumor patients (TGCTs)," *Journal of Clinical Oncology*, vol. 31, no. 15, p. e15599, 2013.

[51] M. Chovanec, M. Mego, D. Cholujova et al., "A cytokine and angiogenic factor (CAF) analysis in plasma in testicular germ cell tumor patients (TGCTs)," *Journal of Clinical Oncology*, vol. 33, no. 15, p. e15552, 2015.

[52] B. E. Lippitz, "Cytokine patterns in patients with cancer: a systematic review," *The Lancet Oncology*, vol. 14, no. 6, pp. e218–e228, 2013.

[53] X. Su, J. Ye, E. C. Hsueh, Y. Zhang, D. F. Hoft, and G. Peng, "Tumor microenvironments direct the recruitment and expansion of human Th17 cells," *Journal of Immunology*, vol. 184, no. 3, pp. 1630–1641, 2010.

[54] D. Svetlovska, V. Miskovska, D. Cholujova et al., "Plasma cytokines correlated with disease characteristics, progression-free survival, and overall survival in testicular germ-cell tumor patients," *Clinical Genitourinary Cancer*, vol. 15, no. 3, pp. 411–416, 2017.

[55] H. Pearce, P. Hutton, S. Chaudhri et al., "Spontaneous CD4+ and CD8+ T-cell responses directed against cancer testis antigens are present in the peripheral blood of testicular cancer patients," *European Journal of Immunology*, vol. 47, no. 7, pp. 1232–1242, 2017.

[56] S. A. Rosenberg, M. T. Lotze, J. C. Yang et al., "Experience with the use of high-dose interleukin-2 in the treatment of 652 cancer patients," *Annals of Surgery*, vol. 210, no. 4, pp. 474–484, 1989.

[57] N. Adra, S. K. Althouse, N. R. Ammakkanavar et al., "Phase II trial of pembrolizumab in patients (pts) with incurable platinum refractory germ cell tumors (GCT)," *Journal of Clinical Oncology*, vol. 35, no. 1, p. 4520, 2017.

[58] S. Zschabitz, F. Lasitschka, B. Hadaschik et al., "Response to anti-programmed cell death protein-1 antibodies in men treated for platinum refractory germ cell cancer relapsed after high-dose chemotherapy and stem cell transplantation," *European Journal of Cancer*, vol. 76, pp. 1–7, 2017.

[59] S. Zschabitz, F. Lasitschka, D. Jager, and C. Grüllich, "Activity of immune checkpoint inhibition in platinum refractory germ-cell tumors," *Annals of Oncology*, vol. 27, no. 7, pp. 1356–1360, 2016.

[60] S. Shah, J. E. Ward, R. Bao, C. R. Hall, B. E. Brockstein, and J. J. Luke, "Clinical response to anti-PD1 immunotherapy in a patient with non-seminomatous germ cell tumor and evaluation of the immune landscape in testicular cancer," *Journal of Clinical Oncology*, vol. 34, p. e16040, 2016.

[61] E. A. Chi and M. T. Schweizer, "Durable response to immune checkpoint blockade in a platinum-refractory patient with nonseminomatous germ cell tumor," *Clinical Genitourinary Cancer*, vol. 15, no. 5, pp. e855–e857, 2017.

[62] C. Albany, M. P. Hever-Jardine, K. M. von Herrmann et al., "Refractory testicular germ cell tumors are highly sensitive to the second generation DNA methylation inhibitor guadecitabine," *Oncotarget*, vol. 8, no. 2, pp. 2949–2959, 2017.

20

CK20 and CK5/6 Immunohistochemical Staining of Urothelial Neoplasms

Mohammed Akhtar, Sameera Rashid, Mohamed Ben Gashir, Noheir Mostafa Taha, and Issam Al Bozom

Department of Laboratory Medicine and Pathology, Hamad Medical Corporation, Doha, Qatar

Correspondence should be addressed to Mohammed Akhtar; dr.mohammed.akhtar@gmail.com

Academic Editor: Mohammad H. Ather

Cytokeratins belong to the family of intermediate filaments. They are expressed in a highly specific manner in epithelial cells where they play a crucial role in the integrity and mechanical stability of the cells. Several types of cytokeratins have been described in normal as well as neoplastic urothelium. In the case of urothelial neoplasms expression of CK20 and CK5/6 has been shown in several studies to have diagnostic and prognostic implications. Thus, low-grade urothelial carcinoma manifests CK expression limited to the umbrella cells, while high-grade tumors usually have an expression in the entire thickness of the urothelium except for the basal layer. CK5/6 expression on the other hand is expressed in the basal cells in all low-grade and some high-grade urothelial carcinomas. Diffuse CK20 staining accompanied by loss of CK5/6-positive basal layer is usually associated with aggressive clinical behavior. Double staining of the slides for these cytokeratins may facilitate proper interpretation and correlation.

1. Introduction

Cytokeratins belong to the family of 10 nm intermediate filament cytoskeleton present in all the cells. Intermediate filament proteins are expressed in a highly cell type-specific manner, and herein keratins represent the typical intermediate filament category present in epithelial cells. These filaments are a complex group of water-insoluble polypeptides, ranging in size from 40,000 to 68,000 Mr. In epithelia, keratin filaments may be bundled as tonofilaments, braid the nucleus, span through the cytoplasm, and attach to the cytoplasmic plaques of the typical epithelial cell-cell junctions, the desmosomes. Thus, keratins play a major functional role in the integrity and mechanical stability of both the single epithelial cells and that of the epithelial tissues and are an inherent part of the continuum of stability from the single cell to the tissue formation [1–6].

The keratin proteins may be divided into small acidic type I and large basic to neutral type II keratins. A unique property of the keratins is that, in contrast to the other intermediate filament proteins, they only can constitute their filamentous stage by pair formation of type I and type II (1 : 1) molecules. Among human keratins, the recent consensus nomenclature comprises the type I keratins K9–K10, K12–K28, and K31–K40 and type II keratins K1–K8 and K71–K86. In the human genome, the keratin genes are clustered at two different chromosomal sites: chromosome 17q21.2 (type I keratins, except K18) and chromosome 12q13.13 (type II keratins and K18). It is thought that the two cytokeratin subfamilies arose through gene duplication and subsequent divergence of the CK8 and CK18 [2–6].

Each type of epithelial cell expresses a characteristic combination of two to ten cytokeratin isotypes. Thus, normal epithelial cells in vivo or in vitro can be identified with respect to their cytokeratin isotype profile. The characteristic cytokeratin profiles of the different normal epithelial cell types tend to be retained following neoplastic transformation and this feature may be exploited in tumor diagnosis. However, cytokeratin profiles of epithelial cells may also reflect functional differentiation, rather than tissue of origin. Thus, metaplastic cells express cytokeratin profile characteristics of their morphology rather than that of their normal counterpart [1].

2. Cytokeratin Expression in Urothelium during Embryologic Development

The cytokeratins are the first intermediate filament type to appear during embryogenesis, and all cells at some stage of fetal development are cytokeratin positive. The first cytokeratin isotypes to be expressed are the CK8 + CK18 pair. During embryological epithelial-mesenchymal transformation, cytokeratin expression is lost by certain lineages of cells, which either remain cytokeratin negative and develop into connective tissue or later re-express cytokeratins of secondary epithelia [1]. Embryologic development of the urinary bladder is from the cloaca, a hindgut structure, that is a common chamber for gastrointestinal and urinary waste. In the 4th–7th weeks of development, the cloaca is divided by the urorectal septum into two parts: posterior anorectal canal and anterior urogenital sinus. The upper part of the urogenital sinus forms the urinary bladder [7].

During the early development of the bladder, the lining epithelium gradually transforms from simple endodermal epithelium to multilayered urothelial lining. As the pattern of the endodermal lining in the GI tract, the developing urothelial lining is initially diffusely positive for CK20 in all layers. During subsequent maturation of the urothelium, a basal layer develops which may be demonstrated by CK5 and CK13 positivity. Further maturation of urothelium involves loss of CK20 in virtually all layers except for the umbrella cells. Thus, there appear to be three distinct phases of urothelial development. The first stage is characterized by a lack of basal cells and CK20 expression in all layers. The second phase is determined by the appearance of the basal layer, but the CK20 expression pattern is still diffuse. In the third and final stages, there is maturation of the CK20 expression pattern which is characterized by CK20 only in the umbrella layer. The basal layer is well developed and can be demonstrated by CK5/6 or CK13 immunostaining [8, 9].

3. Cytokeratin Expression in Normal Urothelium

The urinary bladder is lined by urothelium which is specialized to function as a barrier to urine and to accommodate changes in the intraluminal volume. Urothelium appears as a multilayered epithelium, with three cell zones: (1) a basal cell layer composed of cells in contact with and orientated perpendicularly to the plane of the basement membrane; (2) the intermediate cell zone composed of 2–5 cell layers; (3) a luminal or superficial cell layer composed of late intermediate cells and large, frequently binucleated, "umbrella" cells with their apical surface facing the lumen. The umbrella cells are characterized by a zonula occludens type of cell junctions and by the presence of specialized plaques of the asymmetric unit membrane in the apical cell membrane and within intracellular fusiform vesicles [10]. This appearance is due to the presence of abundant uroplakin within the cell membrane [11].

In the normal adult urothelium, CK7, CK8, CK18, and CK19 are expressed throughout all urothelial cell layers, CK5 is basally expressed, and CK20 is associated with umbrella cells (Figure 1).

There may also be a few CK20-positive cells in the intermediate cell layer of some normal specimens [1].

4. Cytokeratin Expression in Papillary Urothelial Neoplasia

Neoplastic transformation of urothelial cells gives rise to urothelial carcinoma, the commonest form of bladder cancer in most of the countries. Many patients present with superficial tumors which are either noninvasive (pTa) or invade the lamina propria only (pT1). Whilst recurrence is common (50–70%), the disease can usually be controlled by local treatment. Nevertheless, 10–15% of patients with superficial disease eventually progress to muscle-invasive and metastatic disease. An increase in grade, characterized by a loss of differentiation, and the presence of dysplastic changes are both determinants of poor prognosis. In addition, some urothelial carcinomas show basal/squamous differentiation, which has been associated with poorer prognosis [12–14].

The immunohistochemical staining pattern for cytokeratin20 and CK5/6 varies with the type and nature of the urothelial neoplasm. For example, papillary urothelial neoplasms of limited malignant potential (PUNLMP) as well as low-grade papillary carcinomas reveal CK20 limited to the umbrella cells and CK5/6 staining confined to the basal layer, identical to the distribution of these keratins in the normal urothelium (Figure 2).

High-grade urothelial carcinomas, on the other hand, tend to have diffuse immunoreactivity for CK20 involving the umbrella cells as well as the intermediate layer. In addition, the basal layer may be demonstrated by CK5/6 positivity (Figure 3).

Higher grade papillary urothelial carcinoma, on the other hand, reveals CK20 expression in the entire thickness of the urothelium with the absence of basal layer and negative staining for CK5/6 (Figure 4).

This pattern with diffuse full-thickness CK20 staining in the absence of basal layer staining is also a feature encountered in high-grade urothelial carcinomas with lamina propria or muscle invasion [15–18] (Figure 5).

It has been suggested that the pattern of CK20 staining is a useful adjunct to morphology in the diagnosis of urothelial carcinoma. It has also been suggested that CK20 expression can predict malignant potential in low-grade urothelial tumors, and, therefore, CK20 can be useful in defining treatment strategies for patients with these tumors. CK20 expression was retained by most of the pure urothelial carcinomas, retaining the normal superficial localization pattern in some well-differentiated papillary tumors or showing a heterogeneous or uniformly positive reaction throughout all cell layers. Portions of the carcinoma with squamous differentiation reveal a reduction of CK20 expression. These areas, however, react positively for CK5/6

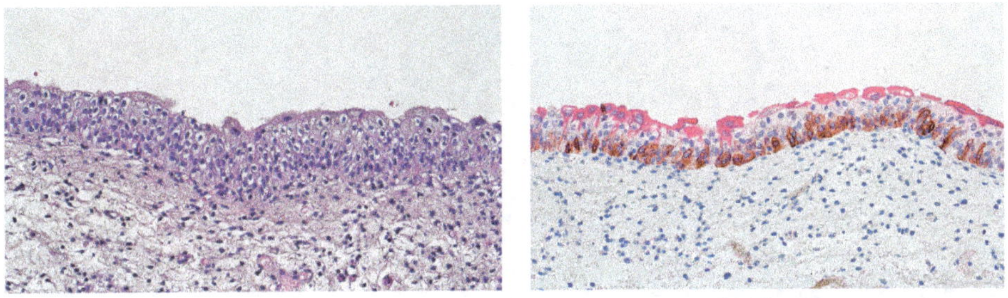

(a) (b)

FIGURE 1: (a) Normal urothelium revealing multiple layers of cells including basal cell, intermediate cells, and umbrella cells. (b) Immunohistochemical stain revealing normal staining pattern of the urothelium. The umbrella cells are decorated by CK20 (magenta). The intermediate cells are unstained. Basal cells are decorated by CK5/6 staining (brown).

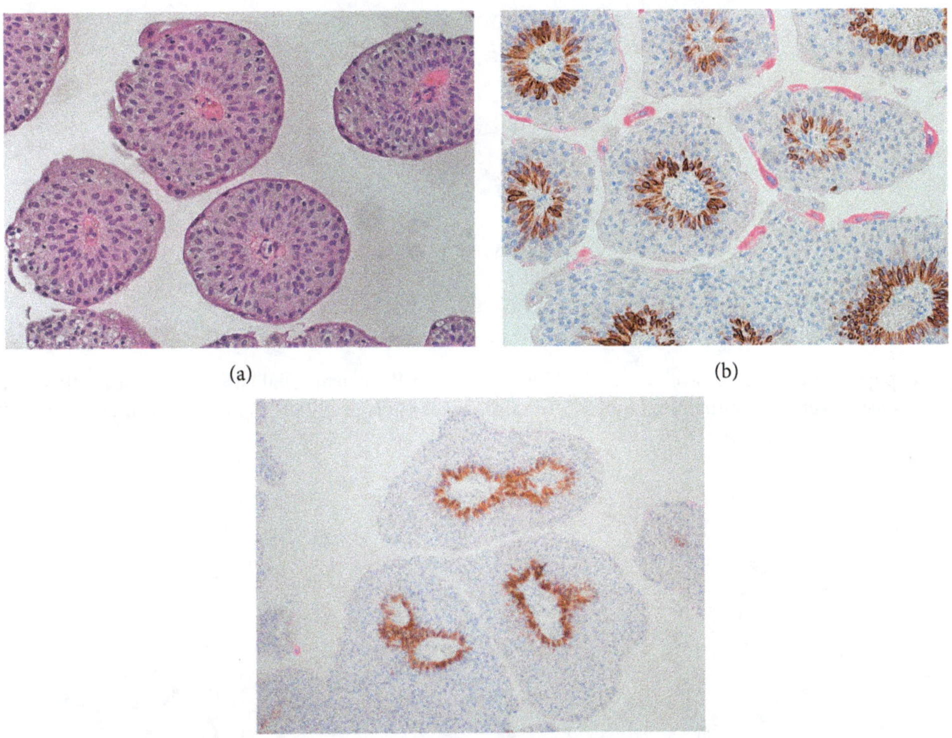

(a) (b) (c)

FIGURE 2: (a) Low-grade papillary urothelial carcinoma. (b) Immunohistochemical stain depicting the CK20 (magenta) expression limited to the umbrella cells and a well-formed basal layer depicted by CK5/6 staining (brown). (c) Low-grade urothelial carcinoma with staining of basal cells but lacking umbrella cells.

(Figures 6(a) and 6(b)) in a pattern that is different from the basal distribution of the basal layer [19–22].

In some cases, the entire carcinoma may show basosquamous features. These cases show strong reactivity for CK5/6 with little or no positivity for CK20 (Figures 6(c) and 6(d)).

Two recently published studies have provided additional evidence regarding the clinical significance of various patterns of immunostaining for CK20 and CK5/6. In one of these studies, tumor samples from 222 patients with upper tract urothelial carcinomas who were treated with radical nephroureterectomy were analyzed for the expression of seven basal/luminal immunohistochemical markers (CK5, EGFR, CD44, CK20, p63, GATA3, and FOXA). By using CK5 and CK20, they defined four subtypes of upper tract urothelial carcinomas:

(i) Exclusively CK20 positive and CK5 negative (CK20+/CK5−)

(ii) Exclusively CK5 positive and CK20 negative (CK20−/CK5+)

(iii) Both markers positive (CK20+/CK5+)

(iv) Both markers negative (CK20−/CK5−)

In multivariate Cox's regression analysis, the CK20+/CK5− subtype was an independent negative prognostic

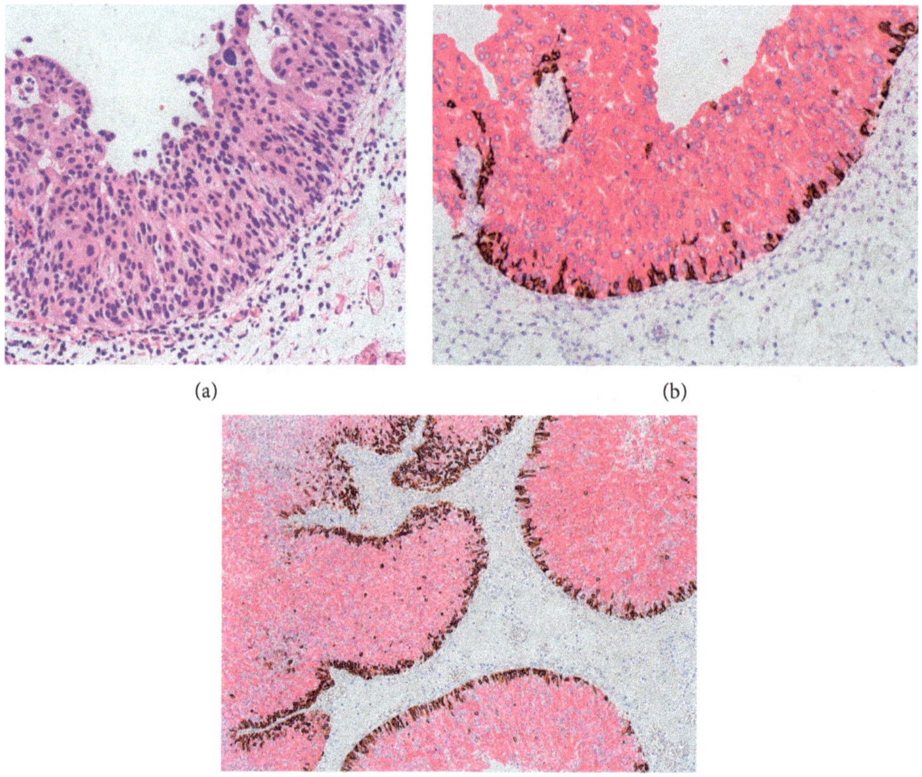

(c)

FIGURE 3: (a) High-grade papillary urothelial carcinoma. (b) High-grade papillary urothelial carcinoma with diffuse full-thickness staining for CK20 and presence of basal layer as demonstrated by CK5/6 staining. (c) High-grade urothelial carcinoma revealing the diffuse presence of basal cells and full-thickness staining for CK20.

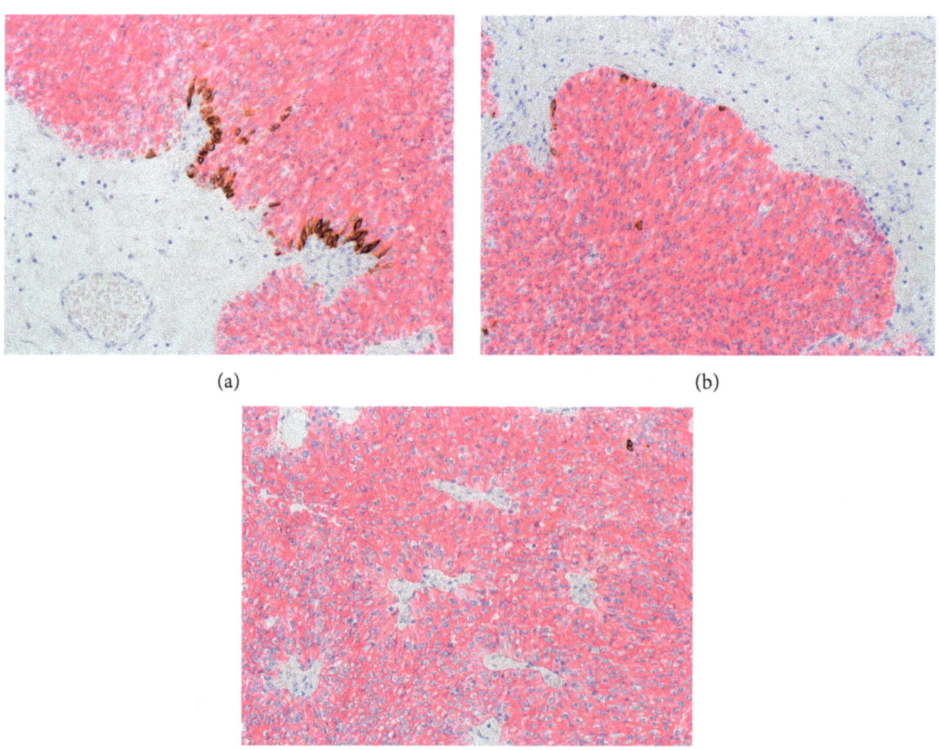

(c)

FIGURE 4: (a) High-grade urothelial carcinoma with partial loss of basal cells but diffuse staining for CK20. (b) High-grade urothelial carcinoma with almost complete loss of basal cells. (c) High-grade papillary urothelial carcinoma revealing diffuse immunohistochemical staining for CK20 and complete absence of basal layer with no staining for CK5/6.

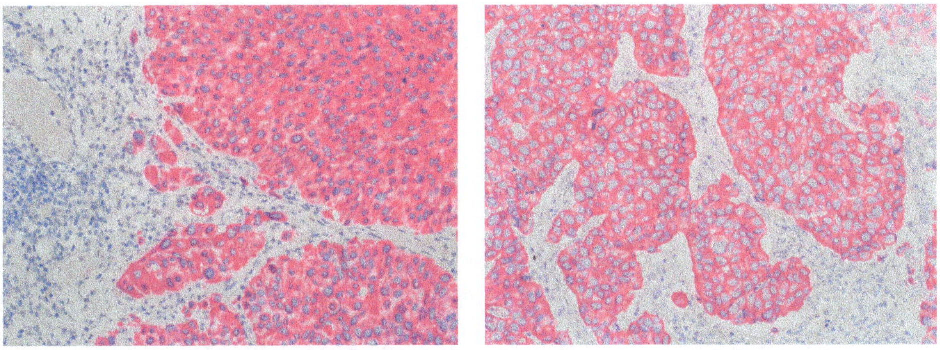

(a) (b)

FIGURE 5: (a) High-grade urothelial carcinoma with early invasion showing strong CK20 cytoplasmic staining and absence of basal cells. (b) High-grade urothelial carcinoma with extensive invasion. The carcinoma cells are diffusely positive for CK20, but the basal layer is absent.

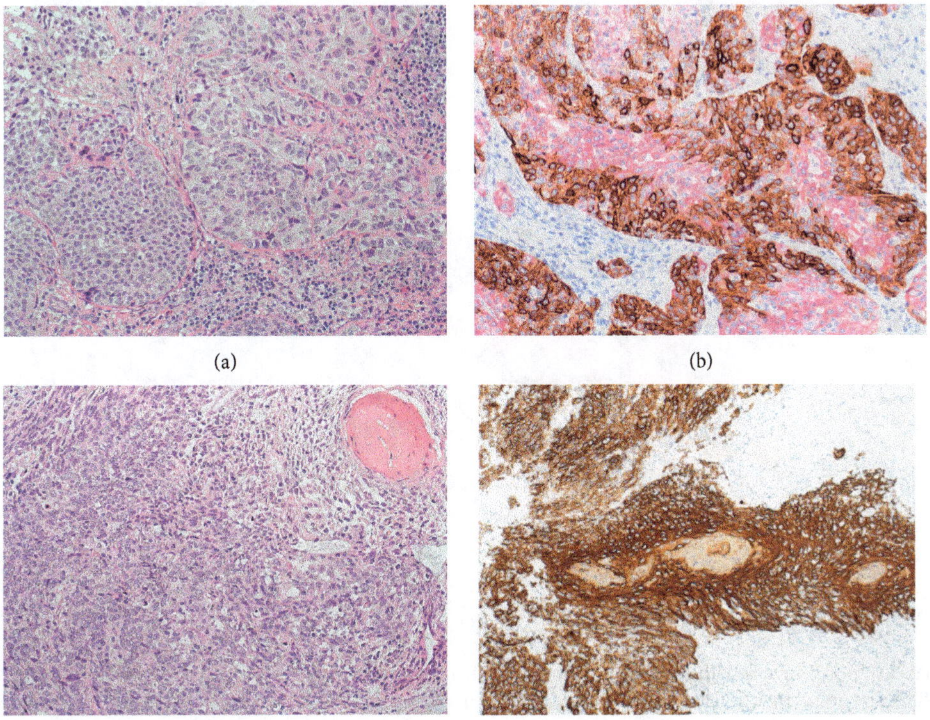

(a) (b) (c) (d)

FIGURE 6: (a) High-grade urothelial carcinoma with focal squamous differentiation. (b) Immunohistochemical staining demonstrating strong CK5/6 staining in the area of squamous differentiation. The remaining part of carcinoma stains for CK20. (c) High-grade urothelial carcinoma with basosquamous morphologic features. (d) Immunohistochemical staining in basosquamous carcinoma featuring strong immunostaining for CK5/6 and complete absence of CK20 positivity.

marker with a 3.83-fold increased risk of cancer-specific death ($p = 0.02$) compared to the other three subtypes [23].

In a second study, immunohistochemical staining for CK5/6 and CK20 was reported to be correlated with the prognosis of early urothelial carcinoma. In addition, the gene expression profiles of subgroups of non-muscle-invasive papillary high-grade upper tract urothelial carcinoma (UTUC) classified by CK5/6 and CK20 expression levels were studied and correlated with clinical outcomes. These subgroups included CK5/6-high/CK20-low, CK5/6-high/CK20-high, and CK5/6-low/CK20-high. The latter group characterized by low expression of CK5/6 and high expression of CK20 was predictive of worse prognosis of non-muscle-invasive papillary high-grade urothelial carcinomas. Transcriptional analysis revealed 308 differentially expressed genes across the subgroups. Functional analyses of the genes identified cell adhesion as a common process differentially enriched in this subgroup compared to the others, which could explain its high-risk phenotype. Late cell cycle/proliferation signatures were also enriched in this subgroup [24]. Thus, it seems that urothelial tumors characterized by diffuse staining for CK20 in the absence of demonstrable

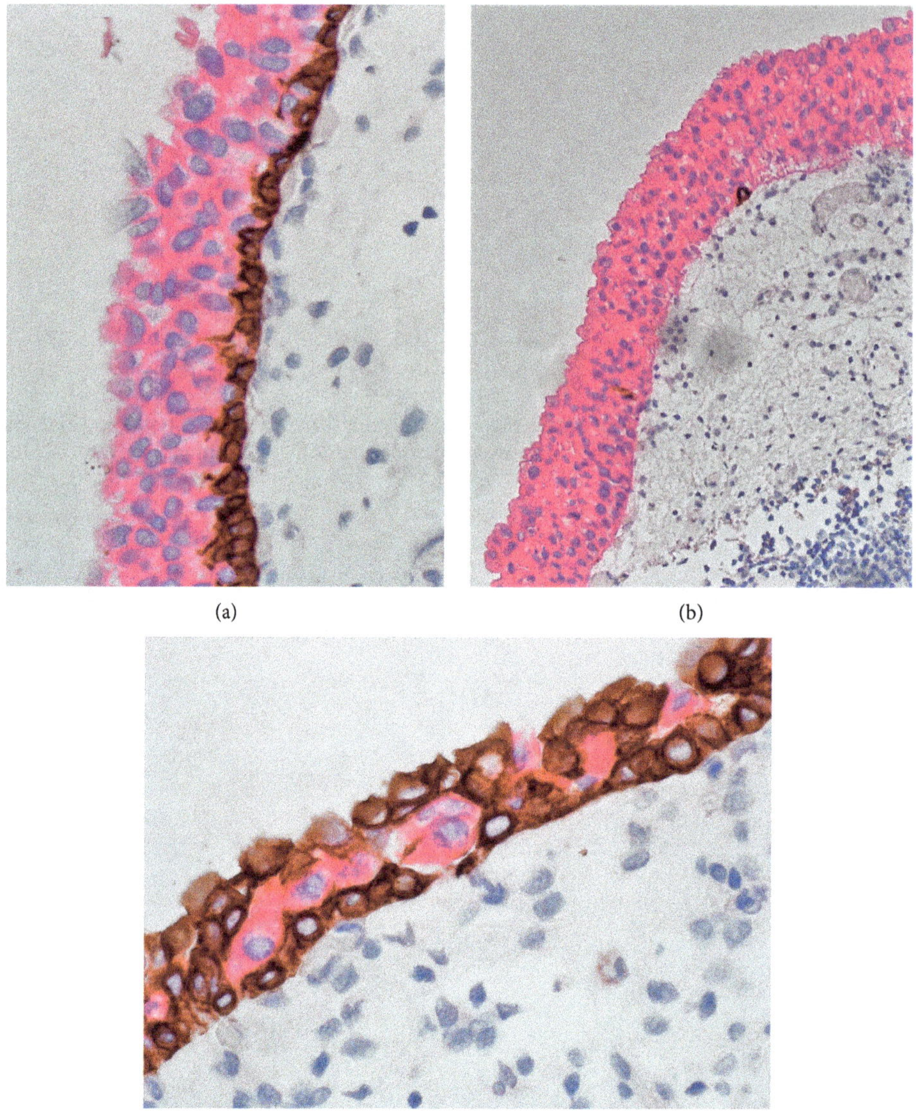

(a) (b) (c)

FIGURE 7: (a) Urothelial carcinoma in situ with strong full-thickness immunostaining for CK20 with a distinct basal cell layer positive for CK5/6. (b) Another urothelial carcinoma in situ featuring strong staining for CK20 and absence of basal layer. (c) Pagetoid extension of urothelial carcinoma demonstrated by strong cytoplasmic staining for CK20 in a background of multiple layers of basal cells reactive for CK5/6.

basal layer represent the most aggressive subtype of papillary urothelial carcinoma.

Cytokeratin 5/6 is present in the normal keratinizing epidermis and squamous mucosal epithelium, as well as in basal cells or myoepithelial cells of the breast, salivary glands, and prostate [25–28]. In prostate and breast biopsies, CK5/6 decorates the basal cell layer and thus is useful in the diagnosis of invasive carcinoma, the latter being devoid of basal cells. The architecture of urothelium is different from that of the prostatic or mammary ductal epithelium with the result that the presence or absence of basal cells cannot be used to stratify urothelial neoplasms into benign or malignant types. However, the absence of basal cells in the urothelial neoplasms may indicate poor prognosis. Thus, a high-grade urothelial carcinoma with a preserved basal layer may behave less aggressively as compared to another high-grade tumor in which the basal layer has been lost. In our laboratory, we use double staining for these cytokeratins which is extremely helpful in the proper interpretation of these stains.

A similar staining pattern may also be seen in urothelial carcinoma in situ [29, 30]. These lesions are usually strongly reactive for CK20 and may or may not retain the CK5/6-positive basal cell layer. Clinging type of urothelial carcinoma in situ and pagetoid extension of carcinoma cells may also be recognized by positive CK20 staining (Figure 7).

In a minority of cases, carcinoma in situ may be reactive for CK5/6 indicating a basaloid differentiation [31].

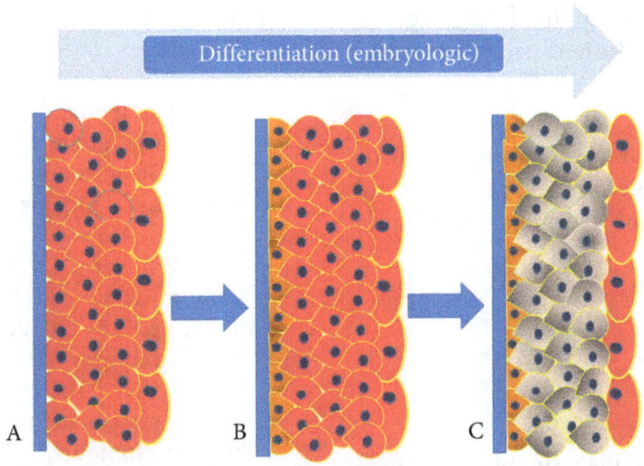

FIGURE 8: (a) Cartoon depicting stages of differentiation during the embryologic development of the urothelium. During the early stages, the developing urothelium retains CK20 expression normally seen in the cloaca. During this stage, no basal layer is present. (b) During the development of urothelium, the basal layer cannot be demonstrated by staining for CK5/6. (c) Final stage of urothelial differentiation with normal expression of CK20 limited to the umbrella cells and presence of normal basal layer manifesting expression of CK5/6.

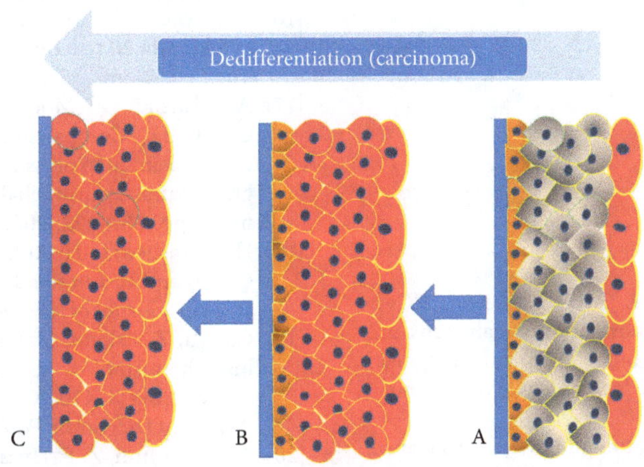

FIGURE 9: (a) Cartoon depicting immunohistochemical staining pattern in a low-grade papillary urothelial carcinoma with CK20 expression limited to the umbrella cells and presence of a well-defined basal layer which expresses CK5/6. (b) High-grade urothelial carcinoma reveals expression of CK20 in all layers of urothelium except for the basal layer which contains CK5/6. This may represent an intermediate stage of dedifferentiation of the tumor. (c) In high-grade urothelial carcinoma, the basal layer may be absent but the diffuse CK20 pattern of staining is maintained. These features may indicate further dedifferentiation of the carcinoma.

5. Embryologic Urothelial Differentiation versus Dedifferentiation in Urothelial Neoplasia

The close correlation between cytokeratin isotype expression patterns and epithelial differentiation suggests that cytokeratins are crucial to epithelial tissue structure and/or function. However, it has been difficult to establish what the precise contributions of individuals or combinations of cytokeratin isotypes are to normal and neoplastic epithelial cell phenotype and behavior. Thus, the changes in CK20 immunolocalization which indicate a higher risk of urothelial carcinoma recurrence probably reflect a secondary change related to dysregulation of the urothelial differentiation program during carcinogenesis rather than indicating that CK20 is directly involved. It may be speculated that the patterns of expression of CK20 and CK5/6 in various urothelial carcinomas tend to mimic the stages of embryologic development and differentiation of urothelium. Thus, high-grade urothelial carcinomas (with or without invasion) which are characterized by diffuse CK20 expression without any basal layer may represent the early stage of urothelial differentiation after the urogenital sinus separates from the cloaca [7–9]. During this stage of development, urothelium manifests diffuse CK20 staining but lacks a basal layer. In some of the high-grade urothelial carcinomas, there is uniform staining of all the layers by CK20, but there is also a well-formed basal layer demonstrable by expression of CK5/6. This may be equivalent to the intermediate stage of embryonic urothelial differentiation. The well-differentiated urothelial carcinomas are characterized by the presence of a mature pattern of CK20 expression where its expression is mostly limited to the umbrella cells, while well-defined basal cell layer immunoreactive for CK5/6 is also present (Figures 8 and 9).

This pattern may be equivalent to the final stage of urothelial development and maturation during the intrauterine period.

In summary, immunohistochemical staining of urothelial carcinoma for CK20 and CK5/6 may provide useful information regarding the nature of urothelial carcinoma and its clinical behavior.

Acknowledgments

The authors would like to acknowledge valuable assistance and technical expertise of the following supervisory and technical staff of our immunohistochemical laboratory in performance of the two-color immunohistochemical staining: MS Rajaa Al Abdulla, supervisor; MS Huda Ahmed Al Hijji, supervisor; and MS Zuhoor Ali, senior technologist.

References

[1] J. Southgate, P. Harnden, and L. K. Trejdosiewicz, "Cytokeratin expression patterns in normal and malignant urothelium: a review of the biological and diagnostic implications," *Histology and Histopathology*, vol. 14, no. 2, pp. 657–664, 1999.

[2] R. L. Haines and E. B. Lane, "Keratins and disease at a glance," *Journal of Cell Science*, vol. 125, pp. 3923–3928, 2012.

[3] P. Awasthi, A. Thahriani, and A. Bhattacharya, "Keratins or cytokeratins—a review article," *Journal of Advanced Medical and Dental Sciences Research*, vol. 4, no. 4, pp. 140–148, 2016.

[4] J. Schweizer, P. E. Bowden, P. A. Coulombe et al., "New consensus nomenclature for mammalian keratins," *Journal of Cell Biology*, vol. 174, no. 2, pp. 169–174, 2006.

[5] R. MaginLane, M. Divo, and L. Langbein, "The human keratins: biology and pathology," *Histochemistry and Cell Biology*, vol. 129, no. 6, pp. 705–733, 2008.

[6] V. Karantza, "Keratins in health and cancer: more than mere epithelial cell markers," *Oncogene*, vol. 30, no. 2, pp. 127–138, 2011.

[7] L. Baskin and G. Cunha, *Embryology of the Human Genitourinary Tract*, M. Campbell and P. Walsh, Eds., Saunders, Philadelphia, PA, USA, 2018.

[8] A. Alonso, U. Ikinger, and J. Kartenbeck, "Staining patterns of keratins in the human urinary tract," *Histology and Histopathology*, vol. 24, no. 11, pp. 1425–1437, 2009.

[9] J. D. L. Rosette, F. Smedts, C. Schoots, H. Hoek, and P. Laguna, "Changing patterns of keratin expression could be associated with functional maturation of the developing human bladder," *The Journal of Urology*, vol. 168, no. 2, pp. 709–717, 2002.

[10] P. Veranic, R. Romih, and K. Jezernik, "What determines differentiation of urothelial umbrella cells?" *European Journal of Cell Biology*, vol. 83, no. 1, pp. 27–34, 2004.

[11] X.-R. Wu, X.-P. Kong, A. Pellicer, G. Kreibich, and T.-T. Sun, "Uroplakins in urothelial biology, function, and disease," *Kidney International*, vol. 75, no. 11, pp. 1153–1165, 2009.

[12] E. M. Comperat, M. Burger, P. Gontero et al., "Grading of Urothelial Carcinoma and the New "World Health Organisation Classification of Tumours of the Urinary System and Male Genital Organs" 2016," *European Urology Focus*, vol. 5, no. 3, pp. 457–466.

[13] R. T. Vollmer, "A review of outcomes for stage Ta bladder tumors," *American Journal of Clinical Pathology*, vol. 146, no. 2, pp. 215–220, 2016.

[14] P. A. Humphrey, H. Moch, A. L. Cubilla, T. M. Ulbright, and V. E. Reuter, "The 2016 WHO classification of tumors of the urinary system and male genital organs—part b: prostate and bladder tumours," *European Urology*, vol. 70, no. 1, pp. 106–119, 2016.

[15] P. Harnden, A. Allam, A. D. Joyce, A. Patel, P. Selby, and J. Southgate, "Cytokeratin 20 expression by non-invasive transitional cell carcinomas: potential for distinguishing recurrent from non-recurrent disease," *Histopathology*, vol. 27, no. 2, pp. 169–174, 1995.

[16] P. Harnden, N. Mahmood, and J. Southgate, "Expression of cytokeratin 20 redefines urothelial papillomas of the bladder," *The Lancet*, vol. 353, no. 9157, pp. 974-977, 1999.

[17] A. Alsheikh, Z. Mohamedali, E. Jones, J. Masterson, and C. B. Gilks, "Comparison of the WHO/ISUP classification and cytokeratin 20 expression in predicting the behavior of low-grade papillary urothelial tumors," *Modern Pathology*, vol. 14, no. 4, pp. 267–272, 2001.

[18] H. E. Rashed, E. H. Abdelbary, and A. R. Ali, "Role of CK20, CK5/6 and P53 in the diagnosis of flat urothelial lesions with atypia," *Journal of American Science*, vol. 10, pp. 29–37, 2014.

[19] C. Wu, Z. Eslami, S. Tanguay et al., "The role of immunohistochemistry in the diagnosis of flat urothelial lesions: a study using CK20, CK5/6, P53, CD138, and Her2/Neu," *Annals of Diagnostic Pathology*, vol. 18, no. 1, pp. 27–32, 2014.

[20] A. A. Hashmi, Z. F. Hussain, M. Irfan et al., "Cytokeratin 5/6 expression in bladder cancer: association with clinicopathologic parameters and prognosis," *BMC Research Notes*, vol. 11, no. 1, p. 207, 2018.

[21] A. Lopez-Beltran, V. Henriques, R. Montironi, A. Cimadamore, M. R. Raspollini, and L. Cheng, "Variants and new entities of bladder cancer," *Histopathology*, vol. 74, no. 1, pp. 77–96, 2019.

[22] O. Kaufmann, E. Fietze, J. Mengs, and M. Dietel, "Value of p63 and cytokeratin 5/6 as immunohistochemical markers for the differential diagnosis of poorly differentiated and undifferentiated carcinomas," *American Journal of Clinical Pathology*, vol. 116, no. 6, pp. 823–830, 2001.

[23] D. Sikic, B. Keck, S. Wach et al., "Immunohistochemiocal subtyping using CK20 and CK5 can identify urothelial carcinomas of the upper urinary tract with a poor prognosis," *PLoS One*, vol. 12, no. 6, Article ID e0179602, 2017.

[24] M. Jung, J. H. Lee, B. Kim, J. H. Park, and K. C. Moon, "Transcriptional analysis of immunohistochemically defined subgroups of non-muscle-invasive papillary high-grade upper tract urothelial carcinoma," *International Journal of Molecular Sciences*, vol. 20, no. 3, p. 570, 2019.

[25] J. I. Epstein, L. Egevad, P. A. Humphrey, and R. Montironi, "Best practices recommendations in the application of immunohistochemistry in the prostate," *The American Journal of Surgical Pathology*, vol. 38, no. 8, pp. e6–e19, 2014.

[26] M. Eckstein, M. R. Wirtz, and M. Gross-Weege, "mRNA-expression of KRT5 and KRT20 defines distinct prognostic

subgroups of muscle-invasive urothelial bladder cancer correlating with histological variants," *International Journal of Molecular Sciences*, vol. 19, no. 11, p. 3396, 2018.

[27] A. Bhalla, M. Manjari, S. Kahlon, P. Kumar, and N. Kalra, "Cytokeratin 5/6 expression in benign and malignant breast lesions," *Indian Journal of Pathology and Microbiology*, vol. 53, no. 4, pp. 676–680, 2010.

[28] P. G. Chu and L. M. Weiss, "Expression of cytokeratin 5/6 in epithelial neoplasms: an immunohistochemical study of 509 cases," *Modern Pathology*, vol. 15, no. 1, pp. 6–10, 2002.

[29] H. E. Rashed, E. H. Abdelbary, and A. R. Ragab Ali, "Role OF CK20, CK5/6 and P53 in the diagnosis of flat urothelial lesions with atypia," *Journal of American Science*, vol. 10, pp. 29–37, 2014.

[30] S. Jung, C. Wu, Z. Eslami et al., "The role of immunohistochemistry in the diagnosis of flat urothelial lesions: a study using CK20, CK5/6, P53, Cd138, and Her2/Neuflat urothelial lesions: a study using CK20, CK5/6, P53, Cd138, and Her2/Neu," *Annals of Diagnostic Pathology*, vol. 18, no. 1, pp. 27–32, 2014.

[31] K. T. Mai, A. Busca, and E. C. Belanger, "Flat intraurothelial neoplasia exhibiting diffuse immunoreactivity for CD 44 and cytokeratin 5 (urothelial stem cell/basal cell markers)," *Applied Immunohistochemistry & Molecular Morphology*, vol. 25, no. 7, pp. 505–512, 2017.

21

Chlamydia trachomatis Growth and Cytokine mRNA Response in a Prostate Cancer Cell Line

Ivan M. Petyaev,[1] Naylia A. Zigangirova,[2] Elena Y. Morgunova,[2] Nigel H. Kyle,[1] Elena D. Fedina,[2] and Yuriy K. Bashmakov[1]

[1]*Lycotec Ltd., Granta Park, Cambridge CB21 6GP, UK*
[2]*Department of Medical Microbiology, Gamaleya National Research Center of Epidemiology and Microbiology, Ministry of Health, 18 Gamaleya Str, Moscow 123098, Russia*

Correspondence should be addressed to Yuriy K. Bashmakov; ybash47926@aol.com

Academic Editor: Kostis Gyftopoulos

In the present paper, we report that *C. trachomatis* can be efficiently propagated and affect mRNA expression for two major cytokines, relevant to tumor progression, in CWR-R1 cells, a malignant prostate cell line. CWR-R1 and McCoy cells, a classic cell line for chlamydial research, were grown and infected with *C. trachomatis* under similar conditions. Cell monolayers were harvested for RNA analysis and immunostaining with major outer membrane protein (MOMP) antibody at 24, 48, and 72 hours of the postinfection (hpi) period. It was shown that the infectious cycle of chlamydial pathogen in CWR-R1 cells resembles the progression of *C. trachomatis* infection in McCoy cells but with a few important differences. First of all, the initial stage of *C. trachomatis* propagation in CWR-R1 cells (24 hpi) was characterized by larger inclusion bodies and more intense, specific immunofluorescent staining of infected cells as compared with McCoy cells. Moreover, there was a corresponding increase in infective progeny formation in CWR-R1 cells along with mRNA for EUO, a crucial gene controlling the early phase of the chlamydial development cycle (24 hpi). These changes were more minimal and became statistically insignificant at a later time point in the infectious cycle (48 hpi). Altogether, these data suggest that the early phase of *C. trachomatis* infection in CWR-R1 cells is accompanied by more efficient propagation of the pathogen as compared with the growth of *C. trachomatis* in McCoy cells. Furthermore, propagation of *C. trachomatis* in CWR-R1 cells leads to enhanced transcription of interleukin-6 and fibroblast growth factor-2, genes encoding two important proinflammatory cytokines implicated in the molecular mechanisms of chemoresistance of prostate cancer and its ability to metastasize. The possible roles of reactive oxygen species and impaired mitochondrial oxidation in the prostate cancer cell line are discussed as factors promoting the early stages of *C. trachomatis* growth in CWR-R1 cells.

1. Introduction

Chlamydia trachomatis (*C. trachomatis*) is an obligate, nonspore-forming intracellular Gram-negative bacterial pathogen able to propagate in epitheliocytes of mucous membranes (urogenital system and eye) and which displays a distinct parasitic cell cycle [1, 2]. *C. trachomatis* is the most prevalent sexually transmitted pathogen causing a wide range of syndromes and diseases, with an alarming growth rate of 100 million newly reported cases annually worldwide [3, 4]. Although most *C. trachomatis* infections are asymptomatic, untreated individuals may develop a variety of genital (urethritis, endocervicitis, salpingitis, endometritis, and pelvic inflammatory disease) and extragenital (arthritis, perihepatitis, and ocular infection) manifestations [5]. There are 17 *C. trachomatis* serovars. All of them have a similar and unique life cycle and exist in two developmental forms—elementary body and reticulate body [6]. Eukaryotic cells are infected with nondividing elementary bodies which form phagolysosomal fusion particles in the cytoplasm of the host cell at the initial stage of infection. Inside, the endosome elementary bodies differentiate into reticulate bodies which divide via binary fission [1, 7]. Once infection progresses and the endosome (otherwise known as the inclusion body) accumulates a significant number of reticulate bodies, a reverse transformation of reticulate bodies into elementary bodies takes place. Newly formed elementary bodies undergo exocytosis after 48–72 hours of postinfection development to initiate a new round of *C. trachomatis* infection in neighboring cells. Such a sophisticated developmental cycle is highly energy dependent and known to be supported by host cell metabolism [8]. All members of Chlamydiaceae rely heavily on the host cell metabolism. The chlamydial genome lacks most of the genes encoding cholesterol biosynthesis although chlamydial species can synthetize some phospholipids, long chain fatty acids and branched fatty acids [8–10]. Chlamydiaceae are completely auxotrophic for purine and pyrimidine nucleotides, most amino acids, and utilize host cell cytosolic ATP for at least the early stages of infection [11].

A large number of nonhematopoietic cells can support *C. trachomatis* growth using in vitro systems. Most of the genital strains grow very efficiently in a McCoy mouse fibroblast cell line, which is a classic cell for stock expansion and maintenance [12]. Ocular strains of the pathogen show preferential growth in conjunctival cells [13]. Epithelial cell lines from the vagina, endocervix, and endometrium have been established to provide physiologically relevant models for the study of pathogenesis in genital forms of *C. trachomatis* infection [14]. There is a continuous pursuit of physiologically relevant in vitro systems for the investigation of pathogenesis and treatment of *C. trachomatis* infection.

In the present paper, we report that *C. trachomatis* can be efficiently propagated and affect host cell mRNA expression for two major cytokines, relevant for tumor progression, in CWR-R1 cells, a malignant prostate cell line.

2. Materials and Methods

2.1. Reagents and Organisms. All reagents were from Sigma-Aldrich (St. Louis, USA) unless specified otherwise. *C. trachomatis* strain L2/Bu434 was kindly provided by Dr. P Saikku (University of Oulu, Finland). CWR-R1 cells (a human prostate cancer epithelial cell line), as well as McCoy cells (a mouse fibroblast cell line), were obtained from the Cultured Cells Depository Collection (Moscow, Russia).

2.2. Cell Culture. C. trachomatis was propagated in McCoy mouse fibroblasts grown in DMEM with 10% HyClone FCS supplemented with 2 mM glutamine, 4.0 mg/ml gentamicin, and 5.0 mg/ml amphotericin B, and further purified by Renografin gradient centrifugation, as previously described [15]. Briefly, elementary bodies were isolated and resuspended in sucrose-phosphate-glutamic acid (SPG) buffer (0.2 M sucrose, 8.6 mM Na2HPO4, 3.8 mM KH2PO4, 5 mM glutamic acid, 0.2 mm-filtered, pH 7.4). Titers were determined by infecting cell monolayers with dilutions of thawed stock suspension (2.5×10^7). Subconfluent McCoy cell monolayers were infected with the suspension of *C. trachomatis* at MOI 1. Plates were centrifuged for 1 hour at 1500 g to synchronize the infection. Nucleic acid-based assay (RT-PCR) was performed at 24, 48, and 72 hours following *C. trachomatis* inoculation of the cultured cells. The infection rate in the McCoy cells and infective progeny formation was estimated as hours of postinfection (hpi) period following pathogen introduction into the incubation medium. To avoid discrepancies, CWR-R1 cells were grown, infected, and monitored under similar conditions.

2.3. Immunofluoresence Staining. Infected McCoy and CWR-R1 cells were grown on coverslips in 24-well plates and used for analysis at 0, 24, 48, and 72 hpi. The cells were fixed with ice-cold methanol, permeabilized with 0.1% Triton X-100, and preblocked for 1 hour at 4°C with 1% bovine serum albumin in PBS. Cell monolayers were stained using FITC-conjugated monoclonal antibody against MOMP, a major outer membrane protein (Bio-Rad, USA). Inclusion-containing cells were visualized using a Nikon Eclipse 50i microscope (Nikon, Japan) at ×1000 or lower magnification. Size of the inclusion bodies was measured using a MicroScan attachment to the microscope with a resolution of 0.1 μm (Protvino, Russia) along with morphometric software (DiagNodus, Cambridge, UK).

2.4. Assessment of Infective Progeny. Infective progeny accumulation was assessed in McCoy and CWR-R1 cell monolayers infected with *C. trachomatis* at different time points. Infected cell monolayers were harvested 48 hours after bacterial inoculation and lysed by freezing/thawing. Serial dilutions of lysates were inoculated into McCoy cells, and plates were centrifuged for 1 hour at 1500 g. The infected cells were visualized at 48 hours of the postinfection period with FITC-conjugated monoclonal antibody against chlamydial MOMP, a major outer membrane protein (BioRad, USA).

2.4.1. Attachment and Internalization Assay. This assay was performed as described in our previous paper [16].

2.5. RNA Extraction and Reverse Transcription. RNA was isolated from *C. trachomatis*-infected McCoy cells or CWR-R1 monolayers grown on 6-well plates using TRIZol (Invitrogen, Waltham MS, USA) at the 24-hour time point of the postinfection period. Total mRNA was pretreated with DNase I (DNA-free™, Ambion, Waltham MS, USA) and quantified on a NanoDrop ND-100 spectrophotometer (Thermo Fisher Scientific, Waltham MS, USA). 1 μg of each RNA sample was converted into cDNA using random hexamer primers and a SuperScript III First-Strand Synthesis kit (Invitrogen, Waltham MS, USA).

2.5.1. Quantitative Real-Time PCR. mRNA levels for *EUO*, a developmental gene of *C. trachomatis*, were analyzed in McCoy and CWR-R1 cells at different hpi by quantitative RT-PCR using a CFX-96 thermocycler and master mixes from Bio-Rad Laboratories (Hercules CA, USA). RT-qPCR Taqman primers were designed using Primer 3 software and were validated by BLAST search and regression plot analysis using Cp values obtained with multiple dilutions of cDNA. Specificity of the designed primers and fluorescent probes was confirmed in different systems using cDNA from *C. trachomatis* Bu434, *C. trachomatis* UW-3/Cx, *C. trachomatis* UW- 31/Cx, and *C. pneumoniae* K-6, as well as from uninfected McCoy and CWR-R1 cells and some other common bacterial pathogens as previously described [15].

The *C. trachomatis*-specific primers used were as follows: for *EUO* gene: Pr-F 5′ TCCCCGACGCTCTCCTTTCA 3′, Pr-R 5′CTCGTCAGGCTATCTATGTTGCT 3′, Probe 5′-ROX- ATG GAC GCC ACT TGT CCC ACG GAA T-BHQ2-3′. Primers for human interleukin-6 (IL-6) were as follows: PR-F 5′-CCAGCTATGAACTCCTTCTC-3′, PR-R 5′-GCTTGTTCCTCACATCTCTC-3′. Primers for human fibroblast growth factor-2 (FGF-2) were: PR-F 5′-GGCTTCTTCCTGCGCATCCA-3′ and PR-R 5′-GCTCTTAGCAGACATTGGAAGA-3′. Primer sequences for eukaryotic beta-actin were used as published previously [15, 16]. All primers were verified and used at 0.4 μM final concentration under thermal cycling conditions of 95°C for 10 min, 50 cycles of 95°C for 15 seconds, 60°C for 1 min, and 72°C for 20 seconds. Serial dilutions of RNA extracted from C. *trachomatis*-infected McCoy and CWR-R1 cells were used as a standard for quantification of chlamydial gene expression. The mRNA expression levels were referenced to Ct values for chlamydial genes detected in uninfected McCoy cells grown under similar conditions. This reference value was taken as 1.00. All mRNA measurements were done in triplicate. All experiments were conducted at least three times. Statistical analysis was performed where possible using Student's *t*-test and calculation of medians as well as 95% confidence intervals. The most representative sets of immunofluorescence images were selected and are shown above.

3. Results

3.1. Morphological Assessment. The morphological characteristics of *C. trachomatis* growth in McCoy and CWR-R1 cells were monitored in immunofluorescence experiments conducted side by side. There was no difference in the attachment/entry of EB into McCoy and CWR-R1 cells at the early time points of infection corresponding to 6, 9, and 12 hpi (results not shown). Almost equal numbers of infected cells were seen in both cells lines at the different MOI used (0.5 and 1.0). Also, there was no statistical difference in the number of infected cells in the cell lines investigated. For example, at 24 hpi, the number of infected cells seen in the McCoy line at MOI = 1 was 26.3 (95% CI : 29.4/22.9), whereas the corresponding infectivity rate in CWR-R1 cells observed under the same conditions was 28.1 (95% CI : 30.1/21.4, $P > 0.05$). Despite the similar number of infected cells assessed by IF at all time points, the inclusion bodies developing in McCoy cells at the initial stage of infection (24 hpi) tended to be less mature, with a patchy and more granular pattern of staining. Moreover, there was greater variability in the pattern of inclusion body staining in McCoy cells. In contrast, the majority of CWR-R1 cells at this time point had a less variable and stronger pattern of staining. They contained more mature inclusion particles with higher IF density and a more globular appearance, suggesting altogether a better synchronization of infection (Figure 1). At the late stage of the infectious cycle (72 hpi), the difference in the intensity of IF staining of the inclusion bodies was less obvious. However, the majority of McCoy cells were disrupted with visible exocytosis of EB, whereas EB in the CWR-R1 cells appeared to be more contained within cell remnants.

The results shown in Figure 2 document the difference in chlamydial inclusion size seen in both cell lines during the infectious cycle. As can be seen, under the culture conditions used, the inclusions in CWR-R1 cells were significantly larger ($P < 0.05$) than the inclusion bodies formed in McCoy cells at 24 and 48 hpi.

3.2. Infective Progeny Formation. Figure 3 shows the difference in infective progeny formation in McCoy and CWR-R1 cells at 24 and 48 hpi. There was a statistically significant ($P < 0.05$) increase in the median reflecting infective progeny formation in CWR-R1 cells (7.7×10^5, 95% CI : 9.1/6.3) in comparison with McCoy cells (4.6×10^5, 95% CI : 5.4/3.7) at the early stage of infection (24 hpi). However, the later stage of chlamydial infection (48 hpi) was not accompanied by a statistically significant difference in infective progeny formation in the cell lines studied ($P > 0.05$).

3.3. EUO Expression. The results reported above reveal that the greatest differences in the infectious cycle of *C. trachomatis* in McCoy and CWR-R1 cells are evident at the initial stage of pathogen propagation in the host cells. Therefore, we decided to investigate next the mRNA levels for *EUO*, a key chlamydial gene controlling multiple gene transcription during the early stage of *C. trachomatis* propagation in eukaryotic cells [16].

As can be seen from Figure 4, the highest level of EUO expression in both cell lines was seen in our experiments at 12 hpi, and especially at 24 hpi. At both time points, *EUO* expression was noticeably higher in CWR-R1 cells than that in McCoy cells (by 2.1- and 1.8-folds, respectively). Interestingly, even at the earliest time point investigated (3 hpi), CWR-R1 cells had a higher level of copies for *EUO* mRNA (by 30%) than that in with McCoy cells. *EUO* mRNA remained almost equally elevated but subsided somewhat from the values measured at 24 hpi (up to 4.1- and 4.5-folds in McCoy and CWR-R1 cells, respectively) at 48 hpi.

3.4. Host Cell Cytokine mRNA Expression. Since *C. trachomatis* is known to affect cytokine gene expression in host cells during the postinfection period [17], we decided to investigate next the mRNA levels of IL-6 and FGF-2, two crucial proinflammatory cytokines, following exposure of McCoy and CWR-R1 cells to the pathogen.

As can be seen from Figure 5, both genes (IL-6 and FGF-2) are constitutively expressed in uninfected McCoy and CWR-R1 cells. Both proinflammatory mRNAs were

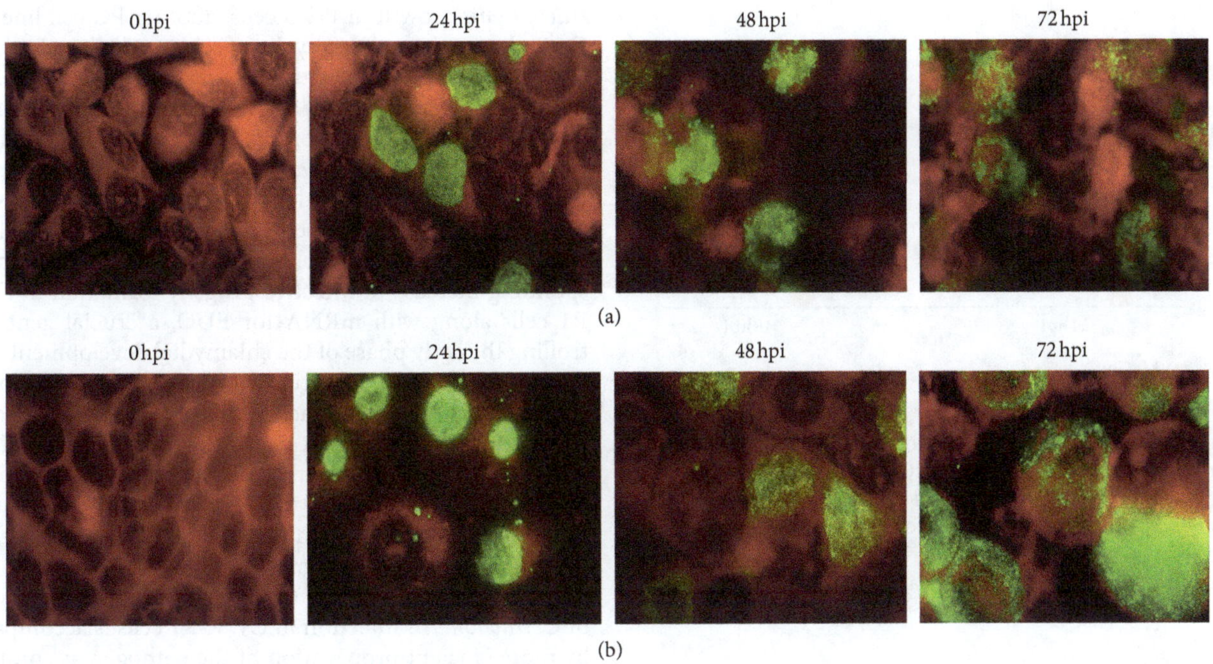

FIGURE 1: Immunofluoresence analysis of *C. trachomatis* propagation in (a) McCoy versus (b) CWR-R1 cells. McCoy and CWR-R1 cells were plated, grown, and harvested at "0", 24, 48, and 78 hours after inoculation of *C. trachomatis*. The cells were stained with MOMP-specific antibody and photographed as described in Material and Methods.

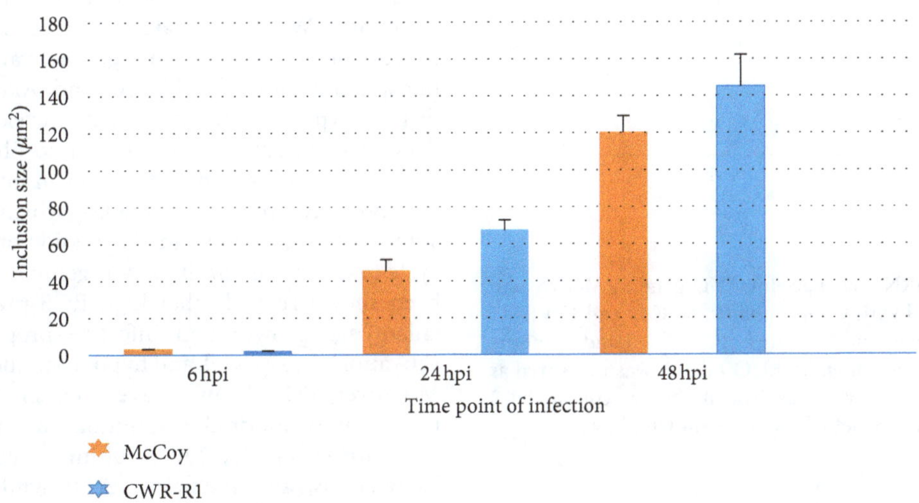

FIGURE 2: Inclusion body size in McCoy and CWR-R1 cells infected with *C. trachomatis*. McCoy and CWR-R1 cells were plated, grown, and harvested at 6, 24, 48, and 78 hours after inoculation of *C. trachomatis*. The cells were stained with MOMP-specific antibody, and inclusion size was measured as described in Material and Methods.

upregulated in infected McCoy cells (up to 1.3- and 1.5-folds for IL-6 and FGF-2, respectively). However, increases were much more pronounced in the infected CWR-R1 cells. The mRNA level for IL-6 went up to 9.7-fold and mRNA for FGF-2 was upregulated by 6.3-fold as compared with mRNA values detected in the uninfected cells. Since the two cell lines used in the studies are of different origin (mouse versus human) and require different primer sets for mRNA quantification with possible differences in annealing efficiency, it would be questionable to conduct direct quantitative assessment of the mRNA responses in McCoy and CWR-R1 cells in terms other than fold increase over basal values detected for each cell line.

4. Discussion

Prostate cancer (PC) is the most common noncutaneous cancer in men and the third most common cause of cancer-related death in males residing in the USA and the UK [18]. Newly diagnosed individuals with localized PC have a high 10-year survival rate and a high chance of complete recovery whereas men with metastatic "aggressive" forms of PC tend

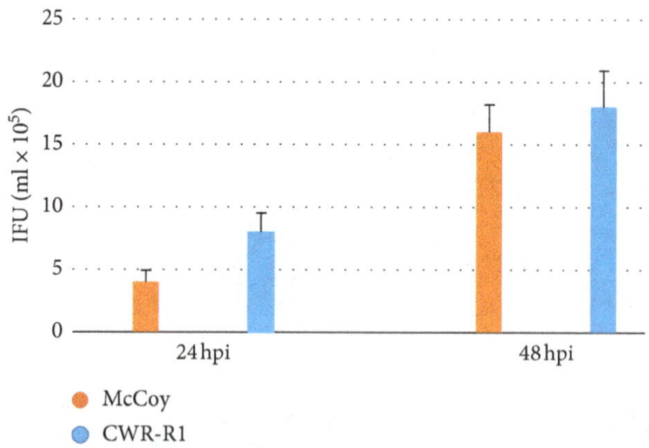

FIGURE 3: Infective progeny formation in McCoy and CWR-R1 cells infected with *C. trachomatis*. McCoy and CWR-R1 cells were plated, grown, and harvested at 24 and 48 hours after inoculation of *C. trachomatis*. Infective progeny formation was measured as described in Material and Methods in five different sets of the experiments, and average data with standard deviations are shown.

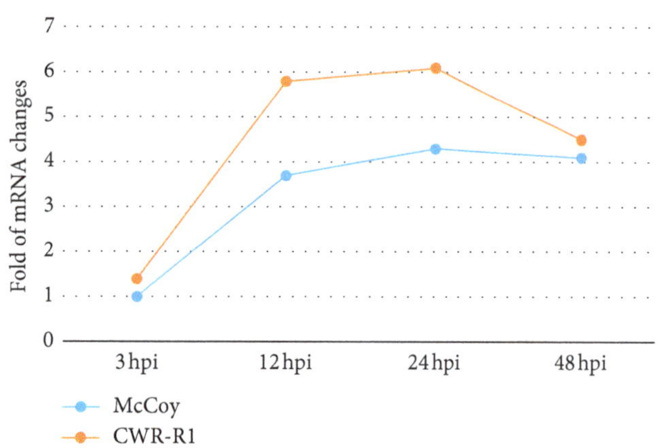

FIGURE 4: Folds of mRNA changes for *EUO* gene in McCoy and CWR-R1 cells infected with *C. trachomatis*. McCoy and CWR-R1 cells were plated, grown, and harvested at 3, 12, 24, and 48 hours after inoculation of *C. trachomatis*. EUO mRNA was measured as described in Material and Methods. The study was conducted 3 times. Most representative set of results is shown above.

to have much poorer outcomes [19, 20]. The molecular and cellular mechanisms of initiation, progression, and outcomes of PC are poorly understood. Chronic prostate inflammation (prostatitis), sedentary lifestyle, obesity, high-fat diet, and smoking are among epidemiological factors predisposing to PC [21, 22]. *Chlamydia trachomatis* is currently considered to be among common and frequent uropathogens causing chronic and difficult to treat bacterial prostatitis [23]. Although the frequency of confirmed cases of chlamydial prostatitis in the general population seems to be low, *C. trachomatis* can ascend the male urogenital tract and affect the bladder, prostate, seminal vesicles, epididymis, and testicles [24, 25].

In the present paper, we report that *C. trachomatis* can efficiently propagate in CWR-R1 cells, a PC cell line. This observation is in good agreement with results describing *C. trachomatis* growth in PC-3 cells, another PC cell line (26). Overall, the infectious cycle of chlamydial pathogen in CWR-R1 cells resembles the progression of *C. trachomatis* infection in McCoy cells, a classic cell line for chlamydial research, with a few important differences. First of all, the initial stage of *C. trachomatis* propagation in CWR-R1 cells (24 hpi) was characterized by larger inclusion bodies and higher intensity of IF staining of the infected cells as compared with McCoy cells. Moreover, there was a corresponding increase in infective progeny formation in CWR-R1 cells along with mRNA for EUO, a crucial gene controlling the early phase of the chlamydial development cycle. It remains an open question now if other developmental chlamydial genes (*incA* and *omcB*) studied in our previous work [15] have a different pattern of expression in McCoy and CWR-R1 cells during the later stages of infectious cycle. Interestingly, the changes in *EUO* expression between two cell lines studied were minimized and became statically insignificant at a later time point in the infectious cycle (48 hpi). Altogether, these data suggest that the early phase of *C. trachomatis* infection in CWR-R1 cells is accompanied by more efficient propagation of the pathogen as compared with the growth of *C. trachomatis* in McCoy cells. This conclusion comprises a novelty in our research. The underlying mechanism of these phenomena may be related to biochemical characteristics of PC cells and the metabolic requirements for *C. trachomatis* growth in the early stages of infection. CWR-R1 cells are known constitutively to express functional elements of mitogen-activated protein kinase, phosphatidylinositol-3 kinase, and Akt pathways and to display hyperactivated Akt which develops due to an Akt-dependent increase in oxidative phosphorylation [26, 27]. These changes are known to cause an intracellular excess of reactive oxygen species (ROS) which are an essential stimulus for initiation and progression of the developmental cycle of *C. trachomatis* in the urogenital system [3, 28]. It has been shown recently that high ROS production promotes chlamydial growth and infective progeny formation via activation of caspase-1 and hypoxia-inducible factor 1α [29]. Moreover, PC cell lines have been shown to have an impaired mitochondrial respiration rate and exemplify the Warburg effect [27, 30], resulting in enhanced glycolysis, lactogenesis, and inefficient ATP synthesis. However, as recently reported, moderate hypoxia is highly beneficial for the chlamydial growth cycle in cultured cells and promotes the infection rate of both *C. trachomatis and C. pneumoniae* [28]. Additionally, as shown lately [11] *C. trachomatis* can sustain its own energy needs during the infectious cycle at least in part via sodium-dependent synthesis of ATP. Therefore, high competition for ATP metabolic pathways in PC cells need not be a limiting factor for chlamydial cycle progression in PC cell lines and seems rather to be a factor activating chlamydial growth.

Another aspect of our results reveals that propagation of *C. trachomatis* in CWR-R1 cells leads to enhanced transcription of IL-6 and FGF-2, genes encoding two important pro-inflammatory cytokines. IL-6 is a well-known inducer of chemoresistance, progression, and metastatic transformation of PC [31, 32]. On the other

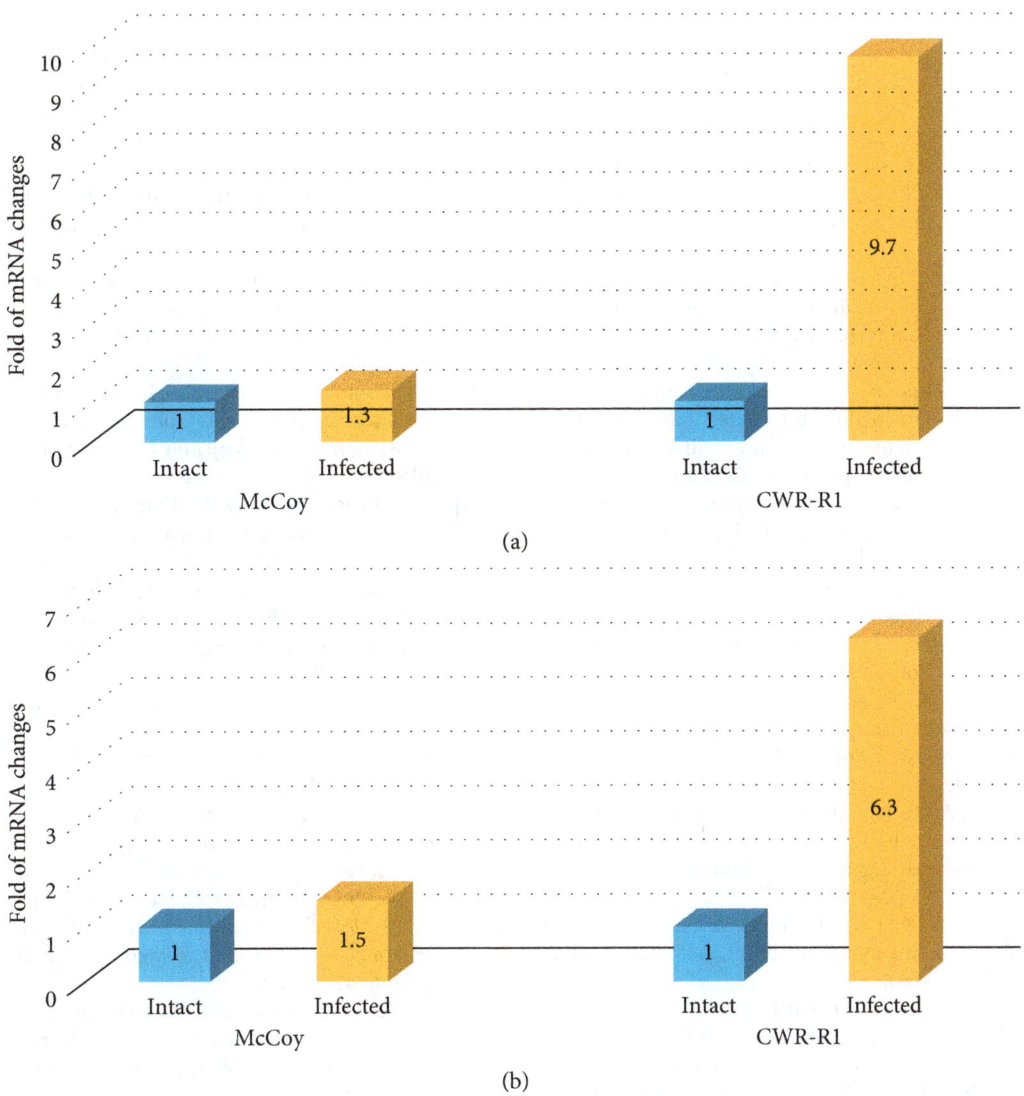

FIGURE 5: mRNA values for interleukin-6 (a) and fibroblast growth factor-2 (b) in McCoy and CWR-R1 cells infected with *C. trachomatis* AT 24 hpi. McCoy and CWR-R1 cells were plated, grown, and harvested 48 hours after inoculation of *C. trachomatis*. mRNAs for IL-6 and FGF-2 were measured as described in Material and Methods. The study was conducted 3 times. Most representative set of results is shown above.

hand, FGF-2 is reported to promote vascularization of primary PC tumors and formation of metastatic lesions [33]. Therefore, the pattern of changes in cytokine mRNA profile seen in CWR-R1 cells infected with *C. trachomatis* clearly leads to predisposition to the advancement of PC. Similar results have been reported by Sellami H et al. who described enhanced transcription of VEGF mRNA in PC-3 cells, another PC cell line, infected with *C. trachomatis* [34]. However, it has to be emphasized that these results are of highly questionable relevance to clinical practice. Although a limited body of epidemiological evidence places past urogenital infections and sexually transmitted infections among the risk factors for PC, there is no proven epidemiological link between chlamydiosis and PC yet [35]. Additional epidemiological analysis is required to evaluate the possible interplay between *C. trachomatis* infection and PC outcomes and to determine the relevance of the observed changes to clinical practice. Nevertheless, the results reported above and the cell culture system proposed in our study could be a useful tool in experiments exploring the role of impaired host cell mitochondrial function in chlamydial growth as well as in understanding the general biology of chlamydial infection.

Acknowledgments

The study was a subject of internal funding by Lycotec Ltd. (UK) and Gamaleya National Research Center of Epidemiology and Microbiology (Russia).

References

[1] I. Haferkamp, "Crossing the border—solute entry into the chlamydial inclusion," *International Journal of Medical Microbiology*, vol. 308, no. 1, pp. 41–48, 2017.

[2] S. S. Witkin, E. Minis, A. Athanasiou, J. Leizer, and I. M. Linhares, "*Chlamydia trachomatis*: the persistent pathogen," *Clinical and Vaccine Immunology*, vol. 24, no. 10, 2017.

[3] K. A. Redgrove and E. A. McLaughlin, "The role of the immune response in *Chlamydia trachomatis* infection of the male genital tract: a double-edged sword," *Frontiers in Immunology*, vol. 5, p. 534, 2014.

[4] N. Ziklo, W. M. Huston, J. S. Hocking, and P. Timms, "*Chlamydia trachomatis* genital tract infections: when host immune response and the microbiome collide," *Trends in Microbiology*, vol. 24, no. 9, pp. 750–765, 2016.

[5] A. B. Lane and C. F. Decker, "*Chlamydia trachomatis* infections," *Disease-a-Month*, vol. 62, no. 8, pp. 269–273, 2016.

[6] C. Elwell, K. Mirrashidi, and J. Engel, "Chlamydia cell biology and pathogenesis," *Nature Reviews Microbiology*, vol. 14, no. 6, pp. 385–400, 2016.

[7] A. Nunes and J. P. Gomes, "Evolution, phylogeny, and molecular epidemiology of Chlamydia," *Infection, Genetics and Evolution*, vol. 23, pp. 49–64, 2014.

[8] N. Käding, M. Szaszák, and J. Rupp, "Imaging of Chlamydia and host cell metabolism," *Future Microbiology*, vol. 9, no. 4, pp. 509–521, 2014.

[9] E. M. Fozo and E. A. Rucks, "The making and taking of lipids: the role of bacterial lipid synthesis and the harnessing of host lipids in bacterial pathogenesis," *Advances in Microbial Physiology*, vol. 69, pp. 51–155, 2016.

[10] L. König, A. Siegl, T. Penz et al., "Biphasic metabolism and host interaction of a chlamydial symbiont," *mSystems*, vol. 2, no. 3, pp. e00202–e00216, 2017.

[11] P. Liang, M. Rosas-Lemus, D. Patel, X. Fang, K. Tuz, and O. Juárez, "Dynamic energy dependency of *Chlamydia trachomatis* on host cell metabolism during intracellular growth: role of sodium-based energetics in chlamydial ATP generation," *Journal of Biological Chemistry*, vol. 293, no. 2, pp. 510–522, 2017.

[12] T. Mestrović, S. Ljubin-Sternak, M Sviben et al., "Antimicrobial sensitivity profile of *Chlamydia trachomatis* isolates from Croatia in McCoy cell culture system and comparison with the literature," *Clinical Laboratory*, vol. 62, no. 3, pp. 357–364, 2016.

[13] T. G. Moffa, F. J. DeToma, S. Ellen Frederick, and M. Howe, "Growth of an ocular strain of *Chlamydia trachomatis* on Chang conjunctival cells," *Ophthalmic Research*, vol. 21, no. 5, pp. 388–391, 1989.

[14] C. Foschi, M. Salvo, R. Cevenini, and A. Marangoni, "*Chlamydia trachomatis* antimicrobial susceptibility in colorectal and endocervical cells," *Journal of Antimicrobial Chemotherapy*, vol. 73, no. 2, pp. 409–413, 2017.

[15] I. M. Petyaev, N. A. Zigangirova, E. Y. Morgunova, N. H. Kyle, E. D. Fedina, and Y. K. Bashmakov, "Resveratrol inhibits propagation of *Chlamydia trachomatis* in McCoy cells," *BioMed Research International*, vol. 2017, Article ID 4064071, 7 pages, 2017.

[16] Y. Cong, L. Gao, Y Zhang et al., "Quantifying promoter activity during the developmental cycle of *Chlamydia trachomatis*," *Scientific Reports*, vol. 6, no. 1, p. 27244, 2016.

[17] S. Jerchel, I. Kaufhold, L. Schuchardt, K. Shima, and J. Rupp, "Host immune responses after hypoxic reactivation of IFN-γ induced persistent *Chlamydia trachomatis* infection," *Frontiers in Cellular and Infection Microbiology*, vol. 4, p. 43, 2014.

[18] R. A. Madan and J. L. Gulley, "Prostate cancer immunotherapy: the path forward," *Current Opinion in Supportive and Palliative Care*, vol. 11, no. 3, pp. 225–230, 2017.

[19] A. Toledano, M. Bourmech, H. Lamallem et al., "Prospective: how will renal, prostatic and urothelial tumours be treated in 10 years?," *Néphrologie & Thérapeutique*, vol. 13, no. 1, pp. S115–S125, 2017.

[20] M. J. Barry and L. H. Simmons, "Prevention of prostate cancer morbidity and mortality: primary prevention and early detection," *Medical Clinics of North America*, vol. 101, no. 4, pp. 787–806, 2017.

[21] R. Eeles and H. N. Raghallaigh, "Men with a susceptibility to prostate cancer and the role of genetic based screening," *Translational Andrology and Urology*, vol. 7, no. 1, pp. 61–69, 2018.

[22] S. D. Brookman-May, R. Campi, J. D. S Henríquez et al., "Latest evidence on the impact of smoking, sports, and sexual activity as modifiable lifestyle risk factors for prostate cancer incidence, recurrence, and progression: a systematic review of the literature by the european association of urology section of oncological urology (ESOU)," *European Urology Focus*, vol. 8, no. 18, pp. 30069–30075, 2018.

[23] J. Videčnik Zorman, M. Matičič, S. Jeverica, and T. Smrkolj, "Diagnosis and treatment of bacterial prostatitis," *Acta Dermatovenerol Alp Pannonica Adriat*, vol. 24, no. 2, pp. 25–29, 2015.

[24] F. M. E. Wagenlehner, W. Weidner, and K. G. Naber, "Chlamydial infections in urology," *World Journal of Urology*, vol. 24, no. 1, pp. 4–12, 2006.

[25] W. Weidner, T. Diemer, P. Huwe, H. Rainer, and M. Ludwig, "The role of *Chlamydia trachomatis* in prostatitis," *International Journal of Antimicrobial Agents*, vol. 19, no. 6, pp. 466–470, 2002.

[26] D. Wu, C. U. Thakore, G. G. Wescott, J. A. McCubrey, and D. M. Terrian, "Integrin signaling links protein kinase Cε to the protein kinase B/Akt survival pathway in recurrent prostate cancer cells," *Oncogene*, vol. 23, no. 53, pp. 8659–8672, 2004.

[27] F. Cutruzzolà, G. Giardina, M Marani et al., "Glucose metabolism in the progression of prostate cancer," *Frontiers in Physiology*, vol. 8, p. 97, 2017.

[28] N. Käding, I. Kaufhold, C Müller et al., "Growth of Chlamydia pneumoniae is enhanced in cells with impaired mitochondrial function," *Frontiers in Cellular and Infection Microbiology*, vol. 7, p. 499, 2017.

[29] A. A. Abdul-Sater, N. Saïd-Sadier, V. M. Lam et al., "Enhancement of reactive oxygen species production and chlamydial infection by the mitochondrial Nod-like family member NLRX1," *Journal of Biological Chemistry*, vol. 285, no. 53, pp. 41637–41645, 2010.

[30] E. Eidelman, J. Twum-Ampofo, J. Ansari, and M. M. Siddiqui, "The metabolic phenotype of prostate cancer," *Frontiers in Oncology*, vol. 7, p. 131, 2017.

[31] M. Esfahani, N. Ataei, and M. Panjehpour, "Biomarkers for evaluation of prostate cancer prognosis," *Asian Pacific Journal of Cancer Prevention*, vol. 16, no. 7, pp. 2601–2611, 2015.

[32] Z. Culig, "Proinflammatory cytokine interleukin-6 in prostate carcinogenesis," *American Journal of Clinical and Experimental Urology*, vol. 2, no. 3, pp. 231–238, 2014.

[33] P. G. Corn, F. Wang, W. L. McKeehan, and N. Navone, "Targeting fibroblast growth factor pathways in prostate

cancer," *Clinical Cancer Research*, vol. 19, no. 21, pp. 5856–5866, 2013.

[34] H. Sellami, N. Said-Sadier, A. Znazen, R. Gdoura, D. M. Ojcius, and A. Hammami, "*Chlamydia trachomatis* infection increases the expression of inflammatory tumorigenic cytokines and chemokines as well as components of the Toll-like receptor and NF-κB pathways in human prostate epithelial cells," *Molecular and Cellular Probes*, vol. 28, no. 4, pp. 147–154, 2014.

[35] S. Caini, S. Gandini, M. Dudas, V. Bremer, E. Severi, and A. Gherasim, "Sexually transmitted infections and prostate cancer risk: a systematic review and meta-analysis," *Cancer Epidemiology*, vol. 38, no. 4, pp. 329–338, 2014.

22

Conventional-Dose versus High-Dose Chemotherapy for Relapsed Germ Cell Tumors

Deaglan J. McHugh[1] **and Darren R. Feldman**[1,2]

[1]*Department of Medicine, Memorial Sloan Kettering Cancer Center, New York, NY, USA*
[2]*Department of Medicine, Weill Medical College of Cornell University, New York, NY, USA*

Correspondence should be addressed to Darren R. Feldman; feldmand@mskcc.org

Academic Editor: Fabio Campodonico

The majority of metastatic germ cell tumors (GCTs) are cured with cisplatin-based chemotherapy, but 20–30% of patients will relapse after first-line chemotherapy and require additional salvage strategies. The two major salvage approaches in this scenario are high-dose chemotherapy (HDCT) with autologous stem cell transplant (ASCT) or conventional-dose chemotherapy (CDCT). Both CDCT and HDCT have curative potential in the management of relapsed/refractory GCT. However, due to a lack of conclusive randomized trials, it remains unknown whether sequential HDCT or CDCT represents the optimal initial salvage approach, with practice varying between tertiary institutions. This represents the most pressing question remaining for defining GCT treatment standards and optimizing outcomes. The authors review prognostic factors in the initial salvage setting as well as the major studies assessing the efficacy of CDCT, HDCT, or both, describing the strengths and weaknesses that formed the rationale behind the ongoing international phase III "TIGER" trial.

1. Background

Germ cell tumors (GCTs), comprising 1% of male cancers and 5% of male genitourinary malignancies, are the most common tumor in young men. Most patients with advanced disease are cured with platinum-based chemotherapy; however, 20–30% patients will fail to achieve a durable response and require salvage treatment [1]. Unfortunately, the majority of patients requiring salvage chemotherapy will ultimately die, with death from GCT accounting for the greatest number of average life years lost of any non-childhood malignancy [2]. Presently, the two major salvage approaches include conventional-dose chemotherapy (CDCT) and high-dose chemotherapy (HDCT) with autologous stem cell transplant (ASCT).

Due to inconsistencies between retrospective and randomized data comparing these two strategies and the rarity of the patient population, a universally recommended approach in the initial salvage setting is lacking. As such, practices vary widely throughout the world and patients are highly encouraged to participate in clinical trials. The objective of this review is to outline the prognostic factors that affect outcome in the salvage setting, the data supporting both salvage chemotherapy strategies (CDCT and HDCT), and an ongoing randomized clinical trial that seeks to definitively establish one of these approaches as the standard of care in the initial salvage setting.

2. Prognostic Factors for Salvage Chemotherapy

For patients with metastatic GCT, prognostic factors at initial diagnosis are universally accepted with the International Germ Cell Cancer Cooperative Group (IGCCCG) classification used to guide first-line chemotherapy. Patients experiencing treatment failure with cisplatin-based first-line chemotherapy, however, represent a highly heterogeneous population. Traditionally, separate prognostic factor analyses were performed for patients undergoing CDCT and HDCT, respectively. Factors consistently associated with favorable outcome to salvage CDCT regimens across multiple series included gonadal primary tumor site, complete response (CR) to first-line chemotherapy, and disease-free interval after first-line chemotherapy of at least several months, whereas burden of disease and tumor marker levels at the time of salvage chemotherapy demonstrated prognostic importance in some but not all series [3–6].

Prognostic factors for outcome to salvage HDCT were initially reported on small number of patients at individual centers treated with one specific regimen limiting the generalizability of the findings. Beyer et al. were the first to develop a multicenter prognostic model for HDCT derived from 310 patients treated with various HDCT regimens at 4 different centers in Europe and the United States. Factors associated with an adverse outcome included primary mediastinal nonseminomatous germ cell tumor (PM-NSGCT), HCG ≥ 1,000 IU/L, progressive disease prior to HDCT, and platinum-refractory disease. A point value was assigned to each of these factors and used to calculate a cumulative score which separated patients into good, intermediate, and poor-risk groups with failure-free survival rates of 51%, 27%, and 5%, respectively.

In a retrospective study of 184 patients with gonadal or retroperitoneal primary GCTs (PM-NSGCT patients were excluded) treated with salvage high-dose carboplatin and etoposide at Indiana University (IU), Einhorn and colleagues identified platinum-refractory disease, IGCCCG poor-risk classification at first-line chemotherapy, and receipt of HDCT as third-line or later to be associated with adverse outcome [7]. Feldman et al. reported on 107 patients treated with salvage HDCT as part of a phase I/II study of the TI-CE regimen at Memorial Sloan Kettering Cancer Center (MSKCC) and observed PM-NSGCT, receipt of HDCT as third-line or later, presence of lung metastases, HCG ≥ 1,000 IU/L, ≥3 metastatic sites and IGCCCG intermediate- or poor-risk classification at first-line chemotherapy as associated with poor outcome [8]. A more recent study from IU of 364 patients treated with high-dose carboplatin and etoposide identified use of HDCT as third-line or later therapy (n = 61, 17%), platinum-refractory disease (n = 122, 34%), PM-NSGCT (n = 20, 5%), nonseminoma histology (n = 285, 78%), IGCCCG intermediate- or poor-risk disease (n = 213, 59%) and HCG ≥ 1000 mIU/ml at HDCT initiation (n = 90, 25%) as associated with adverse progression-free survival (PFS) [9].

Given the variation in prognostic factors reported in these and other studies, the separate focus on CDCT and HDCT, the limited number of patients from which these models were derived, and the small number of chemotherapy (particularly HDCT) regimens used, a collaborative effort, known as the International Prognostic Factor Study Group (IPFSG), was formed to develop a universally accepted prognostic model prior to initial salvage chemotherapy. The IPFSG collected data from a retrospective cohort of nearly 1,600 patients treated in 13 countries who progressed after initial cisplatin-based chemotherapy [10]. Fifty-one percent of these patients received HDCT, justifying the use of the classifier in this population. Prognostic variables on multivariate analysis applicable to the entire population independent of treatment approach (CDCT or HDCT) included primary tumor site, response to first-line treatment, progression-free interval between first-line therapy and relapse, tumor markers at relapse (AFP and HCG), and presence of liver, bone, or brain metastases at relapse. Each of these risk factors was assigned a numerical point value depending on its prognostic significance, with the sum total score (maximum of 10) used to segregate patients into five risk groups (very low, low, intermediate, high, and very high). Two-year PFS varied significantly according to risk group (very low risk: 91%, low risk: 64%, intermediate risk: 53%, high risk: 33%, and very high risk: 22%). Overall survival (OS) was also significantly different across the groups.

3. Salvage Conventional-Dose Chemotherapy

Cisplatin plus ifosfamide-containing regimens form the backbone of salvage CDCT, with studies testing a variety of third drugs to add to this combination. In the 1980s when the combination of cisplatin, vinblastine, and bleomycin (PVB) was the standard first-line regimen, the combination of etoposide, ifosfamide, and cisplatin (VIP) was the most common salvage regimen since it included two drugs not administered in the first-line setting. Once etoposide plus cisplatin (EP) and bleomycin plus EP (BEP) supplanted PVB as standard first-line treatment regimens, vinblastine, ifosfamide, and cisplatin (VeIP) became the most popular salvage regimen. Numerous studies reported on salvage VIP, VeIP, or both used in heterogeneous populations of patients including in the second-, third-, and even later-line setting. CR rates approximated 25–35% with durable remission rates of 5–15% [11–13]. Once activity was demonstrated, VeIP and VIP were moved forward for evaluation in the initial salvage setting with improvement in CR rates to approximately 40–50% and durable remission rates to approximately 25% (Table 1) [4, 5]. In the largest study evaluating VeIP as initial salvage treatment, Loehrer and colleagues treated 135 patients who experienced progressive GCT after first-line chemotherapy but who had remained disease-free for at least 3 weeks from their last chemotherapy dose and observed a CR rate of 50% and durable remission rate of 24% [5].

A subsequent phase I/II study at Memorial Sloan Kettering Cancer Center (MSKCC) evaluated the addition of paclitaxel to ifosfamide plus cisplatin (TIP) as initial salvage treatment of 46 patients [14]. This trial limited eligibility to patients with features predicting a favorable outcome to salvage CDCT including gonadal primary tumor site and either a CR to first-line chemotherapy or a partial response with negative tumor markers (PR-negative markers) lasting ≥6 months. The CR rate was 70%, 2-year PFS rate was 65%, and 63% of patients remained continuously disease-free with median follow-up of nearly 7 years. These significantly improved outcomes compared to initial salvage VeIP can be partially explained by favorable patient selection and a small number of patients included with metastatic disease in the setting of a second gonadal primary GCT. However, the study also included 14 (30%) patients with late relapse (>2

Table 1: Prospective studies examining the use of initial salvage conventional-dose chemotherapy.

Author (year)	N	CDCT Regimen(s)	Notable inclusion or exclusion criteria	EP/BEP as first-line therapy	CR/PR to first-line therapy	IR to first-line therapy	CR	Median f/u (months)	Durable remission
McCaffrey et al. [4]	56	VeIP or VIP	None	53%	36%	64%	36%	52	23%
Loehrerr et al. [5]	135	VeIP	Cisplatin-refractory patients excluded[a]	100%	100%	0%	50%	72[b]	24%
Kondagunta et al. [14]	46	TIP	Included only patients with CR- or PR-negative marker to first line, gonadal primary, and <6 cycles of cisplatin in first line	74%	100%	0%	70%	69	63%
Fizazi et al. [17]	37	GIP	Included only patients with CR or PR-negative marker to first line, gonadal primary, and <6 cycles of cisplatin in first line	86%	100%	0%	54%	53	51%

CDCT, conventional-dose chemotherapy; EP, etoposide plus cisplatin; BEP; bleomycin, etoposide, and cisplatin; IR; incomplete response; CR, complete response; f/u, follow-up; VIP, etoposide, ifosfamide, and cisplatin; VeIP, vinblastine, ifosfamide, and cisplatin; GIP, gemcitabine, ifosfamide, and cisplatin; [a]progression at <3 weeks after completion of first-line chemotherapy; [b]minimal (not median) follow-up.

years from the end of prior chemotherapy), a group with historically poor outcome to salvage CDCT, with 7 achieving durable remissions. TIP has also been studied as salvage therapy in series with less restrictive eligibility criteria and using a lower dose of paclitaxel and in some cases, also ifosfamide [15, 16]. Not surprisingly, these studies did not duplicate the high CR and durable remission rates achieved in the MSKCC TIP series, although Mardiak observed a 65% objective response rate (ORR), 41% CR rate, and 47% 2-year PFS rate, all of which still compare favorably to VeIP [15].

More recently, Fizazi et al. reported on a phase II trial combining gemcitabine with ifosfamide and cisplatin (GIP) in the initial salvage treatment of 37 patients with GCT and the favorable criteria used in the MSKCC TIP study [17]. Although this trial did not reach its primary endpoint of a 65% CR rate, GIP still demonstrated activity with favorable response (e.g., CR or PR-negative markers), CR, and 2-year PFS rates of 78%, 54%, and 51%, respectively. The authors suggested GIP exhibited similar efficacy as TIP in this favorable-risk population but with less febrile neutropenia (22% versus 48%) and severe neurotoxicity (0% versus 7%). However, the durable remission rate was lower with GIP even though none of the patients had experienced a late relapse.

Given the traditional ifosfamide-cisplatin backbone of curative salvage CDCT regimens, use of VIP as an alternative to BEP for first-line treatment of intermediate- and poor-risk patients can make selecting an initial salvage CDCT regimen difficult. This is particularly applicable to patients > 50 years old or those with pulmonary compromise at diagnosis, groups with increased susceptibility to bleomycin lung toxicity in whom bleomycin is often avoided. Potential options include PVB (if patients are now candidates for bleomycin) given neither vinblastine nor bleomycin was used in the first-line setting, or the combination of gemcitabine, oxaliplatin, and paclitaxel (GOP), which can also result in some durable CRs [18]. However, a more common approach seems to be initial salvage HDCT with ASCT.

A lack of phase III studies demonstrating the superiority of any one conventional-dose regimen has led to variation in practice. Nevertheless, TIP appears to be the most commonly used regimen, perhaps because no study has yet to report a higher durable remission rate than the MSKCC TIP series and given the study of GIP did not meet its primary endpoint [17].

4. Salvage High-Dose Chemotherapy

The concept of HDCT stemmed from work in the 1980s, demonstrating that tumor cell resistance acquired after therapy with alkylating agents could be overcome by dose intensification (e.g., increase in dose by multiples of 5–10). To avoid the need for direct bone marrow harvest, growth factor support, typically G-CSF with or without chemotherapy, is used to disrupt adhesions between hematopoietic stem cells (HSCs) and stromal cells in the bone marrow, releasing HSCs into the vasculature for collection.

An early report by Nichols et al. demonstrated the potential for HDCT to salvage some patients with relapsed GCT but at the cost of significant toxicity, including treatment-related mortality (TRM) [19]. With improved supportive care measures, four modern studies provide robust evidence of clinical benefit with salvage HDCT with limited TRM (Table 2) [7–9, 20]. In a retrospective study at IU [7], 184 consecutive patients with testicular or retroperitoneal primary GCT underwent two cycles of high-dose carboplatin and etoposide, each followed by ASCT. Carboplatin dose was calculated using body surface area (BSA), and patients in remission after HDCT received adjuvant oral etoposide for 3 months. At median follow-up of 48 months, 116 (63%) patients had a durable CR with 5-year OS of 65%. Notably, patients with PM-NSGCT and late relapse were excluded from this series.

MSKCC investigators reported outcomes with the TI-CE regimen within a prospective phase I/II trial of 107 patients with relapsed/refractory GCT and unfavorable

Table 2: Studies examining the use of high-dose chemotherapy as initial (or later) salvage therapy.

Author (Year)	Study design	N	Notable I/E criteria	Median f/u (m)	HDCT as initial salvage	HDCT regimen	Cycles	Durable CR	OS
Einhorn et al. [7]	Retrospective	184	I: None E: PM-NSGCT and late relapse	48	73%	Carboplatin 700 mg/m^2 (d 1–3) Etoposide 750 mg/m^2 (d 1–3)	2	58% 2-year DFS	65% at 5 years
Feldman et al. [8]	Prospective, phase I/II	107	I: ≥1 adverse prognostic feature for salvage CDCT[a] E: None	61	76%	Part A (TI): Paclitaxel 200 mg/m^2 (d 1) Ifosfamide 2000 mg/m^2 (d 1–3) Part B (CE): Carboplatin AUC 7-8 (d 1–3) Etoposide 400 mg/m^2 (d 1–3)	2 3	48% 5-year DFS	52% at 5 years
Lorch et al. [20]	Prospective, randomized phase III	211	I: None E: None	90	86%	Arm A: VIP Carboplatin 500 mg/m^2 (d 1–3) Etoposide 500 mg/m^2 (d 1–3) Arm B: VIP Carboplatin 550 mg/m^2 (d 1–4) Etoposide 600 mg/m^2 (d 1–4) Cyclophosphamide 1600 mg/m^2 (d 1–4)	1 3 3 1	52% 2-year PFS 47% 2-year PFS	50% at 5 years 40% at 5 years
Adra et al. [9]	Retrospective	364	I: None E: Late relapse	40	83%	Carboplatin 700 mg/m^2 (d 1–3) Etoposide 750 mg/m^2 (d 1–3)	2	60% 2-year PFS	66% at 2 years

I, inclusion; E, exclusion; HDCT, high-dose chemotherapy; f/u, follow-up; m, months; CR, complete response; OS, overall survival; PM-NSGCT, primary mediastinal nonseminomatous germ cell tumor; d, day; DFS, disease-free survival; AUC, area under the curve; PFS, progression-free survival; VIP, etoposide, ifosfamide, and cisplatin; [a]extragonadal primary site, incomplete response (IR) to first-line therapy, and PD after a salvage CDCT (cisplatin plus ifosfamide-based) regimen.

features for achieving a durable remission to CDCT including an extragonadal primary site, incomplete response to initial therapy or relapse/incomplete response to salvage CDCT [8]. Patients received two cycles of paclitaxel with ifosfamide every two weeks, followed by 3 cycles of high-dose carboplatin and etoposide every three weeks. In contrast to the IU study, carboplatin dose was based on area under the curve (AUC) instead of BSA and patients with late relapses and PM-NSGCT were eligible. Fifty percent ($n = 54$) of patients achieved a CR and 8% ($n = 8$) achieved a PR-negative marker response. At median follow-up of 61 months, 5-year disease-free survival (DFS) and 5-year OS were 47% and 52%, respectively. When only patients who would have met the criteria for HDCT at Indiana University were considered, the 5-year DFS and OS improved to 57% and 62%, respectively [8]. In addition, the data demonstrated that patients with late relapse and PM-NSGCT remain potentially curable with salvage HDCT, albeit with a lower probability.

The IU group recently reported on another 364 patients treated with salvage HDCT and ASCT between 2004 and 2014 [9]. A notable difference from their prior series was inclusion of patients with PM-NSGCT; patients with late relapse were still excluded. Treatment was identical to the prior IU series with two consecutive courses of 700 mg/m^2 carboplatin and 750 mg/m^2 etoposide daily for 3 consecutive days, followed by ASCT. Maintenance oral etoposide was administered to 134 patients who achieved a CR, of whom 105 received three cycles. With median follow-up of 3.3 years, the 2-year PFS and OS were 60% and 66%, respectively. Of 9 treatment-related deaths (2.5%), 6 occurred within 30 days of HDCT completion and three resulted from secondary leukemia. The authors acknowledged the potential for selection bias that is inherent within studies of HDCT-eligible populations.

The German Testicular Cancer Study Group compared sequential HDCT with single HDCT in 211 patients with relapsed or refractory GCT. Patients were randomized to one cycle of VIP plus three cycles of high-dose carboplatin and etoposide (arm A) or three cycles of VIP plus one cycle of high-dose carboplatin, etoposide, and cyclophosphamide (arm B), followed by ASCT. At a median of 7.5 years of follow-up, 5-year PFS and OS rates were 48% versus 46% and 50% versus 40%, respectively, for sequential and single HDCT, respectively. The 10% difference in 5-year OS, which almost reached statistical significance ($p = 0.057$) was attributed to the fewer treatment-related deaths in the sequential HDCT arm (4% versus 16%). When IPFSG scores were applied, the improved outcome with sequential HDCT was most prominent in IPFSG high-risk patients treated in the first salvage setting (3-year OS 56% versus 11%) and those attempting HDCT as second salvage (3-year OS 40% versus 20%) [20].

5. HDCT versus CDCT as First Salvage Therapy

Given the efficacy of both CDCT and HDCT in the salvage setting and in particular, the excellent outcomes with HDCT for patients with unfavorable features, several

TABLE 3: Studies comparing the use of conventional-dose chemotherapy with high-dose chemotherapy as initial salvage therapy.

Author (Year)	Study design	Notable I/E criteria	Treatment regimen	NCDCT versus HDCT	Median f/u	PFS/EFS	OS
Beyer et al. [21]	Retrospective matched-pair analysis[a]	I: NSGCT only E: Pure seminoma	CDCT: Any HDCT: VIP × 2–3 then 1 cycle ICE	55[b] 55[b]	7.5y & 9y[c] 5y	HR 0.72–0.84[d]	HR 0.77–0.83[d]
Pico et al. [24]	Phase III randomized (IT-94)	I: none E: IR to first-line therapy; pure seminoma treated with carboplatin	CDCT: VIP or VeIP × 4 HDCT: VIP or VeIP × 3 then CarboPEC × 1	128 135	45 months	35% at 3y 42% at 3y	47% 47%
Lorch et al. [20]	Retrospective, including IPFSG subgroup analyses	I: ≥3 cycles of EP-based CT E: cisplatin-refractory disease[e]	CDCT: Any HDCT: ≥1 cycle carboplatin + etoposide ± ifosfamide, thiotepa, or cyclophosphamide	773 821	58 months	HR 0.44[d]	HR 0.65[d]

I, inclusion; E, exclusion; CDCT, conventional-dose chemotherapy; HDCT, high-dose chemotherapy; f/u, follow-up; PFS, progression-free survival; EFS, event-free survival; OS, overall survival; NSGCT, nonseminomatous germ cell tumor; VIP, etoposide, ifosfamide, and cisplatin; ICE, ifosfamide, carboplatin, and etoposide; y, years; HR, hazard ratio; CarboPEC, carboplatin, etoposide, and cyclophosphamide; IPFSG, International Prognostic Factor Study Group; [a]matching factors: primary tumor location, response to first-line treatment, duration of response, HCG and AFP levels; [b]fifty-five pairs of patients had full matches on >4 of 5 factors; [c]median follow-up for patients treated at Medical Research Council and Munich, respectively; [d]hazard ratio(s) favoring HDCT; [e]progression within 4 weeks of the first-line cisplatin-based regimen.

studies have attempted to compare these two strategies to establish the optimal initial salvage approach (Table 3). In the first study to address this question, Beyer et al. conducted a retrospective, matched pair analysis comparing initial salvage HDCT and CDCT [21]. Fifty-five pairs of patients with relapsed/refractory NSGCT treated with either initial salvage CDCT or HDCT between 1981 and 1995 had full matches on at least 4 of 5 selected prognostic factors (primary tumor location, response to first-line treatment, duration of response, and serum AFP and serum HCG). Hazard ratios favored HDCT for both event-free survival (EFS; 0.72–0.84) and OS (0.77–0.83). Results remained consistent when restricting analysis to those who received both etoposide and cisplatin as initial therapy. Limitations were acknowledged, including the fact that CDCT patients were treated at multiple institutions as part of a cooperative group trial and from earlier time points, in contrast to HDCT, where patients were treated at a single center and more recently. These differences were previously demonstrated to be of prognostic significance [22, 23]. Furthermore, 18% of CDCT patients did not receive etoposide in their first-line regimen and not all patients received ifosfamide during salvage CDCT. Finally, selection bias leading to patients with better performance status or fewer comorbidities receiving initial salvage HDCT could not be excluded. Collectively, these weaknesses may overinflate the differences favoring HDCT.

In the only randomized phase III study to address this question, a multi-institutional European trial (IT-94) compared four cycles of VIP or VeIP (arm A) with three such cycles followed by one cycle of high-dose carboplatin, etoposide, and cyclophosphamide with ASCT (arm B) [24]. Of 263 eligible patients, 128 and 135 patients were randomized to arms A and B, respectively, with 103 (80%) and 98 (73%) receiving all four chemotherapy cycles, respectively. Among evaluable patients, objective response (OR) rates after 4 cycles were 67% versus 75% ($p = 0.23$). At median follow-up of 45 months, there was no significant difference in EFS or OS, though there was a significant difference in 3-year EFS (55% versus 75%) favoring HDCT among patients achieving a CR. Although the authors concluded that IT-94 demonstrated no clinical benefit with initial salvage HDCT, there are several notable limitations of this study. Accrual was lower than expected with early stoppage of the study negatively impacting the statistical power. Only a single (rather than sequential) HDCT cycle was administered as part of arm B and 27% of patients randomized to HDCT did not receive the fourth (high-dose) cycle. Mortality was also higher than expected at 7% for Arm B (versus 3% for Arm A), potentially obscuring any benefit with HDCT. Furthermore, patients with incomplete response to initial therapy were excluded, a group more likely to benefit from HDCT given historically poor outcomes with salvage CDCT.

In light of these limitations and the small size of the prior Beyer-matched pairs analysis, Lorch et al. used the IPFSG database to retrospectively compare initial salvage HDCT and CDCT among 1594 patients with progression after at least three cisplatin-based cycles in the first-line setting. Two-year PFS was significantly superior after HDCT ($n = 821$) compared with CDCT ($n = 773$), both overall (50% versus 28%, $p < 0.001$) and within each IPFSG risk category. There was also a significant improvement in 5-year OS (53% versus 41%, $p < 0.001$) favoring initial salvage HDCT, overall, and within each IPFSG subgroup with the exception of low-risk patients. Despite the benefit observed for HDCT, numerous biases were acknowledged including patient selection bias (given the nonrandom treatment allocation) potentially favoring HDCT, wide variation in the CDCT regimens used, with some possibly inferior to others (e.g., TIP), and potential investigator bias in considering patients to progress earlier with CDCT than HDCT. Given the inherent methodological limitations of this retrospective, albeit large analysis, this study does not definitively prove the superiority of HDCT over CDCT, but rather underscores the

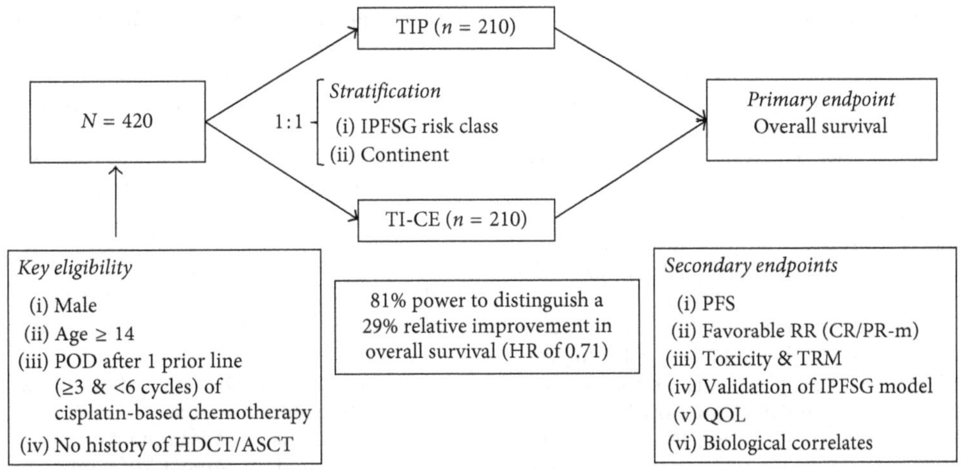

Figure 1: Study design of the TIGER trial (Alliance 0311012; EORTC 1407). POD, progression of disease; HDCT/ASCT, high-dose chemotherapy with autologous stem cell transplant; TIP, paclitaxel, ifosfamide, and cisplatin; TI-CE, paclitaxel and ifosfamide followed by high-dose carboplatin and etoposide; IPFSG, International Prognostic Factors Study Group; PFS, progression-free survival; response rate; CR, complete response; PR-m, partial response with normal tumor markers; TRM, treatment-related mortality; QOL, quality of life.

need for a prospective randomized trial to compare a highly effective CDCT regimen (TIP) to a sequential HDCT regimen (TI-CE), and this ultimately formed the foundation of the TIGER trial.

6. The TIGER Trial

The TIGER trial (A031102, E1407) is an international collaboration among many centers in North America, Europe, and Australia with the goal of determining the optimal initial salvage chemotherapy approach in patients with advanced GCT. Patients with unequivocal disease progression after a minimum of 3 and no more than 6 cisplatin-based chemotherapy cycles, administered in the first-line setting, are randomized 1:1 to receive CDCT with TIP (control arm) or HDCT using TI-CE (experimental arm) as illustrated in Figure 1. The primary endpoint is OS, with secondary endpoints including PFS, favorable response rate, toxicity, quality of life, and biological correlates. Patients will be stratified by a modification of their IPFSG category into low-, intermediate-, and high-risk groups, with prospective evaluation of outcomes by risk group. With a target accrual of 420 patients, the study is powered to detect a 29% difference in OS between the two arms. The study is ongoing and as of 11/1/2017 has accrued 67 (16%) patients. Results are anxiously awaited and will hopefully definitively establish either HDCT or CDCT as the standard of care in the initial salvage setting.

7. Conclusion

Both CDCT and HDCT have curative potential in the salvage management of relapsed/refractory GCT. Common salvage CDCT regimens include VeIP, TIP, and GIP, with no randomized data establishing one clearly superior regimen, although the best results reported to date are with TIP, albeit in a favorably selected patient population. Salvage HDCT regimens can achieve durable remissions even in patients with unfavorable characteristics with low TRM. As a result of conflicting data from retrospective series suggesting improved outcomes with HDCT and the IT-94 randomized study demonstrating no benefit to HDCT over CDCT, the optimal initial salvage approach remains unclear with practices varying widely around the world. The global cooperative group-led TIGER trial (A031102, E1407) is testing TIP versus TI-CE in this setting and seeks to definitively answer this important question.

Acknowledgments

This research was funded through the NIH P30 Cancer Center Support Grant (P30 CA008748).

References

[1] D. R. Feldman, G. J. Bosl, J. Sheinfeld, and R. J. Motzer, "Medical treatment of advanced testicular cancer," *JAMA*, vol. 299, no. 6, pp. 672–684, 2008.

[2] "Stat bite: average years of life lost from cancer," *Journal of the National Cancer Institute*, vol. 93, no. 5, p. 341, 2001.

[3] R. J. Motzer, N. L. Geller, C. C. Tan et al., "Salvage chemotherapy for patients with germ cell tumors. The Memorial Sloan-Kettering Cancer Center experience (1979–1989)," *Cancer*, vol. 67, no. 5, pp. 1305–1310, 1991.

[4] J. A. McCaffrey, M. Mazumdar, D. F. Bajorin, G. J. Bosl, V. Vlamis, and R. J. Motzer, "Ifosfamide- and cisplatin-containing chemotherapy as first-line salvage therapy in germ cell tumors: response and survival," *Journal of Clinical Oncology*, vol. 15, no. 7, pp. 2559–2563, 1997.

[5] P. J. Loehrerr, R. Gonin, C. R. Nichols, T. Weathers, and L. H. Einhorn, "Vinblastine plus ifosfamide plus cisplatin as initial salvage therapy in recurrent germ cell tumor," *Journal of Clinical Oncology*, vol. 16, no. 7, pp. 2500–2504, 1998.

[6] S. D. Fosså, S. P. Stenning, A. Gerl et al., "Prognostic factors in patients progressing after cisplatin-based chemotherapy for

malignant non-seminomatous germ cell tumours," *British Journal of Cancer*, vol. 80, no. 9, p. 1392, 1999.
[7] L. H. Einhorn, S. D. Williams, A. Chamness, M. J. Brames, S. M. Perkins, and R. Abonour, "High-dose chemotherapy and stem-cell rescue for metastatic germ-cell tumors," *New England Journal of Medicine*, vol. 357, no. 4, pp. 340–348, 2007.
[8] D. R. Feldman, J. Sheinfeld, D. F. Bajorin et al., "TI-CE high-dose chemotherapy for patients with previously treated germ cell tumors: results and prognostic factor analysis," *Journal of Clinical Oncology*, vol. 28, no. 10, pp. 1706–1713, 2010.
[9] N. Adra, R. Abonour, S. K. Althouse, C. Albany, N. H. Hanna, and L. H. Einhorn, "High-dose chemotherapy and autologous peripheral-blood stem-cell transplantation for relapsed metastatic germ cell tumors: the Indiana University Experience," *Journal of Clinical Oncology*, vol. 35, no. 10, pp. 1096–1102, 2016.
[10] A. Lorch, J. Beyer, C. Bascoul-Mollevi et al., "Prognostic factors in patients with metastatic germ cell tumors who experienced treatment failure with cisplatin-based first-line chemotherapy," *Journal of Clinical Oncology*, vol. 28, no. 33, pp. 4906–4911, 2010.
[11] P. J. Loehrer, R. Lauer, B. J. Roth, S. D. Williams, L. A. Kalasinski, and L. H. Einhorn, "Salvage therapy in recurrent germ cell cancer: ifosfamide and cisplatin plus either vinblastine or etoposide," *Annals of Internal Medicine*, vol. 109, no. 7, pp. 540–546, 1988.
[12] R. J. Motzer, K. Cooper, N. L. Geller et al., "The role of ifosfamide plus cisplatin-based chemotherapy as salvage therapy for patients with refractory germ cell tumors," *Cancer*, vol. 66, no. 12, pp. 2476–2481, 1990.
[13] A. Harstrick, H. Schmoll, H. Wilke et al., "Cisplatin, etoposide, and ifosfamide salvage therapy for refractory or relapsing germ cell carcinoma," *Journal of Clinical Oncology*, vol. 9, no. 9, pp. 1549–1555, 1991.
[14] G. V. Kondagunta, J. Bacik, A. Donadio et al., "Combination of paclitaxel, ifosfamide, and cisplatin is an effective second-line therapy for patients with relapsed testicular germ cell tumors," *Journal of Clinical Oncology*, vol. 23, no. 27, pp. 6549–6555, 2005.
[15] J. Mardiak, T. Salek, Z. Sycova-Mila et al., "Paclitaxel plus ifosfamide and cisplatin in second-line treatment of germ cell tumors: a phase II study," *Neoplasma*, vol. 52, no. 6, pp. 497–501, 2005.
[16] G. M. Mead, M. H. Cullen, R. Huddart et al., "A phase II trial of TIP (paclitaxel, ifosfamide and cisplatin) given as second-line (post-BEP) salvage chemotherapy for patients with metastatic germ cell cancer: a medical research council trial," *British Journal of Cancer*, vol. 93, no. 2, pp. 178–184, 2005.
[17] K. Fizazi, G. Gravis, A. Flechon et al., "Combining gemcitabine, cisplatin, and ifosfamide (GIP) is active in patients with relapsed metastatic germ-cell tumors (GCT): a prospective multicenter GETUG phase II trial," *Annals of Oncology*, vol. 25, no. 5, pp. 987–991, 2014.
[18] C. Bokemeyer, K. Oechsle, F. Honecker et al., "Combination chemotherapy with gemcitabine, oxaliplatin, and paclitaxel in patients with cisplatin-refractory or multiply relapsed germ-cell tumors: a study of the German Testicular Cancer Study Group," *Annals of Oncology*, vol. 19, no. 3, pp. 448–453, 2007.
[19] C. R. Nichols, G. Tricot, S. D. Williams et al., "Dose-intensive chemotherapy in refractory germ cell cancer–a phase I/II trial of high-dose carboplatin and etoposide with autologous bone marrow transplantation," *Journal of Clinical Oncology*, vol. 7, no. 7, pp. 932–939, 1989.
[20] A. Lorch, A. Kleinhans, A. Kramar et al., "Sequential versus single high-dose chemotherapy in patients with relapsed or refractory germ cell tumors: long-term results of a prospective randomized trial," *Journal of Clinical Oncology*, vol. 30, no. 8, pp. 800–805, 2012.
[21] J. Beyer, S. Stenning, A. Gerl, S. Fossa, and W. Siegert, "High-dose versus conventional-dose chemotherapy as first-salvage treatment in patients with non-seminomatous germ-cell tumors: a matched-pair analysis," *Annals of Oncology*, vol. 13, no. 4, pp. 599–605, 2002.
[22] L. H. Einhorn, *Complicated Problems in Testicular Cancer. Seminars in Oncology*, Elsevier, Amsterdam, Netherlands, 1988.
[23] L. Collette, R. J. Sylvester, S. P. Stenning et al., "Impact of the treating institution on survival of patients with "poor-prognosis" metastatic nonseminoma. European Organization for Research and Treatment of Cancer Genito-Urinary Tract Cancer Collaborative Group and the Medical Research Council Testicular Cancer Working Party," *Journal of the National Cancer Institute*, vol. 91, no. 10, pp. 839–846, 1999.
[24] J. L. Pico, G. Rosti, A. Kramar et al., "A randomised trial of high-dose chemotherapy in the salvage treatment of patients failing first-line platinum chemotherapy for advanced germ cell tumours," *Annals of Oncology*, vol. 16, no. 7, pp. 1152–1159, 2005.

23

Characteristics of Obstetric and Iatrogenic Urogenital Fistulas in Burkina Faso

Fasnéwindé Aristide Kabore[1] **Stéphanie Dominique Amida Nama,**[1] **Boureima Ouedraogo,**[2] **Moussa Kabore**[1] **Adama Ouattara**[3] **Brahima Kirakoya**[1] **and Gilles Karsenty**[4]

[1]*Department of Urology and Andrology, University Hospital Yalgado Ouedraogo of Ouagadougou, Ouagadougou, Burkina Faso*
[2]*Urology Department, University Hospital of Tingandogo, Tingandogo, Burkina Faso*
[3]*Urology Department, Souro Sanou University Hospital of Bobo-Dioulasso, Bobo-Dioulasso, Burkina Faso*
[4]*Aix-Marseille Université, Marseille, France*

Correspondence should be addressed to Fasnéwindé Aristide Kabore; kaborefamd@icloud.com

Academic Editor: Kostis Gyftopoulos

Objective. To compare the sociodemographic, clinical, and therapeutic characteristics of obstetric urogenital fistulas (OF) and iatrogenic urogenital fistulas (IF) treated in seven centers in Burkina Faso. *Material and Methods.* We carried out a cross-sectional study over a seven years' period (January 1, 2010 to December 31, 2016). We considered as iatrogenic all urogenital fistulas (UGF) occurred after elective caesarean section, gynecologic surgery (hysterectomy, myomectomy, and prolapse repair), or induced abortion. UGF following vaginal delivery after prolonged labor without obstetric maneuvers or caesarean section were considered as obstetric. UGF caused by other mechanisms (emergency caesarian section, congenital, and traumatic) were excluded from this study. The statistical analysis was carried out using version 14 of the STATA software. A logistic regression model was used to compare the two groups. *Results.* 310 cases of UGF were included. IF accounted for 25.8% ($n = 80$) versus 74.2% ($n = 230$) for OF. The median age was 35 years for IF and 35.38 years for OF. The vesicovaginal fistulas were predominant (74.5%) in the two groups. All circumferential fistulas were found in the OF group. OF were frequently associated with residence in rural areas (OR = 1.8; CI = [1.05–3.1]), low level of education (OR = 5.4; CI = [2.3–12.9]), and a height under 158 cm (OR = 3.4 CI = [1.7–6.6]). Vaginal sclerosis was less common among IF (OR = 2.2; CI = [1–4.6]). The failure of surgical treatment after 3 months was more associated with OF (OR = 4.7; CI = [1.1–20.5]). *Conclusion.* OF were the most common, frequently affecting short women living in rural area and with low level of schooling. Fistulas were also more severe in the OF group. IF gave better results after surgical repair.

1. Introduction

Urogenital fistula (UGF) is an abnormal communication between the urinary and the genital tracts leading to involuntary loss of urine through the vagina. This society scourge mostly affects sub-Saharan Africa and South Asia regions with an incidence of 1.13 women in 1000 of childbearing age [1]. The social, economic, and psychological handicap caused by the UGF places them as a major public health problem [1–4]. The most common etiologies of UGF are obstetric (OF) and iatrogenic (IF). Previous studies in high-resource countries reported a majority of IF (83.2%) caused by pelvic surgery or radiation therapy [3–5]. On the other hand, OF concern the developing world resulting from obstructed labor and inadequate obstetric care. OF represent 87% to 95.6% of all UGF in low-resource countries [2, 3, 6]. Both OF and IF lead to an uncomfortable loss of urines but have different physiopathological mechanisms. Are their sociodemographic, clinical, and therapeutic aspects so different? There are studies on each of these two etiological types of UGF in Africa, but accounting for available data, there is a lack of comparative studies concerning the patterns of IF and OF. Most studies deal with factors associated with OF because of their predominance [2, 7]. However, according to Hilton [8], specialists of the field perceived a change of trend in developing countries, revealing an increasing proportion of IF. In Burkina Faso, OF's estimated prevalence is 23.1 per 100,000 births [9] and to our knowledge no study comparing OF and IF has been published. We hypothesized that IF differ from OF in both clinical and therapeutic characteristics. The present study aims to compare the sociodemographic, clinical, and therapeutic characteristics of IF and OF in Burkina Faso through a multicenter cross-sectional study. This will help to identify women at risk for each type of fistula and plan prevention strategies. It will also allow planning the surgery according to each type of fistula and predicting the results. Finally, it will draw the attention of health care providers to their responsibility in the prevention of IF.

2. Material and Methods

We carried out a cross-sectional study of hospital records on patients who had surgical repair for UGF in seven fistula treatment centers in Burkina Faso over a seven years' period (January 1, 2010 to December 31, 2016). The seven fistula treatment centers are University Hospital Yalgado Ouedraogo of Ouagadougou, Regional Hospital of Fada N'Gourma, Regional Hospital of Dori, Saint Camille Hospital in Ouagadougou, New Polyclinic of the Center in Ouagadougou, Medical Center with Surgical Antenna in Boromo, and Medical Center with Surgical Antenna of Schipphra in Ouagadougou. These seven centers are not the only urogenital fistulas treatment centers in Burkina Faso. Patients were followed up by a surgeon in each of the 7 centers. The survey was conducted by a single surgeon who collected data from the other surgeons in each of the 7 urogenital fistula centers. Two groups of UGF were individualized in this study: OF and IF. We considered as iatrogenic all UGF that occurred after prophylactic caesarean section, gynecologic surgery (hysterectomy, myomectomy, and prolapse repair), or induced abortion. UGF following vaginal delivery after prolonged labor without obstetric maneuvers or caesarean section were considered as obstetric [10]. We included patients with OF or IF and with a complete medical record. UGF caused by other mechanisms (emergency caesarian section, congenital, and traumatic) were excluded from this study. Figure 1 shows the flowchart of how we selected subjects for the study.

The method of treatment of all fistulas was delayed repair after 3 months.

After approval of the local staff, data were collected on an individual and anonymous data sheet preserving patients' confidentiality at all centers. Information was collected on sociodemographic, obstetric, and previous surgeries history, fistula characteristics and history, intraoperative procedures, and surgical outcomes three months after discharge. The classification of UGF was performed through the Goh classification [11]. A dye test was performed whenever the patients reported for continuous urine leaking to determine the outcome of repair. Patients were followed for 3 months. Three surgical outcomes were considered: (i) failed or unclosed fistulas, (ii) closed fistula without stress urinary incontinence (SUI), and (iii) closed fistula with stress urinary incontinence.

Data entry and statistical analysis were performed using the software STATA 14 (StataCorp 2015, College Station, TX, USA). The dependent variable was the cause of the fistula. The modalities were the iatrogenic cause and the obstetric cause. Qualitative variables were presented in terms of numbers and percentages. Quantitative variables were presented as percentage (%), number (n), and average, with their standard deviation (SD), maximum (Max) and minimum (Min), or median values. Statistical analysis was performed to compare the two groups. Chi^2 test or Fisher's exact test (where cell sizes were <5) were used to compare the frequencies. For the comparison of the averages in the two groups, we used the independent t-test. Odd Ratios (OR) with 95% confidence intervals (CI) were calculated from univariate tests to search for links between obstetric or iatrogenic causes and independent variables. In order to determine the significant differences between the two groups, we created a logistical regression model by including variables which have less than 10% missing data and with a disparity in the distribution. All P values less than 0.05 were considered statistically significant.

3. Results

During the study period, 497 cases of UGF were registered and 310 (62.4%) cases matched our inclusion criteria. The proportion of IF was 25.8% ($n = 80$) versus 74.2% ($n = 230$) for OF. The mean age of the patients at the time of diagnosis for the two groups was 37.2 ± 12.7 years. The mean age of IF and OF was, respectively, 37.8 ± 12.2 (min 19, max 70) and 36.9 ± 12.9 years (min 15, max 72). Most of these patients had no formal education (78.75% for IF and 95.6% for OF). The majority of patients in the OF group were from rural areas (58%) when the majority in IF group were from urban areas (58.75%). The mean duration of fistula was 65.8 ± 105.9 months and 116 ± 117.4 months, respectively, for IF and OF. The other sociodemographic characteristics and medical history of the patients are resumed in Table 1.

The majority of fistula was vesicovaginal in our two groups (Figure 2). Among these vesicovaginal fistulas (VVF), the most frequent location was supratrigonal (58%) in the two groups (Figure 3).

The mean size of the IF was 1.5 ± 1.3 cm (min: 0.2; max: 0.7) and 1.9 ± 1.6 cm (min: 0.2; max: 10) for the OF ($P = 0.02$). The perifistula sclerosis was most frequent in the OF group 23.9% ($n = 55$) versus 12.5% ($n = 10$) in IF group ($P = 0.01$). Using the Goh classification, 260 (83.9%) fistulas were classified as type 1-2 (Table 2).

All the OF followed obstructed labor in our study. Prophylactic caesarean section was the main etiology of IF in this study (63.8%, $n = 51$) (Table 3). The surgical procedures

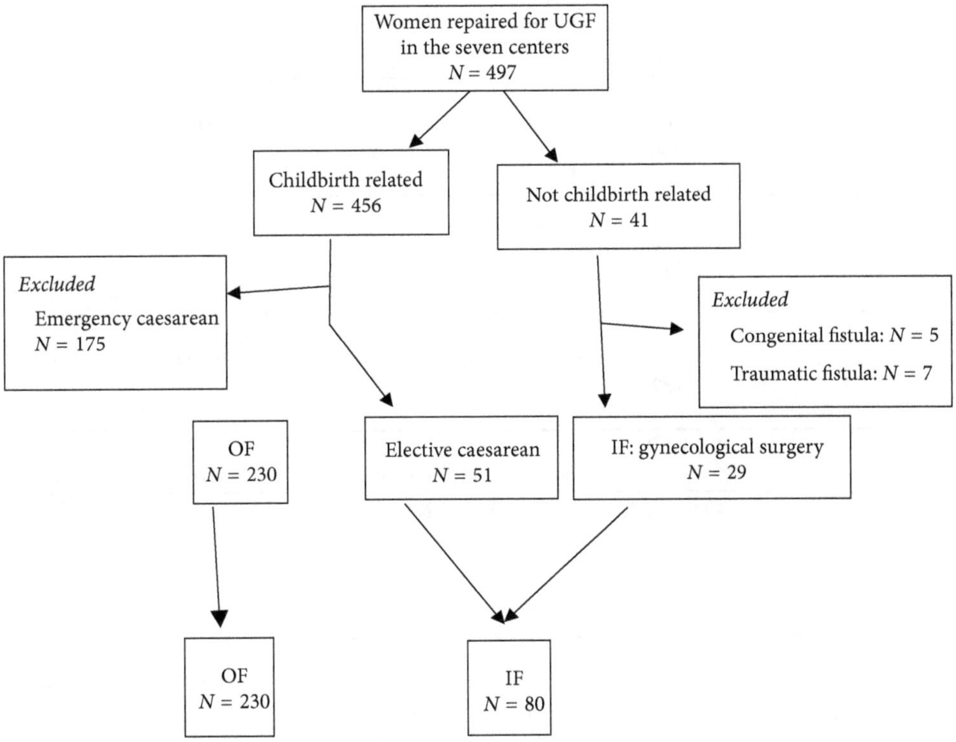

Figure 1: Flowchart of how we selected subjects for our study.

Table 1: Sociodemographic, clinical, and therapeutic characteristics of patients.

	OF (*n*)	IF (*n*)	*P*	OR	IC = 95%
Patient's age at diagnosis	36.9 ± 12.9 years	37.8 ± 12.2 years	0.77	—	—
Area of residence					
Rural	124	29	0.04	1.8	1.05–3.1
Urban	99	42			
Missing: 16					
Educational level					
Less than primary school	183	63	<0.001	5.4	[2.3–12.9]
Higher than primary school	9	17			
Missing: 38					
Marital status before fistula					
Married	183	56	0.057	—	
Not married	0	2			
Missing: 69					
Height					
≤158 cm	103	45	<0.001	3.4	[1.7–6.6]
158 cm	20	30			
Missing: 112					
Duration of fistula					
>2 years	60	22	0.002	3.48	[1.5–7.6]
<2 years	18	233			
Missing: 187					
Circumferential fistula					
Yes	28	80	<0.001	—	
No	202	0			
Missing: 0					
Number of fistulas					
1	226	30	<0.001	0.25	[0.07–0.87]
>1	4	19			
Missing: 0					

Table 1: Continued.

	OF (n)	IF (n)	P	OR	IC = 95%
Ureteral lesion					
Yes	0	73	<0.001	5.41	[1.5–19]
No	230	7			
Missing: 0					
Perifistula fibrosis					
Yes	55	10	0.01	2.2	[1–4.6]
No	175	70			
Missing: 0					
Urethral lesion					
Yes	48	73	0.004	3.2	[1.3–7.8]
No	182	6			
Missing: 0					
Fistula size	1.5 ± 1.3 cm				
Missing: 0		1.9 ± 1.6 cm	0.02	—	—
Labor duration	49.8 ± 32.5 h	N/A			
Surgical failure at 3 months					
Yes	25	2	0.02	4.7	[1.1–20.5]
No	205	78			
Missing: 0					
RSUI					
Yes	27	12	0.69	—	
No	178	66			
Missing: 27					

RSUI: residual stress urinary incontinence.

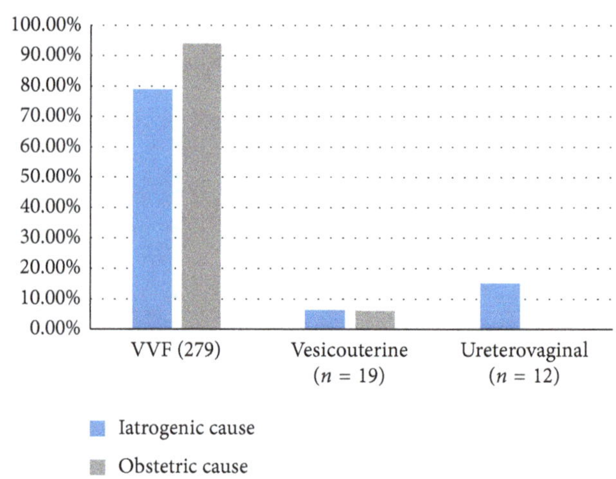

Figure 2: Type of UGF.

at the origin of IF have been performed by trained gynecologists in 53% ($n = 42$) of cases and by a general practitioner in 47% ($n = 38$).

Three months after surgery, the overall successful closure rate of the two groups was 79% ($n = 245$), failure of the repair represented 8.4% ($n = 26$), and residual stress urinary incontinence (RSUI) rate was 12.6% ($n = 39$). Failure of the repair occurred for 2.5% ($n = 2$) in the IF group and for 11% ($n = 25$) in OF ($P = 0.02$). The fistula was closed without SUI in 66 (82.5%) cases in the IF group and 178 (77.3%) cases in the OF group. Residual SUI represented 15% ($n = 12$) and 11.7% ($n = 27$) for IF and OF, respectively ($P = 0.69$). Logistic regression model is summarized in Table 4.

4. Discussion

Although during the last decade the number of IF treated in developing countries is increasing, the main etiology of UGF remains the obstetric cause [2, 3, 8, 12]. In our study, OF are three times more frequent than IF. Prolonged labor is the primary risk factor of OF. The current study with an average of labor duration over than two days (49.8 hours) confirms the results of previous reports from Africa [6,12–14]. The

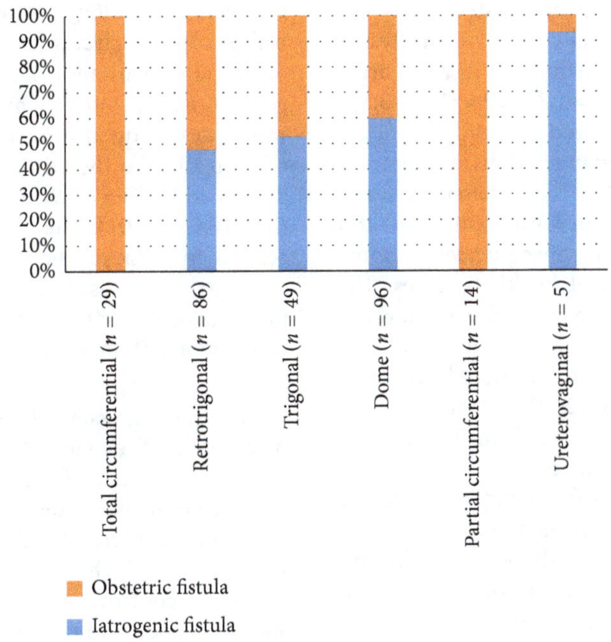

FIGURE 3: Seat of the vaginal fistula.

TABLE 2: The Goh classification of UGF.

	Iatrogenic fistula $N = 80$	Obstetric fistula $N = 230$
Goh's classification		
T1	38.75% ($n = 31$)	49.13% ($n = 113$)
T2	42.5% ($n = 34$)	35.65% ($n = 82$)
T3	18.75% ($n = 15$)	15.22% ($n = 35$)

TABLE 3: Etiologies of iatrogenic fistulas.

Etiologies	n	%
Prophylactic caesarean section	51	63.75
Hysterectomies	23	28.75
For uterine fibroids	19	23.75
For obstetric complications	3	3.75
For cervical neoplasia	1	1.25
Abortion	1	1.25
Prolapse repair	2	2.5
Uterine myomectomy	3	3.75

TABLE 4: Logistic regression model.

	OR	Std err	z	$P > \|z\|$	CI = 95%
Age (≤35 years/>35 years)	0.90	0.28	−0.34	0.732	[0.49–1.66]
Fistula size (≤1 cm/>1 cm)	0.35	0.15	−2.46	0.014	[0.15–0.8]
Sclerosis (yes/no)	1.16	0.55	0.32	0.752	[0.45–2.94]
Urethra lesion (yes/no)	0.26	0.18	−1.95	0.051	[0.07–1.008]
T1 of Goh's classification (yes/no)	0.078	0.06	−3.52	<0.001	[0.02–0.32]
T2 of Goh's classification (yes/no)	0.3	0.18	−2.01	0.045	[0.09–0.97]
Retrotrigonal fistula (yes/no)	1.8	1.07	1.00	0.318	[0.56–5.77]
Trigonal fistula (yes/no)	1.55	0.89	0.76	0.444	[0.50–4.79]
Bladder dome fistula (yes/no)	2.51	1.53	1.52	0.129	[0.76–8.27]
Area of residence (rural/urban)	0.45	0.15	−2.47	0.014	[0.24–0.85]
RSUI	0.51	0.3	−1.20	0.229	[0.17–1.53]

RSUI: residual stress urinary incontinence.

logistical difficulty to access to emergency obstetric care is a main trouble for women living in rural area. In our study, the obstetric cause was two times more common in rural areas than the iatrogenic cause (OR = 1.8, CI = [1.05–3.1]). According to rural residents interviewed in a study about OF in Burkina Faso, "it would be an endangered disease that was much more common at the time when there were no medical recourse" [15]. Traditional practices in rural populations and low medical literacy concerning the consequences of home births do not promote attendance at health facilities. The lack of medical literacy is a consequence of the low level of education in developing countries. In our study, patients with low level of schooling were four times more likely to be exposed to OF (OR = 5.4, CI = [2.3–12.9]). Tebeu et al. [13] reported an illiteracy rate ranging from 19 to 96% among patients with OF in sub-Saharan Africa.

In developing countries, the IF's frequency is increasing [8, 12, 16]. This is related to the increasing accessibility to surgery, especially caesarean section. Indeed, the World Health Organization (WHO) advocated for a caesarean section rate of 5 to 15% in developing countries to reduce the maternal mortality rate [17]. So, developing countries have initiated strategies to facilitate accessibility to caesarean section. But most of these caesarean sections often cause an additional risk to have an UGF because they are performed in ischemic tissues after a prolonged labor or when the fetus death in utero is recorded for several days [6, 14].

In Burkina Faso, the caesarean section's rate is 0.6% and a considerable number of UGF occurs after caesarean section [18]. In our series, elective caesarean was incriminated for 63.75% of IF. These results can be explained by the insufficiency of trained specialized medical doctors added to the lack of health infrastructures. In fact, concerning the IF, a gynecologist was the operator in only 42 cases (53%) in our study. Clinical officers and physician trained in basic surgery were involved in 38 cases (47%). Raassen et al. [6] reported 26.5% of IF cases for which a gynecologist was incriminated; the other UGF were caused by clinical officers and physician trained in basic surgery. In Burkina Faso, only 46% of caesarean sections are performed by a gynecologist, and amongst all caesareans performed, 12% are classified by experts as medically unjustified. Those are mostly carried out by nonspecialist agents [18]. We warn against these risky interventions because, as with any surgical procedure, caesareans are associated with short- and long-term risks for health. These risks are higher for women with limited access to appropriate obstetric care.

The most common type of UGF in our study was vesicovaginal (90%) according to the data reported in the medical literature [4, 6, 8, 16]. The high prevalence of VVF comes from the close adherence between the bladder and the vagina and the large contact area between its two organs. Depending on the etiology, the most affected anatomical area may vary. Studies report that, in IF, VVF are often high situated at the bladder dome, whereas in OF they are low situated with frequently cervical–urethral circumferential lesion [16]. Our results report an absence of correlation between the etiology of the UGF and the seat in the bladder wall except for circumferential lesions which are exclusively obstetric and ureteric lesions, which are exclusively iatrogenic. Onsrud et al. [16] also report that uterovaginal fistulas were more frequently iatrogenic. The diameter of the UGF is often related to the etiology. A large diameter is frequently described in OF [7, 19]. In our study, OF tended to be larger than IF ($P = 0.02$). The high propensity for OF to be large is related to their mechanism of occurrence. The size is determined by the ischemic zone, from which is removed the pressure ulcer giving way to the UGF. This ischemic area will cause tissue changes leading to fibrosis [14].

Logistic regression showed a high propensity for IF to be type 1 or 2 of the Goh classification. This testifies to the simplicity of most IF leading to the best successful fistula closure. Three months after the surgical repair, OF were almost five times more associated with failure of the repair of UGF in our study ($P = 0.02$). The predictive factors of treatment's failure are subject to controversies. Some authors reported only clinical and therapeutic implications while others pointed out the importance of the psychosocial status of the patient [7, 14, 20]. In our study, factors which can be regarded as predictive factors of failure are sclerosis, the loss of tissue, and the urethral destruction. These items were frequently associated with obstetric origin. That explained why the failure of the closure is more often seen in the obstetric group.

4.1. Limitations. One of the limitations of our study was the cases of fistula related to operative delivery for prolonged obstructed labor. It is difficult to tell if the fistula is due to surgery or prolonged ischemia. Raassen et al. reported the same difficulty [6]. For this reason, we excluded 175 cases of fistula from our study in order to have an homogeneous study population. However, this exclusion has considerably reduced the size of our population. Our data do not include all fistula treatment centers in Burkina Faso, so our results cannot be generalized to the entire population of Burkina Faso. Also because of the retrospective nature of this study, some data were missing.

5. Conclusion

Our study demonstrated that there are some important differences between IF and OF in Burkina Faso. OF mostly affected women living in rural areas, having a low level of education. OF give worst treatment's result than IF. IF are tiny, from type 1 or 2 of the Goh classification, less surrounded by sclerosis. IF are more frequent among women with at least a primary schooling level, living in urban areas. Although IF are looking less serious than OF, it is necessary to pay special attention to them because they lead to a loss of confidence from patients in health providers.

References

[1] A. J. Adler, C. Ronsmans, C. Calvert, and V. Filippi, "Estimating the prevalence of obstetric fistula: a systematic review and meta-analysis," *BMC Pregnancy and Childbirth*, vol. 13, no. 1, p. 246, 2013.

[2] F. A. Kabore, T. Kambou, A. Ouattara et al., "Epidemiology, etiology and psychosocial impact of urogenital fistulas in a cohort of 170 consecutive patients managed in three treatment centers in Burkina Faso," *Progres en Urologie*, vol. 24, no. 8, pp. 526–532, 2014.

[3] C. J. Hillary, N. I. Osman, P. Hilton, and C. R. Chapple, "The aetiology, treatment, and outcome of urogenital fistulae managed in well- and low-resourced countries: a systematic review," *European Urology*, vol. 70, no. 3, pp. 478–492, 2016.

[4] O. Singh, S. S. Gupta, and R. K. Mathur, "Urogenital fistulas in women: 5-year experience at a single center," *Urology Journal*, vol. 7, no. 1, pp. 35–39, 2010.

[5] M. J. Wong, K. Wong, A. Rezvan, A. Tate, N. N. Bhatia, and T. Yazdany, "Urogenital fistula," *Female Pelvic Medicine & Reconstructive Surgery*, vol. 18, no. 2, pp. 71–78, 2012.

[6] T. J. I. P. Raassen, C. J. Ngongo, and M. M. Mahendeka, "Iatrogenic genitourinary fistula: an 18-year retrospective review of 805 injuries," *International Urogynecology Journal*, vol. 25, no. 12, pp. 1699–1706, 2014.

[7] S. Rajaian, M. Pragatheeswarane, and A. Panda, "Vesicovaginal fistula: review and recent trends," *Indian Journal of Urology*, vol. 35, no. 4, pp. 250–258, 2019.

[8] P. Hilton, "Urogenital fistula in the UK: a personal case series managed over 25 years," *BJU International*, vol. 110, no. 1, pp. 102–110, 2012.

[9] I. Sombié, T. Kambou, S. Conombo et al., "Retrospective study of urogenital fistula in Burkina Faso from 2001 to 2003," *Médecine Tropicale: Revue Du Corps De Santé Colonial*, vol. 67, pp. 48–52, 2007.

[10] J. Goh, L. Romanzi, S. Elneil et al., "An international continence society (ICS) report on the terminology for female pelvic floor fistulas," *Neurourology and Urodynamics*, vol. 39, no. 8, pp. 2040–2071, 2020.

[11] J. T. W. Goh, "A new classification for female genital tract fistula," *The Australian and New Zealand Journal of Obstetrics and Gynaecology*, vol. 44, no. 6, pp. 502–504, 2004.

[12] T. J. I. P. Raassen, E. G. G. Verdaasdonk, and M. E. Vierhout, "Prospective results after first-time surgery for obstetric fistulas in East African women," *International Urogynecology Journal*, vol. 19, no. 1, pp. 73–79, 2008.

[13] P. M. Tebeu, J. N. Fomulu, S. Khaddaj, L. de Bernis, T. Delvaux, and C. H. Rochat, "Risk factors for obstetric fistula: a clinical review," *International Urogynecology Journal*, vol. 23, no. 4, pp. 387–394, 2012.

[14] D. Mukwege, L. Peters, C. Amisi, A. Mukwege, A. R. Smith, and J. M. Miller, "Panzi score as a parsimonious indicator of urogenital fistula severity derived from Goh and Waaldijk classifications," *International Journal of Gynecology & Obstetrics*, vol. 142, no. 2, pp. 187–193, 2018.

[15] L. P. Freedman, "Using human rights in maternal mortality programs: from analysis to strategy," *International Journal of Gynecology & Obstetrics*, vol. 75, no. 1, pp. 51–60, 2001.

[16] M. Onsrud, S. Sjøveian, and D. Mukwege, "Cesarean delivery-related fistulae in the Democratic Republic of Congo," *International Journal of Gynecology & Obstetrics*, vol. 114, no. 1, pp. 10–14, 2011.

[17] World Health Organization, *Monitoring Emergency Obstetric Care: A Handbook*, World Health Organization, Geneva, Switzerland, 2009.

[18] S. Kouanda, A. Coulibaly, A. Ouedraogo, T. Millogo, B. I. Meda, and A. Dumont, "audit of cesarean delivery in Burkina Faso," *International Journal of Gynecology & Obstetrics*, vol. 125, no. 3, pp. 214–218, 2014.

[19] B. T. Sambo, C. Missikpode, K. Salifou, A. Hodonou, and E. Mensah, "Developing a simple proof of concept clinical decision-making tool for predicting surgical outcomes after obstetric fistula repair in a developing country," *Tropical and Medicine Surgery*, vol. 4, no. 2, pp. 1–7, 2016.

[20] G. M. Ghoniem and H. A. Warda, "The management of genitourinary fistula in the third millennium," *Arab Journal of Urology*, vol. 12, no. 2, pp. 97–105, 2014.

24

Alexis Wound Retractor for Radical Cystectomy: A Safe and Effective Method for Retraction

Ajaydeep S. Sidhu,[1] **Eric Marten**,[2] **Nikita Bodoukhin**,[2] **George Wayne**,[1] **Elizabeth Nagoda**,[1] **Akshay Bhandari**,[1] **and Alan M. Nieder**[1]

[1]*Columbia University Division of Urology, Mount Sinai Medical Center, Miami Beach 33140, FL, USA*
[2]*Herbert Wertheim College of Medicine, Florida International University, Miami 33199, FL, USA*

Correspondence should be addressed to Alan M. Nieder; anieder@msmc.com

Academic Editor: Fabio Campodonico

Surgical site infection rates remain a common postoperative problem that continues to affect patients undergoing urologic surgery. Our study seeks to evaluate the difference in surgical site infection rates in patients undergoing open radical cystectomy when comparing the Bookwalter vs. the Alexis wound retractors. After institutional review board approval, we performed a retrospective chart review from February 2010 through August 2017 of patients undergoing open radical cystectomy with urinary diversion for bladder cancer. We then stratified the groups according to whether or not the surgery was performed with the Alexis or standard Bookwalter retractor. Baseline characteristics and operative outcomes were then compared between the two groups, with the main measure being incidence of surgical site infection as defined by the CDC. We evaluated those presenting with surgical site infections within or greater than 30 postoperatively. Of 237 patients who underwent radical cystectomy with either the Alexis or Bookwalter retractor, 168 patients were eligible to be included in our analysis. There was no statistical difference noted regarding surgical site infections (SSIs) between the two groups; however, the trend was in favor of the Alexis (3%) vs. the Bookwalter (11%) at less than 30 days surgery. The Alexis wound retractor likely poses an advantage in reducing the incidence in surgical site infections in patients undergoing radical cystectomy; however, multicenter studies with larger sample sizes are suggested for further elucidation.

1. Introduction

Self-retaining retractors fixed to the operating table have traditionally been used in major open operations. The Bookwalter retractor has been in use for several decades and is frequently used during major open operations, including open urologic surgery. More recently, combined wound-edge protectors and retractors are being used in operations at risk for surgical wound complications, including colorectal and gynecologic surgery [1, 2]. To our knowledge, the use of wound-edge protectors/retractors has not been studied in open urologic operations, though its feasibility was recently evaluated for robotic-assisted cystectomy [3].

The Alexis dual-ring wound protector/retractor (Applied Medical, Rancho Santa Margarita, CA) is a useful tool for open surgery including radical cystectomy with urinary diversion. The advantages of using this particular retractor include adequate and atraumatic wound retraction, protection from bowel contents and spillage, and potentially reduced incidence of surgical site infection (SSI).

We routinely use the Alexis retractor at our institution, where, in our experience, it provides adequate exposure during radical cystectomy. Though surgeon preference largely dictates retraction modality, it is important to consider whether such choices influence patient outcomes. Thus, we present our institution's initial perioperative outcomes while using the Alexis wound retractor for radical cystectomy and compare these cases to a similar cohort of cases using a traditional Bookwalter retractor.

2. Methods

After institutional review board approval, we performed a nonrandomized, retrospective chart review of 237 patients undergoing open radical cystectomy with a urinary diversion from February 2010 through August 2017. Of these, 168 patients were included in this study. Patients who underwent robotic cystectomy (15), simple cystectomy (11), and aborted cystectomies (11) were excluded from the analysis. In addition, 4 cases were excluded due to an intraoperative change to a different retractor. Finally, 28 cases were excluded due to insufficient data. The remaining 168 patients underwent radical cystectomy with a urinary diversion using either a Bookwalter or an Alexis wound retractor for the entirety of the operation. Different surgeons did indeed utilize the Alexis retractor in a nonrandomized fashion. Importantly, while the Bookwalter retractor was used predominantly in the first half of our radical cystectomy series, it was mostly utilized in our morbidly obese patients during the second half of the series when most of the surgeons had converted to the Alexis.

We evaluated the baseline characteristics of the two groups and compared their perioperative outcomes. Baseline characteristics included age, gender, history of diabetes, history of pelvic or abdominal radiation, smoking status, body mass index (BMI), and American Society of Anesthesiologists Physical Status Classification (ASA). All patients underwent preoperative medical clearance and, if indicated, cardiopulmonary clearance. Patients received a preoperative mechanical bowel preparation with polyethylene glycol or ERAS protocol. Our more contemporary patients received heparin 5000 units subcutaneously and oral alvimopan 12 mg preoperartively. All patients received intravenous antibiotic prophylaxis prior to incision with cefoxitin 2 g or clindamycin 900 mg as well as postoperative prophylaxis for up to 24 hours. Upon entering the peritoneum and reflecting the colon cephalad, the decision was made by the surgeon to use either the Alexis wound retractor or a traditional Bookwalter retractor. Fascial incisions were closed with a running loop 0-PDS suture (Ethicon), and primary skin closure was performed with staples.

Perioperative outcomes evaluated included estimated blood loss (EBL), operative time (OR time), type of urinary diversion performed (ileal conduit, orthotopic neobladder, or cutaneous ureterostomy), intraoperative complications, length of stay (LOS), and SSI stratified by time of presentation. SSI was defined using Centers for Disease Control (CDC) guidelines: "Any infection of the superficial or deep tissues or the organ/space affected by surgery, and which occurs within 30 days of surgery when no prosthesis is implanted" [4]. Differences between the two groups were assessed using standard statistical methods, including independent sample t-tests, Pearson chi-squared tests, and the Mann–Whitney U-test using RStudio version 1.0.153.

3. Results

We identified 168 patients who were included in our study. 95 operations were performed entirely with the Alexis retractor and 73 with the Bookwalter. Besides average BMI, baseline characteristics were similar between the two groups with no statistically significant differences (Table 1).

There was no statistically significant difference in the incidence of SSI between the Alexis and Bookwalter retractor groups (Table 2). There were no differences in surgical site infections at either more than 30 days or less than 30 days postoperatively. Overall, 9 (12%) patients in the Bookwalter group and 4 (4%) patients in the Alexis group presented with a SSI. A statistically significant difference was observed regarding operative time: the mean operative time for those patients in the Alexis vs Bookwalter cohort was 219 min vs. 242 min, respectively ($p < 0.05$). We also identified a median length of stay in favor of the Alexis vs Bookwalter cohort, 5 vs 6 days ($p < 0.05$). Also, ASA score was lower for the Alexis group.

4. Discussion

In our single-center, retrospective study, we found that the Alexis provides appropriate exposure during radical cystectomy, with a decreased operative time and a possible trend towards reduced wound infection. The Alexis wound retractor/protector was developed in 2000 and combines wound retractor with wound barrier protection. It is comprised of two plastic rings with a plastic sleeve connecting the rings. The inner ring is placed underneath the body wall, and the outer ring is placed on top of skin. The plastic sleeve is rolled over the outer ring to retract the body wall circumferentially outward, theoretically applying equal force throughout the wound.

The Alexis wound retractor is currently and frequently used at our institution for performing open cystectomies (as well as during extracorporeal diversions during robotic cystectomies) with outcomes comparable to those operations where a Bookwalter retractor is used. Combined retractors and wound-edge protectors, such as those incorporated in the design of the Alexis wound retractor, have been studied in other open abdominal operations, particularly in colorectal and obstetric/gynecologic procedures [1, 2]. The authors from these fields have reported mixed results with such technologies, but their studies appear to lend overall support to the anecdotally efficient and adequate anatomic exposure, improvement in SSI rate, and reduction in trauma to retracted tissues. SSIs are an important cause of morbidity following radical cystectomy with urinary diversion. This is especially concerning in obese and diabetic patients who often suffer from comorbid metabolic and immunologic impairment, as well as in patients with a history of radiation or smoking.

Clean-contaminated (Class II) operations as a category, which includes cystectomy with diversion, have an overall SSI rate of 3–11% [5]. Lavallée et al. reported the incidence of SSI after radical cystectomy to be 8% [6]. In our study, while there was a trend towards lower SSI between the Alexis and Bookwalter retractor groups (4% and 12% total, respectively), this difference was not statistically significant. The Alexis retractor may indeed provide the benefit of lower SSI rates; however, further studies are needed with more

Table 1: Patient demographics for those undergoing radical cystectomy with either the Bookwalter retractor or the Alexis retractor.

	Alexis		Bookwalter		p value	
Age (years), SD	73	8	71	9	0.23	*
Gender					0.28	**
Male	76	80%	63	86%		
Female	19	20%	10	14%		
BMI mean (kg/m^2), SD	25.9	4.2	27.6	4.4	0.027	*
BMI count 25–29.99	60	63%	51	70%	0.60	**
BMI count >30	17	18%	19	26%	0.31	**
History of diabetes	17	18%	18	25%	0.40	**
Current smokers	14	15%	4	5%	0.12	**
Prior Radiation/brachytherapy	6	6%	11	15%	0.12	**

*Independent sample t-test, **Pearson's chi-squared test, ***Mann–Whitney U-test.

Table 2: Operative measures and outcomes for patients undergoing radical cystectomy with either the Alexis retractor or the Bookwalter retractor.

	Alexis		Bookwalter		p value	
ASA, SD	2.7	0.5	2.8	0.4	0.034	***
EBL (mL), SD	386	241	375	157	0.77	*
OR time (min), SD	219	42	246	60	0.0004	*
Diversion						
Radical cystectomy/IC	92	97%	66	90%	0.82	**
Radical cystectomy/neobladder	1	1%	5	7%	0.11	**
Radical cystectomy/cutaneous ureterostomy	2	2%	2	3%	1.00	**
Median LOS (days)	5		6		0.027	***
SSI						
<30 days	3	3%	8	11%	0.092	**
30–60 days	1	1%	1	1%	1.00	**

patients to confirm this finding. In addition, it appears that the Alexis retractor may provide the advantage of less operative time and be associated with a lower length of hospital stay. Several nonurological studies have produced similar findings in regards to postoperative wound infection rates when using the Alexis wound retractor. Mihalijevic et al. demonstrated a reduction in superficial SSI when using Alexis wound retractors in open abdominal surgery [7]. Further, Reid et al. demonstrated a reduced incidence of surgical site infection with the use of barrier retraction wound protection in colorectal surgery [8]. Within the colorectal surgery literature, Cheng et al. [2] found that the use of the Alexis retractor has an absolute risk reduction of SSI of 20% and that the use of 5 Alexis O-ring wound retractors is needed to prevent one probable SSI. Scolari Childress et al. [1] demonstrated significantly fewer episodes of uterine exteriorization with the use of the Alexis wound retractor, facilitating hysterectomy repair in situ, which the authors suggest may be due to improved surgical visualization using the retractor. Likely, such improved visualization contributes to the shorter operative times observed when using the Alexis retractor in our practice. Hinkson et al. [9] reported a significantly lower incidence of SSI in the Alexis group, which the authors postulate is due to the circumferential coverage the device offers, thus protecting the wound edges. Another study involving Huynh et al. [3] reviewed 15 cases where the Alexis retractor was used for the bowel diversion, and did not report any wound-related complications. Though their study had a limited sample size, the authors did draw similar conclusions regarding the safety and efficacy of using the Alexis retractor as opposed to traditional retraction methods.

Though our study does not demonstrate a statistically significant difference in wound infection rate between Alexis and Bookwalter retractors, our results do suggest that infection rates favor the use of the Alexis wound retractor. Given our smaller cohort, in combination with the relatively low rates of SSI, we were not able to detect a statistical difference in our study, as it was likely underpowered. Anecdotally, we have noted retractor setup and breakdown to be much easier than with fixed body-wall retractors. We have also found it to be faster and easier for our OR staff when counting instruments. As surgeons strive to contain operative costs, decreasing operative time is advantageous. In our study, the operative time of the Alexis cohort was 23 minutes shorter compared to that of the Bookwalter cohort. This time saved is likely related to multiple causes including increased surgeon experience, though we do believe that the Alexis setup and removal do indeed save time compared to a standard fixed retractor.

Our study does have significant limitations: most importantly that it is a single-center, non-randomized, and retrospective study. Multiple unknown biases could have thus affected which cases utilized which retractors. As mentioned, most contemporary patients in our study underwent radical cystectomy with the Alexis retractor. Therefore, our improved results in the Alexis cohort may indeed have been related to improved surgeons' experience. Finally, retraction in very obese patients is always difficult and thus standard retractors are typically used, at least in our experience.

5. Conclusion

The Alexis retractor is a safe and effective tool for retraction and wound protection during open radical cystectomy and may potentially reduce wound-related complications, improve operative time, and lead to lower length of stay among patients. The Alexis retractor likely provides the benefit of lower surgical site infections compared to traditional retraction methods; however, further, larger, prospective multicenter trials should be initiated to confirm our findings.

References

[1] K. M. Scolari Childress, J. A. Gavard, D. G. Ward, K. Berger, and G. A. Gross, "A barrier retractor to reduce surgical site infections and wound disruptions in obese patients undergoing cesarean delivery: a randomized controlled trial," *American Journal of Obstetrics and Gynecology*, vol. 214, no. 2, p. 285, 2016.

[2] K. Cheng, A. Roslani, K. Arumugam et al., "ALEXIS O-Ring wound retractor vs conventional wound protection for the prevention of surgical site infections in colorectal resections," *Colorectal Disease*, vol. 14, no. 6, pp. e346–e351, 2012.

[3] D. Huynh, A. Henderson, T. Haden et al., "Feasibility and safety study for the use of wound protectors during robotic radical cystectomy and ileal conduit," *Journal of Robotic Surgery*, vol. 11, no. 2, pp. 187–191, 2016.

[4] A. J. Mangram, T. C. Horan, M. L. Pearson, L. C. Silver, and W. R. Jarvis, "Guideline for prevention of surgical site infection, 1999," *American Journal of Infection Control*, vol. 27, no. 2, pp. 97–132, 1999.

[5] G. Ortega, D. S. Rhee, D. J. Papandria et al., "An evaluation of surgical site infections by wound classification system using the ACS-NSQIP," *Journal of Surgical Research*, vol. 174, no. 1, pp. 33–38, 2012.

[6] L. T. Lavallée, D. Schramm, K. Witiuk et al., "Peri-operative morbidity associated with radical cystectomy in a multicenter database of community and academic hospitals," *PLoS One*, vol. 9, no. 10, Article ID e111281, 2014.

[7] A. L. Mihaljevic, T. C. Müller, V. Kehl, H. Friess, and J. Kleeff, "Wound edge protectors in open abdominal surgery to reduce surgical site infections: a systematic review and meta-analysis," *PLoS One*, vol. 10, no. 3, Article ID e0121187, 2015.

[8] K. Reid, P. Pockney, B. Draganic, and S. R. Smith, "Barrier wound protection decreases surgical site infection in open elective colorectal surgery: a randomized clinical trial," *Diseases of the Colon and Rectum*, vol. 53, no. 10, pp. 1374–1380, 2010.

[9] L. Hinkson, J.-P. Siedentopf, A. Weichert, and W. Henrich, "Surgical site infection in cesarean sections with the use of a plastic sheath wound retractor compared to the traditional self-retaining metal retractor," *European Journal of Obstetrics and Gynecology and Reproductive Biology*, vol. 203, pp. 232–238, 2016.

25

Are Technology-Driven Mobile Phone Applications (Apps) the New Currency for Digital Stent Registries and Patient Communication: Prospective Outcomes Using Urostentz App

B. M. Zeeshan Hameed,[1,2] Milap J. Shah,[1] Nithesh Naik,[3] Mohan Amaresh,[1] Padmaraj Hegde,[1] Rahil Hussein Beary,[4] Suraj Jayadeva,[1] and Bhaskar K. Somani[5]

[1]*Department of Urology, Kasturba Medical College and Hospital, Manipal Academy of Higher Education, Manipal, India*
[2]*Chief of Innovation Centre, Kasturba Medical College, Manipal Academy of Higher Education, Manipal, India*
[3]*Faculty of Engineering, Manipal Institute of Technology, Manipal Academy of Higher Education, Manipal, India*
[4]*Kasturba Medical College, Manipal Academy of Higher Education, Manipal, India*
[5]*Department of Urology, University Hospital Southampton NHS Trust, Southampton, UK*

Correspondence should be addressed to Nithesh Naik; nithesh.naik@manipal.edu

Academic Editor: Mohammad H. Ather

Background. Forgotten ureteral stents (FUS) and stent-related symptoms (SRS) lead to increased postprocedural emergency department visits and add to the psychological and financial burden of the patients. *Purpose.* To review the usage and benefits of ureteral stent tracking and symptom monitoring through a single smartphone-based application (App) platform with 2-way clinician-patient communication. This study also compared the features with other smartphone apps used for stent tracking. *Materials and Methods.* 100 patients were included in this single-center prospective study conducted between September 2019 and December 2019. Patients who had metallic or long-term indwelling stents, noncomprehensible patients, and those not willing to share their data were excluded from the study. *Results.* Of 100 patients, 92 downloaded the Urostentz application, and 72 (78.2%) patients answered the pictorial symptom questionnaire. Symptom score analysis suggested that 62 patients (86.1%) had stent-related symptoms of which 3 required readmission and underwent early stent removal. The mean stent duration was 17.2 + 3.5 days (range: 11–23 days), with 69% of patients having their stent removed on the scheduled date and 25% of patients requesting a change of their appointment via the App. *Conclusion.* In this study, there was no case of FUS encountered. The "Urostentz" App is a freely available patient safety stent tracking application that provides a secure and simplified interface, which can significantly reduce the incidence of FUS and provide digital remote assistance in the management of stent-related symptoms.

1. Introduction

Ureteral stents are a vital part of the present-day endourological practice. The indications for ureteral stent insertion consist of operative interventions involving the kidney or ureter as well any condition causing internal or external obstruction of the ureter [1–4]. According to the literature, 12% of all stents remain indwelling beyond their maximal safe life [2]. Such stents are termed as forgotten ureteral stent (FUS). FUS can be associated with complications such as migration, infection, encrustation, stent fracture, renal failure, and sepsis [3]. More than 75% of stents are found to be encrusted when removed after 12 weeks of insertion [2, 3]. Stent-related symptoms (SRS) such as dysuria, loin pain, haematuria, urinary incontinence, and lower urinary tract symptoms (LUTS) are observed in nearly 80% of stented cases [4]. The removal of FUS also posed a challenge to urologists. Multiple endourological procedures may be required for the removal of infected, fractured, or encrusted FUS. In addition to the increased costs of post-procedure-related events (PRE) such as multiple clinic appointments, readmissions, and emergency department visits, there is also an added burden of medicolegal issues associated with it. This adds to an increased physical, psychological, and economic burden on the patients [4, 5].

One of the important components of using ureteral stents is creating an effective structure to track and monitor these stents and ensure their timely removal. At present, there is no standard universally accepted protocol regarding their follow-up and retrieval. Despite the existence of few stent registries, mishaps continue to happen and there are significant patient and financial benefits to be sought from engendering the use of a robust system. Few stent tracking applications are available but none of them addresses the issues related to the SRS or allows 2-way communication with the patients. Hence, we developed a smartphone application that helps in tracking the ureteral "stents" as well as monitoring the "symptoms" associated with these stents via a 2-way clinician-patient communication.

In this study, we aimed to evaluate the usefulness of the "Urostentz" application in ureteral stent tracking, SRS monitoring, and compare the features with other smartphone applications used for stent tracking.

2. Materials and Methods

2.1. Patients. This was a single-center study conducted in our university teaching hospital. Institutional Ethics Committee clearance and certificate was obtained for the study (IEC: 651/2019). Over 4 months between September 2019 and December 2019, prospective outcomes were recorded for consecutive patients in whom ureteral stenting was done for any urological indication. All procedures performed in studies involving human participants were in accordance with the ethical standards of the institutional and/or national research committee and with the 1964 Helsinki declaration and its later amendments or comparable ethical standards.

The inclusion criteria were all patients having ureteral stent insertion (polyurethane) and patients or their immediate relatives having a smartphone or analog phone willing to participate in the study. Patients who had metallic or long term indwelling stents, non-comprehensible patients, and those not willing to share their data were excluded from the study. The total number of patient recruitment was limited to the first 100 patients for this pilot study.

2.2. Mobile Phone Application (App). In 2019, "Urostentz" was developed to streamline the tracking of ureteral stents and stent-related symptoms, improve patient safety by creating an effective medium of communication, and improve the quality of data collection. Urostentz is one of its kind smartphone applications, which also provides the facility to track the SRS of the patients and provide digital remote assistance for the same. It is freely available to download on Google Playstore. It can also be accessed on the computer by visiting the website http://www.urostentz.com. The iOS application is submitted and the same shall be available soon on the App store.

2.2.1. Protocol. After double J stent insertion for urological procedures, the application was downloaded in the patient's or relative's smartphone, linked to a profile that was created under the treating surgeon, containing the details related to the procedure and the stent insertion.

All patients were registered under the experienced treating surgical team. Once the patient was registered, the details were protected as only the treating surgeon could access the data. All information obtained was encrypted and kept secure. In each case, details such as patient demographics, indication for stent insertion, stent size, length, date of its insertion, and scheduled removal date were entered as shown in Figures 1(a)–1(c). This information was stored in the database which could be accessed for audit and gave the entire information with search options as per the requirement.

The patient could log in from their smartphone or web browser and access information regarding the scheduled date of stent removal (Figure 2(a)). In the case of SRS, the patient could also access the pictorial questionnaire and submit details regarding their symptoms to the clinician. The decision to include the stent-related symptoms was derived using a "Delphi" method involving six experienced endourologists.

This questionnaire was based on the pictorial depiction of the symptoms from the Ureteral Stent Symptom Questionnaire (USSQ) to improve patient compliance (Figures 2(b)–2(d)) [6]. The application also provided the patient with the facility to request a change in the scheduled appointment.

The clinician received notifications regarding the patient queries and responded with a message accordingly. The patient received reminders regarding the stent removal date as scheduled by the clinician. The clinician was also notified regarding the total patients scheduled for stent removal on a day-to-day basis to plan their stent removals (Figure 3(a)). When a patient reported for stent removal, the entry was updated as "removed" in the stent dashboard (Figure 3(b)).

A patient who did not return for stent removal within 3 months of their scheduled date was categorized as FUS. A patient could only have 1 profile but could have more than 1 ureteral stent care plan during the study period. Bilateral stent placement done in the same sitting was considered as a single stent care plan. As per standard protocol, all stents were removed after 2-3 weeks from the date of insertion after confirming the stone-free status with X-ray or ultrasound for radioopaque stones and NCCT (noncontrast computerized tomography) scan of the KUB (kidneys ureter bladder) for radiolucent stones.

2.2.2. Outcome Measures. The primary outcome measures were the incidence of FUS and stent-related symptom

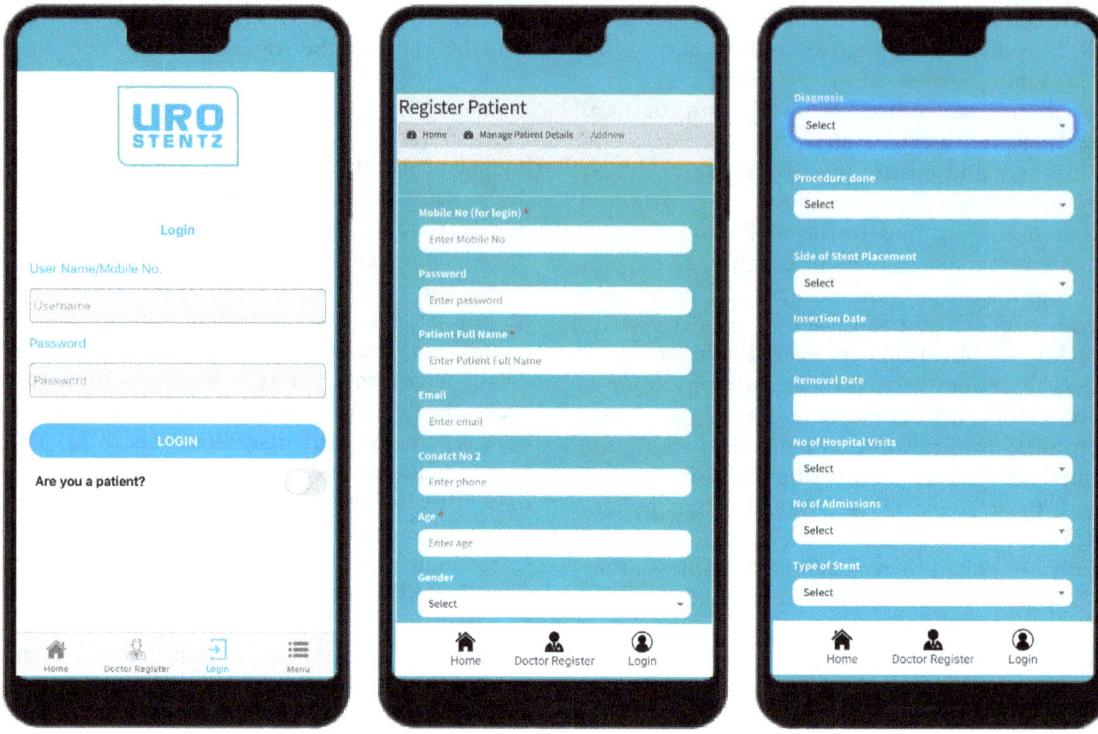

(a) (b) (c)

Figure 1: (a) Doctor and patient login. (b) and (c) Patient registration details including demographics, indication for stent insertion, stent size, length, date of its insertion, and scheduled removal date (reproduced with the permission of developers of the application (RAYZ CHARTERED)).

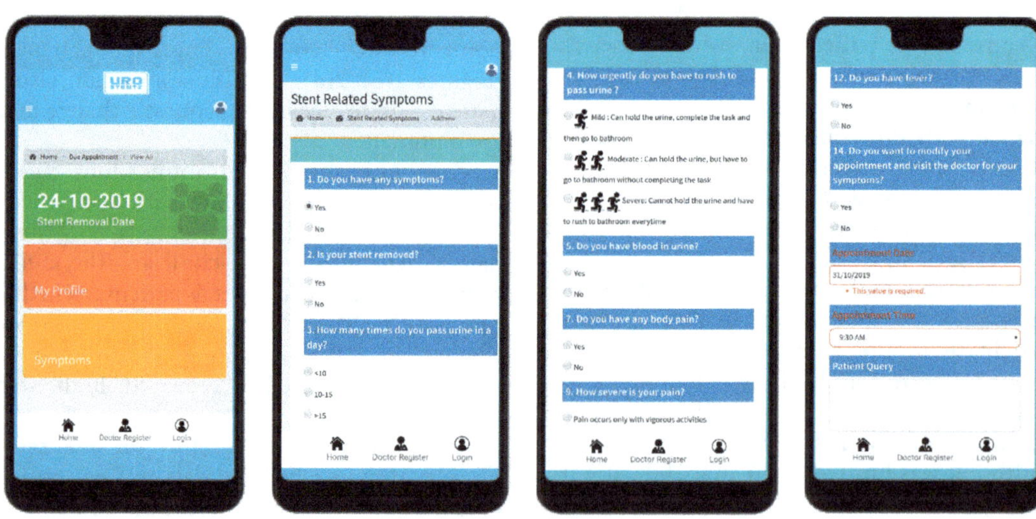

(a) (b) (c) (d)

Figure 2: (a) Patient dashboard showing the scheduled date of stent removal, access to symptom questionnaire, and personal profile. (b–d) Pictorial symptom questionnaire for patients with stent-related symptoms and symptoms even after stent removal (reproduced with the permission of developers of the application (RAYZ CHARTERED)).

analysis based on the questionnaire answered. The secondary outcome measures were adherence to the scheduled date of removal, rate of outpatient visits, and readmissions. The number of patient communication episodes was also captured.

2.3. Statistical Analysis. Data extracted included patient demographics, diagnosis, procedure, stent characteristics, use of smartphones or web browsers, stent-related questionnaire response, and adherence to the scheduled appointment. Descriptive statistics were performed to calculate

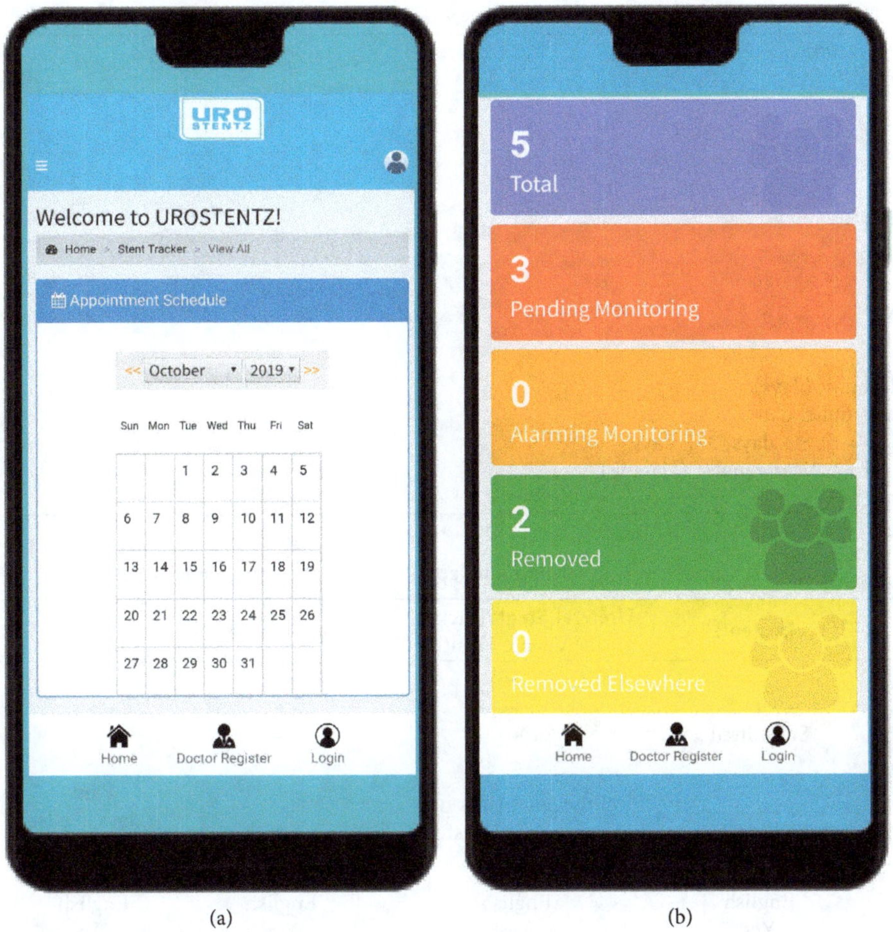

FIGURE 3: (a) Clinician dashboard to receive notifications regarding the total patients scheduled for stent removal on a day-to-day basis. (b) Clinician dashboard: updates regarding patient's ureteral stent removal status (reproduced with the permission of developers of the application (RAYZ CHARTERED)).

mean, standard deviation, and range using IBM SPSS Statistics for Windows, Version 24 (IBM Corp., Armonk, NY).

3. Results

An initial group of 100 patients underwent ureteral stent placement for various indications and were subsequently tracked using the "Urostentz" application. The details regarding patient demographics, symptom score analysis, and adherence to the schedule are described in Table 1.

The mean patient age was 42.3 ± 13.7 years (range: 14–80 years), with a male : female ratio of 2 : 1. Stent placement was done after percutaneous nephrolithotomy (PCNL) ($n = 44$), after ureterocopy (URS) ($n = 48$), and other procedures ($n = 8$). Of 100 patients, 92 had smartphone access and were able to download the Urostentz application while the other 8 patients were registered through the website. 72 (78.2%) patients answered the pictorial symptom questionnaire through the Urostentz application. Based on the answers, the symptom score analysis suggested that 10 patients (13.8%) had no symptoms and 62 patients (86.1%) had stent-related symptoms. Three (3%) patients required readmission due to severe loin pain ($n = 2$) and pyelonephritis ($n = 1$). All 3 patients underwent early stent removal. 15 (15%) patients were managed conservatively for their symptoms on an outpatient department (OPD) basis. 69% of patients had their stent removed on the scheduled date while 25% of patients requested a change in appointment. Overall, 6 (6%) cases had delayed stent removal. The mean stent duration was 17.25 ± 3.5 days (range: 11–23 days). There was no case of FUS encountered in the study.

4. Discussion

To our knowledge, this is the first study on ureteral stent tracking and symptom monitoring through a single smartphone-based app platform. The preliminary data from this pilot study suggest that the Urostentz application is an effective mode to track the patients with indwelling ureteral stents and monitor their stent-related symptoms.

Smartphones have become an integral part of our routine life. Various smartphone-based applications have been developed for tracking patients with indwelling ureteral stents. In 2016, Boston Scientific in partnership with Visible Health launched the Ureteral Stent Tracker (UST) application. Other smartphone-based applications launched in

Table 1: Patient demographics, symptom score analysis, and adherence to the schedule.

Patient demographics (N = 100)	
Age (mean ± SD) in years	42.3 ± 13.76 (range: 14–80)
Male : female	2 : 1
Right: left: bilateral	52 (52%): 40 (40%): 8 (8%)
PCNL : URS : others	44 (44%): 48 (48%): 8 (8%)
Smartphones: website	92 (92%): 8 (8%)
Symptom score analysis	
No symptoms	10 (13.8%)
Symptoms present	62 (86.1%)
Readmissions	03 (3%)
OPD visits only	15 (15%)
Adherence to the stent removal schedule	
Mean (+/−SD) stent duration (days)	17.25 ± 3.54 (range: 11–23)
Stent removal on the scheduled date	69
Delayed stent removal ($n = 6$): ≤3 days, 3–7 days	4 patients, 2 patients
Stent postponed as per the patient request (via app)	25 patients
Forgotten ureteral stent (SUF)	Nil

Table 2: Comparison of smartphone applications for ureteral stent tracking.

Features	Urostentz	Ureteral Stent Tracker * by Visible Health	Stent Tracker	Double J Tracker	Stone MD
Platforms available					
Android	+	+	+	+	+
iOS	Submitted	+	+	—	+
Web browser	+	+	—	—	—
Access	Free	Withdrawn (was only accessible to registered doctors)	Free	Paid 14 days of a free trial Rs 7900/year	Free
Languages	English	English	English	English	English
Doctors dashboard	Yes	Yes	Yes	NA	No
Patient dashboard	Yes	No	No	NA	Yes
Patient education dashboard	Yes	No	No	NA	Yes
Symptom tracking	Yes	No	No	NA	No
Two-way communication between the doctor and the patient	Present	Absent	Absent	Absent	Absent
Personalized message facility	Yes	No	No	NA	No
Notifications/reminders	Yes	Yes	Yes	NA	Self-reminder
Medium of notifications	Short messaging service (SMS) E-mail (if provided)	E-mail	NA	NA	NA
Timing of reminders	1 week before the scheduled date On the day of the scheduled date 1 day after the scheduled date (if the patient does not follow-up)	Daily or weekly as per requirement	NA	NA	On the day of the scheduled date
Facility for change in appointment	Yes	No	No	NA	NA
Record of total hospital visits/consultations/readmissions	Yes	No	No	NA	NA

Table 2: Continued.

Features	Urostentz	Ureteral Stent Tracker * by Visible Health	Stent Tracker	Double J Tracker	Stone MD
Limitations	Not integrated to institutional EMR	Limited to physicians who are registered and preauthorized by Boston Scientific Not integrated to institutional EMR No monitoring of SRS Withdrawn by the company	Single language No SRS monitoring facility Not available on the web browser No automated reminders or messages for stent removal Limited to the users defined by the pharma company	Single language No SRS monitoring facility Not available on the web browser Only available on iOS Paid services	Single language No reminders to the doctors No two-way communication for stent removal No SRS monitoring facility Not available on the web browser

* The app was withdrawn from both iOS and Android platforms.

2019 were Stent Tracker, Stone MD, and Double J Tracker. The authors have discussed the features of the different available applications and their limitations and given a comprehensive comparison of the same in Table 2. Urostentz app is the only smartphone application with stent tracking as well as stent-related symptom tracking. This is a unique application that helps in two-way objective communication between patients and the urologist.

Various studies have been conducted using the UST application to check its clinical application. In 2017, Molina et al. reported their retrospective study using the UST. In this study, 77% of stents were removed on time while 9% were overdue. Only 1 out of 194 patients were lost to follow-up [7]. Ziemba et al. (2017) reported that 3 out of 115 patients (3%) who did not return for their scheduled stent removal could be identified only through the UST application [8]. Ulker et al. [9] used UST and compared it with the appointment card registry to track patients with indwelling ureteric stents. The results showed that patients could easily be recalled through UST [9]. Similar to these studies, in our series using the Urostentz application there was no incidence of FUS.

In literature, SRS include storage and voiding symptoms such as urgency (57–60%), frequency (50–60%), incomplete emptying (76%), dysuria (40%), suprapubic pain (30%), flank pain (19–32%), haematuria (25%), and incontinence [10–17]. Stent placement is also associated with increased postprocedure-related events (PREs) including phone calls, extraclinic appointments, and emergency department visits [18]. This adds to increased psychological as well as an economic burden on the patients. The clinicians also have the burden to attend to these extra calls and patient visits. There is no system or software designed to help reduce these stent-related issues. Urostentz is the first smartphone-based application that addresses this issue where the App is applied clinically to track and monitor SRS. We monitored the SRS of patients who answered the pictorial questionnaire through the App. Out of 72 patients who answered the questionnaire, only 18 patients had to revisit the hospital for the same while the rest of the patients were reassured and none of them reported any further complaints or complications.

Although our sample size was small and based on a single institution, it is a pilot study and the objective was to check the efficacy and usefulness of Urostentz application. The authors plan to further evaluate the effectiveness of this application in reducing the incidence of FUS and SRS by utilizing this application in a larger cohort through a multi-institutional global study. The impact of this application in reducing the economic burden on patients having stent-related symptoms also needs to be evaluated. Since the Urostentz app is currently available only on Google Playstore, the wider application of this App after its availability on iOS phones needs to be evaluated.

5. Conclusion

The "Urostentz" App is a freely available patient safety stent tracking application that provides a secure and simplified interface, which can significantly reduce the incidence of FUS and provide digital remote assistance in the management of stent-related symptoms. In case of patients who have passed their scheduled date of stent removal, this application can provide an effective medium for 2-way clinician-patient communication to notify the patients and also avoid unnecessary hospital visits in case of insignificant SRS thereby reducing the financial burden on the patients.

Abbreviations

FUS: Forgotten ureteral stents
SRS: Stent-related symptoms
LUTS: Lower urinary tract symptoms
PRE: Postprocedure-related events
USSQ: Ureteral Stent Symptom Questionnaire
PCNL: Percutaneous nephrolithotomy
OPD: Outpatient department
UST: Ureteral Stent Tracker
NCCT: Noncontrast computerized tomography
KUB: Kidneys ureter bladder.

Consent

Informed consent was obtained from all individual participants included in the study.

Authors' Contributions

All authors contributed to this work and read and approved the final version of the manuscript.

References

[1] H. K. Mardis, R. M. Kroeger, J. J. Morton, and J. M. Donovan, "Comparative evaluation of materials used for internal ureteral stents," *Journal of Endourology*, vol. 7, no. 2, pp. 105–115, 1993.

[2] S. R. El-Faqih, A. B. Shamsuddin, A. Chakrabarti et al., "Polyurethane internal ureteral stents in treatment of stone patients: morbidity related to indwelling times," *Journal of Urology*, vol. 146, no. 6, pp. 1487–1491, 1991.

[3] N. Divakaruni, C. J. Palmer, P. Tek et al., "Forgotten ureteral stents: who's at risk?" *Journal of Endourology*, vol. 27, no. 8, pp. 1051–1054, 2013.

[4] M. Monga, E. Klein, W. R. Castaneda-Zuniga, and R. Thomas, "The forgotten indwelling ureteral stent: a urological dilemma," *Journal of Urology*, vol. 153, no. 6, pp. 1817–1819, 1995.

[5] P. Tenke, B. Kovacs, M. Jäckel, and E. Nagy, "The role of biofilm infection in urology," *World Journal of Urology*, vol. 24, no. 1, pp. 13–20, 2006.

[6] H. B. Joshi, N. Newns, A. Stainthorpe, R. P. Macdonagh, F. X. Keeley, and A. G. Timoney, "Ureteral stent symptom questionnaire: development and validation of a multidimensional quality of life measure," *Journal of Urology*, vol. 169, no. 3, pp. 1060–1064, 2003.

[7] W. R. Molina, R. Pessoa, R. Donalisio da Silva et al., "A new patient safety smartphone application for prevention of "forgotten" ureteral stents: results from a clinical pilot study in 194 patients," *Patient Safety in Surgery*, vol. 11, no. 1, 2017.

[8] J. B. Ziemba, W. W. Ludwig, L. Ruiz, E. Carvalhal, and B. R. Matlaga, "Preventing the forgotten ureteral stent by using a mobile point-of-care application," *Journal of Endourology*, vol. 31, no. 7, pp. 719–724, 2017.

[9] V. Ulker, H. A. Atalay, O. Cakmak, C. Yucel, O. Celik, and Z. Kozacioglu, "Smartphone-based stent tracking application for prevention of forgotten ureteral double-J stents: a prospective study," *International Brazilian Journal of Urology*, vol. 45, no. 2, pp. 376–383, 2019.

[10] B. H. Chew, B. E. Knudsen, and J. D. Denstedt, "The use of stents in contemporary urology," *Current Opinion in Urology*, vol. 14, no. 2, pp. 111–115, 2004.

[11] G. Haleblian, K. Kijvikai, J. De la Rosette, and G. Preminger, "Ureteral stenting and urinary stone management: a systematic review," *Journal of Urology*, vol. 179, no. 2, pp. 424–430, 2008.

[12] H. B. Joshi, A. Okeke, N. Newns, F. X. Keeley, and A. G. Timoney, "Characterization of urinary symptoms in patients with ureteral stents," *Urology*, vol. 59, no. 4, pp. 511–516, 2002.

[13] P. Hao, W. Li, C. Song, J. Yan, B. Song, and L. Li, "Clinical evaluation of double-pigtail stent in patients with upper urinary tract diseases: report of 2685 cases," *Journal of Endourology*, vol. 22, no. 1, pp. 65–70, 2008.

[14] R. Thomas, "Indwelling ureteral stents: impact of material and shape on patient comfort," *Journal of Endourology*, vol. 7, no. 2, pp. 137–140, 1993.

[15] R. L. Sur, G. E. Haleblian, D. A. Cantor, W. P. Springhart, D. M. Albala, and G. M. Preminger, "Efficacy of intravesical ropivacaine injection on urinary symptoms following ureteral stenting: a randomized, controlled study," *Journal of Endourology*, vol. 22, no. 3, pp. 473–478, 2008.

[16] A. Rane, A. Saleemi, D. Cahill, S. Sriprasad, N. Shrotri, and R. Tiptaft, "Have stent-related symptoms anything to do with placement technique?" *Journal of Endourology*, vol. 15, no. 7, pp. 741–745, 2001.

[17] F. H. Smedley, J. Rimmer, M. Taube et al., "168 double J (pigtail) ureteric catheter insertions: a retrospective review," *Annals of the Royal College of Surgeons of England*, vol. 70, no. 6, p. 377, 1988.

[18] C. J. Paul, N. A. Brooks, G. M. Ghareeb, and C. R. Tracy, "Pilot study to determine optimal stent duration following ureteroscopy: three versus seven days," *Current Urology*, vol. 11, no. 2, pp. 97–102, 2017.

26

Microbiota, Prostatitis and Fertility: Bacterial Diversity as a Possible Health Ally

Jenniffer Puerta Suárez and Walter D. Cardona Maya

Reproduction Group, Department of Microbiology and Parasitology, School of Medicine, University of Antioquia-UdeA, Medellin, Colombia

Correspondence should be addressed to Walter D. Cardona Maya; wdario.cardona@udea.edu.co

Academic Editor: Mohammad H. Ather

Background. In health, microorganisms have been associated with the disease, although the current knowledge shows that the microbiota present in various anatomical sites is associated with multiple benefits. *Objective.* This study aimed to evaluate and compare the genitourinary microbiota of chronic prostatitis symptoms patients and fertile men. *Materials and Methods.* In this preliminary study, ten volunteers have included 5 volunteers with symptoms of chronic prostatitis (prostatitis group) and five fertile volunteers, asymptomatic for urogenital infections (control group) matched by age. Bacterial diversity analysis was performed using the 16S molecular marker to compare the microbiota present in urine and semen samples from chronic prostatitis symptoms and fertile volunteers. Seminal quality, nitric oxide levels, and seminal and serum concentration of proinflammatory cytokines were quantified. *Results.* Fertile men present a greater variety of operational taxonomical units-OTUs in semen (67.5%) and urine (17.6%) samples than chronic prostatitis symptoms men. Chronic prostatitis symptoms men presented a higher concentration of IL-12p70 in seminal plasma. No statistically significant differences were observed in conventional and functional seminal parameters. The species diversity in semen samples was similar in healthy men than prostatitis patients, inverted Simpson index median 5.3 (5.0–10.7) vs. 4.5 (2.1–7.8, $p = 0.1508$). Nevertheless, the microbiota present in the semen and urine samples of fertile men presents more OTUs. Less microbial diversity could be associated with chronic prostatitis symptoms. The presence of bacteria in the genitourinary tract is not always associated with the disease. Understanding the factors that affect the microbiota can implement lifestyle habits that prevent chronic prostatitis. *Conclusion.* Chronic prostatitis does not seem to affect male fertility; however, studies with a larger sample size are required. Our preliminary results strengthen the potential role; the greater bacterial diversity is a protective factor for chronic prostatitis.

1. Introduction

Chronic prostatitis is a frequent and multicausal condition. Among the causes of prostatitis that include infections [1], mainly bacterial, however, identifying the causative agent is not always possible, and in addition, the gland can harbour microbiota. With sequencing techniques, it is possible to identify a great variety of microbiota, its effects on health, and its effect on the immune system [2]. In chronic bacterial prostatitis men, an improvement in symptoms, life quality, and less antibiotic consumption have been described with the oral administration of *Lactobacillus casei* [3], suggesting the close relationship between gastrointestinal and urogenital microbiota [4].

Prostatitis is the most common urological diagnosis in young men under 50 years after benign prostatic hyperplasia and prostate cancer [5]. The primary causes of the illness such as infections, immunologic status, urine reflux, and mental stress have been identified as primary causes [1]. Clinically, prostatitis is classified into four types: (i) acute bacterial prostatitis, (ii) chronic bacterial prostatitis, (iii) chronic pelvic pain syndrome, and (iv) asymptomatic inflammatory prostatitis [6–8]. Chronic bacterial prostatitis is responsible for 5–10% of total prostatitis cases, of which at least 30% is associated with recurrent urinary infections [8]. Up to 90% of patients are classified as having chronic pelvic pain syndrome because the cause cannot be identified. The gold standard for prostatitis is the four-vessel test [9]; however, at present, it is not performed routinely due to the risk of causing bacteremia [7].

Furthermore, this test only detects those culturable microorganisms, so new techniques are necessary to identify all the organisms in the gland responsible for the disease. The use of next-generation sequencing (NGS) techniques could improve the understanding of the microbiome [10], especially dysbiosis caused by prostatitis and its impact on health. Bacterial diversity analysis (metataxonomics) uses the 16S molecular marker (variable regions V3–V4) to assess men's microbiota. Besides, the semen sample has higher sensitivity than expressed prostatic excretion (EPS) for diagnosing chronic bacterial prostatitis [11], and it is also practical and comfortable for the patient. Therefore, this preliminary study aimed to determine men's microbiota with prostatitis-like symptoms and their impact on seminal quality.

2. Materials and Methods

2.1. Study Participants. The protocol and informed consent form were approved by the Bioethics Committee for Research in Humans at the Institute of Medical Research, School of Medicine, University of Antioquia (act number 006), in April 2018. All patients provided written informed consent regarding their participation and publication of their clinical data. Five chronic prostatitis symptoms and five fertile men asymptomatic for urogenital infections volunteers were included. All men were generally in good health, without sexually transmitted diseases. None was under antibiotic treatment at the time of the sampling. National Institute of Health of Chronic Prostatitis Symptoms Index (NIH–CPSI [12]) translated and validated into Spanish [13] was employed to select the volunteers according to the criteria reported by Nickel et al., [5].

Each volunteer gave a semen sample and a midstream urine sample; both samples replaced the prostate fluid sample obtained through stimulation of the gland through the rectum [14]. In addition, a blood sample was taken by qualified personnel in a nonanticoagulated vacutainer tube (Becton Dickinson, NJ, USA) to obtain the serum. The donors also filled out a survey with sociodemographic factors, lifestyle, urinary symptoms, and other relevant aspects of sexual and reproductive health to identify factors associated with prostatitis symptoms.

2.2. Semen and Seminal Parameters. Prior to semen analysis, all donors were asked to abstain from sexual intercourse or masturbation for 3–5 days before semen collection and delivered to the laboratory within 1 hour of ejaculation.

2.3. Conventional Seminal Parameters. After semen liquefaction was completed, each semen sample was analyzed for conventional parameters: sperm motility, vitality, concentration, total sperm concentration, and sperm morphology according to those established by the World Health Organization in the fifth edition of its Human Semen Processing Manual, while the sperm concentration was evaluated using the Makler chamber [15, 16].

2.4. Functional Seminal Parameters. Sperm mitochondrial membrane potential [17], sperm membrane integrity [18], chromatin structure assay [19], sperm membrane lipoperoxidation [20], and intracellular levels of reactive oxygen species (ROS) [17] were evaluated by flow cytometry (Fortessa, Becton Dickinson, NJ, USA), according to previously established protocols, analyzing between 5,000 and 10,000 sperm cells. Data analysis was carried out with FlowJo 7.6 (TreeStar Inc., Oregon, USA).

2.5. Seminal Plasma Total Antioxidant Capacity. For this test, 3 mL of DPPH (2,2-diphenyl-1-picrylhydrazyl) was mixed with 200 μL of the sample. After one hour of incubation, the sample was read in a spectrophotometer (Spectronic 20 spectrophotometer®, Genesys, Rochester, NY, USA) at 515 nm, used ascorbic acid as a positive control [21].

2.6. Prostate-Specific Antigen (PSA). According to the manufacturer's instructions, PSA was quantified using the commercial total PSA kit (DiaMetra, Perugia, Italy). Prostate antigen values greater than 4 ng/mL were considered positive.

2.7. Nitric Oxide Quantification. Nitrite quantification was performed using the commercial Griess reagent kit for nitrite determination (Molecular probes, Oregon, USA) according to the manufacturer's instructions and after deproteinization of the semen and serum samples according to the Serafini method [22].

2.8. Cytokine Quantification. Quantification of the cytokines IL-12p70, IL-10, IL-1β, IL-6, IL-8, TNF, IL-2, IL-4, IL-10, IL-17, and INF-γ was performed using the kits BD Cytometric Bead Array (CBA) Human Inflammatory Cytokines and Human Th1/Th2/Th17 Cytokine Kit (Becton Dickinson, NJ, USA). The analysis was carried out in the FlowJo 7.6.

2.9. Bacterial Diversity Analysis. DNA extraction was performed using the Stool DNA Isolation Kit (Norgen) to identify the microbiota, and gDNA quantification was performed by the PicoGreen colourimetric method. Subsequently, control of 16S gene amplification was performed using the primers 27F (AGAGTTTGATCCTGGCTCAG) and 1492R (TACGGYTACCTTGTTACGACTT), and a 1500 base pair (bp) fragment was successfully amplified for all samples. For sequencing, the 16S ribosomal gene variables V3 and V4, the Bakt_341F (CCTACGGGNGGCWGCAG), and Bakt_805R (GACTACHVGGGTATCTAATCC) oligonucleotides were used. Sequencing was performed on the platform MiSeq Illumina, generating paired reads 300 bases each. Sequence quality analysis and classification were developed in

TABLE 1: NIH–CPSI classification of volunteers.

Domain (score)	Symptoms classification, median (range)		P value
	Fertile group, control	Prostatitis-like symptoms	
Pain (0–21)	0 (0-1)	11 (7–11)	0.0079
Urinary symptoms (0–10)	1 (0–3)	7 (6–10)	0.0079
Quality of life impact (0–12)	0 (0–2)	4 (2–5)	0.0159
Total score (0–43)	1 (0–5)	20 (20–26)	0.0079

TABLE 2: Seminal quality and oxidative stress in prostatitis-like symptoms men and fertile men.

	Fertile group, control, median (range)	Prostatitis-like symptoms, median (range)	P value
Seminal volume (mL)	4 (1.5–4.5)	3 (1.5–7.5)	0.7460
Progressive motility (%)	55.5 (41.5–81.0)	57 (6.0–64.0)	0.6667
Nonprogressive motility (%)	6.5 (2.0–16.0)	6.0 (1.0–25.0)	0.9524
Immotile spermatozoa (%)	39.0 (17.0–45.0)	42.0 (29.0–90.0)	0.8016
Concentration/mL (10^6/mL)	80.0 (40.5–270.0)	205.0 (7.0–254.0)	0.9444
Total concentration (10^6/ejaculate)	178.2 (115.5–1080.0)	431.8 (22.4–1538.0)	0.8016
Viability (%)	79.0 (77.0–90.0)	70.0 (49.0–85.0)	0.1667
Sperm with normal morphology (%)	4.8 (4.2–8.6)	4.4 (2.8–6.8)	0.8016
Teratozoospermia index	1.4 (1.1–1.5)	1.2 (1.1–1.5)	0.2222
High mitochondrial membrane potential (%)	63.2 (44.2–7.5)	50.0 (12.3–55.5)	0.0556
Plasma membrane integrity (%)	64.8 (48.1–84.4)	35.8 (6.2–69.7)	0.1508
ROS production (%)	64.3 (50.5–86.2)	55.7 (17.7–61.9)	0.0556
DNA fragmentation index (%)	10.6 (10.4–11.4)	11.1 (10.5–14.3)	0.3889
Membrane lipid peroxidation (%)	49.8 (9.1–80.5)	67.0 (44.9–93.3)	0.4127
Antioxidant capacity of seminal plasma %)	61.0 (45.3–81.4)	62.0 (9.5–69.3)	0.5317
Serum nitric oxide (μM)	3.7 (2.1–13.0)	3.0 (1.7–4.1)	0.5000
Plasma nitric oxide (μM)	1.5 (0.6–1.7)	0.5 (0.2–1.9)	0.3016
PSA (ng/mL)	0.0 (0.0–1.4)	0.9 (0.0–120.0)	0.3651

Mann–Whitney test. Data indicate median and range.

MetaCoMET (Metagenomics Core Microbiome Exploration Tool, MetaCoMET).

2.10. Statistical Analysis. A chi-square and a Mann–Whitney test were used to compare the dichotomous and numerical variables between both groups. The data were analyzed using the statistical program GraphPad Prism 6.0 (GraphPad, San Diego, CA, USA), and a value of $p < 0.05$ was considered significant.

3. Results

The median and range of age, abstinence period, and body mass index of the fertile group and prostatitis-like symptoms patients included in the study was 34 (21–44) years and 34 (21–44) years ($p > 0.999$), 2 (2–5) and 3 (2–5) days ($p = 0.9206$), and 26.4 (24.4-30.9) and 22.9 (19.7–26.8) kg/m^2 ($p = 0.0952$), respectively.

Semen and urine microbiota of five fertile volunteers and five chronic prostatitis symptoms volunteers matched by age, and classified using the NIH–CPSI were compared (Table 1).

When comparing the conventional and functional semen analyses of prostatitis-like symptoms men and fertile men matched by age, we did not find statistically significant differences (Table 2). All conventional seminal parameters were in both groups above the lower limit of reference according to the WHO [23]. In addition, no PSA serum concentration differences were observed (Table 2). The median level of IL-12p70 in seminal plasma was significantly increased in chronic prostatitis symptoms volunteers compared to the fertile group. Also, there was no difference in other cytokine concentrations between both groups (Table 3).

When evaluating the genitourinary microbiota, it is observed that the species diversity in semen samples was similar in healthy men than prostatitis patients, inverted Simpson index median 5.3 (5.0–10.7) vs. 4.5 (2.1–7.8, $p = 0.1508$). Nevertheless, the microbiota present in the semen and urine samples of fertile men presents 67.5% and 17.6% more OTUs, respectively, than prostatitis-like symptoms volunteer (Figure 1). We also observe men with prostatitis and fertile men share 144 operational taxonomic units (OTU). We also found no differences in the urine sample (inverted Simpson index median control 6.2 (4.5–6.8) vs. prostatitis 4.8 (4.3-12.2), $p = 0.8016$). Finally, we observed statistically significant differences in 14 OTUs in the different samples of the groups (Figure 2).

4. Discussion

This preliminary study evaluated some factors associated with chronic prostatitis by comparing fertile men with no urogenital infections and men with chronic prostatitis in a

TABLE 3: Concentrations of seminal cytokines in seminal and serum samples of the control group and prostatitis-like symptoms.

	Cytokine (pg/mL)	IL-12p70	IL-10	IL-1β	IL-6	IL-8	TNF	IL-2	IL-4	IL-10	IL-17	IFN-γ
Seminal samples	Fertile group	0[a] (0–1.9)	0 (0–0.8)	0 (0–4.5)	2.2 (0–32.7)	1812.0 (997.9–3299)	0 (0–7.1)	0 (0–27.09)	0 (0–6.3)	1.5 (0.0–18.3)	5.9 (5.3–10.2)	ND
	Prostatitis-like symptoms group	45.5 (0–252.8)	1.0 (0–29.4)	1.6 (0–31.6)	6.0 (01–100.9)	1230.0 (684.1–2533)	47.75 (0–127.5)	0.0 (0.0–116.3)	0 (0–20.25)	0.9 (0.0–21.3)	8.1 (5.5–48.1)	0 (0–22.1)
Serum samples	Fertile group	0 (0–210.3)	0 (0–199.1)	0 (0–455.7)	0 (0–304.2)	24.4 (0–313.5)	0 (0–50.8)	1.0 (0.0–176.1)	2.0 (0–13.5)	0.0 (0.0–7.3)	10.4 (9.1–24.8)	0 (0–5.3)
	Prostatitis-like symptoms group	ND	ND	ND	ND	2.2 (0.0–11.5)	0.0 (0.0–1.4)	0.0 (0.0–21.9)	4.5 (0–10.5)	0 (0–3.1)	17.1 (11.2–53.7)	0 (0–27.3)

Data indicate median (range). ND, not detected. [a]Significantly different from the control group: $p < 0.05$ (Mann–Whitney U test).

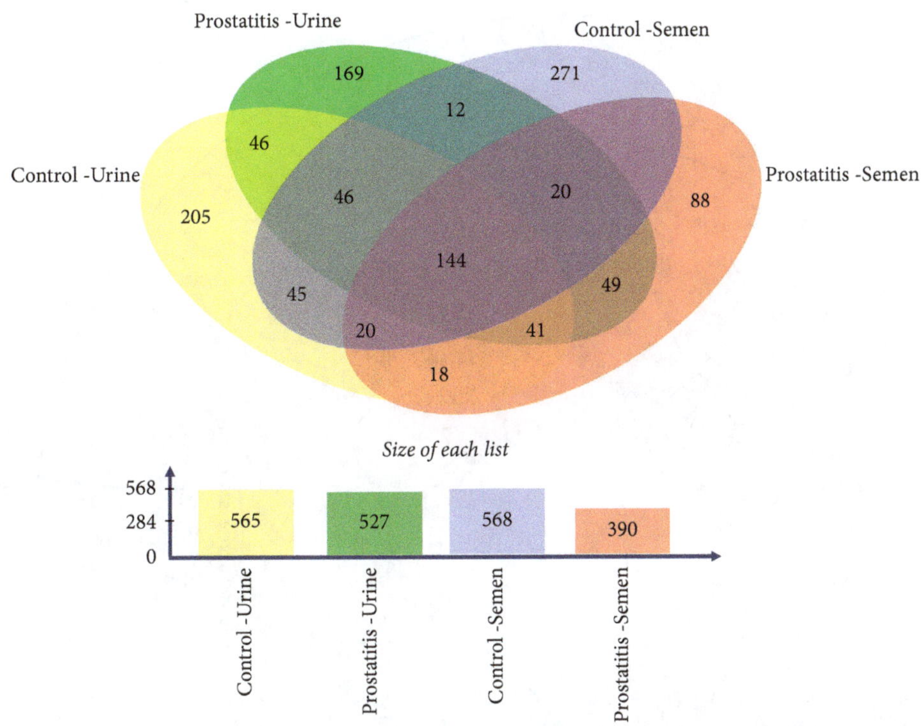

FIGURE 1: Venn diagram of OTU overlapping in urine and semen samples. (a) Venn diagram obtained with semen and urine samples from chronic prostatitis symptoms and fertile men showing that both types of samples in both groups share 144 OTUs. (b) Semen and urine samples from volunteers with chronic prostatitis showing a lower amount of OTU than samples from fertile men in the control group.

small sample of volunteers. We explored the microbial content of the semen and urine of men to evaluate the prostatitis effect on seminal parameters and fertility. We compared the conventional and functional seminal parameters of prostatitis symptoms with men who had a pregnant partner or children under two years of age.

We observed no differences in semen quality between both groups. In fact, the seminal parameters of the volunteers in both groups were higher than the WHO lower reference limit. Additionally, men with prostatitis also presented higher seminal concentration and high concentrations of IL-12p70 in serum. This proinflammatory cytokine is secreted mainly by macrophages and monocytes, stimulating the production of IFN-γ, which suggests a predominance of Th1 lymphocyte activation, facilitating the establishment of an inflammatory environment that becomes chronic [24].

The microbiome is composed of genetic material and microorganisms. It is also considered more complex than the human genome, and the microbiota refers to the population of bacteria present in various anatomical sites [10]. Although prostatitis is a multicausal condition, genitourinary infections are included among its causes, and the majority of bacterial prostatitis follows a urinary tract infection [1, 6]. However, the presence of microorganisms does not always imply disease, and caution is required in interpreting the microbiological results of urinary tract samples until the microbiota of this anatomical site is correctly established. An adequate association between symptoms and the detection of microorganisms should contribute to the diagnosis of prostatitis.

Bacterial diversity is a crucial factor in preventing the appearance of genitourinary diseases. The urine of prostatitis-like symptoms men presented 17.6% less diversity of OTUs than fertile men. This result was higher in the semen sample since 67.5% fewer OTUs were observed in the semen of prostatitis-like symptoms men. The urogenital tract microbiota of men with and without symptoms of prostatitis includes bacteria *Rhizobiaceae, Burkholderia, Achromobacter, Delftia, Campylobacter, Ezakiella, Anaerococcus, Prevotella, Haemophilus*, and *Porphyromonas*. Specifically, in urine, the most common bacterial genera in men with and without symptoms of prostatitis are *Pantoea, Geobacillus, Kocuria, Veillonella, Brevibacterium, Pseudomonas, Acetobacteraceae, Neisseria, Chryseobacterium*, and *Dialister* and in semen are *Weissella, Proteobacteria, Burkholderiales, Achromobacter, Campylobacter*, and *Prevotella* because today's available technique makes that some microorganisms are uncultivable in traditional microbial evaluation methods that are obsolete. *Prevotella* appeared to exert a negative effect on sperm quality [10]. *Firmicutes* (especially *Lactobacilli*), *Bacteroidetes, Proteobacteria*, and *Actinobacteria* comprise the highest proportion of the seminal microbiome [25].

In this preliminary study, we only found statistically significant differences in the presence of fourteen OTUs. These fourteen OTUs explain the difference in the microbiota of prostatitis-like symptoms and fertile men: *Burkholderiaceae, Achromobacter, Aerococcus, Blautia, Burkholderiales, Propionibacterium, Betaproteobacteria, Haemophilus, Burkholderia, Massilia, Rhizobiaceae*, and *Neorhizobium*. In general, they are little-known microorganisms in the clinical

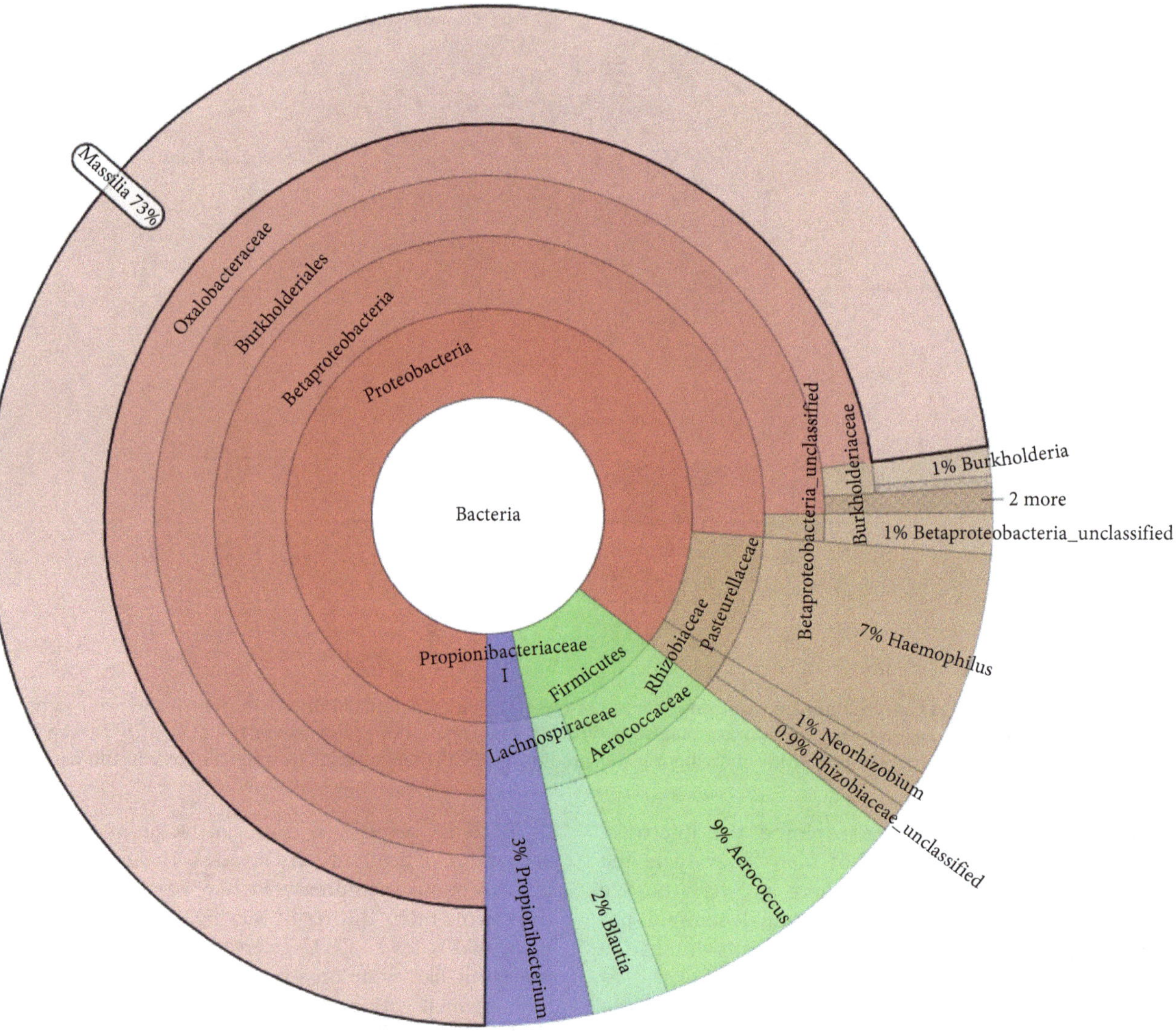

FIGURE 2: Different OTUs between prostatitis-like symptoms men and fertile men. Semen and urine samples from chronic prostatitis symptoms and fertile men differ statistically in 14 OTU. Most of them are not detectable by traditional culture techniques, which show the importance of sequencing in the study of prostate disease.

field, so sequencing is a powerful tool that allows us to discover the world surrounding enigmatic infectious diseases such as prostatitis [26–28]. Culture-based studies detected fewer anaerobic bacteria than NGS [10]. Few are the cases described for prostatitis caused by the *Burkholderia* genus. However, pulmonary infections by this microorganism that spread through the hematogenous route can reach the prostate causing chronic prostatitis [29]. The particularities in the microbial culture have made the accurate diagnosis of genitourinary infections difficult, as in *Corynebacterium urealyticum*, a Gram-positive, facultative anaerobic bacillus that is difficult to grow, responsible for prostatitis that is also associated with calcifications in the prostate [30]. Molecular tools allow the diagnosis of hidden infections in the light of traditional microbiological culture techniques.

Nevertheless, sequencing costs today are higher than traditional bacteriological methods; the microorganism's effect on fertility is still under discussion. Much more research is required to establish the microbiota of health and disease and validate powerful tools such as sequencing for daily use in the clinic. Microbiota studies are novel and have shown bacteria as a protective factor against disease; it should not be forgotten that bacteria can negatively impact sperm function [10]. However, studies evaluating the microbiota have used semen or urine samples, which could be biased by contaminating the sample collection [31].

Prostatitis is associated with affected male fertility, during illness can be affected semen quality, especially sperm concentration, motility, vitality, and morphology [25]. Semen and vaginal discharge are not sterile. The bacterial microbiome impacts on fertility and pregnancy [10], and this microbiome can be changed all the time, depending on such environmental factors and interaction with other organisms [31].

In addition to aerobic bacteria, anaerobes can also cause chronic bacterial prostatitis, mainly due to microorganisms such as *Peptostreptococcus* spp. and *Bacteroides* spp.

Knowledge about these infections is limited by the diagnostic methods, causing underestimating of the natural role of anaerobes [6].

The main limitations that affected the study quality included selecting participants using the NIH–CPSI without diagnostic imaging techniques, digital rectal examination, the use of the four-vessel test, and the limited number of participants in both groups. The selection of participants and the similarities of the patients, primarily in terms of age and most of the evaluated characteristics, allow us to somehow rule out the impact of lifestyle habits, features, and sexual behaviours over genitourinary microbiota.

5. Conclusion

Chronic prostatitis does not seem to affect seminal quality; however, more studies are required. The greater bacterial diversity of the genitourinary microbiota could be a protective factor for chronic prostatitis in men. Studying the factors associated with this greater microbial diversity will allow the establishment of healthy behaviours that limit the appearance of genitourinary diseases in men.

Acknowledgments

The authors acknowledge the valuable contributions of the volunteers. Puerta-Suárez J was supported by a fellowship from Minciencias (785-2017).

References

[1] C. E. Ejike and L. U. Ezeanyika, "Prevalence of chronic prostatitis symptoms in a randomly surveyed adult population of urban-community-dwelling Nigerian males," *International Journal of Urology*, vol. 15, no. 4, pp. 340–343, 2008.

[2] Y. Chen, K. M. Guo, T. Nagy, and T. L. Guo, "Chronic oral exposure to glycated whey proteins increases survival of aged male NOD mice with autoimmune prostatitis by regulating the gut microbiome and anti-inflammatory responses," *Food & Function*, vol. 11, no. 1, pp. 153–162, 2020.

[3] T. Cai, L. Gallelli, E. Cione, G. Perletti, F. Ciarleglio, and G. Malossini, "The use of Lactobacillus casei DG® prevents symptomatic episodes and reduces the antibiotic use in patients affected by chronic bacterial prostatitis: results from a phase IV study," *World Journal of Urology*, 2021.

[4] S. D. Lundy, N. Sangwan, N. V. Parekh, M. K. P. Selvam, S. Gupta, and P. McCaffrey, "Functional and taxonomic dysbiosis of the gut, urine, and semen microbiomes in male infertility," *European Urology*, vol. 76, 2021.

[5] J. C. Nickel, J. Downey, D. Hunter, and J. Clark, "Prevalence of prostatitis-like symptoms in a population based study using the national institutes of health chronic prostatitis symptom index," *The Journal of Urology*, vol. 165, no. 3, pp. 842–845, 2001.

[6] J. Videcnik Zorman, M. Maticic, S. Jeverica, and T. Smrkolj, "Diagnosis and treatment of bacterial prostatitis," *Acta Dermatovenerologica Alpina Pannonica et Adriatica*, vol. 24, no. 2, pp. 25–29, 2015.

[7] S. Kumar, A. Dave, B. Wolf, and E. V. Lerma, "Urinary tract infections," *Disease-A-Month*, vol. 61, no. 2, pp. 45–59, 2015.

[8] Y. Shang, C. Liu, D. Cui, G. Han, and S. Yi, "The effect of chronic bacterial prostatitis on semen quality in adult men: a meta-analysis of case-control studies," *Scientific Reports*, vol. 4, no. 1, p. 7233, 2014.

[9] E. M. Meares Jr. and T. A. Stamey, "The diagnosis and management of bacterial prostatitis," *British Journal of Urology*, vol. 44, no. 2, pp. 175–179, 1972.

[10] L. Farahani, T. Tharakan, T. Yap, J. Ramsay, C. Jayasena, and S. Minhas, "The semen microbiome and its impact on sperm function and male fertility: a systematic review and meta-analysis," *Andrology*, vol. 9, 2020.

[11] A. Budía, J. Luis Palmero, E. Broseta et al., "Value of semen culture in the diagnosis of chronic bacterial prostatitis: a simplified method," *Scandinavian Journal of Urology and Nephrology*, vol. 40, no. 4, pp. 326–331, 2006.

[12] M. S. Litwin, M. McNaughton-Collins, F. J. Fowler et al., "The national institutes of health chronic prostatitis symptom index," *The Journal of Urology*, vol. 162, no. 2, pp. 369–375, 1999.

[13] M. M. Collins, M. P. O'Leary, E. A. Calhoun et al., "The Spanish national institutes of health-chronic prostatitis symptom index," *The Journal of Urology*, vol. 166, no. 5, pp. 1800–1803, 2001.

[14] L. R. Zegarra Montes, A. A. Sanchez Mejia, C. A. Loza Munarriz, and E. C. Gutierrez, "Semen and urine culture in the diagnosis of chronic bacterial prostatitis," *International Brazilian Journal of Urology*, vol. 34, no. 1, pp. 30–40, 2008.

[15] World Health Organization, *WHO Laboratory Manual for the Examination and Processing of Human Semen*, World Health Organization, Geneva, Switzerland, 2010.

[16] W. Cardona-Maya, J. Berdugo, and A. Cadavid, "Comparación de la concentración espermática usando la cámara de Makler y la cámara de Neubauer," *Actas Urológicas Españolas*, vol. 32, no. 4, pp. 443–445, 2008.

[17] B. J. M. Mayorga-Torres, W. Cardona-Maya, Á. Cadavid, and M. Camargo, "Evaluation of sperm functional parameters in normozoospermic infertile individuals," *Actas Urológicas Españolas*, vol. 37, no. 4, pp. 221–227, 2013.

[18] F. Martínez-Pastor, M. Mata-Campuzano, M. Álvarez-Rodríguez, M. Álvarez, L. Anel, and P. de Paz, "Probes and techniques for sperm evaluation by flow cytometry," *Reproduction in Domestic Animals*, vol. 45, no. 2, pp. 67–78, 2010.

[19] D. P. Evenson, K. L. Larson, and L. K. Jost, "Sperm chromatin structure assay: its clinical use for detecting sperm DNA fragmentation in male infertility and comparisons with other techniques," *Journal of Andrology*, vol. 23, no. 1, pp. 25–43, 2002.

[20] R. J. Aitken, J. K. Wingate, G. N. De Iuliis, and E. A. McLaughlin, "Analysis of lipid peroxidation in human spermatozoa using BODIPY C11," *MHR: Basic science of reproductive medicine*, vol. 13, no. 4, pp. 203–211, 2007.

[21] A. M. Gil-Villa, W. Cardona-Maya, A. Agarwal, R. Sharma, and Á. Cadavid, "Assessment of sperm factors possibly involved in early recurrent pregnancy loss," *Fertility and Sterility*, vol. 94, no. 4, pp. 1465–1472, 2010.

[22] M. Serafini, G. Maiani, and A. Ferro-Luzzi, "Alcohol-free red wine enhances plasma antioxidant capacity in humans," *Journal of Nutrition*, vol. 128, no. 6, pp. 1003–1007, 1998.

[23] W. Cardona Maya, "World Health Organization manual for the processing of human semen-2010," *Actas Urológicas Españolas*, vol. 34, no. 7, pp. 577-578, 2010.

[24] Y. Liu, R. Mikrani, D. Xie et al., "Chronic prostatitis/chronic pelvic pain syndrome and prostate cancer: study of immune cells and cytokines," *Fundamental & Clinical Pharmacology*, vol. 34, no. 2, pp. 160–172, 2020.

[25] R. Mändar, M. Punab, P. Korrovits et al., "Seminal microbiome in men with and without prostatitis," *International Journal of Urology*, vol. 24, no. 3, pp. 211–216, 2017.

[26] M. Zhang, Y. Liu, J. Chen, L. Chen, J. Meng, and C. Yang, "Single-cell multi-omics analysis presents the landscape of peripheral blood T-cell subsets in human chronic prostatitis/chronic pelvic pain syndrome," *Journal of Cellular and Molecular Medicine*, vol. 24, 2020.

[27] X. Cui, M. Naveed, M. M. F. A. Baig et al., "Therapeutic effects of Qianlie Tongli decoction on chronic prostatitis/chronic pelvic pain syndrome induced by peptide T2 in mice," *Journal of Pharmacy and Pharmacology*, vol. 72, no. 10, pp. 1436–1444, 2020.

[28] R. D. Motrich, M. L. Breser, R. I. Molina, A. Tissera, J. J. Olmedo, and V. E. Rivero, "Patients with chronic prostatitis/chronic pelvic pain syndrome show T helper type 1 (Th1) and Th17 self-reactive immune responses specific to prostate and seminal antigens and diminished semen quality," *BJU International*, vol. 126, no. 3, pp. 379–387, 2020.

[29] S. Bahal, N. Verma, S. Tadros, D. M. Lowe, and S. O. Burns, "A case of Burkholderia prostatitis in a patient with chronic granulomatous disease," *Journal of Clinical Immunology*, vol. 40, no. 8, pp. 1204–1206, 2020.

[30] D. Nicolosi, C. Genovese, M. A. Cutuli, F. D'Angeli, L. Pietrangelo, and S. Davinelli, "Preliminary in vitro studies on Corynebacterium urealyticum pathogenetic mechanisms, a possible candidate for chronic idiopathic prostatitis?" *Microorganisms*, vol. 8, no. 4, 2020.

[31] V. Mouraviev and M. McDonald, "An implementation of next generation sequencing for prevention and diagnosis of urinary tract infection in urology," *The Canadian Journal of Urology*, vol. 25, no. 3, pp. 9349–9356, 2018.

Experience with Renal Autotransplantation: Typical and Atypical Indications

Ali Bourgi, Rana Aoun, Elias Ayoub, and Maroun Moukarzel

Department of Urology, Hotel-Dieu de France University Hospital, Boulevard Alfred Naccache, Achrafieh, P.O. Box 166830, Beirut, Lebanon

Correspondence should be addressed to Ali Bourgi; alibourgi@gmail.com

Academic Editor: Miroslav Djordjevic

Introduction and Objectives. Renal autotransplantation is a kidney-saving surgical procedure used in selected patients. The purpose of this report is to review nine typical and atypical indications for kidney autotransplantation and evaluate its effectiveness in maintaining kidney function and avoiding cancer recurrence. *Materials and Methods.* From 1999 till 2014, nine renal autotransplantations were performed in our center. A retrospective case review was done. Four of nine patients had a solitary functioning kidney. Typical indications for autotransplantation included extended ureteric disease in 5 patients, intrasinusal tumor on a solitary kidney in 1 patient, and renal artery aneurysm in 1 patient. Atypical indications consisted in bilateral urothelial tumors in 1 patient and interrupted live kidney transplantation in 1 patient. Mean cold ischemia time was 209 minutes. Demographic factors, indications, renal function before and after surgery, and in the long term, cancer recurrence and disease-free survival were evaluated. *Results.* Renal function was maintained in 8 patients during the early follow-up. No serious complications occurred in the postoperative period. Median duration of follow-up was 50 months. In 4 patients with a normal contralateral kidney, mean preoperative and at discharge creatinine clearance were 105.45 ml/min and 121.02 ml/min, respectively. Although values showed an improvement in the kidney function, the difference was not significant (p value 0.3). In the other 4 patients with a solitary kidney, mean discharge creatinine clearance was 99.24 ml/min surprisingly higher than the preoperative value 96.92 ml/min. At the last follow-up, kidney function was preserved for the two groups (normal contralateral kidney/solitary kidney) with relatively stable creatinine clearance values: 108.45 ml/min and 85.9 ml/min, respectively. No patients required secondary dialysis. *Conclusion.* Renal autotransplantation is a rare, safe, and effective surgical procedure for the treatment of complex urologic conditions. In some instances, it may be of great utility for kidney salvage in some carefully selected patients.

1. Introduction

Renal autotransplantation (RA) is a rare, safe, and effective surgical procedure for the treatment of complex urologic conditions. It was first reported by J. D. Hardy in 1963 when he repaired a high ureteric injury following aortic surgery by reimplanting the repaired organ into the ipsilateral iliac fossa.

Hardy's accomplishment was made possible, thanks to allotransplantation techniques developed by Dr Murray and colleagues in Boston a decade earlier. Managing renal disease via a "benchwork" approach soon became a novel idea pursued worldwide by surgeons [1].

After this landmark surgery, RA has been steadily improved to a safe and effective procedure and has been used in the treatment of different complex urologic diseases like extensive ureteric injuries, complex nephrolithiasis, loin-pain syndrome, renovascular diseases (stenotic lesions of distal renal arteries, intrarenal aneurysms, and arteriovenous malformations), tumors of the kidney and ureter, and retroperitoneal fibrosis [2], even more in rare and unusual critical situations.

As minimal invasive surgery has started to take the lead, decrease in surgical morbidity is now seen with laparoscopic and even completely intracorporeal robotic surgery [3].

The purpose of this report is to present nine typical and atypical indications for kidney autotransplantation in order to evaluate its effectiveness in maintaining kidney function and avoiding cancer recurrence and to review the current literature.

Table 1: Demographic and preoperative data in study population.

Patient	Age	Sex	BMI (kg/m^2)	Indication for autotransplantation	Contralateral kidney
1	42	M	27.42	Extended left ureteral injury	Right kidney agenesis
2	52	F	27.34	Extended left ureteral injury	Nonfunctioning right kidney due to neglected ureteropelvic junction
3	60	F	22.8	Interrupted living kidney donor due to perioperative cardiac failure in the recipient	Normal
4	60	M	33.4	5.5 right hilum tumor (ex vivo repair)	Left nephrectomy for familial living donor
5	61	M	31.31	Right ureter fibrosis after radiotherapy for prostate cancer	Chronic renal failure
6	32	F	21.48	Left ureteral injury (stripping during ureteroscopy)	Normal
7	38	F	21.03	Right extended ureteral stenosis	Normal
8	38	F	22.58	Left renal artery aneurysm (ex vivo repair)	Normal
9	65	M	20.28	Bilateral ureteral and pelvic tumor	Nephroureterectomy for right ureteral and pelvic tumor

Table 2: Perioperative and postoperative parameters.

	Patient 1	Patient 2	Patient 3	Patient 4	Patient 5	Patient 6	Patient 7	Patient 8	Patient 9
Operating time (hours)	8	8	6.5	8.5	10	9	6	7.5	11
Duration of ischemia (min)	70	180	215	270	230	230	145	240	300
Duration of hospitalization (days)	17	8	7	16	12	18	9	7	14
Pre-op creatinine clearance (ml/min)	139.77	108.54	113.33	79.37	60.03	57.01	106.1	145.3	59.5
Creatinine clearance at discharge (ml/min)	157.27	109.4	123.19	40.26	90.04	76.69	153.2	131	23.6
Duration of follow-up (months)	120	6	12	60	24	72	24	120	48
Creatinine clearance at the last follow-up (ml/min)	154.29	91.52	107.24	61.6	36.21	72.68	127.78	126.1	41.93

2. Materials and Methods

From 1999 till 2014, nine renal autotransplantations were performed in our center (Hotel Dieu de France University Hospital). A retrospective case review was done. The series included five females and four males with a mean age of 49.8 years. 4/9 patients had a solitary functioning kidney. Typical indications for autotransplantation included extended ureteric disease in 5 patients, intrasinusal tumor on a solitary kidney in 1 patient, and renal artery aneurysm in 1 patient. Atypical indications consisted in bilateral urothelial tumors in 1 patient and interrupted live kidney transplantation in 1 patient.

The kidneys were removed through a flank incision over the 11th rib or laparoscopically and transplanted to the iliac fossa. In all patients, the ureter was reimplanted in the bladder using the Lich–Gregoir technique. Mean cold ischemia time was 209 minutes.

Demographic factors, indications, renal function before and after surgery, and in the long term, cancer recurrence and disease-free survival were evaluated (Tables 1–3).

3. Results

Renal function was evaluated by creatinine clearance estimate using the Cockcroft–Gault equation. This was maintained in 8 patients during the early follow-up (Figure 1).

No serious complications occurred in the postoperative period. Median duration of follow-up was 50 months. In 4 patients with a normal contralateral kidney, mean preoperative and at discharge creatinine clearance were 105.45 ml/min and 121.02 ml/min, respectively. Although values showed an improvement in the kidney function, the difference was not deemed significant (p value 0.3).

In the other 4 patients with a solitary kidney, mean discharge creatinine clearance was 99.24 ml/min surprisingly higher than the preoperative value 96.92 ml/min. Note that the difference between these means was not significant (p value 0.72). At the last follow-up, kidney function was preserved for the two groups (normal contralateral kidney/solitary kidney) with relatively stable creatinine clearance values: 108.45 ml/min and 85.9 ml/min, respectively. No patients required secondary dialysis. The patient with bilateral pelvic and ureteric tumors is still cancer free, 7 years after surgery, with no recurrence on the annual CT scan. Finally, the patient with solitary kidney and intrasinusal tumor is also cancer free after 10 years of follow-up.

4. Discussion

The main reason for the use of kidney autotransplantation is to preserve renal parenchyma. RA is generally reserved to severe situations and is often the last option before nephrectomy. Previous studies have emphasized AR as a highly effective surgical procedure for the treatment of renal pathologies.

The most common indications of RA are the extensive ureteral lesions. In fact, it allows a direct pelvivesical anastomosis. Indeed RA is a viable option for complicated ureteral lesions and

Table 3: Perioperative and postoperative complications.

Patient	Complications
1	Immediate renal artery thrombosis necessitating retransplantation of the kidney in the contralateral iliac fossa
2	Urinary infection
3	None
4	Acute tubular necrosis, pneumonia
5	Intestinal occlusion medically resolved
6	Urinary infection
7	None
8	Urinary infection
9	None

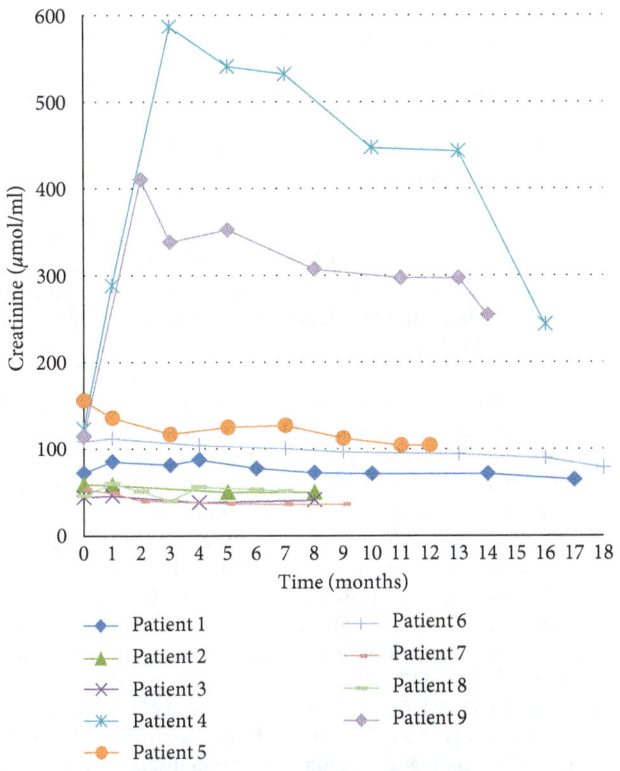

Figure 1: Early outcome: renal function.

is an alternative to known methods not limited to psoas Hitch procedure, Boari flap, and transureteroureterostomy [4].

In the oncological setting, no study aimed at comparing the oncological outcome after autotransplantation versus radical surgery, but in most published papers, low recurrence rate and few complications were reported with autotransplantation in patients with renal or ureteral tumors.

The first paper was published in 1984 by Pettersson et al. [4] who performed nephroureterectomy, renal autotransplantation, and pyelocystostomy in eight patients with upper urinary tract urothelial carcinoma. Five of eight patients remained cancer free after 32 months of follow-up. Radical surgery had to be done in one patient after 4.5 years because of infiltrating tumor recurrence, and transurethral endoscopic resection was done successfully in three patients with calyceal recurrence. Pettersson et al. concluded that this procedure implies increased radicality compared with conventional conservative treatment and simplified follow-up. It may be considered in patients with bilateral tumors or tumors of a solitary kidney and in selected patients with unilateral low-grade, low-stage tumors [5].

The longest follow-up was reported by Holmang and Johansson in 2005 [6]. His study was conducted on 23 patients with urothelial neoplasm in the upper urinary tract, operated with resection and autotransplantation than followed for 7 to 20 years. Of the nine patients who had solitary kidney or bilateral tumors, three patients survived with no recurrences and no dialysis after 238 and 127 months, respectively, three patients required dialysis 2 to 9 years later, and 3 patients died of the disease. Concerning patients with normal contralateral kidney, Holmang and Johansson argued that resection and renal autotransplantation are not indicated and might even be harmful, compared to standard nephroureterectomy [6].

Ex vivo nephron-sparing surgery for renal carcinoma is also an option in solitary kidney or in bilateral tumors.

The term "bench surgery" is used to describe reconstructive surgery on diseased kidneys receiving asanguineous perfusion outside the body. The first uses of bench surgery were reported by Corman et al. in 1973. Their report and subsequent ones about bench surgery have shown how this sophisticated approach is a significant advance in urologic operative procedures.

In their report, Putnam et al. [7] reported two uses of bench surgery (staghorn calculi in a solitary kidney and abdominal aortic aneurysm with abnormalities of both renal arteries and early renal failure).

One study published in 1985 by Mayo Clinic showed similar rates of nonprogression (76%) and survival (87%) in patients with low-grade (1 or 2), low-stage (I or II), bilateral or solitary renal cell carcinoma treated with conservative surgical treatment (in situ enucleation, in situ partial nephrectomy, or an extracorporeal operation) compared to radical surgery after 5 years of follow-up [8].

Two recent studies on ex vivo nephron-sparing surgery for renal carcinoma were published in 2014.

The first series included 9 patients. The absolute indications were organ saving and technical impossibility of renal tumor resection in situ. The mean duration of operation was 297.8 minutes, and the mean period of hypothermic ischemia consisted of 112.6 minutes. A postoperative follow-up (maximum 4 years) revealed that there is not noted dissemination of the tumor, and functional condition of the transplanted kidney was satisfactory [9].

The second series included 3 patients. Two patients had complex renal cell carcinoma, and 1 patient had bilateral large angiomyolipoma. All 3 patients did not have renal replacement therapy and currently live a good quality of life. According to the authors, the advantage of this procedure over renal replacement therapy is better quality of life and cost-effectiveness [10].

In this new era of minimal invasive surgery, laparoscopic renal harvest for autotransplantation provided an opportunity to decrease morbidity. Fabrizio et al. performed the first laparoscopic nephrectomy with open autotransplantation (kidney extraction was done through a periumbilical incision followed by a transplantation through a Gibson incision) [11].

Gill et al. described retroperitoneoscopic laparoscopic nephrectomy followed by open autotransplantation using a Gibson incision for both extraction and subsequent transplantation [12].

One of the largest series of laparoscopic nephrectomies for autotransplantation was reported by Tran et al. in 2015 including 52 patients with more than 90% success rate over a 6-year follow-up period [13].

Also, although a very challenging procedure, completely intracorporeal robot-assisted nephrectomy with RA is now a feasible approach to renal preservation after major ureteral injury [3].

Finally, a randomized study comparing RA to another approach like "bowel interposition" is necessary to determine the differences in benefits and risks associated with these procedures.

Analysis of values and changes in renal clearance revealed that the majority of patients had an improvement in renal function, with the exception of two patients with a postoperative clearance of <60 ml/min (36.21 and 41.5 ml/min, resp.), knowing that these 2 patients had some degree of kidney failure before surgery (preoperative clearance of 60.5 and 59.5 ml/min, resp.). This reflects the improvement in renal function and the rarity of delayed complications.

In our study, the patient with pelvic and bilateral ureteral tumors showed remission, without any recurrence on the annual scan even 7 years after the surgery, as well as for the patient with a solitary and an intrasinusal tumor who is disease free after 10 years of follow-up.

In this study, the relatively long follow-up (average of 55 months) empowers the study and explains RAs validity and effectiveness. However, a retrospective study like ours could be criticized. The limited number of patients enrolled, the one center-one surgeon experience are some of the limitations of this study.

5. Conclusion

Renal autotransplantation is a rare, safe, and effective surgical procedure for the treatment of complex urologic conditions. In some instances, it may be of great utility for kidney salvage in some carefully selected patients. Our center's experience in renal autotransplantation showed low complications rate, preserved kidney function, and no cancer recurrence on the early and late follow-up.

Ethical Approval

All procedures performed in studies involving human participants were in accordance with the ethical standards of the institutional and/or national research committee and with the 1964 Helsinki Declaration and its later amendments or comparable ethical standards.

Consent

Informed consent was obtained from all individual participants included in the study.

Authors' Contributions

Ali Bourgi performed project development and manuscript writing. Rana Aoun was involved in data collection. Elias Ayoub did manuscript writing. Maroun Moukarzel was responsible for data analysis and manuscript editing.

References

[1] R. H. Dean, P. W. Meacham, and F. A. Weaver, "Ex vivo renal artery reconstructions: indications and techniques," *Journal of Vascular Surgery*, vol. 4, no. 6, pp. 546–552, 1986.

[2] A. M. Meraney, I. S. Gill, J. H. Kaouk, M. Skacel, and G. T. Sung, "Second prize (Co-winner): laparoscopic renal autotransplantation," *Journal of Endourology*, vol. 15, no. 2, pp. 143–149, 2001.

[3] Z. N. Gordon, J. Angell, and R. Abaza, "Completely intracorporeal robotic renal autotransplantation," *The Journal of Urology*, vol. 192, no. 5, pp. 1516–1522, 2014.

[4] S. Pettersson, H. Brynger, C. Henriksson, S. L. Johansson, A. E. Nilson, and T. Ranch, "Treatment of urothelial tumors of the upper urinary tract by nephroureterectomy, renal autotransplantation, and pyelocystostomy," *Cancer*, vol. 54, no. 3, pp. 379–386, 1984.

[5] S. Pettersson, H. Brynger, S. Johansson, and A. E. Nilson, "Extracorporeal surgery and autotransplantation for carcinoma of the pelvis and ureter," *Scandinavian Journal of Urology and Nephrology*, vol. 13, no. 1, pp. 89–93, 1979.

[6] S. Holmäng and S. L. Johansson, "Tumours of the ureter and renal pelvis treated with resection and renal autotransplantation: a study with up to 20 years of follow-up," *BJU International*, vol. 95, no. 9, pp. 1201–1205, 2005.

[7] C. W. Putnam, C. G. Halgrimson, D. P. Stables et al., "Ex vivo renal perfusion and autotransplantation in treatment of calculous disease or abdominal aortic aneurysm," *Urology*, vol. 5, no. 3, pp. 337–342, 1975.

[8] H. Zincke, D. E. Engen, K. M. Henning, and M. W. McDonald, "Treatment of renal cell carcinoma by in situ partial nephrectomy and extracorporeal operation with autotransplantation," *Mayo Clinic Proceedings*, vol. 60, no. 10, pp. 651–662, 1985.

[9] B. K. Komiakov, S. A. Zamiatnin, S. V. Popov, V. V. Shlomin, A. V. Tsygankov, and I. S. Gonchar, "Extracorporal surgical treatment of patients with renal cell carcinoma," *Vestnik Khirurgii Imeni II Grekova*, vol. 173, no. 4, pp. 53–56, 2013.

[10] G. P. Abraham, A. T. Siddaiah, K. Ramaswami, D. George, and K. Das, "Ex-vivo nephron-sparing surgery and autotransplantation for renal tumours: Revisited," *Canadian Urological Association Journal*, vol. 8, no. 9-10, p. E728, 2014.

[11] M. D. Fabrizio, L. R. Kavoussi, S. Jackman, D. Y. Chan, E. Tseng, and L. E. Ratner, "Laparoscopic nephrectomy for autotransplantation," *Urology*, vol. 55, no. 1, p. 145, 2000.

[12] I. S. Gill, R. G. Uzzo, M. G. Hobart, S. B. Streem, D. A. Goldfarb, and M. J. Noble, "Laparoscopic retroperitoneal live donor right nephrectomy for purposes of allotransplantation and autotransplantation," *The Journal of Urology*, vol. 164, no. 5, pp. 1500–1504, 2000.

[13] G. Tran, K. Ramaswamy, T. Chi, M. Meng, C. Freise, and M. L. Stoller, "Laparoscopic nephrectomy with autotransplantation: Safety, efficacy and long-term durability," *Journal of Urology*, vol. 194, no. 3, pp. 738–743, 2015.

28

Antibiotic Prophylaxis with Trimethoprim-Sulfamethoxazole versus No Treatment after Mid-to-Distal Hypospadias Repair

Elizabeth B. Roth, John V. Kryger, Charles T. Durkee, Melissa A. Lingongo, Ruth M. Swedler, and Travis W. Groth

Division of Pediatric Urology, Department of Urology, Medical College of Wisconsin, Children's Hospital of Wisconsin, Milwaukee, WI, USA

Correspondence should be addressed to Travis W. Groth; tgroth@chw.org

Academic Editor: Kostis Gyftopoulos

Purpose. To evaluate the impact of prophylactic antibiotics after distal hypospadias repair on postoperative bacteriuria, symptomatic urinary tract infection, and postoperative complications in a prospective, randomized trial. *Materials and Methods.* Consecutive patients aged 6 months to 2 years were enrolled at our institution between June 2013 and May 2017. Consenting patients were randomized to antibiotic prophylaxis with trimethoprim-sulfamethoxazole versus no antibiotic. Patients had catheterized urine samples obtained at surgery and 6–10 days postoperatively. The primary outcome was bacteriuria and pyuria at postoperative urine collection. Secondary outcomes included symptomatic urinary tract infection and postoperative complications. *Results.* 70 patients consented to the study, of which 35 were randomized to receive antibiotics compared to 32 who did not. Demographics, severity of hypospadias, and type of repair were similar between the groups. Patients in the treatment group had significantly less pyuria (18%) and bacteriuria (11%) present at stent removal compared to the nontreatment group (55% and 63%; $p = 0.01$ and $p < 0.001$, resp.). No patient had a symptomatic urinary tract infection. There were 11 postoperative complications. *Conclusions.* Routine antibiotic prophylaxis appears to significantly decrease bacteriuria and pyuria in the immediate postoperative period; however, no difference was observed in symptomatic urinary tract infection or postoperative complications.

1. Introduction

Hypospadias occurs in at least 1/300 live births [1], making it one of the most common entities treated by pediatric urologists. A 2010 report of practice patterns among pediatric urologists in North America showed that >90% place patients on routine antibiotic prophylaxis after single-stage hypospadias repair requiring use of a urethral stent [2]. As such, this represents a significant utilization of antibiotics in the pediatric urology practice. While antibiotic prophylaxis has been extensively studied in patients with other urologic conditions, including hydronephrosis and vesicoureteral reflux, less is known about the efficacy and necessity of antibiotic prophylaxis in the setting of hypospadias repair.

Three studies in the literature have previously examined this question [3–5] but reached different conclusions regarding the efficacy of prophylaxis. Meir and Livne showed support for prophylaxis, with increased bacteriuria and a clinical urinary tract infection rate of 24% in children who did not receive postoperative antibiotic prophylaxis as compared to those that did [3]. Conversely, a study by Kanaroglou et al. showed no difference in symptomatic urinary tract infections or postoperative complications between two retrospective cohorts of patients, one receiving antibiotic prophylaxis and one not receiving prophylaxis [4]. A more recent study in Sweden reported a higher complication rate (26% versus 15%) and a similar infection rate (5% versus 4%) in children receiving a decreased two-dose antibiotic course as compared to full-dose TMP-SMX in children who underwent tubularized incised plate repair [5]. To date, no published study has prospectively examined the efficacy of antibiotics at a prophylactic dose in the acute postoperative setting after single-stage primary repair of mid-to-distal hypospadias. Our study aims to address this question with regard to urine characteristics in the postoperative period as well as clinical outcomes of postoperative complications and symptomatic UTIs.

2. Materials and Methods

After approval by our institutional review board, we prospectively enrolled patients between 6 months and 2 years of age with mid-to-distal shaft hypospadias scheduled for elective primary hypospadias repair at our institution between June 2013 and May 2017. Children with proximal hypospadias or a history of previous hypospadias repair were excluded, as were children with allergies to trimethoprim-sulfamethoxazole (TMP-SMX). Children were randomized into treatment (TMP-SMX prophylaxis at 3 mg/kg trimethoprim daily) versus nontreatment. Simple randomization using a random number generator was used to assign patients to treatment versus nontreatment groups. Surgeons were not aware of the patient's randomization at the time of surgery, and the surgical technique was not standardized. Patients did not routinely receive IV antibiotics perioperatively, and the treatment group was instructed to begin TMP-SMX on the evening of surgery and continue until the evening prior to catheter removal in the clinic. Postoperative care was standardized for all patients utilizing the same 6 Fr Kendall-type hydrophilic urethral stent (Covidien Dover Hydrogel Coated Urethral Catheter 6 Fr #6006) and double diaper urinary drainage for 6–10 days following surgery. All children had urine samples obtained intraoperatively and at the first postoperative clinic visit prior to catheter removal. Patients in the treatment group were asked to return study medication at their first postoperative clinic visit, and residual TMP-SMX was measured to assess compliance with the regimen.

The postoperative urine sample was obtained by cleaning the catheter hub with alcohol followed by clamping the catheter for 15–30 minutes to allow an adequate amount of urine to collect in the bladder. The catheter hub was then reprepped with alcohol and urine obtained prior to catheter removal.

Our primary endpoints were bacteriuria and pyuria at the time of the first postoperative visit. We defined bacteriuria as the presence of >50,000 colony-forming units on postoperative urine culture. These were chosen as primary endpoints due to the wide range of symptomatic UTIs in the postoperative period after hypospadias repair in previous studies (0–24%) and due the subjective nature of determining positive symptoms in this nonverbal population [3–5]. Power calculations based on published symptomatic UTI after hypospadias repair in the literature estimated 160 patients, 80 in each study arm to achieve 80% power with 95% confidence. Power calculations based on our primary endpoints were not performed as the prevalence of bacteriuria and pyuria in this population is not well established.

Secondary endpoints were symptomatic UTI, defined as fever, pain, or other clinical symptoms consistent with UTI along with a urine culture of >50,000 CFU, and postoperative complications. Positive cultures without symptoms were not routinely treated to avoid exposure of either group to additional antibiotics. Measured postoperative complications included wound infection, urethrocutaneous fistula, wound dehiscence, and meatal stenosis. Data analysis was completed using standard, 2-tailed univariate statistical tests with significance of $p < 0.05$. Continuous variables were assessed with Student's t-test, and categorical variables were assessed utilizing the Fisher exact test.

3. Results

Of 113 consecutive eligible patients, 70 consented to the study. Thirty-five were randomized to receive TMP-SMX prophylaxis at 3 mg/kg daily, and 32 received no antibiotics. Three patients who enrolled in the study were unable to be randomized, one due to finding a proximal hypospadias during reexam under anesthesia at the time of operative repair and two due to lack of pharmacy support to provide the study drug should they be randomized to treatment with TMP-SMX. One patient in the nontreatment group had bacteria present on urinalysis in the OR and was excluded from further analysis (Figure 1).

Demographic and clinical data about hypospadias severity and type of repair were similar between both groups. Treatment group patients presented for surgery at 9.8 ± 3.1 months of age compared to 10.5 ± 4.7 months in the nontreatment group ($p = 0.45$). Weight, presence of chordee, urethral deficit length, glans size, and type of repair were not significantly different between the two groups (Table 1). Study medication was returned by 31/35 patients, and 30 patients returned an amount consistent with >90% compliance with the prescribed regimen.

Postoperative urine samples were successfully obtained on 30/35 patients in the treatment group and 22/32 patients in the nontreatment group ($p = 0.14$). Among the 15 patients unable to provide postoperative urinalysis or culture, 6 patients experienced premature catheter removal outside the clinic, 4 specimens were unable to be processed by the lab, 3 patients were unable to retain urine in the bladder during the clamping period, 1 parent refused specimen collection at postoperative visit, and 1 was excluded due to the presence of bacteria in urine at the time of surgery.

Leukocyte esterase was detected in 18% (5/28) of samples in the treatment group and 55% (11/20) of samples in the nontreatment group ($p = 0.01$). Similarly, bacteriuria on urine microscopy was present in 11% (3/25) patients in the treatment group and 63% (7/19) of the nontreatment group ($p < 0.001$). Urine culture was positive for a single organism of at least 50,000 colony-forming units in 7% (2/30) of the treatment group and 64% (10/22) of the nontreatment group ($p < 0.001$). Organisms isolated from the cultures are reported in Table 2. Of 17 isolated organisms isolated from no treatment group tested against TMP-SMX, resistance was reported in 2/17 organisms (*E. coli* × 2) compared to 3/3 organisms (*E. coli* and *Enterococcus* species × 2) in the treatment group ($p = 0.009$).

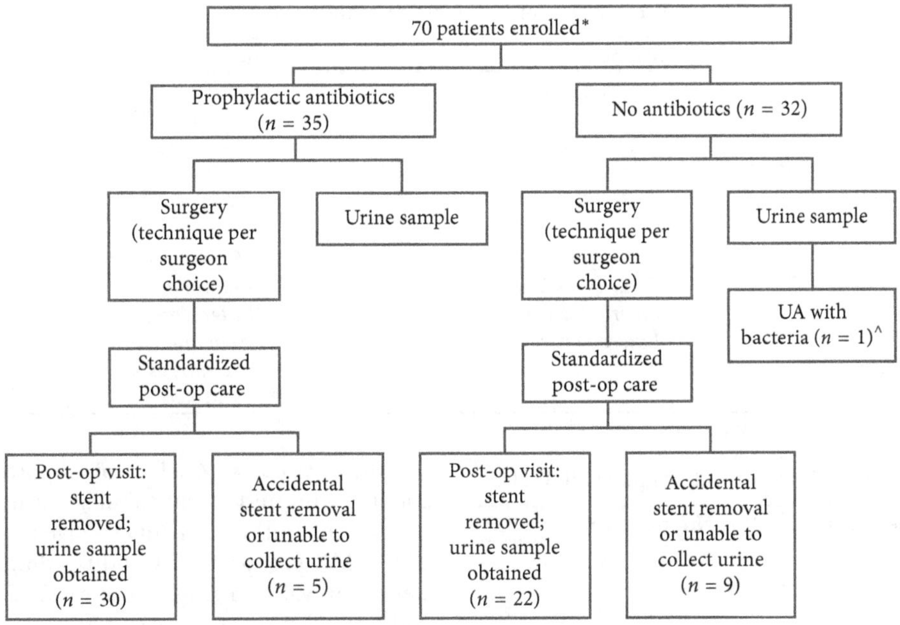

Figure 1: Study design. *3 patients withdrawn after enrolling in the study: 1 with proximal hypospadias on reexam at the time of surgery and 2 patients due to lack of pharmacy support to dispense the study drug if randomized to the treatment group. ^The patient excluded from further analysis due to bacteriuria at surgery.

Table 1: Patient and hypospadias characteristics and repair type in treatment and nontreatment groups.

	Treatment ($n = 35$)	Nontreatment ($n = 32$)	p value
Age (months)	9.8 (±3.1)	10.5 (±4.7)	0.45
Weight (kg)	9.2 (±1.3)	9.3 (±2.0)	0.68
Type of hypospadias			
Midshaft	2	2	0.90
Distal shaft	27	26	
Megameatus	6	4	
Chordee present	20/33	19/31	0.96
Preop testosterone	5	2	0.43
Type of surgery			
TIP repair	17	18	0.74
Matthieu	4	4	
MAGPI	7	4	
Pyramid repair	6	4	
Urethral advancement	1	2	
Meatus to the tip of glans (mm)	8.0 (±2.6)	9.4 (±2.6)	0.05
Glans size (mm)	13.9 (±3.1)	14.6 (±2.3)	0.36

Postoperative complications were reported in 5/35 patients in the treatment group and 6/32 patients in the nontreatment group ($p = 0.75$). Median follow-up of patients in the study was 25.5 months (2.4–39.9 months). Postoperative complications are summarized in Table 3. No patient in the study met the definition for a symptomatic UTI.

4. Discussion

While it remains common practice among pediatric urologists, the use of perioperative and postoperative antibiotics in hypospadias has not been well characterized in terms of postoperative urine studies or in terms of clinical outcomes. In the absence of true evidence-based guidelines, most providers rely heavily on tradition and on clinical pathways learned during residency and fellowship training when determining whether or not to give antibiotics in this situation.

Based on our data, prophylactic antibiotics do decrease bacteriuria and markers of inflammation within the urine in the acute postoperative period (Table 2). The exact role that urinary tract inflammation and bacterial colonization play in overall surgical outcomes remains unclear, since no patient in the study met criteria for a clinical UTI, and surgical complications were similar between the groups (Table 3). Inadvertent stent removal and failure to obtain the postoperative urine sample were more common in the nontreatment group, though the difference failed to meet statistical significance. While it may be due to random chance, it is possible that antibiotic use may be protective against stent-related complications. Conversely, TMP-SMX

Table 2: Postoperative urine characteristics.

	Treatment (n = 28)	Nontreatment (n = 22)	p value
Leukocyte esterase	18% (5/28)	55% (11/20)	**0.01**
Nitrites	7% (2/28)	40% (8/20)	**0.01**
Bacteria	11% (3/27)	63% (12/19)	**<0.001**
White blood cells	4% (1/27)	47% (9/19)	**<0.001**
Culture with >50K CFU	7% (2/28)	64% (14/22)	**<0.001**
Organisms	*E. coli* × 1 *Enterococcus* × 1 *Enterobacter* × 1	*E. coli* × 7 *K. oxytoca* × 3 *Enterobacter* × 3 *Enterococcus* × 1 *Pseudomonas* × 1 *S. aureus* × 2 Mixed × 2	

Table 3: Postoperative complications and symptomatic UTIs.

Complications	Treatment (n = 35)	Nontreatment (n = 32)
Any	5	6
Fistula	1	2
Glans dehiscence	1	1
Wound infection	2	1
Meatal stenosis	1	2
Symptomatic UTI	0	0

resistance was significantly higher when bacteriuria was present in the postoperative urine sample in the treatment group as compared to the nontreatment group.

Our study aims to add to the body of evidence regarding postoperative antibiotic prophylaxis in patients undergoing mid-to-distal shaft hypospadias repair. Review of the previous study by Meir and Livne demonstrates a higher rate of bacteriuria and higher rate of urinary tract infection in children not receiving postoperative antibiotics but did not show significant differences in noninfectious postoperative complication rates [3]. Two important methodological differences exist between the Meir and Livne study and our study. First, the patients in the Meir study routinely received intravenous antibiotics at the time of surgery and were admitted to the hospital for 24 hours after the procedure. Patients in our study did not routinely receive intraoperative antibiotics, based on more recent evidence that IV antibiotics may not confer benefit in these patients [6] and all surgeries were performed as an outpatient. Second, while the Meir regimen was termed prophylactic, it consisted of treatment-dose antibiotics (cephalexin three times daily) given prophylactically to prevent bacteriuria, rather than prophylactic dosing of antibiotics according to standards for vesicoureteral reflux as utilized in our study.

Kanaroglou et al. studied this issue in a more contemporary patient population in a retrospective manner and found no difference in postoperative outcomes or postoperative UTI [4]. Similar to our patient population, children received prophylactic dosing of antibiotic with TMP-SMX at 2 mg/kg daily or appropriate alternative for sulfa-allergic patients. Again, all patients received intraoperative IV antibiotics at the time of surgery. Urine studies were not performed in this cohort, making comparisons to previous literature difficult.

More recently, Zeiai et al. reported a cohort of 113 patients who underwent tubularized incised plate repair at a single institution. Patients received either twice daily oral TMP-SMX preoperatively and continued on this dose until stent removal or a single dose of IV TMP-SMX at surgery and an oral dose at catheter removal. While complications were decreased in the reduced antibiotic group, this did not achieve statistical significance. Approximately 20% of this cohort had penoscrotal hypospadias, and this subset was responsible for nearly 50% of the reported complications in the group. Again, urine studies and antibiotic-resistance patterns were not examined in this cohort [5].

Our study represents the first published study to report both postoperative urine characteristics and postoperative outcomes in a prospective cohort of patients randomized to treatment with 3 mg/kg/day of TMP-SMX versus no treatment. Additionally, our study is the first to report on postoperative prophylaxis in a series of patients who did not receive routine IV antibiotics at the time of surgery.

While symptomatic UTI and skin infection are certainly the gold standard of clinical outcomes in this population, they are rare events and their prevalence is not agreed upon in the literature. For example, the previous 3 studies on antibiotic prophylaxis reported 0%, 5%, and 24% UTI rates in children, not on continuous antibiotic prophylaxis [3–5]. This makes ensuring adequate power difficult using these two endpoints and makes designing a study to address this issue definitively challenging within a single institution.

Bacteriuria and pyuria are objective endpoints that give a glimpse into the effects of antibiotic prophylaxis on the urinary milieu during initial healing in the acute postoperative phase. We thus felt that these were excellent endpoints to determine the effect of antibiotics on the patients and also that it was an important point to correlate urinary findings with UTI/skin infection in the same patient population, as this has not been done previously with regard to antibiotic prophylaxis. Additionally, we are the first to report a difference in resistance patterns among bacteria cultured from children with or without prophylaxis after hypospadias repair.

Despite its prospective nature, our study is not without limitations. First of all, our sample size is relatively small, despite 40 months of enrolling patients at a tertiary pediatric center with 4 pediatric urologists. Only 50% of parents approached about the study consented to be enrolled.

This mainly served to highlight many of the difficulties inherent in performing randomized, prospective studies in a pediatric surgical setting. As detailed by Vemulakonda and Jones [7], randomization is a challenge for both patients and pediatric providers in a perioperative setting due to the perception that it takes some of the control of the perioperative course away from both parties and serves to emphasize the randomness that may occur in postoperative outcomes. We also experienced difficulties maintaining patients on the defined study protocol, with 22% (15/67) of patients unable to provide a urine sample at postoperative follow-up, mostly due to inadvertent early removal of urethral stent or due to difficulty processing specimens in the lab. Additionally, while we report postoperative outcomes for UTI and complications in our patient population, our follow-up time is limited (median: 25.5 months) and our study is not sufficiently powered to detect small differences in complications between the two groups. Despite these limitations, we believe this study to be an important contribution to the literature in an area where evidence-based recommendations are currently lacking.

5. Conclusions

In a prospective, randomized study of prophylactic antibiotics versus no antibiotics in patients undergoing mid-to-distal hypospadias repair with postoperative urethral stent, patients treated with TMP-SMX at 3 mg/kg/day experienced significantly lower rates of bacteriuria and pyuria at 6–10 days postoperatively than patients not treated with antibiotics. Additionally, organisms cultured from children on prophylaxis were significantly more likely to be resistant to the prophylactic agent. Despite this significant difference, no clinical differences between symptomatic UTI and postoperative complications were observed between the groups. Although limited by sample size and protocol deviation, our study lends credence to the growing body of literature that suggests that postoperative prophylaxis may not improve clinical outcomes in patients undergoing uncomplicated single-stage mid-to-distal hypospadias repair. Further study, likely a multi-institutional prospective trial, is indicated to determine if these outcomes are truly similar over a longer period of time.

Ethical Approval

All procedures performed in this study involving human participants were in accordance with the ethical standards of the institutional and/or national research committee and with the 1964 Helsinki Declaration and its later amendments or comparable ethical standards (Institutional Review Board #485668; CHW 13/140).

Consent

Informed consent was obtained from all individual participants included in the study.

Acknowledgments

Pharmacy and publishing support for this study was provided through a research grant from the Children's Research Institute at Children's Hospital of Wisconsin.

References

[1] W. Snodgrass, "Hypospadias," in *Campbell-Walsh Urology*, A. J. Wein, L. R. Kavoussi, A. C. Novick et al, vol. 4, pp. 3485–3506, Elsevier Saunders, Philadelphia, PA, USA, 10th edition, 2011.

[2] M. H. Hsieh, P. Wildenfels, and E. T. Gonzales, "Surgical antibiotic practices among pediatric urologists in the United States," *Journal of Pediatric Urology*, vol. 7, no. 2, pp. 192–197, 2011.

[3] D. B. Meir and P. M. Livne, "Is prophylactic antimicrobial treatment necessary after hypospadias repair?," *Journal of Urology*, vol. 171, pp. 2621-2622, 2004.

[4] N. Kanaroglou, E. Wehbi, A. Alotay et al., "Is there a role for prophylactic antibiotics after stented hypospadias repair?," *Journal of Urology*, vol. 190, no. 4, pp. 1535–1539, 2013.

[5] S. Zeiai, A. Nordenskjold, and M. Fossum, "Advantages of reduced prophylaxis after tubularized incised plate repair of hypospadias," *Journal of Urology*, vol. 196, no. 4, pp. 1244–1249, 2016.

[6] E. Baillargeon, K. Duan, A. Brzezinski et al., "The role of prophylactic antibiotics in hypospadias repair," *Canadian Urological Association Journal*, vol. 8, no. 7-8, p. 236, 2014.

[7] V. M. Vemulakonda and J. Jones, "Barriers to participation in surgical randomized controlled trials: a qualitative study of key stakeholder perspectives," *Journal of Pediatric Urology*, vol. 12, no. 3, pp. 180.e1–180.e7, 2016.

Microbiome within Primary Tumor Tissue from Renal Cell Carcinoma May Be Associated with PD-L1 Expression of the Venous Tumor Thrombus

Michael A. Liss,[1] Yidong Chen,[2] Ronald Rodriguez,[1] Deepak Pruthi,[1] Teresa Johnson-Pais,[3] Hanzhang Wang,[1] Ahmed Mansour,[1] James R. White,[4] and Dharam Kaushik[1]

[1]*Department of Urology, University of Texas Health San Antonio, San Antonio, TX, USA*
[2]*Greehey Children's Cancer Research Institute, University of Texas Health San Antonio, San Antonio, TX, USA*
[3]*Department of Cell and Molecular Biology, University of Texas Health San Antonio, San Antonio, TX, USA*
[4]*Resphera Biosciences, Baltimore, MD, USA*

Correspondence should be addressed to Michael A. Liss; mliss008@gmail.com

Academic Editor: Daniel W. Lin

Objective. To perform a proof of concept microbiome evaluation and PD-L1 expression profiling in clear-cell renal cell carcinoma (cc-RCC) with associated tumor thrombus (TT). *Methods.* After IRB approval, six patients underwent radical nephrectomy (RN) with venous tumor thrombectomy (VTT). We collected fresh tissue specimens from normal adjacent, tumor, and thrombus tissues. We utilized RNA sequencing to obtain PD-L1 expression profiles and perform microbiome analysis. Statistical assessment was performed using Student's *t*-test, chi-square, and spearman rank correlations using SPSS v25. *Results.* We noted the tumor thrombus to be mostly devoid of diverse microbiota. A large proportion of *Staphylococcus epidermidus* was detected and unknown if this is a surgical or postsurgical contaminant; however, it was noted more in the thrombus than other tissues. Microbiome diversity profiles were most abundant in the primary tumor compared to the thrombus or normal adjacent tissue. Differential expression of PD-L1 was examined in the tumor thrombus to the normal background tissue and noted three of the six subjects had a threshold above 2-fold. These three similar subjects had foreign microbiota that are typical residents of the oral microbiome. *Conclusion.* Renal tumors have more diverse microbiomes than normal adjacent tissue. Identification of resident oral microbiome profiles in clear-cell renal cancer with tumor thrombus provides a potential biomarker for thrombus response to PD-L1 inhibition.

1. Introduction

The United States anticipates more than 62,000 new renal cell carcinoma (RCC) to be diagnosed each year [1]. RCC can develop intravascular venous invasion commonly referred to as a tumor thrombus, projecting into the inferior vena cava in approximately 4–10% of renal cancer cases [2]. Unfortunately, the five-year overall survival can range from 32 to 69% depending on the presence or absence of metastasis [3–5]. If renal thrombus tumors are left untreated, nearly 87% of these patients will die of renal cancer within a median of 5 months [6]. The tumor thrombus level may not directly affect disease-specific survival; however, the anatomic level of the thrombus can significantly impact surgical complexity [7]. Therefore, new therapy targeting tumor thrombus reduction is needed.

Reports indicate that neoadjuvant chemotherapy with tyrosine kinase inhibitors (TKIs) does not reduce tumor thrombus to improve surgical morbidity [8, 9]. Immunotherapy is quickly being incorporated into advanced kidney cancer protocols with several trials underway [10]. The concept of precision medicine is to target individual tumors with specific therapy, yet requires tumor tissue and knowledge of a particular target [11]. For instance, PD-L1 expression profiling may predict the response of anti-PD-L1 therapy [12], and we have demonstrated that the primary tumor and tumor thrombus have differing PD-L1 expression and that a biopsy of the primary tumor in the kidney is unlikely to predict the PD-L1 expression profile of the tumor thrombus [13]. We hypothesize that the immune function is within the tumor microenvironment. Based on the types of bacteria living within tumors, they may promote intravascular growth of kidney cancer via assisting with immune protection of cancer.

Additionally, bacteria make a variety of compounds that may affect the microenvironment effecting epigenetic signaling. Several groups have discovered that the intestinal microbiome has developed cross-talk with PD-1 and PD-L1 profiling [14]. In this proof of consent study, we investigate the association of various microbiome profiles within the renal tumor tissue associated with specific PD-L1 expression profiles of the tumor thrombus to determine not only the mechanisms to which tumors develop intravascular extension but also potential biomarkers to inform therapy.

2. Methods

2.1. Population. Six patients were identified with tumor thrombus and consented prior to nephrectomy and thrombectomy. No patient received neoadjuvant chemotherapy. We collected tissue prospectively by flash frozen processing for preservation using standard protocols. The tissue included normal adjacent renal parenchyma, tumor, and thrombus. Additionally, our pathologists performed standard processing as per standard of care. We obtained and recorded data that included demographic, surgical, and clinical outcomes.

2.2. RNA-Seq. We performed sequencing with an Illumina HiSeq 3000 system using 100 bp paired-end protocol following the manufacturer's protocol to attain mRNAs of all samples. After we obtained short sequence reads, we aligned them to the UCSC human genome build hg19 using TopHat2 [15]. The bam files from alignment were processed using HTSeq-count to compute the counts per gene in all samples [16].

2.3. Bioinformatics and Statistical Analysis. Raw paired-end RNA-seq reads were first filtered for quality (target error rate < 0.25%), Illumina adaptor sequences, and minimum length (95 bp) using Trimmomatic. Bowtie2 searches of the NCBI RefSeq database were performed including fungal, eukaryotic, bacterial, archaeal, and viral members [17, 18]. Pathoscope was extended to include total genome coverage estimates for taxonomic assignment [19, 20]. After assessment of total genome-specific coverage by mapped reads, those microbial members with less than 0.1% average genome coverage were removed from consideration. Additionally, assignments made to the PhiX-174 control genome and *Cutibacterium acnes* were determined to be representatives of contamination and were removed prior to downstream statistical analysis. The paired *t*-test and paired Mann–Whitney *U* test were employed to evaluate statistical significance of differences in taxonomic percentage abundance between groups of interest. The Programmed death-ligand 1 (PD-L1) expression profile cutoff was a two-fold change over adjacent normal kidney tissue. We utilized Student's *t*-test for continuous variables and Fisher's exact test for categorical variables.

3. Results

3.1. Demographics. Six patients presented with tumor thrombus and underwent nephrectomy with tumor thrombectomy. We display patient demographics in Table 1. All tumors with pT3 and varying levels of tumor thrombus are present. The majority of patients in this small population were of Hispanic ancestry. There were no intraoperative or postoperative deaths. We also show the corresponding PD-L1 expression of the tumor thrombus compared to normal adjacent background expression along with corresponding presence of oral microbiota within the primary renal tumor.

3.2. Microbiome Analysis. We analyzed a total of 18 samples from 6 patients. Within our taxonomic profiling, 53.5% of reads were mapped to a reference microbial genome. We removed *PhiX* and *Cutibacterium acnes* as known dominant contaminants prior to analysis. Overview of microbial members detected in each sample is shown as a waterfall plot in Figure 1. We excluded *Cutibacterium acnes* because it was highly represented in each sample and we could then display more clearly the other species identified in the tissues.

Alpha diversity findings (Figure 2) note statistically significant differences between groups over the three locations (normal, adjacent tumor and thrombus; $P = 0.05$). We analyzed the findings of both >1% bacterial abundance and >5% bacterial abundance, both noting the tumor with the highest diversity between samples. We note that microbial diversity within tumors is the greatest. We specifically identified *Micrococcus luteus*, *Fusobacterium nucleatum*, *Streptococcus agalactieae*, and *Corynebacterium diphtheriae* to be more abundant within the tumor specimens, as compared to normal adjacent kidney and tumor thrombus. Specifically noting the microbes traditionally assigned to the oral microbiome, oral microbial members of interest are displayed in Figure 3. We noted a single tumor sample with high *Fusobacterium nucleatum* (patient 1330), who also had the highest PD-L1 expression within the tumor thrombus. We identified three subjects with oral microbiome aggregates located within the tumor which were noted to have high PD-L1 expression within the tumor thrombus.

3.3. PD-L1 Expression. Examining tumor compared to adjacent normal using a two-fold change or higher cutoff from the normal adjacent PD-L1 expression, we noted three tumors (ID# 0,7, and 8) were of high PD-L1 expression in the tumor thrombus noting 5.3-, 4.9-, and 2.7-fold differences, respectively (Figure 3). We compared the fold-change differences in those with or without the presence of the oral microbiome composite and noted a statistical difference regarding PD-L1 expression specifically in the thrombus (*T*-test, $P = 0.015$).

Table 1: Demographics.

ID*	Age	Ethnicity	Laterality	BMI	Tumor size (cm)	Stage	Mayo thrombus level	Fuhrman grade	Thrombus PD-L1 expression**	Oral microbiome present
5	46	Hispanic	Right	29.1	10.5	T3b, N0, M1	L1	3	0.833	No
7	55	Hispanic	Left	36.7	4	T3a, N0, M0	L1	2	4.874	Yes
8	39	Hispanic	Right	21.6	6.5	T4, N0, M1	L2	4	2.705	Yes
9	69	White	Left	35.6	11	T3a, N0, M0	L1	2	1.092	No
0	46	Hispanic	Left		15	T3b, N0, M1	L2	4	5.304	Yes
1	85	White	Left	26.3	8	T3c, N0, M0	L4	3	1.083	No

*ID is the last digit from patient ID (e.g, TB31325). **Thrombus PD-L1 expression is a fold-change compared to normal adjacent tissue.

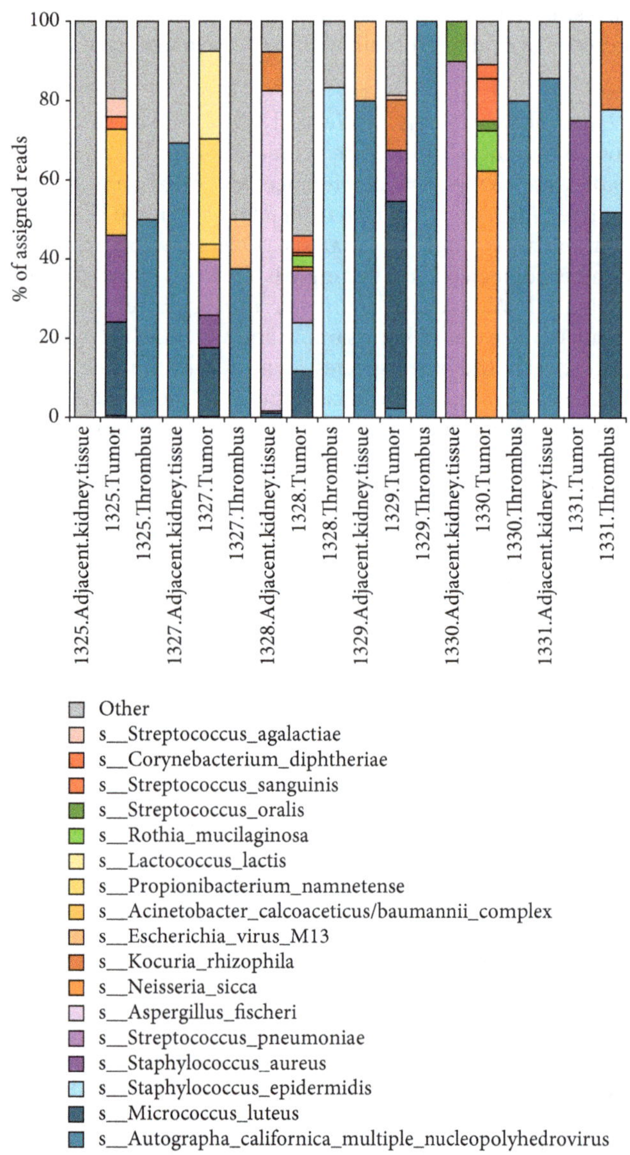

Figure 1: Pathoscope results. Waterfall plot displaying the Pathoscope results identifying the most common microbial genes present in each sample after the removal of PhiX and C. acnes as contaminants.

Overall, all 3 of those subjects with oral microbiome aggregates located within the tumor were noted to have high PD-L1 expression within the tumor thrombus (Fisher's exact, one-tailed *t*-test; $P = 0.05$).

4. Discussion

We have discovered a low detectable rate of microbiome profiles within tumor thrombus and higher diversity of microbes within kidney cancer tissue. We have identified that incongruous oral microbiota within primary renal cancers have an association with PD-L1 expression in the propagated intravascular component of renal cancer. If corroborated, this finding could not only serve as a biomarker for PD-L1 in RCC tumor thrombus patients, but may provide insight regarding tumor thrombus formation and the microenvironment. Our small sample size does not allow for extensive analysis or causal inference, but does provide a new potential biomarker to explore in a larger population. The intravascular portion of the renal tumor is not typically biopsied and would be invasive, which is why we focused on the intratumor microbiota profile. Primary renal tumor tissue can be biopsied, but does suffer from genetic heterogeneity and is one of the controversies regarding renal biopsy accuracy for precision medicine and stratification in clinical trials [21–23].

Gut microbiome has been shown to influence tyrosine kinase therapy in renal cancer [24]. However, there is also an evolving landscape of immune checkpoint inhibitors currently undergoing clinical trials in kidney cancer. Several studies in other cancers have reported response rates could be altered by gut microbiome interactions [14, 25–27]. We did not study the gut microbiome; however, previous investigations have shown that intestinal microbiome may have influence on immune therapy. Our investigation focuses on microbiota identified within the tumor. Given the presence of gastrointestinal tract bacteria within a tumor microenvironment, we hypothesize there may be an immunologic cross-talk occurring within that environment. We do not assume that bacteria cause kidney cancer, but it is interesting that migration of nonresident bacteria can accumulate in the tumor microenvironment. The interaction

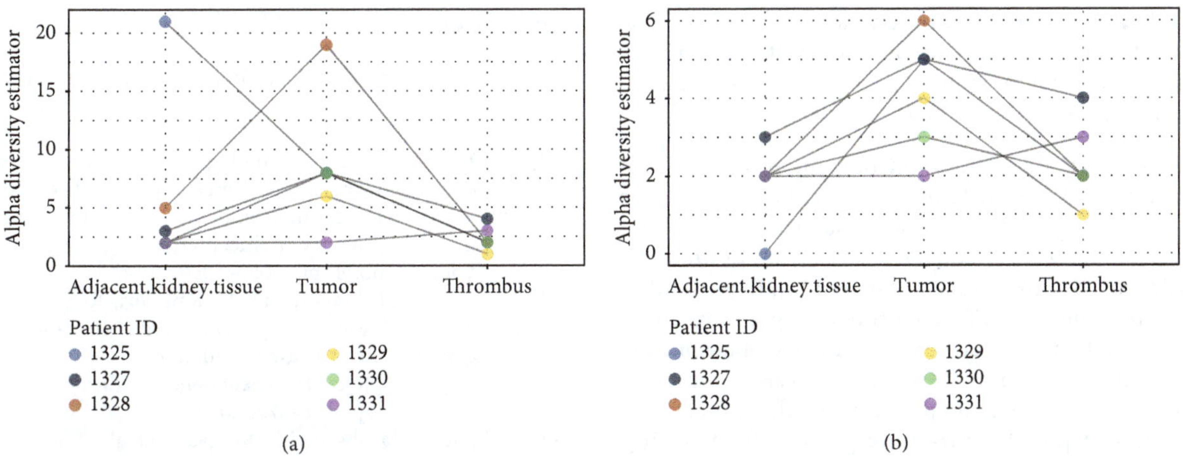

FIGURE 2: Alpha diversity analysis between locations. (a) shows alpha diversity with an abundance of >1% using an alpha diversity estimator as the comparator. In (b), we display the alpha diversity with an abundance of >5%.

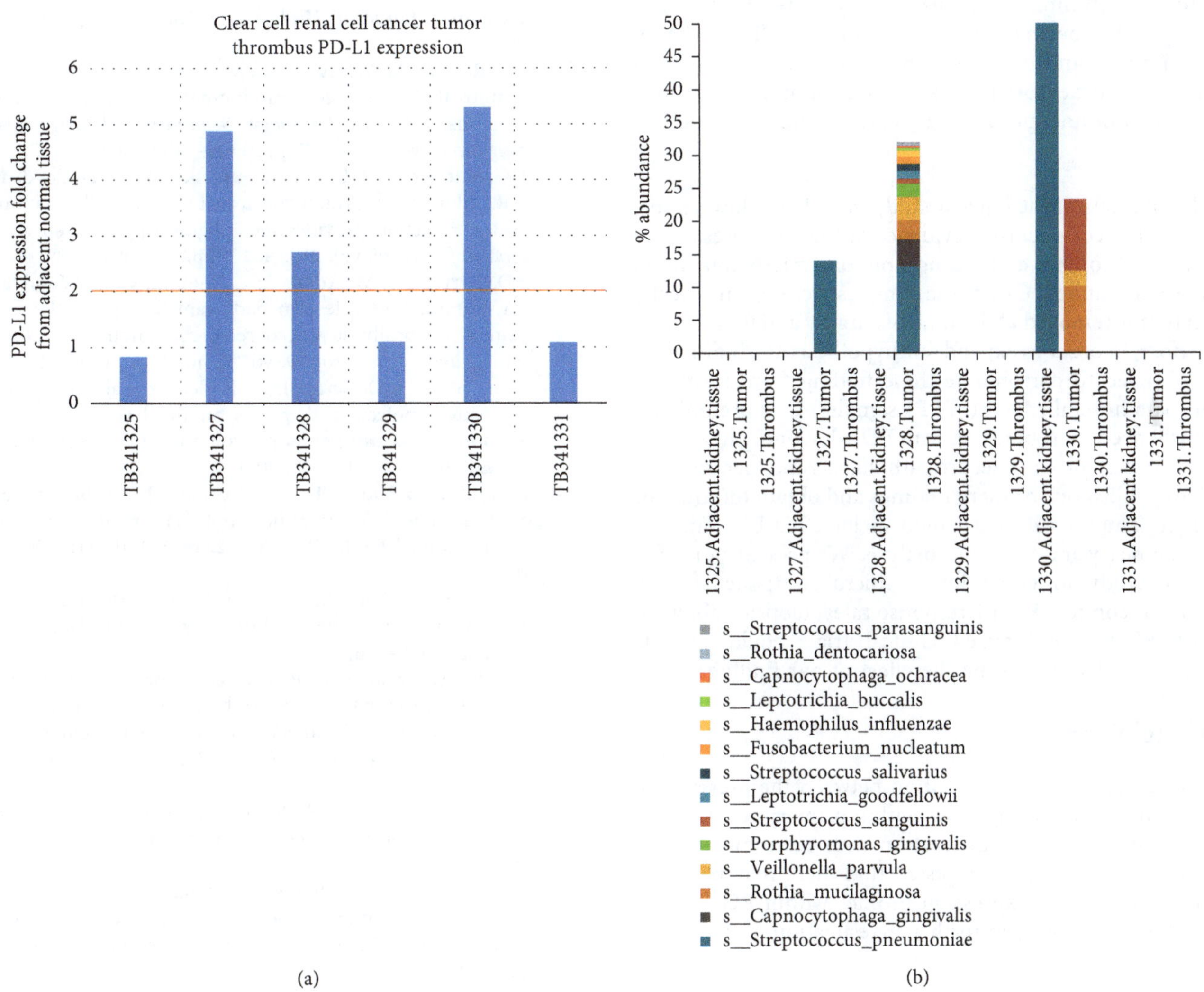

FIGURE 3: Thrombus PD-L1 expression profile in relation to the presence of oral microbiome within the primary tumor. The top bar graph represents the PD-L1 expression within a renal tumor thrombus compared to background normal adjacent tissue. A two-fold difference is demarcated by the red line. The lower bar graph represents the same tumor specimen's oral microbiome abundance.

of these bacteria with the immune system may provide insights into how cancer and or microbiota can inhibit immune cell function to create an environment conducive to intravascular propagation of renal cancer.

The identification of resident oral microbiota within tumors is not unique to kidney cancer. Oral pathogens considered in aggregates such as *Fusobacterium nucleatum*, *Parvimonas micra*, and *Peptostreptococcus stomatis* are highly enriched in colorectal cancer [28]. In particular, *F. nucleatum* induced CCL20 protein expression in in vitro colorectal cancer cells and stimulated macrophage activation and migration [29]. *Fusobacterium* was also found in the urine of patients with bladder cancer and considered as a possible protumorigenic pathogen [30]. The authors confirmed 26% ($n = 11/42$) bladder cancer tissues had *Fusobacterium nucleatum* within the tumor. In our sample, we identified two patients with Fusobacterium and both had more than 2-fold expression of PD-L1 within their tumor thrombus. We hypothesize that oral resident microbes have enhanced ability to live in harsh environments and interact with the host immune system better than other organisms. This communication may enhance immune privilege in certain tumor thrombus patients.

Limitations of the current study include the low sample size to produce conclusive evidence of PD-L1 expression of the tumor thrombus and incongruous oral microbiota found in the renal tumor. Our tissue samples were taken directly from tumor removed at the time of surgery and flash frozen. Therefore, in order to expand our hypothesis as a biomarker, we will need to corroborate these finding from formalin-fixed paraffin-embedded (FFPE) samples. Our preliminary data will need corroboration with PDL-1 staining in a larger sample size. In order to secure pathologists and materials, we seek to publish our primary findings and obtain funding for a larger samples size that would include PD-L1 immunohistochemistry and RNA-seq analysis. We present a proof of concept study to guide future microbial tissue studies. Ideally, to confirm PD-L1 response rates, biopsies obtained before PD-L1 randomized clinical trials could provide preliminary data regarding the effect of our findings.

5. Conclusion

We have described an association between the presence of the oral microbiome aggregate within primary renal cancer tumors and a potential interaction with the tumor microenvironment. We have suggested that there may be interactions with PD-L1 expression profiles within RCC tumor thrombus that will need further investigation.

Acknowledgments

This study was supported by Roger L. and Laura D. Zeller Foundation and UT Health San Antonio Cancer Center (support grant P30 CA054174).

References

[1] R. L. Siegel, K. D. Miller, and A. Jemal, "Cancer statistics, 2017," *CA: A Cancer Journal for Clinicians*, vol. 67, no. 1, pp. 7–30, 2017.

[2] A. Q. Haddad, C. G. Wood, E. J. Abel et al., "Oncologic outcomes following surgical resection of renal cell carcinoma with inferior vena caval thrombus extending above the hepatic veins: a contemporary multicenter cohort," *Journal of Urology*, vol. 192, no. 4, pp. 1050–1056, 2014.

[3] G. Ciancio, M. Manoharan, D. Katkoori, R. De Los Santos, and M. S. Soloway, "Long-term survival in patients undergoing radical nephrectomy and inferior vena cava thrombectomy: single-center experience," *European Urology*, vol. 57, no. 4, pp. 667–672, 2010.

[4] L. Lund, J. Jacobsen, M. Nørgaard et al., "The prognostic impact of comorbidities on renal cancer, 1995 to 2006: a Danish population based study," *Journal of Urology*, vol. 182, no. 1, pp. 35–40, 2009.

[5] B. Wagner, J.-J. Patard, A. Méjean et al., "Prognostic value of renal vein and inferior vena cava involvement in renal cell carcinoma," *European Urology*, vol. 55, no. 2, pp. 452–460, 2009.

[6] A. C. Reese, J. M. Whitson, and M. V. Meng, "Natural history of untreated renal cell carcinoma with venous tumor thrombus," *Urologic Oncology: Seminars and Original Investigations*, vol. 31, no. 7, pp. 1305–1309, 2013.

[7] D. G. Skinner, T. R. Pritchett, G. Lieskovsky, S. D. Boyd, and Q. R. Stiles, "Vena caval involvement by renal cell carcinoma: surgical resection provides meaningful long-term survival," *Annals of Surgery*, vol. 210, no. 3, pp. 387–394, 1989.

[8] L. D. Borregales, M. Adibi, A. Z. Thomas, C. G. Wood, and J. A. Karam, "The role of neoadjuvant therapy in the management of locally advanced renal cell carcinoma," *Therapeutic Advances in Urology*, vol. 8, no. 2, pp. 130–141, 2016.

[9] N. G. Cost, S. E. Delacroix Jr., J. P. Sleeper et al., "The impact of targeted molecular therapies on the level of renal cell carcinoma vena caval tumor thrombus," *European Urology*, vol. 59, no. 6, pp. 912–918, 2011.

[10] A. Rodriguez-Vida, T. E. Hutson, J. Bellmunt, and M. H. Strijbos, "New treatment options for metastatic renal cell carcinoma," *ESMO Open*, vol. 2, no. 2, Article ID e000185, 2017.

[11] Y. Riazalhosseini and M. Lathrop, "Precision medicine from the renal cancer genome," *Nature Reviews Nephrology*, vol. 12, no. 11, pp. 655–666, 2016.

[12] A. Prat, A. Navarro, L. Paré et al., "Immune-related gene expression profiling after PD-1 blockade in non-small cell lung carcinoma, head and neck squamous cell carcinoma, and melanoma," *Cancer Research*, vol. 77, no. 13, pp. 3540–3550, 2017.

[13] M. A. Liss, Y. Chen, R. Rodriguez et al., "Immunogenic heterogeneity of renal cell carcinoma with venous tumor thrombus," *Urology*, vol. 124, pp. 168–173, 2018.

[14] A. Botticelli, I. Zizzari, F. Mazzuca et al., "Cross-talk between microbiota and immune fitness to steer and control response to anti PD-1/PDL-1 treatment," *Oncotarget*, vol. 8, pp. 8890–8899, 2017.

[15] D. Kim, G. Pertea, C. Trapnell, H. Pimentel, R. Kelley, and S. L. Salzberg, "TopHat2: accurate alignment of transcriptomes in the presence of insertions, deletions and gene fusions," *Genome Biology*, vol. 14, no. 4, p. R36, 2013.

[16] S. Anders, P. T. Pyl, and W. Huber, "HTSeq—a Python framework to work with high-throughput sequencing data," *Bioinformatics*, vol. 31, no. 2, pp. 166–169, 2015.

[17] A. M. Bolger, M. Lohse, and B. Usadel, "Trimmomatic: a flexible trimmer for Illumina sequence data," *Bioinformatics*, vol. 30, no. 15, pp. 2114–2120, 2014.

[18] B. Langmead and S. L. Salzberg, "Fast gapped-read alignment with Bowtie 2," *Nature Methods*, vol. 9, no. 4, pp. 357–359, 2012.

[19] O. E. Francis, M. Bendall, S. Manimaran et al., "Pathoscope: species identification and strain attribution with unassembled sequencing data," *Genome Research*, vol. 23, no. 10, pp. 1721–1729, 2013.

[20] J. Oh, NISC Comparative Sequencing Program, A. L. Allyson et al., "Biogeography and individuality shape function in the human skin metagenome," *Nature*, vol. 514, no. 7520, pp. 59–64, 2014.

[21] E. Lopez-Fernandez and J. I. Lopez, "The impact of tumor eco-evolution in renal cell carcinoma sampling," *Cancers*, vol. 10, no. 12, p. 485, 2018.

[22] K. Saeed, P. Ojamies, T. Pellinen et al., "Clonal heterogeneity influences drug responsiveness in renal cancer assessed by ex vivo drug testing of multiple patient-derived cancer cells," *International Journal of Cancer*, vol. 144, no. 6, pp. 1356–1366, 2018.

[23] S. Turajlic, H. Xu, K. Litchfield et al., "Deterministic evolutionary trajectories influence primary tumor growth: TRACERx renal," *Cell*, vol. 173, no. 3, pp. 595.e11–610.e11, 2018.

[24] S. K. Pal, S. M. Li, X. Wu et al., "Stool bacteriomic profiling in patients with metastatic renal cell carcinoma receiving vascular endothelial growth factor-tyrosine kinase inhibitors," *Clinical Cancer Research*, vol. 21, no. 23, pp. 5286–5293, 2015.

[25] V. Gopalakrishnan, B. A. Helmink, C. N. Spencer, A. Reuben, and J. A. Wargo, "The influence of the gut microbiome on cancer, immunity, and cancer immunotherapy," *Cancer Cell*, vol. 33, no. 4, pp. 570–580, 2018.

[26] N. Chaput, P. Lepage, C. Coutzac et al., "Baseline gut microbiota predicts clinical response and colitis in metastatic melanoma patients treated with ipilimumab," *Annals of Oncology*, vol. 28, no. 6, pp. 1368–1379, 2017.

[27] B. Routy, E. Le Chatelier, L. Derosa et al., "Gut microbiome influences efficacy of PD-1-based immunotherapy against epithelial tumors," *Science*, vol. 359, no. 359, pp. 91–97, 2018.

[28] J. L. Drewes, J. R. White, C. M. Dejea et al., "High-resolution bacterial 16S rRNA gene profile meta-analysis and biofilm status reveal common colorectal cancer consortia," *NPJ Biofilms Microbiomes*, vol. 3, no. 1, p. 34, 2017.

[29] X. Ye, R. Wang, R. Bhattacharya et al., "Fusobacterium nucleatum subspecies animalis influences proinflammatory cytokine expression and monocyte activation in human colorectal tumors," *Cancer Prevention Research*, vol. 10, no. 7, pp. 398–409, 2017.

[30] V. Bucevic Popovic, M. Situm, C. T. Chow, L. S. Chan, B. Roje, and J. Terzic, "The urinary microbiome associated with bladder cancer," *Scientific Reports*, vol. 8, no. 1, 2018.

30

Prevalence of Age-Associated Testosterone Deficiency Syndrome in Indian Population

Ghanendra Kumar Yadav, Mrinal Pahwa, Mahendra Singh, Vipin Tyagi, and Sudhir Chadha

Department of Urology, Sir Ganga Ram Hospital, New Delhi, India

Correspondence should be addressed to Mrinal Pahwa; drmrinalpahwa@gmail.com

Academic Editor: Darius J. Bagli

Testosterone deficiency syndrome (TDS) is a gradual age-related phenomenon that occurs in a large proportion of the aging male population. This current prospective study was done with the objective to estimate the prevalence of age-associated TDS in India and its clinical profile. A total of 800 male patients aged ≥40 year were approached to participate in the study. A brief history and focused examination was done. Based on our exclusion criteria, 55 patients were excluded. Androgen deficiency in aging male (ADAM) questionnaire was administered to all remaining 745 patients. Out of these 745 patients, ADAM-positive (symptomatic TDS) patients were found to be 359 and enrolled in the study. In all ADAM-positive patients, serum testosterone levels were measured. Prevalence of symptomatic TDS in study population was found to be 48.18%. Mean total and free testosterone level of symptomatic TDS population were 3.287 ± 1.494 ng/ml (1.12–9.61) and 7.476 ± 2.902 pg/ml (2.18–21.76), respectively. Prevalence of biochemically confirmed TDS among symptomatic TDS population was 60.17%. Prevalence of TDS increases progressively with each decade of life ($p = 0.034$). Prevalence was higher in patients with diabetes, hypertension, coronary artery disease, obesity, and metabolic syndrome. TDS is a real phenomenon with a prevalence of 28.99% in our study population.

1. Introduction

Normal aging frequently results in a progressive functional dwindling of hypothalamic-pituitary-gonadal axis. This results in progressive decline in serum testosterone in men after age of forty between 0.4 and 2.6% per year [1–4], which exhibits significant interindividual variability in age of onset, speed, and depth of decline [1]. This decline of the serum testosterone level is clinically termed as partial androgen deficiency of the aging male (PADAM) or late-onset hypogonadism (LOH) or more accurately testosterone deficiency syndrome (TDS), but the time of onset varies and the epidemiological status is unclear [5].

TDS is defined as a clinical and biochemical syndrome associated with advancing age and characterized by symptoms with or without signs and a deficiency in serum testosterone levels. This condition may result in significant detriment in the quality of life and adversely affect the function of multiple organ systems [1]. The presence of symptoms, however, is a sine qua non for diagnosis and should be coupled with a low or borderline-low objective biochemical measure of serum testosterone [5–8].

The main emphasis of healthcare in the 21st century is to improve the quality of life of the elderly. In women, hormone replacement therapy is a widely accepted concept. Age-associated TDS and the use of exogenous testosterone to treat decreasing testosterone levels in older men is a relatively new concept [6], and most literature is from European or American continents [7, 8].

In Indian subcontinent, this syndrome has been considered as a general phenomenon associated with aging and very few studies have been carried out to document its true prevalence and clinical profile, resulting in a lack of objective treatment for elderly men [9, 10].

2. Materials and Methods

This prospective study was conducted in accordance with the hospital ethical committee requirements in the Department of Urology at a tertiary hospital in New Delhi. A total of 800 male patients aged ≥40 year admitted or attending outpatient department in our department were approached to participate in the study. They were given written information about the study, and informed consent was obtained. A brief history and focused examination was done. Patients with a history of suboptimal pubertal development, medical or surgical castration, dyslipidemia, and chronic liver disease, undergoing androgen supplement therapy, and using drugs which interfere with testosterone levels were excluded. Based on our exclusion criteria, 55 patients were excluded.

ADAM questionnaire was administered to all remaining 745 patients. Symptomatic TDS was considered to be present if at least question numbers 1 or 7 or any 3 other questions of the questionnaire were positive (Table 1).

Out of these 745 patients, 359 patients were found to be suffering from symptomatic TDS based on the ADAM questionnaire and enrolled in the study. In all these ADAM-positive patients, serum total testosterone (TT) and serum free testosterone (FT) levels were measured by the radioimmunoassay method between 07 : 00 and 10 : 00 AM with overnight fasting. The most widely used method for measurement of free testosterone in clinical laboratories is direct RIA. In general, this assay uses a 125I-labeled testosterone analog that has very low affinity for SHBG and albumin and competes with free testosterone for binding sites on an immobilized specific testosterone antibody. Although this approach provides a simple and rapid test for quantifying free testosterone, it has been pointed out that the assay method has several deficiencies; these include low antibody affinity, major biasing effects resulting from dilution of serum samples, significant binding of the analog to serum proteins, and lack of parallelism between measurements of serially diluted serum samples and free testosterone. For these reasons, the reliability of the assay that utilizes the analog-based free testosterone RIA kit has been questioned. [11–13] Other relevant evaluation was also done as needed.

2.1. Statistical Method. Descriptive statistics was analyzed with SPSS version 17.0 software. Continuous variables were presented as mean ± SD. Categorical variables were expressed as frequencies and percentages. Nominal categorical data between the groups were compared using the chi-squared test or Fisher's exact test as appropriate. $P < 0.05$ was considered as statistically significant.

3. Results

In our study, prevalence of symptomatic TDS was 48.18% (359/745). Maximum number of participants were in the 40–49 year group and least in more than 80 years group with a mean age of 54.48 ± 10.679 years (R = 40–93 years) (Table 2).

Table 1: Saint Louis University androgen deficiency in aging male (ADAM) questionnaire.

1	Do you have a decrease in libido or sex drive?	Yes/no
2	Do you have a lack of energy?	Yes/no
3	Do you have a decrease in strength and/or endurance?	Yes/no
4	Have you lost weight?	Yes/no
5	Have you noticed a decreased "enjoyment of life"?	Yes/no
6	Are you sad and/or grumpy?	Yes/no
7	Are your erections less strong?	Yes/no
8	Have you noticed a recent deterioration in your ability to play sports?	Yes/no
9	Are you falling asleep after dinner?	Yes/no
10	Has there been a recent deterioration in your work performance?	Yes/no

Table 2: Prevalence of symptomatic and biochemically confirmed TDS in different age groups.

Age group	ADAM +ve	Biochemically +ve	Prevalence (%)
40–49 years	136	73	53
50–59 years	121	75	61.98
60–69 years	67	44	65
70–79 years	25	17	68
>80 years	10	7	70

In our study, a significant correlation was found between aging and decline of the TT level ($r = -0.153$, p value = 0.004). Significant correlation was also found between aging and decline of the FT level ($r = -0.121$, $p = 0.002$). Prevalence of TDS increases progressively with each decade of life, and it was found to be statistically significant ($p = 0.034$). Most commonly reported ADAM questionnaire symptom was lack of energy followed by decreasing frequency by poor erection and loss of libido, and the least reported symptom was loss of height.

Mean TT level of our symptomatic TDS population was 3.287 ± 1.494 ng/ml (1.12–9.61). Overt TDS (TT < 2.50 ng/ml) and borderline TDS (TT = 2.50–3.46 ng/ml) were found in 34.82% (125/359) and 27.85% (100/359) subjects, respectively. Mean FT level of our symptomatic TDS population was 7.476 ± 2.902 pg/ml (2.18–21.76). Prevalence of biochemically confirmed TDS among symptomatic TDS population was 60.17% on the basis of FT levels.

In our study, association between TT and FT levels was found to be statistically significant (p value < 0.001) (Figure 1). 96.8% participants with overt TDS (total T < 2.50 ng/ml) were found to have the FT level <8.690 pg/ml. The prevalence of symptomatic + biochemical TDS in our study population was 28.99% (216/745) on the basis of FT levels.

Mean body mass index (BMI) of symptomatic TDS population was 24.82 ± 2.59 (18.29–32.59). Obese (BMI > 30) and overweight (BMI = 25–30) patients made up 4.45% and

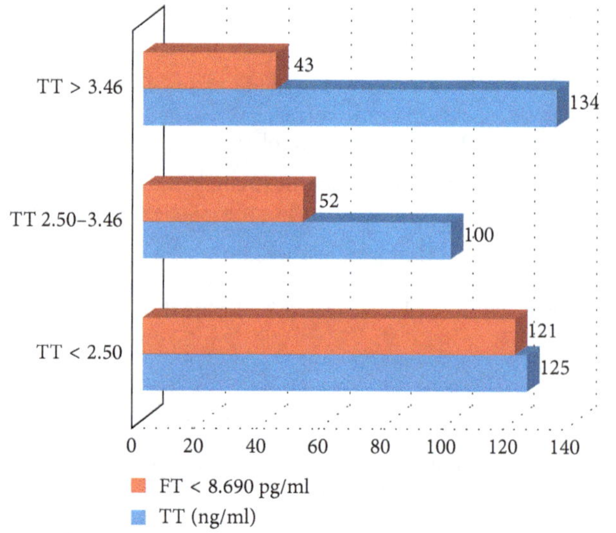

FIGURE 1: Graph showing association between TT and FT levels in the study population.

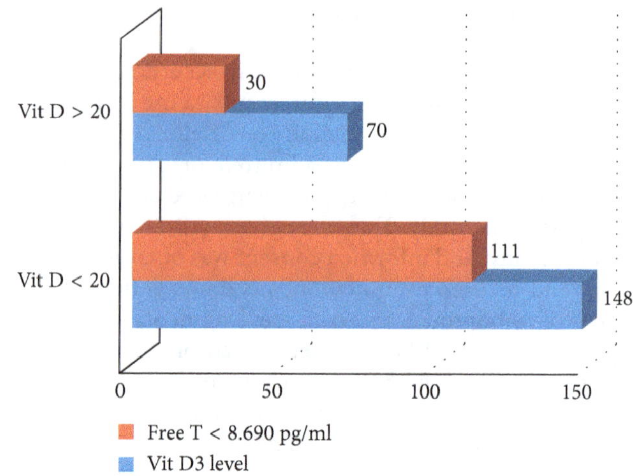

FIGURE 2: Division of study population in two groups based on vitamin D_3 levels ($n = 218$) and prevalence of FT levels in the two subgroups (FT = free testosterone).

37.6% (135/359) of study population. Increasing BMI has a significant correlation with TDS ($r = -0.156$, $p = 0.003$).

Prevalence of TDS in diabetic population was significantly higher as compared to nondiabetics (71.03% vs 52.8%, $p = 0.001$). Similarly, significantly higher number of hypertensive patients were found to have TDS as compared to normotensives (72.89% vs 54.86%, $p = 0.001$). In our study, 11.42% (51/359) of symptomatic TDS were to have metabolic syndrome (MetS). 80.39% (41/51) of participants with MetS were found to have TDS with a statistically significant association ($p = 0.003$). 84.30% (27/32) participants with coronary artery disease (CAD) were found to have TDS, suggesting that patients having TDS should be evaluated for CAD/MetS, and vice versa ($p = 0.003$). In our study, a significant association was found between vitamin D_3 deficiency and TDS ($p < 0.001$), as shown in Figure 2.

4. Discussion

In our study, the ADAM questionnaire was administered among 745 males having aged ≥40 year. Prevalence of symptomatic TDS among study population was found to be 48.18% (359/745). Overt TDS (TT < 2.50 ng/ml) was present in 34.82% (125/359) subjects. Prevalence of biochemically confirmed TDS among symptomatic TDS population was 60.17%. Prevalence of symptomatic + biochemically confirmed TDS in study population was 28.99% (216/745). A preliminary cross-sectional study conducted by Goel et al. on 157 healthy volunteers found that the prevalence of symptomatic LOH was (67.5%) on the ADAM questionnaire [9]. Another Indian study conducted by Ashat et al. reported 40% prevalence of symptomatic andropause among men with age of 40 or above [10]. Goel et al. reported prevalence of biochemical TDS among symptomatic TDS population of male workers between ages 40 and 60 as 38.67%, and prevalence of overt TDS was 30.18% [9]. Mulligan et al. in the HIM study reported prevalence of hypogonadism to be 36.3% among men >45 years attending general clinical practice [10]. In the current study, mean serum TT levels of symptomatic TDS population was 3.287 ng/ml (SD = 1.494, range = 1.12–9.61). Mean TT level was reported to be 1.5 ng/ml by Goel et al. [9] and 3.46 ng/ml by Mulligan et al. [11].

In the current study, maximum number of symptomatic TDS participants was in the 40–49 year group and least in the >80 year group with a mean age of 54.48 ± 10.679 years (40–93 years). Similar age profile for symptoms of TDS was reported by Ashat et al. [10]. This reflects the general assumption in our Indian society that symptoms of TDS are general phenomenon of aging. Most commonly reported ADAM questionnaire symptom was lack of energy followed by decreasing frequency by poor erection and loss of libido, and the least reported symptom was loss of height. Kelleher et al. in their study found that most reported symptoms of androgen deficiency were lack of energy and reduced libido [12].

Significant correlation was also found between aging and decline of the FT level ($r = -0.121$, $p = 0.002$). Prevalence of TDS increases progressively with each decade of life, and it was found to be statistically significant ($p = 0.034$). Similar findings were reported in the HIM study [11]. In the current study, mean BMI of symptomatic TDS population was 24.82 ± 2.59 (18.29–32.59). In a cross-sectional pilot study, mean BMI was 22.9 in patients with TDS [9]. Increasing BMI has a significant correlation with TDS ($r = -0.156$, $p = 0.003$). Similar finding was reported in the HIM study [11]. The odds ratio (2.38) for having hypogonadism was significantly higher in men with obesity, as calculated in the HIM study [11].

In the current study, prevalence of TDS in diabetic population was significantly higher as compared to nondiabetics (71.03% vs 52.8%, $p = 0.001$). Khan et al. also found that testosterone levels are frequently low in men with T2DM, and the majority of these men have symptoms of hypogonadism [13]. 72.89% (78/107) hypertensive patients were found to have TDS with a prevalence of 72.89% which was significantly higher than normotensive ($p = 0.001$) patients. The HIM study also calculated that the odds ratio for having hypogonadism was 2.09 and 1.84, respectively, in diabetic and hypertensive patients [11].

In our study, 11.42% (51/359) of symptomatic TDS were to have MetS based on three of the five criteria (elevated WC, elevated TGs, reduced HDL-C levels, elevated BP, and elevated FBG levels) by a new joint statement from a number of professional organizations such as IDF, the National Heart, Lung, and Blood Institute (NHLBI), WHO, the International Atherosclerosis Society, and the American Heart Association (AHA) for the clinical diagnosis of MetS [14]. 80.39% (41/51) of participants with MetS were found to have TDS with a statistically significant association ($p = 0.003$). Similar association between TDS and MetS has been found by Salam et al. [14].

In our study, 84.30% (27/32) of participants with CAD were found to have TDS and association was found to be statistically significant ($p = 0.003$). In their study, Seth M. et al. found that the mean testosterone levels (241–827 ng/dl) were significantly lower in CAD patients than the controls ($p < 0.05$) [15]. In our study, a significant association was found between vitamin D_3 deficiency and TDS ($p < 0.001$). Tak YJ et al. have found similar association in a cross-sectional study. In the multiple linear regression model, $25(OH)D_3$ showed positive association with TT ($\beta = 0.137$, $p < 0.001$) and FT ($\beta = 0.103$, $p = 0.008$). Vitamin D_3 deficiency ($25(OH)D_3 < 20$ ng/ml) was associated with an increased risk of deficiencies of TT (<2.30 ng/ml) (odds ratio (OR): 2.65; CI: 1.21–5.78, $p = 0.014$) and free testosterone (<6.50 $pg{\cdot}ml^{-1}$) (OR: 1.44; 95% CI: 1.01–2.06, $p = 0.048$) [16]. Patients with hypogonadism have frequently low levels of 25-hydroxyvitamin D due to impairment of the hydroxylating enzyme CYP2R1 in the testis [17].

5. Conclusion

Testosterone deficiency syndrome (TDS) is a clinical and biochemical syndrome associated with aging and characterized by symptoms affecting multiple organ systems. The prevalence of symptomatic TDS and biochemically confirmed TDS is 60.17% and 28.99%, respectively. Its prevalence increases progressively with each decade of life. Prevalence was higher in patients with diabetes, hypertension, obesity, metabolic syndrome, and coronary artery disease. A significant association was found between vitamin D_3 deficiency and TDS.

References

[1] H. A. Feldman, C. Longcope, C. A. Derby et al., "Age trends in the level of serum testosterone and other hormones in middle-aged men: longitudinal results from the Massachusetts male aging study," *Journal of Clinical Endocrinology & Metabolism*, vol. 87, no. 2, pp. 589–598, 2002.

[2] S. M. Harman, E. J. Metter, J. D. Tobin, J. Pearson, and M. R. Blackman, "Longitudinal effects of aging on serum total and free testosterone levels in healthy men," *Journal of Clinical Endocrinology & Metabolism*, vol. 86, no. 2, pp. 724–731, 2001.

[3] J. M. Kaufman and A. Vermeulen, "Declining gonadal function in elderly men," *Baillière's Clinical Endocrinology and Metabolism*, vol. 11, no. 2, pp. 289–309, 1997.

[4] J. M. Zmuda, J. A. Cauley, A. Kriska, N. W. Glynn, J. P. Gutai, and L. H. Kuller, "Longitudinal relation between endogenous testosterone and cardiovascular disease risk factors in middle-aged men: a 13-year follow-up of former multiple risk factor intervention trial participants," *American Journal of Epidemiology*, vol. 146, no. 8, pp. 609–617, 1997.

[5] A. Morales, "Androgen deficiency in the aging male," in *Campbell-Walsh Urology*, A. J. Wein, Ed., pp. 810–822, Elsevier, Philadelphia, PA, USA, 10th edition, 2012.

[6] C. Wang, E. Nieschlag, R. Swerdloff et al., "Investigation, treatment and monitoring of late-onset hypogonadism in males: ISA, ISSAM, EAU, EAA and ASA recommendations," *European Journal of Endocrinology*, vol. 159, pp. 507–514, 2008.

[7] E. Nieschlag, R. Swerdloff, H. M. Behre et al., "Investigation, treatment and monitoring of late-onset hypogonadism in males. ISA, ISSAM, and EAU recommendations," *European Urology*, vol. 48, pp. 1–4, 2005.

[8] B. Lunenfeld, G. Mskhalaya, M. Zitzmann et al., "Recommendations on the diagnosis, treatment and monitoring of hypogonadism in men hypogonadism in men," *The Aging Male*, vol. 18, no. 1, pp. 5–15, 2015 Mar.

[9] A. Goel, R. J. Sinha, D. Dalela, S. Sankhwar, and V. Singh, "Andropause in Indian men: a preliminary cross-sectional study," *Journal of Urology*, vol. 6, pp. 40–46, 2009.

[10] M. Ashat, M. Puri, A. Singh, S. S. Sarpal, N. K. Goel, and B. Kaushal, "Awareness of andropause in males, a north Indian study," *Indian Journal of Medical Sciences*, vol. 65, no. 9, pp. 379–386, 2011.

[11] J. E. Morley, H. M. Perry, R. T. Kevorkian, and P. Patrick, "Comparison of screening questionnaires for the diagnosis of hypogonadism," *Maturitas*, vol. 53, no. 4, pp. 424–429, 2006.

[12] S. Kelleher, A. J. Conway, and D. J. Handelsman, "Blood testosterone threshold for androgen deficiency symptoms," *Journal of Clinical Endocrinology & Metabolism*, vol. 89, no. 8, pp. 3813–3817, 2004.

[13] I. Khan, C. Kant, and A. Samaria, "Assessment of hypogonadism with reference to clinical features and serum testosterone levels in Asian-Indian male type 2 diabetics," *Indian Journal of Clinical Practice*, vol. 23, no. 2, pp. 92–99, 2012.

[14] R. Salam, A. S. Kshetrimayum, and R. Keisam, "Testosterone and metabolic syndrome: the link," *Indian Journal of Endocrinology and Metabolism*, vol. 16, no. 1, pp. 12–19, 2012.

[15] M. Seth, A. Sachdeva, P. Saharoy, S. Seth, and H. Madaan, "Relationship of testosterone levels in males with coronary Heart DIsease," *International Journal of Pharma and Bio Sciences*, vol. 2, no. 2, pp. 566–570, 2011.

[16] Y. J. Tak, J. G. Lee, Y. J. Kim et al., "Serum 25-hydroxyvitamin D levels and testosterone deficiency in middle-aged Korean men: a cross-sectional study," *Asian Journal of Andrology*, vol. 17, no. 2, pp. 324–328, 2015.

[17] C. Foresta, A. Calogero, F. Lombardo, A. Lenzi, and A. Ferlin, "Late-onset hypogonadism: beyond testosterone," *Asian Journal of Andrology*, vol. 17, no. 2, pp. 236–238, 2015.

Novel Use of Household Items in Open and Robotic Surgical Skills Resident Education

Keri Rowley,[1] Deepak Pruthi,[1] Osamah Al-Bayati,[1] Joseph Basler,[1,2,3] and Michael A. Liss[1,2,3,4]

[1]*University of Texas Health San Antonio, Department of Urology, San Antonio, USA*
[2]*University of Texas Health San Antonio Cancer Center, San Antonio, USA*
[3]*South Texas Veterans Healthcare System, Department of Surgery, Division of Urology, San Antonio, USA*
[4]*University of Texas, College of Pharmacy, Austin, USA*

Correspondence should be addressed to Michael A. Liss; mliss008@gmail.com

Academic Editor: Jason M. Hafron

Background. The aim of this study was to investigate the effectiveness of surgical simulators created using household items and to determine their potential role in surgical skills training. *Methods.* Ten urology residents attended a surgical skills workshop and practiced using surgical simulators and models. These included a wound closure model, an open prostatectomy model, a delicate tissue simulation, a knot-tying station, and a laparoscopic simulator. After the workshop, the residents completed a 5-point Likert questionnaire. Primary outcome was face validity of the models. Secondary outcomes included usefulness as a training tool and ability to replicate the models. *Results.* All models were easily created and successfully represented the surgical task being simulated. Residents evaluated the activities as being useful for training purposes overall. They also felt confident that they could recreate the simulators. *Conclusion.* Low-fidelity training models can be used to improve surgical skills at a reasonable cost. The models will require further evaluation to determine construct validity and to determine how the improvements translate to OR performance. While high-fidelity simulators may continue to be utilized in formal surgical training, residents should be encouraged to supplement their training with innovative homemade models.

1. Background

Today's surgical trainees are increasingly challenged to improve their technical skills in an environment with reduced work hours [1]. In a field where hands-on experience is paramount to developing competency, the solution has been the utilization of surgical simulators. Many models are available for endourology as well as laparoscopic and robot-assisted urology; however, few simulators exist for open urological surgery [2, 3]. This creates additional challenges for surgical trainees, who are exposed to fewer open surgery cases due to increasing use of minimally invasive surgery techniques [4].

The current options for high-fidelity open urological surgery simulation are costly, and those that are affordable are limited to bench models for simple and suprapubic catheterization, adult male circumcision, and vasectomy [5]. Some programs have pioneered cadaveric training programs for various operations such as circumcision, vasectomy, and hydrocele repair while others have proposed improving open surgical experience by incorporating organ procurement and transplantation into the curriculum [6, 7]. While such methods are beneficial, they do not allow for repeated independent practice.

Inexpensive open urological surgery models may provide residents further opportunities to improve their open surgical skills. Urology requires mastery of both open and robotic surgical skills. Therefore, we sought to design simulators that could be easily replicated by surgical trainees at a low cost and evaluated the validity of the models for training purposes in open and robotic simulation.

2. Materials and Methods

2.1. Study Design and Data Collection. The simulators and models were used to teach surgical techniques to urology trainees at the Audie L. Murphy Memorial VA Hospital as part of a skills workshop. After the workshop, the trainees completed a 5-point Likert questionnaire to assess the models on face validity, usefulness as a training tool, and perceived ability to replicate the models (Table 1).

2.2. Simulators

2.2.1. Wound Closure Model. The model for wound closure was created using cardboard, T-pins, and a ripe banana. The fruit was removed from the peel and secured to the cardboard surface using T-pins. Trainees practiced suturing the banana using various techniques and angles of approach (Figure 1).

2.2.2. Open Prostatectomy Model. The model was created using a plastic 1-gallon milk or juice container and a large orange. The plastic container simulates the surgical space and abdominal cavity, and the orange represents the prostate. The bottom of the plastic container was cut out, and then, the container was inverted. Using a hot glue gun, the orange was glued into the neck of the inverted container, and the container was glued to a flat surface. The trainees were instructed to practice suturing across the surface of the orange in a straight line using DeBakey forceps and DeBakey needle holder (Figure 2). Residents also practiced knot tying in this simulated confined surgical space.

2.2.3. Delicate Tissue Simulation. Delicate tissue was simulated using various types of boiled pasta coated in olive oil. The pasta was cooked for varying lengths of time to simulate the variation in tissue consistency. Trainees were instructed to anastomose the pasta using sutures strong enough to hold but not tear through the pasta (Figure 3). They were also advised to consider the force applied to their forceps when gripping the pasta. Cooked pasta has been previously utilized to simulate microsurgery for plastic surgery trainees [8].

2.2.4. Knot-Tying Station. This exercise utilizes cooked spaghetti noodles coated in olive oil to help trainees determine the amount of force needed to advance a knot. Trainees used one strand of noodle to tie surgical knots around various objects (Figure 4). If the noodle broke before they were able to throw a significant number of knots, they restarted with a new strand.

2.2.5. Robotic Simulator. The dual console Da Vinci Xi (Intuitive Surgical, Sunnyvale, CA) was used for surgical training. One console was used for practice on the Da Vinci Surgical Skills Simulator (DVSSS) and was included to contrast the expensive high-fidelity models (Figure 5). The DVSSS uses the Mimic software program to evaluate skill competency through various exercises. Residents performed the "Thread the Rings" exercise, which primarily focuses on improving needle control. To practice robotic anastomosis, we also had the residents attempt the "tubes" function, an exercise that has been published as a sensitive marker for robotic skill [9]. The other console was connected to the robot and used in a laparoscopic pelvic trainer model (Figure 6). The learners then performed a robotic anastomosis with a Van Velthoven suture (double armed 3-0 Monocryl) using the LapED 4 : 1 model as previously described [10, 11].

3. Results

3.1. Ease of Model Construction. The cost of the open urological surgery simulators is minimal, and the supplies can be purchased at a local grocery store. The prostatectomy model and wound closure model may be reused for simulation settings, although repeated use may necessitate replacing the orange and banana components for the models, respectively.

3.2. Assessing the Models. Ten urology resident trainees attended the session; 7 urology resident trainees completed the questionnaire, ranging from postgraduate year (PGY) two to five. Trainees felt overall that the activities were helpful in practicing their surgical skills (median Likert score 4/5, range 4-5) and that they would recommend these activities to others interested in practicing their surgical skills (median Likert score 4/5, range 4-5). They also felt confident they could easily replicate the activities, excluding the DVSSS, for personal use (median Likert score 4/5, range 4-5). Face validity is typically demonstrated by a Likert score of 4/5 [12]. When assessing the models individually, trainees felt positive about the prostatectomy model's relative realism (median Likert score 4, range 4-5) and its ability to improve their confidence in suturing a prostate (median Likert score 4, range 3-4). They felt ambivalent about the usefulness of the wound closure station in improving their confidence performing the task (median Likert score 3/5, range 3-4). Trainees also felt neutral about the knot-tying station (median Likert score 3.5/5, range 3-4).

4. Discussion

Simulators currently available for urology training range from low-fidelity bench models to high-fidelity virtual reality models. The models used during the skills workshop for this study may be considered low fidelity, but have the advantage of being affordable, replicable, and portable for trainee use. Additionally, the simulators in this study focused on improving techniques for open urological procedures, which contrasts the more widely available simulators for laparoscopic and robot-assisted procedures [13].

Options for open technique training are limited; however, there are some other models being developed. An open pyeloplasty model using chicken skin demonstrated effectiveness in improving knot tying and suturing ability among medical students [14]. This model is inexpensive and sufficiently replicates living tissue, but there was significant preparation required in producing the model, though it could easily be reproduced by urology resident trainees.

Table 1: Distribution of responses to face validity questionnaire.

	Strongly disagree	Disagree	Neutral	Agree	Strongly agree	Median Likert score
(1) The orange-in-milk-jug prostate model provided a reasonable representation of an open prostatectomy.				3	2	4
(2) The orange-in-milk-jug prostate model improved my confidence in suturing the prostate during an open prostatectomy.			2	3		4
(3) The banana peel suturing station provided a reasonable representation of tissue behavior.			2	3		4
(4) The banana peel suturing station improved my confidence in suturing for wound closure.			3	1		3
(5) The cooked pasta provided a reasonable representation of delicate tissue behavior.			1	3		4
(6) Suturing the cooked pasta improved my confidence in suturing delicate tissue.			1	3		4
(7) Tying knots with cooked spaghetti helped me determine the appropriate amount of force to apply when advancing a knot.			1	1		3.5
(8) Performing the thread the rings exercise on the Da Vinci skills simulator improved my confidence in controlling a needle laparoscopically.			1	3		4
(9) Overall, I found the activities to be helpful in practicing my surgical skills.				3	2	4
(10) I feel confident that I could easily replicate the activities for personal use (excluding the Da Vinci skills simulator).				3	2	4
(11) I would recommend these activities to others interested in practicing their surgical skills.				3	2	4

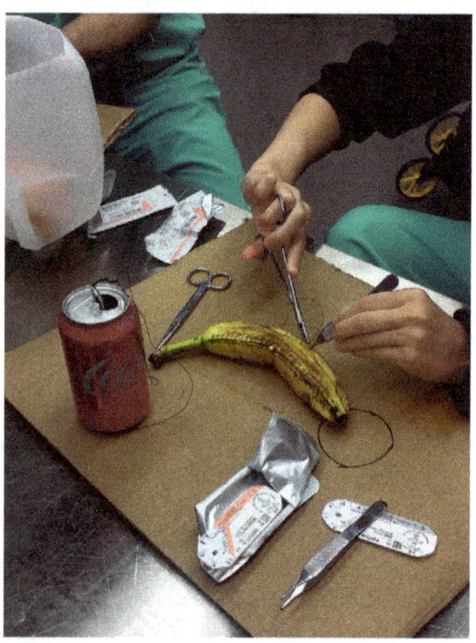

Figure 1: Wound closure model. Learners utilize old banana peels to practice surgical wound closure. Standard running suture and running horizontal mattress. Cola can top can be used to practice knot tying with added difficulty by reducing fluid in the can and not allowing the learner to lift the can as they lead down the knot.

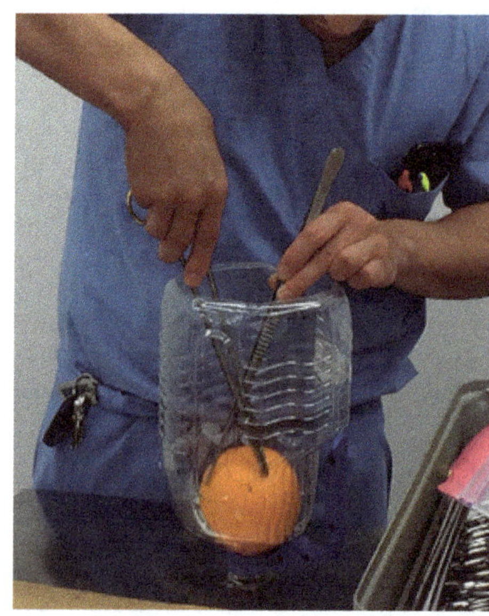

Figure 2: Open prostatectomy model. The orange represents the prostate, and the bottle represents a deep pelvis. Learners can use this model to practice suturing and tying in the pelvis. If the orange is glued down, the learner could also perform a simple prostatectomy by cutting the peel and removing the flesh within the orange as the transitional zone.

Low-fidelity models have also been produced for radical prostatectomy using ballistics gel to reproduce neurovascular bundle dissection [15]. The model was significant for its correct anatomy and for emphasizing the anatomical relationships between the fascia, prostatic capsule, and neurovascular bundle. Preparing low-fidelity models may require more preparation but can be performed by attending physicians and their learners at low cost. The same

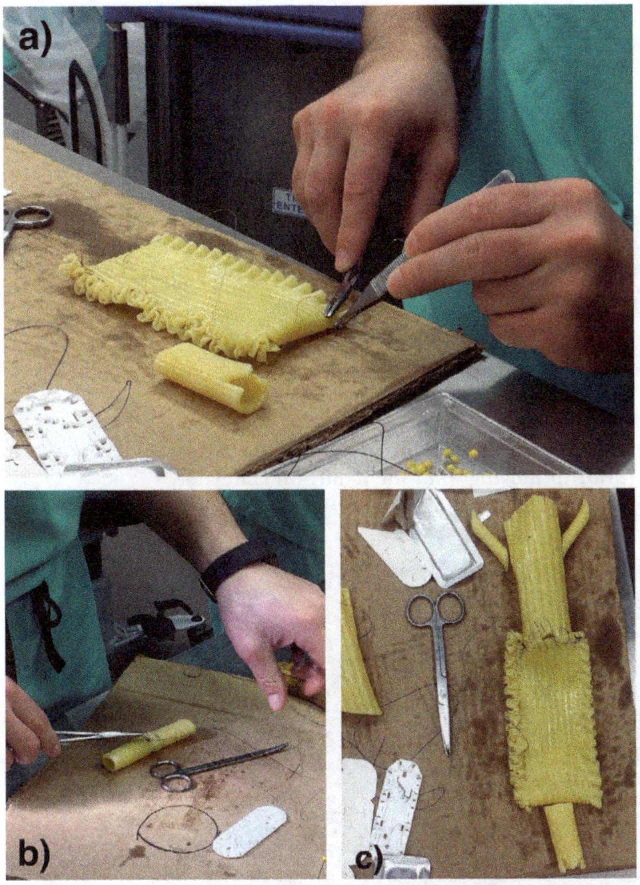

Figure 3: Delicate tissue simulation. (a) Resident suturing cooked pasta al dente. (b) Practicing anastomoses. (c) Neobladder recreation.

study created a simple prostatectomy model similar to the one utilized in our surgical skills workshop. The model utilized citrus fruit to simulate the prostate and included a balloon pulled through the neck of the fruit to form the prostatic urethra. In addition to the balloon urethra, the model also differed from ours, in that the fruit was sutured to a foam board rather than being fixed within a milk carton to replicate the surgical field. Both the neurovascular bundle model and the simple prostatectomy model demonstrated high Likert scores (4.75/5 and 4.5/5, respectively) for overall learning experience.

Suture simulators may be homemade like those utilized in this workshop, or they may be commercially purchased. Homemade simulators are often made of foam, cloth, fruit, or raw chicken, which either lack realism or are difficult to store long term [16]. Commercial simulators are high fidelity but are often ten-fold more expensive than homemade simulators. The suture simulators used in this workshop included a banana (to replicate wound closure) and cooked pasta (to replicate delicate tissue). Cooked pasta has been used in training plastic surgery trainees for microsurgical techniques and has been demonstrated to be a cost-effective, ethical, and suitable simulator [8]. To the best of the authors' knowledge, the use of cooked pasta for urological training

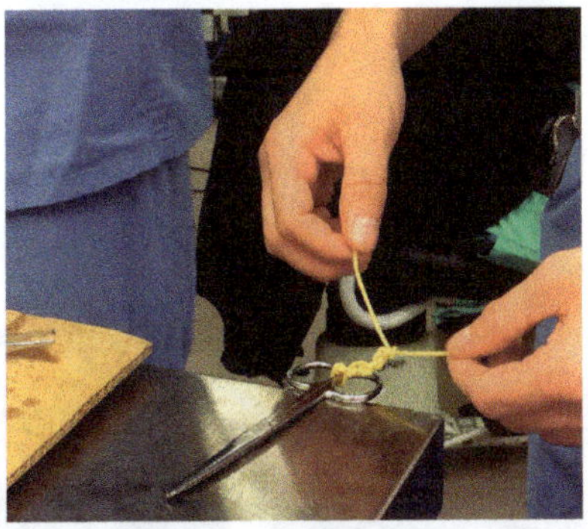

(a)

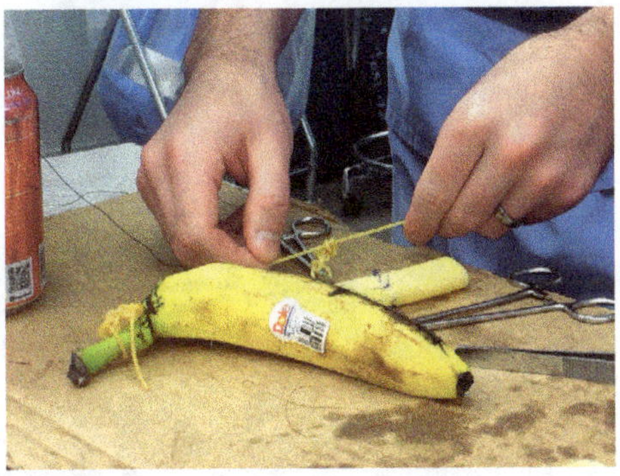

(b)

Figure 4: Knot tying. Utilizing overcooked and al dente spaghetti pasta to perform knot tying will allow the learner to tie a knot with appropriate pressure and confirm square knots.

purposes has not been published and may be a viable option for practicing anastomoses of the fragile tissue.

Overall, the trainees considered the various models used in the workshop to be realistic and the activities useful for training purposes. Some activities such as the knot-tying station and wound closure model might be better utilized in the earlier years of surgical training. Only one respondent was a PGY-2 trainee; so, the lower Likert score for these activities may be because the participants had adequate training and self-confidence prior to the workshop.

Despite evaluating face validity, this study did not assess construct validity. Before using the models and exercises for training, it would be advisable to have them assessed by urology experts to evaluate construct validity. This study also did not investigate if training with the simulator translates to improved trainee performance in the operating room. In future studies, we will test improvement on the robot simulator and improved suturing skills in surgery based on performance evaluations.

5. Conclusions

This study provides support for exploring innovative methods for surgical skills simulation as it establishes face validity while minimizing costs. The models demonstrated reasonable realism, and the residents endorsed use of the models and activities for improving surgical skills. While

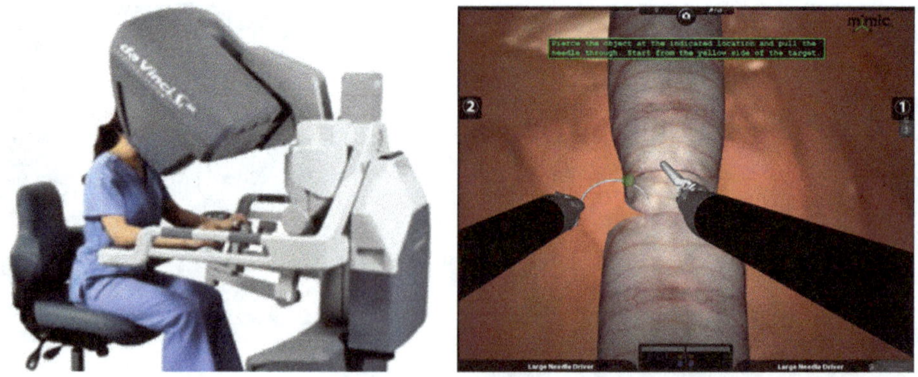

(a) (b)

Figure 5: Robotic simulator by mimic technologies. The robotic simulator attaches to the back of the robot operative cart and connects to the video cable. We use the simulator function "tubes" for two rounds prior to moving onto the hands-on simulator.

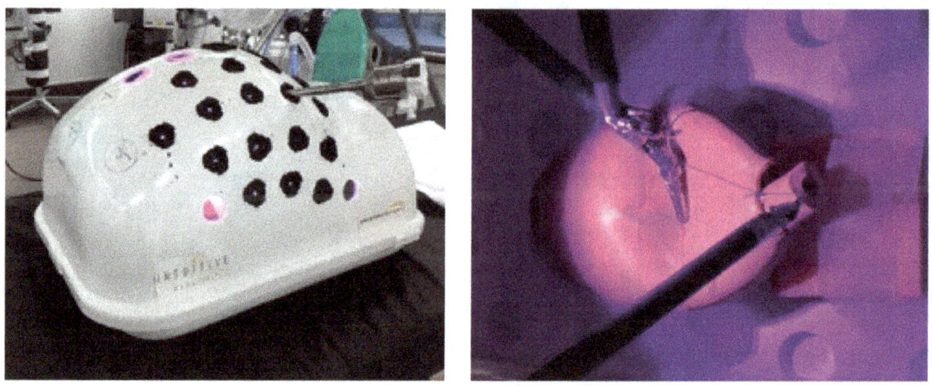

(a) (b)

Figure 6: Robotic simulation (hands-on). Using the standard pelvic Da Vinci trainer and the Da Vinci Xi robot, we perform standard vesicourethral anastomosis using the LapED 4 : 1 silicone training model.

these simulators may not fully replace the use of other costlier training options, the authors hope urology residents will take advantage of these affordable alternatives to supplement their training.

Acknowledgments

This work was supported by the Office of the Assistant Secretary of Defense for Health Affairs through the Prostate Cancer Research Program under Award no. W81XWH-15-1-0441. Additional funding for this work was provided by the Roger L and Laura D. Zeller Foundation.

References

[1] R. K. Reznick and H. MacRae, "Teaching surgical skills—changes in the wind," *New England Journal of Medicine*, vol. 355, no. 25, pp. 2664–2669, 2006.

[2] A. Aydin, A. M. A. Shafi, M. Shamim Khan, P. Dasgupta, and K. Ahmed, "Current status of simulation and training models in urological surgery: a systematic review," *Journal of Urology*, vol. 196, no. 2, pp. 312–320, 2016.

[3] M. A. Liss and E. M. McDougall, "Robotic surgical simulation," *The Cancer Journal*, vol. 19, no. 2, pp. 124–129, 2013.

[4] D. A. Duchene, A. Moinzadeh, I. S. Gill, R. V. Clayman, and H. N. Winfield, "Survey of residency training in laparoscopic and robotic surgery," *Journal of Urology*, vol. 176, no. 5, pp. 2158–2167, 2006.

[5] A. Aydin, N. Raison, M. S. Khan, P. Dasgupta, and K. Ahmed, "Simulation-based training and assessment in urological surgery," *Nature Reviews Urology*, vol. 13, no. 9, pp. 503–519, 2016.

[6] J. W. Gunter III, J. D. Simmons, M. E. Mitchell, and N. Ahmed, "A solution to the decreased resident exposure to open operations in the era of minimally invasive surgery and restricted duty hours may be with organ procurement and transplantation surgery," *Journal of Surgical Education*, vol. 69, no. 5, pp. 575–579, 2012.

[7] K. Ahmed, A. Aydin, P. Dasgupta, M. S. Khan, and J. E. McCabe, "A novel cadaveric simulation program in urology," *Journal of Surgical Education*, vol. 72, no. 4, pp. 556–565, 2015.

[8] L. S. S. Patel and M. Maher, "0011 simulating microsurgery for plastic surgey trainees using boiled pasta—a cost effective,

accessible idea preventing de-skilling," *BMJ Simulation and Technology Enhanced Learning*, vol. 1, no. S1, 2014.

[9] M. A. Liss, C. J. Kane, T. Chen, J. Baumgartner, and I. H. Derweesh, "Virtual reality suturing task as an objective test for robotic experience assessment," *BMC Urology*, vol. 15, p. 63, 2015.

[10] R. F. Van Velthoven, T. E. Ahlering, A. Peltier, D. W. Skarecky, and R. V. Clayman, "Technique for laparoscopic running urethrovesical anastomosis:the single knot method," *Urology*, vol. 61, no. 4, pp. 699–702, 2003.

[11] J. B. A. Abraham, C. S. Abdelshehid, H. J. Lee et al., "LapED 4-In-1 silicone training aid for practicing laparoscopic skills and tasks: a preliminary evaluation," *Journal of Endourology*, vol. 22, no. 6, pp. 1351–1358, 2008.

[12] B. M. A. Schout, A. J. M. Hendrikx, F. Scheele, B. L. H. Bemelmans, and A. J. J. A. Scherpbier, "Validation and implementation of surgical simulators: a critical review of present, past, and future," *Surgical Endoscopy*, vol. 24, no. 3, pp. 536–546, 2010.

[13] R. Khan, A. Aydin, M. S. Khan, P. Dasgupta, and K. Ahmed, "Simulation-based training for prostate surgery," *BJU International*, vol. 116, no. 4, pp. 665–674, 2015.

[14] J. Ooi, N. Lawrentschuk, and D. L. Murphy, "Training model for open or laparoscopic pyeloplasty," *Journal of Endourology*, vol. 20, no. 2, pp. 149–152, 2006.

[15] N. Lawrentschuk, U. Lindner, and L. Klotz, "Realistic anatomical prostate models for surgical skills workshops using ballistic gelatin for nerve-sparing radical prostatectomy and fruit for simple prostatectomy," *Korean Journal of Urology*, vol. 52, no. 2, pp. 130–135, 2011.

[16] N. Uppal and S. Saldanha, "Low-cost suturing training model for use in developing nations," *British Journal of Oral and Maxillofacial Surgery*, vol. 50, no. 1, pp. e13–e14, 2012.

32

Comparison of Oxidative Effects of Two Different Administration Form of Oxybutynin in the Potential Target Tissues

Kaan Kaltalioglu,[1] **Fatmanur Tugcu-Demiroz**,[2] **Fusun Acarturk**,[2] **Barbaros Balabanli**,[3] **and Sule Coskun-Cevher**[3]

[1]*Espiye Vocational School, Giresun University, 28600 Giresun, Turkey*
[2]*Pharmaceutical Technology Department, Pharmacy Faculty, Gazi University, 06330 Ankara, Turkey*
[3]*Biology Department, Science Faculty, Gazi University, 06500 Ankara, Turkey*

Correspondence should be addressed to Kaan Kaltalioglu; kaan.kaltalioglu@gmail.com

Academic Editor: Matthew Rutman

Oxybutynin is an important anticholinergic agent that prevents uncontrolled contractions in the treatment of overactive bladder (OAB). However, drugs containing oxybutynin have significant side effects such as dry eyes, dry mouth, increased heart rate, constipation, blurred vision, and confusion. In recent years, new delivery methods for this agent are being searched. One of them is vaginal delivery. In this study, we aimed to compare the effects of oxybutynin on oxidative parameters in the potential target tissues of the oral and vaginal delivery. Female New Zealand white rabbits ($n = 12$) were divided into two groups: oral delivery and vaginal delivery. The animals were sacrificed 48 h after administration and nitric oxide (NOx), thiobarbituric acid-reactive substances (TBARs), and glutathione (GSH) levels were determined spectrophotometrically in the aorta, salivary gland, and small intestine tissue samples. Vaginal delivery significantly decreased NOx levels in all tissue samples as compared to oral delivery ($p < 0.05$). Moreover, it reduced TBARs levels in salivary gland and aorta tissue samples ($p < 0.05$). In the light on these findings, it can be said that vaginal delivery may decrease the oxidant-induced side effects of oxybutynin as compared to oral delivery.

1. Introduction

Overactive bladder (OAB) is a syndrome that occurs owing to the spontaneous activity of the detrusor muscle during the filling of bladder and marked by urinary urgency, with/without urge incontinence, usually accompanied by nocturia and frequency [1, 2]. OAB is common in both men and women, and negatively affects the quality of life (QOL) [3]. Recent reports showed that the prevalence of OAB is 35.15% in United States [4], and 20% in Asia (men and women aged ≥40 years) [5]. Two main classes of drugs have been used for the treatment of OAB: antimuscarinics (anticholinergics) and β3-adrenoreceptor agonists [6].

The detrusor muscle contractility is generally orchestrated by the parasympathetic nervous system, which acetylcholine (ACh) is the primary neurotransmitter in these actions [7]. Antimuscarinics inhibits the binding of acetylcholine at M_2 and M_3 muscarinic receptors on bladder smooth muscle to show their effects on OAB. Antimuscarinics has demonstrated efficacy for the treatment of OAB, but they affect the potential target organs or tissues, and they can cause side effects for some people [7]. These side effects such as dry mouth, dry eyes, increased heart rate, constipation, confusion, and blurred vision are related to dose [8].

Oxybutynin, a tertiary amine, is an antimuscarinic agent used widely in the treatment of OAB for many years [6]. Oxybutynin has an antimuscarinic and a direct muscle relaxant effect, as well as local anesthetic actions [9]. Nevertheless, it can cause side effects and is discontinued in over 60% of patients due to adverse effects [10]. Oxybutynin have major side effects include dry eyes, dry mouth, blurred vision, and constipation [2]. Oxybutynin is highly lipophilic molecule to have the ability of penetrate the blood-brain barrier [6]. *N*-desethyloxybutynin, which is the major metabolite of oxybutynin, may cause systemic side effects. Oxybutynin and *N*-desethyloxybutynin have similar impacts on the detrusor smooth muscle. But, *N*-desethyloxybutynin is more vigorous in the salivary glands (leads to dry mouth) [11].

Vaginal drug delivery systems promise remarkable potential in pharmacy. The major advantages of this route include a considerable surface area, good blood supply, relatively high permeability to many drugs, and the ability to bypass first-pass liver metabolism [2]. Previous works suggested that the vaginal delivery of oxybutynin may have serious advantages over the oral delivery with relation to long duration of action, consistent blood levels, and reduction of side effects [2].

The imbalance between oxidants and antioxidants (called as oxidative stress) is involved in the etiology and/or pathogenesis of a number of disorders [12]. Reactive oxygen species (ROS) and reactive nitrogen species (RNS) generate a harmful process that can alter the cell membranes and other structures such as proteins, lipids, proteins, and DNA and trigger various diseases [13, 14]. For instance, Sjögren's Syndrome (SS) is an autoimmune disorder, which leads to dry eye and dry mouth. It has been proposed that oxidative stress plays a role in the pathogenesis of SS [15]. It has also been reported that oxidative stress may cause changes in the structure of the salivary gland and may involve in hyposalivation [16]. In addition, nitric oxide may also affect saliva secretion [17].

In this study, we compared the effects of oral and vaginal delivery of oxybutynin on some oxidative parameters (NOx, TBARs, and GSH) on the aorta, salivary gland, and small intestine, organs where oxybutynin may cause side effects.

2. Material and Methods

2.1. Drugs and Chemicals. In this study, oxybutynin hydrochloride was obtained from Sigma (USA). Also, Üropan® (Koçak Farma, Turkey) tablet (5 mg oxybutynin) was purchased from markets, and all other chemicals unless until mentioned were of analytical grade.

2.2. Experiment. The protocol of this study was confirmed by the Animal Ethical Committee of Gazi University, Turkey (G.Ü.ET-04.033). Twelve female New Zealand white rabbits weighing 2.5–3.5 kg were housed them in a controlled environment. During the experimental period animals were allowed free access to food and water. They fasted for 24 h before application. The animals were divided randomly into two groups: oral delivery ($n = 6$) and vaginal delivery ($n = 6$). Vaginal solution (containing 10 mg oxybutynin/1.5 mL pH 4.5 phosphate buffer) was administered through the vaginal route with an applicator as a single dose every 48 h. Üropan® tablets (5 mg oxybutynin) were also administered orally through an oral gavage as a single dose every 24 h. After 48 h from administration, the animals were killed with intracardiac blood aspiration under ketamine/xylazine anesthesia (intramuscularly, 75 and 5 mg/kg, respectively). The aorta, salivary gland, and small intestine tissue samples were collected, frozen and kept in −80° until assay.

2.3. Determination of NOx, TBARs, and GSH. The reactive nitrogen oxide species (NOx) levels were measured spectrophotometrically at 540 nm by Griess reaction. NOx are stable end products of nitric oxide. Sodium nitrite was considered as the standard [18]. Lipid peroxidation was determined spectrophotometrically according to the method detailed before at 535 nm. This method based on the principle that the generation of malondialdehyde (MDA) as an end product of lipid peroxidation, which interacts with thiobarbituric acid producing thiobarbituric acid-reactive substance (TBARs). Tetraethoxypropane solution was considered as a standard for this assay [18]. Levels of glutathione (GSH) were measured spectrophotometrically according to a modified version of the Ellman method at 412 nm. In this method, 5,5′-dithiobis(2-nitrobenzoic acid) (DTNB) reacts with reduced GSH to form a yellow-colored compound [18].

2.4. Statistical Analysis. All results were defined as the mean ± standard deviation. One-way ANOVA (with posthoc Tukey test) was used to compare mean differences. Results of $P < 0.05$ were considered to be statistically significant.

3. Results and Discussion

The amounts of the NOx, TBARs, and GSH in the aorta, salivary gland, and small intestine tissue samples are presented in Figure 1. Our results showed that in the vaginal delivery groups, the levels of NOx are significantly lower in all tissue samples (aorta (140.54 ± 4.63 nmol/g tissue), salivary gland (195.99 ± 24.03 nmol/g tissue), and small intestine (154.29 ± 7.37 nmol/g tissue)) as compared to oral delivery groups (228.63 ± 20.13 nmol/g tissue, 343.42 ± 18.33 nmol/g tissue, 198.69 ± 7.23 nmol/g tissue, respectively) ($p < 0.05$) (Figure 1). Nitric oxide, a highly reactive gas molecule, has multiple physiological roles in both intra- and extracellular signal transduction pathways with relations for health and disease [19]. The concentration of NO is critical since it acts as a signaling molecule at low concentrations, although, at high concentrations, NO or RNS can exert toxic effects on the cell; it is damage to proteins, lipids, and DNA and can lead to cell death or tissue injury [14, 20]. Salivation is dependent on cholinergic stimulation via autonomic nerves and intracellular signals in acinar cells [21]. NO and acetylcholine (ACh) function in salivation. NO can stimulate salivary gland cells to secrete fluid, but a prolonged exposure has a detrimental effect on the cells [22]. Konttinen et al. reported that NO is an important factor in altering salivation in SS, which is characterized by dry mouth and dry eye. Nitrite is present at high concentrations in saliva of these patients, and inducible NO synthase (iNOS) expression is elevated in various cells in salivary glands [23]. Also, dry mouth is an important side effect of the administration of oxybutynin. Therefore, the

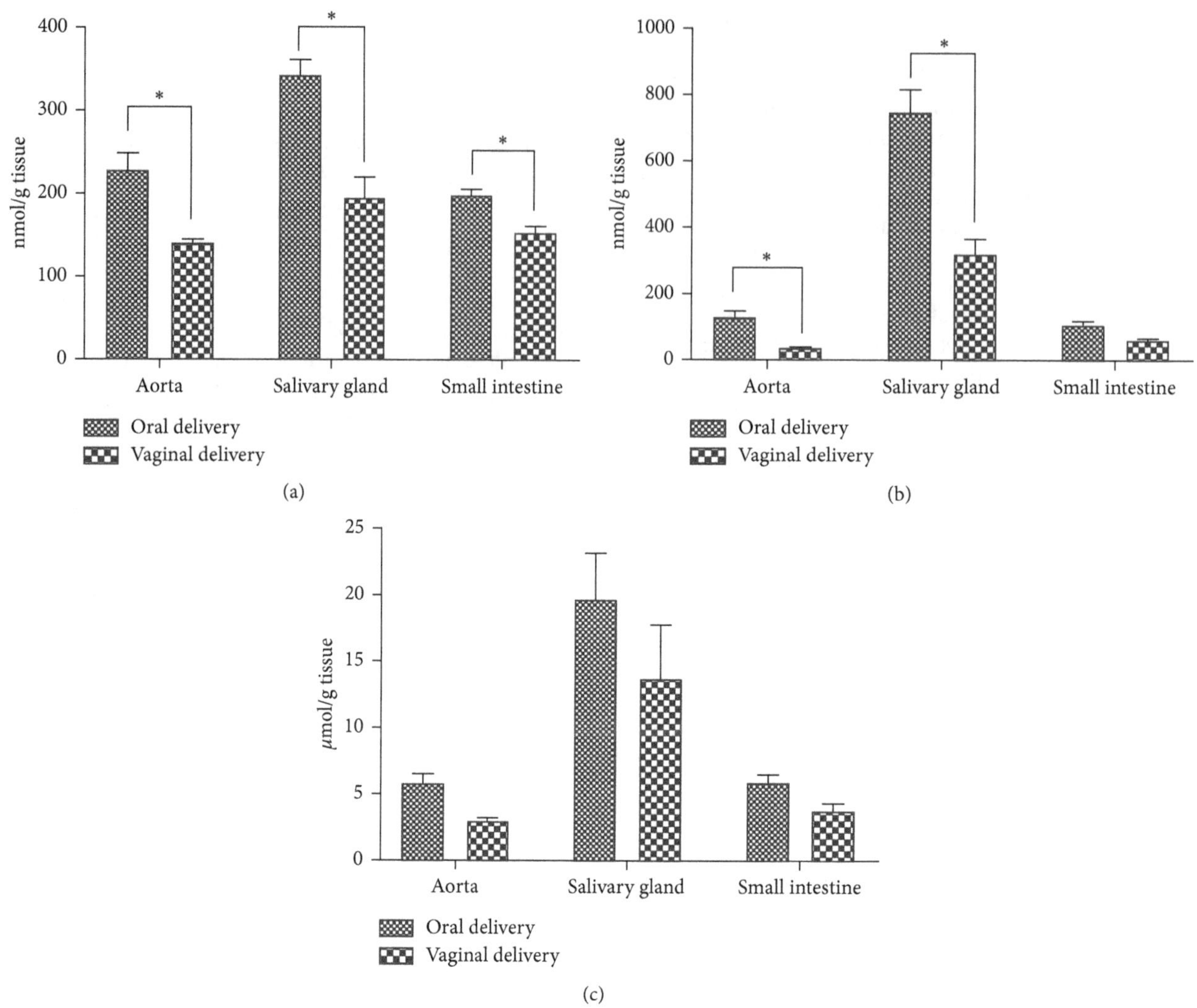

FIGURE 1: Effects of the oral and vaginal delivery of oxybutynin on NOx (a), TBARs (b), and GSH (c) levels in various tissues. $p < 0.05$ compared to the oral and vaginal delivery group.

preference for vaginal delivery may be beneficial for salivation as it reduces NO concentration.

Otherwise, another side effect of oxybutynin is increased heart rate. NO plays an important role in heart contraction response, heart rate, and regulation of vascular tone [24]. The effects of NO on the heart rate are complex. But, in general, NO has a positive chronotropic effect, and NOS inhibition causes a reduction of heart rate [25]. The different effects of NO might be dependent on its concentration. As shown in Figure 1, the level of NOx in the aorta tissue samples of the vaginal delivery group was significantly lower than oral delivery group ($p < 0.05$).

Constipation is a common side effect that may potentially appear with the use of oxybutynin. Another important function of NO is that it affects the gastrointestinal tract (via relaxation of the enteric smooth muscle). A previous study suggested that NO supports maintain gastric mucosal integrity and has a protective effect [20]. In contrast, in cirrhotic rats, L-NAME (a nonselective inhibitor of NOS) alleviate inhibited-gastrointestinal motility. Wang et al. reported that NO may play an important role in the inhibition of gastrointestinal motility [26]. In another study, Tomita et al. found that NO has a significant function in the dysmotility detected in the STC patients' colons [27]. Taken together, the above results suggest that instead of oral delivery, vaginal delivery may be beneficial in attenuating deleterious effects of NO by reducing the concentration of NO.

A significant decrease in TBARs levels of aorta (36.86 ± 3.88 nmol/g tissue) and salivary gland tissues (322.72 ± 43.17 nmol/g tissue) was observed in the vaginal delivery groups when compared with oral delivery groups (131.41 ± 16.66 nmol/g tissue, 749.15 ± 67.50 nmol/g tissue, respectively) ($p < 0.05$) (Figure 1). Lipid peroxidation products are markers for oxidative stress status *in vivo* and its related diseases. Malondialdehyde (MDA) is an important oxidation product, which is considered as the main marker in lipid peroxidation, and can be measured via TBARs assay [28–30]. Some metabolites are formed by the metabolism of oxybutynin by the cytochrome P450 enzyme system. One of these, *N*-desethyloxybutynin, is a stable and toxic metabolite [31]. This oxybutynin derived toxic metabolite can alter oxidative stability. Oxidative stress may lead to dysfunction of salivary gland [32]. Several studies have shown oxidative stress effects secretion and components (calcium, protein, etc.) of saliva [33, 34]. Additionally, it has been suggested that ROS concerned with the onset and pathology of SS [15, 34, 35]. Similarly to salivation, heart failure may also be associated with oxidative stress. Studies of the causes responsible for the progression of heart failure have shown that reactive oxygen species (ROS) play an important pathological role [36]. Overall, these findings indicate that vaginal delivery may be beneficial as it reduces TBARS levels and hence oxidative stress.

In all tissue samples, the level of GSH in the oral delivery group (aorta ($5.83 \pm 0.67\,\mu$mol/g tissue), salivary gland ($19.72 \pm 3.45\,\mu$mol/g tissue), and small intestine ($5.95 \pm 0.56\,\mu$mol/g tissue)) was found to be higher than vaginal delivery group ($2.98 \pm 0.23\,\mu$mol/g tissue, $13.77 \pm 3.97\,\mu$mol/g tissue, $3.86 \pm 0.48\,\mu$mol/g tissue, respectively), but it was not statistically significant ($p > 0.05$) (Figure 1). GSH is a tripeptide acts as a free radical scavenger and is an important member of antioxidant defense system. The reason for this is not clear, but a possible explanation may be that the organism may have increased the level of GSH in order to strengthen the antioxidant defense system in response to increasing oxidative stress (parallel with TBARs result).

4. Conclusion

Oxidants, especially nitric oxide, play an important role in the pathophysiology of many diseases. Instead of orally administration, vaginal administration of oxybutynin can alleviate oxidant-induced side effects. These results can contribute to pharmaceutical studies.

References

[1] R. Vozmediano-Chicharro, B. Madurga, and P. Blasco, "Efficacy of transdermal oxybutynin in the treatment of overactive bladder syndrome: does it make sense using it in 2017?," *Advances in Urology*, vol. 2018, Article ID 6782736, 7 pages, 2018.

[2] F. Tuğcu-Demiröz, F. Acartürk, and D. Erdoğan, "Development of long-acting bioadhesive vaginal gels of oxybutynin: formulation, in vitro and in vivo evaluations," *International Journal of Pharmaceutics*, vol. 457, no. 1, pp. 25–39, 2013.

[3] R. Eapen and S. Radomski, "Review of the epidemiology of overactive bladder," *Research and Reports in Urology*, vol. 2016, pp. 71–76, 2016.

[4] K. S. Coyne, C. C. Sexton, V. Vats, C. Thompson, Z. S. Kopp, and I. Milsom, "National community prevalence of overactive bladder in the United States stratified by sex and age," *Urology*, vol. 77, no. 5, pp. 1081–1087, 2011.

[5] Y. C. Chuang, S. P. Liu, K. S. Lee et al., "Prevalence of overactive bladder in China, Taiwan and South Korea: results from a cross-sectional, population-based study," *Lower Urinary Tract Symptoms*, pp. 1–8, 2017.

[6] V. Hopkinson and I. Pearce, "Pharmacotherapy in overactive bladder," *Journal of Clinical Urology*, vol. 11, no. 1, pp. 38–47, 2017.

[7] P. Abrams and K.-E. Andersson, "Muscarinic receptor antagonists for overactive bladder," *BJU International*, vol. 100, no. 5, pp. 987–1006, 2007.

[8] J. Jayarajan and S. B. Radomski, "Pharmacotherapy of overactive bladder in adults: a review of efficacy, tolerability, and quality of life," *Research and Reports in Urology*, vol. 6, pp. 1–16, 2014.

[9] A. Athanasopoulos and K. Giannitsas, "An overview of the clinical use of antimuscarinics in the treatment of overactive bladder," *Advances in Urology*, vol. 2011, Article ID 820816, 8 pages, 2011.

[10] J. I. Ivanova, E. Hayes-Larson, R. A. Sorg, H. G. Birnbaum, and T. Berner, "Healthcare resource use and costs of privately insured patients who switch, discontinue, or persist on antimuscarinic therapy for overactive bladder," *Journal of Medical Economics*, vol. 17, no. 10, pp. 741–750, 2014.

[11] J. A. Cohn, E. T. Brown, W. S. Reynolds, M. R. Kaufman, D. F. Milam, and R. R. Dmochowski, "An update on the use of transdermal oxybutynin in the management of overactive bladder disorder," *Therapeutic Advances in Urology*, vol. 8, no. 2, pp. 83–90, 2016.

[12] V. Kumar, A. A. Khan, A. Tripathi et al., "Role of oxidative stress in various diseases: relevance of dietary antioxidants," *Journal of Phytopharmacology*, vol. 4, no. 2, pp. 126–132, 2015.

[13] A. Phaniendra, D. B. Jestadi, and L. Periyasamy, "Free radicals: properties, sources, targets, and their implication in various diseases," *Indian Journal of Clinical Biochemistry*, vol. 30, no. 1, pp. 11–26, 2014.

[14] E. Birben, U. M. Sahiner, C. Sackesen, S. Erzurum, and O. Kalayci, "Oxidative stress and antioxidant defense," *World Allergy Organization Journal*, vol. 5, no. 1, pp. 9–19, 2012.

[15] K. Ryo, A. Takahashi, Y. Tamaki, M. Ohnishi-Kameyama, H. Inoue, and I. Saito, "Therapeutic effects of isoflavones on impaired salivary secretion," *Journal of Clinical Biochemistry and Nutrition*, vol. 55, no. 3, pp. 168–173, 2014.

[16] Y. Yamauchi, T. Matsuno, K. Omata, and T. Satoh, "Relationship between hyposalivation and oxidative stress in aging mice," *Journal of Clinical Biochemistry and Nutrition*, vol. 61, no. 1, pp. 40–46, 2017.

[17] M. L. Breseghelo, L. A. Guillo, T. E. Nogueira et al., "Nitric oxide concentration and other salivary changes after insertion of new complete dentures in edentulous subjects," *International Journal of Dentistry*, vol. 2016, Article ID 8351427, 6 pages, 2016.

[18] B. Dindar, K. Kaltalioglu, and S. Coskun-Cevher, "Effect of dual growth factor administration on oxidative markers during acute stage wound healing in rats," *Turkish Journal of Zoology*, vol. 41, pp. 841–847, 2017.

[19] P. Domingos, A. M. Prado, A. Wong, C. Gehring, and J. A. Feijo, "Nitric oxide: a multitasked signaling gas in plants," *Molecular Plant*, vol. 8, no. 4, pp. 506–520, 2015.

[20] P. Gul, H. Alp, A. Kiziltunc, and N. Akgul, "Effects of composite restorations on nitric oxide and uric acid levels in saliva," *Contemporary Clinical Dentistry*, vol. 6, no. 3, pp. 381–385, 2015.

[21] G. B. Proctor and G. H. Carpenter, "Salivary secretion: mechanism and neural regulation," in *Saliva: Secretion and Functions*, A. J. M. Ligtenberg and E. C. I. Veerman, Eds., vol. 24, pp. 14–29, 2014.

[22] J. Malone, "Inflammation, nitric oxide and Sjögren's syndrome," *British Sjögren' Syndrome Association Today Magazine*, vol. 25, no. 2, pp. 2-3, 2010.

[23] Y. T. Konttinen, L. A. M. Platts, S. Tuominen et al., "Role of nitric oxide in Sjögren's syndrome," *Arthritis and Rheumatism*, vol. 40, no. 5, pp. 875–883, 1997.

[24] G. Özcan, E. A. Şahin, and E. Demirel Yilmaz, "Effect of nitric oxide on cardiac functions: review," *Turkiye Klinikleri Cardiovascular Sciences*, vol. 28, no. 3, pp. 99–117, 2016.

[25] A. Gamboa, L. E. Okamoto, S. R. Raj et al., "Nitric oxide and regulation of heart rate in patients with postural tachycardia syndrome and healthy subjects," *Hypertension*, vol. 61, no. 2, pp. 376–381, 2013.

[26] X. Wang, Y.-X. Zhong, Z.-Y. Zhang et al., "Effect of L-NAME on nitric oxide and gastrointestinal motility alterations in cirrhotic rats," *World Journal of Gastroenterology*, vol. 8, no. 2, pp. 328–332, 2002.

[27] R. Tomita, S. Fujisaki, T. Ikeda, and M. Fukuzawa, "Role of nitric oxide in the colon of patients with slow-transit constipation," *Diseases of the Colon and Rectum*, vol. 45, no. 5, pp. 593–600, 2002.

[28] E. Niki, "Lipid peroxidation products as oxidative stress biomarkers," *BioFactors*, vol. 34, no. 2, pp. 171–180, 2008.

[29] T. M. Potter, B. W. Neun, and S. T. Stern, "Assay to detect lipid peroxidation upon exposure to nanoparticles," *Methods in Molecular Biology*, vol. 697, pp. 181–189, 2010.

[30] A. Zeb and F. Ullah, "A simple spectrophotometric method for the determination of thiobarbituric acid reactive substances in fried fast foods," *Journal of Analytical Methods in Chemistry*, vol. 2016, Article ID 9412767, 5 pages, 2016.

[31] R. K. Malcolm, S. D. McCullagh, and R. J. Morrow, "Vagina and uterus as drug-absorbing organs," in *Enhancement in Drug Delivery*, E. Touitou and B. W. Barry, Eds., vol. 1, p. 429, 2006.

[32] M. Choromańska, A. Klimiuk, P. Kostecka-Sochoń et al., "Antioxidant defence, oxidative stress and oxidative damage in saliva, plasma and erythrocytes of dementia patients. Can salivary AGE be a marker of dementia?," *International Journal of Molecular Sciences*, vol. 18, no. 10, p. 2205, 2017.

[33] M. Pande and S. J. S. Flora, "Lead induced oxidative damage and its response to combined administration of α-lipoic acid and succimers in rats," *Toxicology*, vol. 177, no. 2-3, pp. 187–196, 2002.

[34] T. Yamada, K. Ryo, Y. Tai et al., "Evaluation of therapeutic effects of astaxanthin on impairments in salivary secretion," *Journal of Clinical Biochemistry and Nutrition*, vol. 47, no. 2, pp. 130–137, 2010.

[35] K. Okabayashi, T. Narita, Y. Takahashi et al., "Effect of oxidative stress on secretory function in salivary gland cells," in *Oxidative Stress-Environmental Induction and Dietary Antioxidants*, V. Lushchak, Ed., pp. 189–200, 2012.

[36] H. Nojiri, T. Shimizu, M. Funakoshi et al., "Oxidative stress causes heart failure with impaired mitochondrial respiration," *Journal of Biological Chemistry*, vol. 281, no. 44, pp. 33789–33801, 2006.

33

A Review of the Literature on Primary Leiomyosarcoma of the Prostate Gland

Anthony Kodzo-Grey Venyo

Department of Urology, North Manchester General Hospital, Delaunays Road, Manchester, UK

Correspondence should be addressed to Anthony Kodzo-Grey Venyo; akodzogrey@yahoo.co.uk

Academic Editor: In Ho Chang

Primary leiomyosarcoma of the prostate (PLSOP) is rare, with less than 200 cases reported so far. PLSOPs present with lower urinary tract symptoms, haematuria, and perineal pain; may or may not be associated with a history of previous treatment for adenocarcinoma of prostate by means of radiotherapy and or hormonal treatment; may afflict children and adult male. Examination may reveal benign enlarged prostate and hard enlarged mass. PLSOPs may be diagnosed by histological examination findings of spindle-shaped carcinoma cells in prostate specimens. Immunohistochemical staining tends to be positive for vimentin, CD44, smooth muscle actin, and calponin, focally positive for desmin, and at times positive for keratin. They stain negatively for PSA, S-100, CD34, CD117, and cytokeratin. Cytogenetic study on primary leiomyosarcoma of the prostate gland may show clonal chromosomal rearrangement involving Chromosomes 2, 3, 9, 11, and 19. On the whole the prognosis is poor. Surgery with or without chemotherapy would appear to be the mainstay of treatment for PLSOPs that are operable, but generally there is no consensus opinion on the best therapeutic approach. Most cases of PLSOPs are diagnosed in an advanced stage of the disease. A global multicenter trial is required to find therapies that would improve the prognosis.

1. Introduction

Sarcoma of the prostate gland is rare and this accounts for only 0.1% of all malignant tumours of the prostate gland [1]. Leiomyosarcoma of the prostate gland is rare and globally less than 200 cases have been reported in the literature and less than 100 PLSOPs have been reported in the English literature [2]. Leiomyosarcoma accounts for approximately 25% of all sarcomas of the prostate gland. [3] Leiomyosarcoma of the prostate was first described in 1853 by Sambert as stated by Riba et al. [4] in 1950. Leiomyosarcoma of the prostate gland is an aggressive tumour which most clinicians globally have not encountered; in view of this most clinicians would not be familiar with its biological behaviour. The ensuing literature review on primary leiomyosarcoma of the prostate gland is divided into two parts: (A) an overview and (B) miscellaneous narrations and discussions from some reported cases of leiomyosarcoma of the prostate gland.

2. Methods

Various internet data bases were searched, including Google, Google Scholar, PubMed, and Educus, for information on primary leiomyosarcoma of the prostate gland. The search terms used included primary leiomyosarcoma of the prostate gland; leiomyosarcoma of the prostate gland; leiomyosarcoma of prostate; prostatic leiomyosarcoma; primary prostatic leiomyosarcoma. Fifty-five references related to case reports, case series, and other types of the literature related to primary leiomyosarcoma of the prostate gland were identified suitable for writing the literature review.

3. Literature Review

(A) Overview

General Comments

Primary leiomyosarcoma of the prostate gland (PLSOP) is the commonest sarcoma affecting the prostate gland, even though on the whole it is a rare tumour [5].

PLSOPs cause obstruction and tend to involve adjacent organs [5].

PLSOPs tend to recur [5].

PLSOP metastasizes to the liver and lung [5].

PLSOP tends to be associated with a mean survival of 3 to 4 years [5].

Definition. Sarcoma of the prostate is a rare type of malignancy of mesenchymal origin that can rarely afflict the prostate gland. Various types of sarcoma of the prostate gland can occur including leiomyosarcoma, which is a smooth muscle sarcoma, and rhabdomyosarcoma, a skeletal muscle-type sarcoma.

Aetiology of Sarcoma of the Prostate Gland. On the whole the aetiology of PLSOP is unknown or not well understood.

Sarcomatous Dedifferentiation [6]. A number of cases of leiomyosarcoma of the prostate gland develop a number of years after patients had undergone treatment by means of radiotherapy and/or hormonal treatment for adenocarcinoma of the prostate gland. Even though there may be absence of any residual adenocarcinoma of the prostate, evidence of a new malignancy in the form of leiomyosarcoma of the prostate could be conjectured to be a sequel of dedifferentiation of totipotential cells in the prostate gland as an emanation from previous effect of the radiotherapy or hormonal therapy on the totipotential cells.

Li-Fraumeni Syndrome [6–8]. Li-Fraumeni syndrome has been postulated to be associated with mutation of p53 tumour suppressor gene and this leads in some children to the development of sarcomas and their mothers tend to have an increased risk of carcinoma of the breast with siblings having an increased risk for the development of malignancy [7, 8].

Age Distribution. Leiomyosarcoma of the prostate gland has been reported in children and adults whose ages have ranged from 2.5 years to 80 years (see the case of the 2.5-year-old boy in [9]).

Presentation. Patients with PLSOPs tend to present with the following (see [2, 10, 11] for some of the presentations):

(1) "Lower urinary tract symptoms" including urinary frequency, poor flow, hesitancy, urinary urgency, and inability to void. The presentation of lower urinary tract symptoms may mimic benign prostatic hypertrophy clinically in that rectal examination findings may indicate benign prostatic hypertrophy and the diagnosis is established after the patient has undergone transurethral resection of prostate and the histology result would indicate leiomyosarcoma of the prostate.

(2) Haematuria: sometimes a history of previous treatment for adenocarcinoma of prostate by means of hormonal therapy and/or radiotherapy in the form of external beam radiotherapy or brachytherapy may be obtained

(3) Retention of urine may occur.

(4) They may present with an exophytic mass of prostate projecting towards or infiltrating the rectum or a perineal mass.

(5) Leiomyosarcomas of the prostate may manifest with metastases to the liver and lung [12].

Clinical Findings. Digital rectal examination may reveal the following:

(1) An enlarged prostate which may feel benign.

(2) An enlarged/firm prostate gland.

(3) A hard prostate which has extended to the capsule or distorted the capsule.

(4) An enlarged hard mass arising from the prostate and extending to the rectum, pelvic side wall, perineum, and seminal vesicle or involving the base of the urinary bladder.

(5) An enlarged mass arising in the prostate gland in a child with voiding symptoms.

Laboratory Investigations. The following investigations tend to be undertaken in cases of PLSOP:

(1) Urine: urinalysis may be normal or may show evidence of visible or nonvisible haematuria and these are not specific for a diagnosis of leiomyosarcoma of the prostate but form part of the general assessment of the patient. Urine microscopy and culture may or may not show evidence of infection and this examination is used as part of the general assessment of the patient.

(2) Blood tests: routine blood tests are undertaken in the assessment of the patient including full blood count, serum urea and electrolytes, liver function tests, serum glucose, and coagulation screen. If the patient is anaemic, then the appropriate management is undertaken to correct the anaemia. Furthermore attempts tend to be made to correct any impairment noticed in the blood test results to improve upon the general management of the patient. Serum PSA may be normal or raised, but this would not be diagnostic of leiomyosarcoma of the prostate and the level of serum PSA would not be helpful to determine the progress of leiomyosarcoma of the prostate following treatment (see [13], e.g., when serum PSA was normal).

Radiological Investigations. Radiological investigations which may be undertaken in PLSOP include the following:

(1) Ultrasound scan (see [14] when ultrasound scan of abdomen and pelvis was done): ultrasound scan of the abdomen and pelvis would assess whether or not the patient has hydronephrosis; it can also indicate whether or not there is thickening of the bladder wall or trabeculation or sacculation or if there is a blood clot in the urinary bladder. Infiltration of

the base of the bladder or any part of the bladder can be illustrated by ultrasound scan. Enlargement of the prostate as well as the characteristic features of the prostate gland and its relationship to nearby structures can be illustrated by ultrasound scan.

(2) Transrectal ultrasound scan of prostate (TRUSP) and biopsies (see [10, 15] in which transrectal ultrasound scan of prostate and biopsies were undertaken): transrectal ultrasound scan of prostate is a useful technique for the assessment of the characteristics of the prostate gland which may show enlargement of the whole or part of the prostate gland involved. It may show heterogeneous hypoechoic lesions in the prostate, invasion of the capsule or extension into the rectum, pelvic side wall, seminal vesicle, ejaculatory duct, or protrusion into the urinary bladder or infiltration of the wall of the urinary bladder. Transrectal ultrasound-guided biopsy tends to be the usual approach for obtaining specimens of the prostatic lesion for histological examination which would establish the diagnosis of leiomyosarcoma of the prostate. A patient who had previously undergone radiotherapy by means of external beam method or brachytherapy or who has been having hormonal treatment for adenocarcinoma of prostate gland upon subsequent development of relapse and further enlargement of prostate may undergo a further ultrasound-guided biopsy of the prostate gland and its histological examination on the second occasion may reveal leiomyosarcoma of the prostate.

(3) Computed tomography (CT) scan (see [10, 11, 13] in which CT scan was used): CT scan of abdomen, pelvis, and thorax can be used to assess the features of the prostatic lesion, the relation of the lesion to nearby structures, and the extent of the disease locally. It can also show whether or not there is lymphadenopathy or metastases in the abdomen or within the thorax. CT scan can also be used in the follow-up assessment of the patient following treatment.

(4) Magnetic resonance imaging (MRI scan) (see [15] in which MRI scan was used): MRI scan of abdomen, pelvis, and thorax can be used to assess the features of the prostatic lesion, the relation of the lesion to nearby structures, and the extent of the disease locally. It can also show whether or not there is lymphadenopathy or metastases in the abdomen or within the thorax. MRI scan can also be used in the follow-up assessment of the patient following treatment.

(5) Isotope bone scan (see [10] in which isotope bone scan was used): isotope bone scan can be used in the initial as well as follow-up assessment of the patient to ascertain whether or not there is bone metastasis.

Cystoscopy Findings

(i) Cystoscopy may be undertaken in the assessment of the patient and this may show an enlarged prostate gland. Cystoscopy may at times show enlarged necrotic or bleeding median lobe of the prostate; it may also show protrusion or invasion of the prostatic lesion into the urinary bladder as well as trabeculation of the urinary bladder or blood clot in the urinary bladder. Nevertheless, these findings are not specific to leiomyosarcoma of the prostate gland.

(ii) Transurethral resection biopsy of a bleeding or necrotic median lobe can be undertaken after cystoscopy for histological examination which may lead to a diagnosis of leiomyosarcoma of the prostate.

(iii) At the end of cystoscopy transurethral resection of the prostate gland may be done for a presumed benign prostatic hypertrophy requiring resection to improve urinary flow or to relieve urinary retention and the histological examination may incidentally reveal leiomyosarcoma of the prostate gland.

Macroscopic Features

(i) Leiomyosarcomas of the prostate tend to be large tumours arising from the prostate and breaching the capsule of the prostate, extending into the perineum, towards the side wall of the pelvis or projecting into or invading the urinary bladder. When the median lobe is involved necrotic areas and bleeding areas may be seen of the median lobe of the prostate. The macroscopic features of leiomyosarcoma of the prostate gland are not specific features.

(ii) The size of PLSOPs tends to vary from 3 cm to 21 cm and infiltrative [2].

(iii) Macroscopic examination of PLSOPs tends to reveal a non-well-defined mass which may be fleshy with areas of necrosis and bleeding.

Microscopic Features

(i) Microscopic examination of leiomyosarcoma of the prostate tends to reveal spindle cells with enlarged hyperchromatic nuclei with evidence of increased mitotic activity [10].

(ii) Most cases of PLSOP tend to have high-grade features on microscopic examination associated with areas of viable tumour which comprise hypercellular, intersecting bundles of eosinophilic, spindle-shaped cells that have variable degrees of nuclear mitotic activity as well as nuclear atypia. Some cases may have low-grade features [13].

Immunohistochemistry

Positive Immunohistochemistry. Leiomyosarcomas of the prostate tend to stain positively for the following:

(i) Vimentin [2, 13].

(ii) CD44 [13].

(iii) Smooth muscle actin—about 63% may stain positive for actin [2].

(iv) Calponin—focally positive [11].

(v) Desmin—20% of cases may stain weakly for desmin [2].

(vi) Keratin—27% of cases may stain positive for keratin [2].

Negative Immunohistochemistry. Leiomyosarcomas of the prostate gland tend to stain negatively for the following:

(i) S-100 [13].

(ii) Cytokeratin [13].

(iii) CD117 (c-kit) [13].

(iv) PSA [11].

(v) CD34 [11].

Cytogenetics/Molecular Genetic Tests. Cytogenetic study on primary leiomyosarcoma of the prostate gland may show clonal chromosomal rearrangement involving Chromosomes 2, 3, 9, 11, and 19 [16].

Electron Microscopic Features. Electron microscopic examination of specimens of leiomyosarcoma of the prostate gland may show the bulk of the cytoplasm to be filled with microfilaments which are arranged on a long axis [15].

Differential Diagnoses. The differential diagnoses of PLSOP include the following:

(i) Nodular hyperplasia of prostate with atypical changes: in this case microscopic examination would reveal no evidence of invasion and no evidence of mitotic figures [2]. In nodular hyperplasia of the prostate gland microscopic examination of the specimen of the prostate tends to show hyperplasia of stroma and glandular tissue with evidence of papillary buds; in-folding and cysts, associated with squamous metaplasia and necrosis; the microscopic features which tend to begin around the urethra where the ejaculatory ducts enter the prostate gland (in the transitional and periurethral zone); the basal layer which tends to be continuous, evidence of stromal changes including increased smooth muscle, lymphocytes, and ducts which in the majority of cases are not associated with infectious process of prostatitis, reduced elastic tissue; various other features including sclerosing adenosis, fibroadenoma-like and phyllodes-like hyperplasia, leiomyoma-like nodules, and fibromyxoid nodules associated with infarct [17]. Nodular hyperplasia of prostate gland on immunohistochemistry tends to be positive for CD10 [18]. It has been stated that in nodular hyperplasia of the prostate gland no well-organized fascicles are seen on microscopic examination of the prostatic lesion and also there is hyalinization, no necrosis, and no calcification on microscopic examination [12].

(ii) Postoperative spindle cell nodules: diagnosis of this condition could be based upon history of previous prostatic operation and microscopic examination tends to reveal no evidence of invasion and no evidence of mitotic figures [2]. Microscopic examination of the prostate specimen involved with postoperative spindle cell nodule tends to show evidence of cellular tissue with high mitotic activity, interlacing fascicles of spindle cells with extravasation of red blood cells which resemble Kaposi's sarcoma, minimal nuclear pleomorphism, and no atypical mitosis, and the size of the lesion tends to be relatively small [19].

(iii) Gastrointestinal stromal tumour of rectum (Rectal GIST): it has been stated that there may be difficulties differentiating between PLSOP and Rectal GIST [20]. In Rectal GIST microscopic examination tends to show transmural, usually plump, spindle cells with eosinophilic cytoplasm within stroma that tend to be variably hyalinised or oedematous, skeinoid fibres which are extracellular globules tend to be commonly seen, muscle infiltration may also be seen, there may be evidence of epithelioid morphology, and one to two mitotic figures may be seen per ten high-power fields [21]; on rare occasions there may be evidence of osteoclast-like giant cells [21, 22]. In Rectal GIST immunohistochemistry tends to reveal positive staining with CD117, CD34, and vimentin; immunohistochemistry also tends to show positive staining in 30% to 40% of cases for alpha smooth muscle actin and in 5% of cases for S100. Variable weak positive staining for keratin may also be seen in Rectal GIST [21]. In Rectal GIST electron microscopic examination of the specimen tends to show predominantly features of smooth muscle differentiation including long interdigitating cytoplasmic processes, intercellular junctions, and dense core granules [21]. In Rectal GIST electron microscopic examination also tends to show features of predominant neural differentiation including neuron-like cells which have axonal cytoplasmic processes, synapse-like structures, and dense core neurosecretory granules [21].

(iv) Some PLSOPs mimic stromal sarcoma of the prostate and sarcomatoid carcinoma of the prostate. Macroscopic examination of stromal sarcoma of the prostate specimen may reveal a whitish-yellow multinodular appearance with focal necrosis; microscopic examination of the specimen may show sarcomatoid oval to spindle cells; immunohistochemical staining of the specimen tends to show the membrane of the tumour cells to be positive with CD56, focal positivity in the cytoplasm of the tumour cells for synaptophysin, and positive staining on the cell membrane of the tumour cells for CD99 [23]. Microscopic examination of sarcomatoid carcinoma of the prostate gland (carcinosarcoma of the prostate) tends to reveal a biphasic tumour with adenocarcinoma and recognizable sarcoma components including chondrosarcoma, rhabdomyosarcoma, angiosarcoma, osteosarcoma, and leiomyosarcoma [24]. Immunohistochemistry of sarcomatoid carcinomas of the prostate tends to exhibit positive staining for the epithelial component for cytokeratin and PAP but negative staining for PSA [25]. Immunohistochemistry of the sarcoma component of sarcomatoid carcinoma of the prostate tends to reveal negative staining for PSA, EMA, and keratin [24].

(v) Other PLSOPs may mimic leiomyomas. In leiomyomas of the prostate gland microscopic examination of the prostate tends to show well-organized fascicles of spindle cells [12]. In leiomyoma of the prostate the lesion tends to be normocellular with no or rare mitotic activity and no or rare nuclear atypia, but there may be evidence of atypical bizarre stromal cells [26, 27]. Leiomyomas of the prostate gland tend to stain positively with desmin, actin, and androgen receptor on immunohistochemical staining [12]. On the other hand, leiomyosarcomas of the prostate gland microscopic examination of the prostatic lesion tend to show hypercellularity, evidence of infiltration, variable atypia, definite mitotic activity, and necrosis [12].

Treatment. Treatment options that can be undertaken in cases of leiomyosarcoma of the prostate gland include the following:

(1) Radical surgery in the form of radical prostatectomy or exenteration alone or plus or minus chemotherapy alone or plus radiotherapy (see, e.g., [15, 28]).

(2) Chemotherapy and radiotherapy (see, e.g., [29]).

(3) Chemotherapy alone (see, e.g., [10]).

(4) Radiotherapy alone (see, e.g., [13]).

(5) Palliative care including pain control and overall supportive care by a multidisciplinary team approach.

(6) Patients who have stomas in the form of ileal conduit or colostomies in cases where the rectum is involved and colostomy performed would require support from the stoma nurse.

Outcome. The outcome of the disease may be summarized as follows:

(1) On the whole the prognosis of leiomyosarcoma of the prostate is poor, but variable survival rates have been reported (see [2]), but it has been stated that the best survival occurs following curative surgery without evidence of residual or metastatic disease. It would appear that curative surgery together with multimodal therapy with chemotherapy would be the best form of treatment if the patient is fit to undergo multimodal treatment, but this approach may be hampered by the advanced stage of the disease at presentation and the general condition of the patients who may not be fit for multimodal treatment.

(2) There is no consensus opinion on the best therapeutic approach in view of the rarity of leiomyosarcoma of the prostate; therefore there is need for a global multicentre trial on management of leiomyosarcoma of the prostate in order to form an opinion on the best treatment option that would improve the prognosis.

(3) Perhaps if leiomyosarcoma of the prostate is diagnosed at an early stage, then the prognosis may improve following treatment. It may be that if patients who had previously undergone radiotherapy and/or hormonal therapy for adenocarcinoma of prostate are made to undergo prostate biopsies early when there is evidence of relapse or recurrence of their prostate carcinomas those whose tumours may have dedifferentiated into leiomyosarcoma of the prostate would be detected early, but this is conjectural.

(4) Leiomyosarcomas of the prostate gland are aggressive tumours with a median survival of 3 to 4 years and they tend to recur as well as metastasize to the liver and the lungs [5].

(B) Miscellaneous Narrations and Discussions from Some Reported Cases (See Table 1 for a List of Some of the Reported Cases and Case Series). Cheville et al. [2] undertook a clinicopathological study of all of the cases of leiomyosarcoma of prostate that had been managed in their institution from 1929 to 1994. They had retrieved twenty-three cases from their files and out of these clinical follow-up data were available for 14 patients. Immunohistochemical studies had been undertaken including actin, desmin, S-100 protein, keratin, and vimentin. With regard to the results, Cheville et al. [2] reported the following:

(i) The ages of the patient had ranged between 41 years and 78 years and their mean age was 61 years.

(ii) All of the patients (100%) presented with urinary obstruction. Twenty-five percent of the patients presented with perineal pain. Seven percent of the patients had presented with burning on ejaculation and seven percent of the patients had presented with weight loss.

(iii) The dimensions of the prostatic tumours had ranged from 3.3 cm to 21 cm in the greatest dimension with a mean dimension of 9 cm.

(iv) The tumours quite often were associated with necrosis.

(v) With regard to the histological grading of the tumours 7 tumours were assigned grade 2; 10 tumours were assigned grade 3 and 6 tumours were assigned grade 4. The grading of the tumours was based upon Broder's grading system (scale, 1–4).

(vi) The mitotic figure counts had varied between 2 and 24 per 10 high-power fields.

Table 1: List of some of the reported cases of primary leiomyosarcoma of the prostate gland.

Authors and reference	Year of publication	Number of cases
Dotan et al. [30]	2006	8
Talapatra et al. [31]	2006	1
Sexton et al. [32]	2001	12
Cheville et al. [2]	1995	23
Dundore et al. [33]	1995	5
Russo et al. [34]	1993	1
Ahlering et al. [35]	1988	4
Vandoros et al. [13]	2008	1
Singh et al. [10]	2013	1
Dubey et al. [11]	2010	1
Chen et al. [15]	2000	1
Vakilha et al. [29]	2004	1
Horiguchi et al. [28]	2014	1
Sastri et al. [14]	2002	1
Germiyanoglu et al. [9]	1994	1
Barone and Joelson [36]	1950	1
Yee et al. [37]	2009	1
Lida et al. [38]	1998	2 cases, but they also reviewed 57 cases in the Japanese literature previously published
Palma et al. [39]	1983	1
Stallwoodand Davidson [40]	1977	1
Moreira et al. [41]	2004	1
Limon et al. [16]	1986	1
Cambronero et al. [42]	1999	1
Cuesta Alcaca et al. [43]	2000	1
Chen et al. [44]	2005	1
Camuzzi et al. [45]	1981	1
Kuroda et al. [46]	1994	1
Tazi et al. [47]	2001	2
Mansouri et al. [48]	2001	1 (14-year-old boy)
Mondaini et al. [49]	2005	3

(vii) With regard to immunohistochemistry, fifteen of 15 (100%) of the tumours were immunohistochemically positively stained for vimentin, 10 out of 16 (63%) were positively stained for actin, and 3 out of 15 (20%) were weakly reactive for desmin. Immunohistochemical expression was observed for keratin in 15 (27%) of the cases and, furthermore, all of the tumours (100%) were negatively stained for S-100.

(viii) With regard to treatment, the patients underwent various types of treatment which usually included a combination of radiotherapy, chemotherapy, and radical prostatectomy or cystoprostatectomy.

(ix) The follow-up of the patients had ranged from 2 months to 72 months and the mean follow-up was 19 months.

(x) With regard to the outcome of the patients, 10 patients had died 3 months to 72 months (mean, 22 months) pursuant to their diagnosis and 4 patients were alive at the time of publication of the paper which included three patients who had residual tumour and one patient who did not have any evidence of tumour at 1 month, 4 months, 30 months, and 4.5 months, respectively. Ten out of 11 patients had developed local recurrence which included 5 patients who had gross residual tumour present after their surgery. Metastases had developed up to 40 months pursuant to their surgery (with a mean time of 10.3 months after their surgeries) and most of the metastases had involved the lungs.

Cheville et al. [2] made the ensuing conclusions:

(i) Their findings indicated that leiomyosarcoma of the prostate gland has a variable histological appearance which ranges from spindle cell tumours reminiscent of smooth muscle to pleomorphic sarcoma.

(ii) Epithelioid characteristics may be present in the tumours.

(iii) The majority of the tumours on immunohistochemical staining were positively stained with vimentin and actin and immunoreactivity with antikeratin antibodies would not exclude the diagnosis of leiomyosarcoma.

(iv) Leiomyosarcoma of the prostate gland has a poor prognosis, even though the duration of survival has been variable.

(v) Radical surgery had been the treatment modality of choice in their series, but it was difficult to achieve complete excision of tumour in the majority of cases and the surgical operations did not result in cure.

Vandoros et al. [13] reported an 80-year-old man who had presented with urinary frequency, dysuria, poor urinary stream, and nocturia. His rectal examination showed a firm nodular mass of 3 cm to 4 cm diameter which had involved the left lobe of the prostate gland and which had extended to the edge of the gland. The right lobe of the prostate gland was noted to be diffusely firm. His serum prostate specific antigen (PSA) level at presentation was 2.7 ng/mL and this had not changed over 3 years. He underwent transurethral resection of prostate (TURP) and histological examination of the specimen showed a dominant population neoplastic spindle cells which were intermingled with giant neoplastic cells and multifocal necrosis which had involved almost the entire tumour (see Figures 1(a) and 1(b)). Immunohistochemical staining of the tumour was reported to have confirmed the diagnosis of leiomyosarcoma of the prostate gland in that the tumour cells on immunohistochemistry expressed

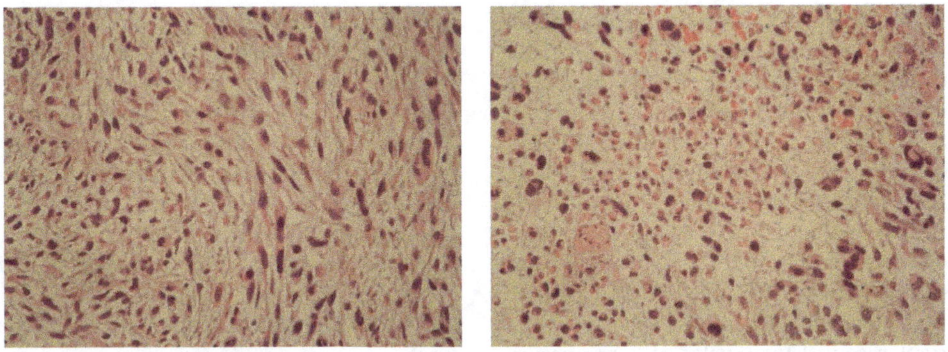

(a) (b)

FIGURE 1: (a) Leiomyosarcoma composed of a dominant population of neoplastic spindle cells: (a) intermingled with giant neoplastic cells and multifocal and multifocal necrosis (b). Reproduced from [13].

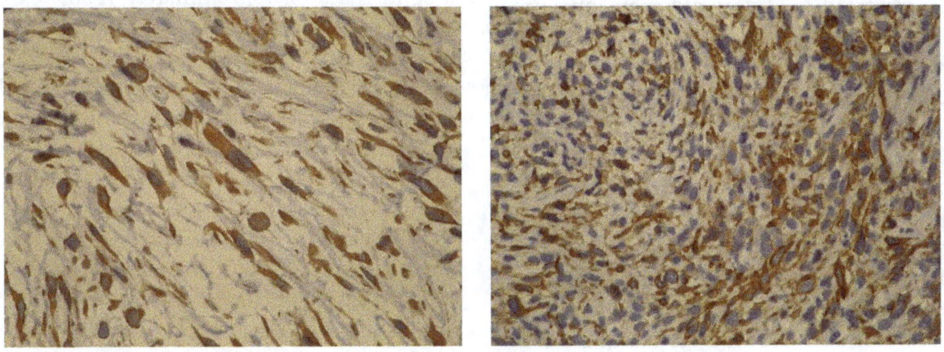

(a) (b)

FIGURE 2: (a) and (b) Immunohistochemistry demonstrates that tumour cells express smooth muscle actin (a) and vimentin (b). Reproduced from [13].

positive staining with smooth muscle actin (see Figure 2(a)), vimentin (see Figure 2(b)), and CD44, and the tumours on immunohistochemistry exhibited negative staining for S-100, cytokeratins, and CD117 (c-KIT). He had computed tomography (CT) scan of the abdomen and thorax which had revealed two hypodense liver lesions, multiple pulmonary nodules, and mediastinal and left hilar lymphadenopathy, which were all considered to be suspicious of metastases. He also had CT scan of the brain which did not show any metastasis. He did not want any intervention; therefore, he was treated symptomatically. Three months subsequently, he presented with retention of urine and acute renal failure for which a long-term urinary catheter was inserted and for which palliative external beam radiotherapy was recommended, but he refused to undergo radiotherapy, so he was discharged home with hospice care. He died 2 months later. Vandoros et al. [13] stated that they had reviewed 54 cases of leiomyosarcoma which had been reported prior to the publication of their case and their review had revealed the following:

(i) The mean survival of leiomyosarcoma of the prostate gland was estimated at 17 months (95% CI, 20.7–43.7 months).

(ii) The 1-, 3-, and 5-year actuarial survival rates were 68%, 34%, and 26%, respectively.

(iii) The only factors predictive of long-term survival were negative surgical margins and absence of metastatic disease at the time of initial presentation.

Vandoros et al. [13] concluded that a multidisciplinary approach to the management of leiomyosarcoma of the prostate gland is necessary for the appropriate management of this dire (aggressive) disease.

Singh et al. [10] reported a 35-year-old man who had presented with lower urinary tract symptoms and progressive perineal pain. He was found on examination to have a palpable urinary bladder and a nontender, lobulated asymmetrically enlarged, prostate gland of variegated consistency. His serum PSA level was slightly raised at 5.31 ng/mL. His urine analysis and the rest of his serum biochemical analyses were normal. He had transrectal ultrasound scan of prostate which revealed an enlarged prostate gland with a heterogeneous mass on the left posterolateral aspect of the prostate gland. He had transrectal ultrasound-guided biopsies of the prostate gland and histological examination of the specimens had revealed the tumour to be composed of spindle-shaped cells, with elongated, plump nuclei, nuclear pleomorphism, and brisk bizarre multipolar mitotic activity. A diagnosis of leiomyosarcoma of the prostate gland was made. He had a CT scan of abdomen, pelvis, and thorax which had shown a heterogeneous mass arising from the left posterolateral aspect of the prostate gland with an area of infiltration in the base of the urinary bladder, anterior wall of the rectum, and left posterolateral wall of the pelvis. The CT scan also showed multiple enlarged presacral lymph nodes and small nodules on the base of the lung on the left side. He had isotope bone scan which was normal with no evidence of bone metastasis. The patient received two cycles of combination chemotherapy which consisted of ifosfamide (1600 mg/m^2) and epirubicin at 40 mg/m^2 for three days at three-weekly intervals. However, he died one month after receiving his second cycle of chemotherapy.

Dubey et al. [11] reported a 73-year-old man who presented with memory loss. His wife reported that he had been having problems with his bowel movements and at times he had had episodes of severe rectal burning. He had also been having lower urinary tract symptoms. He had colonoscopy which was on the whole normal but which showed a benign polyp at 35 cm. His serum biochemistry tests were normal except for evidence of hyponatraemia which was considered to be the reason for his confusion. His serum PSA at initial manifestation was 2.7 ng/mL and this had not changed over 3 years. He had a CT scan of brain, thorax abdomen, and pelvis which had shown a very large nodular prostate gland of about 6 cm in size and which had projected into the left posterior inferior aspect of the urinary bladder and had indented into the lumen of the rectum and this was adjudged to have almost obstructed the lumen of the rectum at the level of the dentate line. There was no evidence of lymphadenopathy or metastasis. He had a digital rectal examination which had revealed a very large, hard, nodular prostate gland projecting into the lumen of the rectum and almost causing obstruction of the lower gastrointestinal tract. He could not tolerate transrectal ultrasound-guided biopsy of the prostate under local anaesthesia because it was too painful. He underwent trocar needle biopsy of prostate under sedation in the operating theatre. During assessment at the time of the prostate biopsy upon assessment of the prostate gland it was felt that the tumour was far more advanced than was previously envisaged. The histopathological findings of the biopsy specimens showed malignant spindle cell tumour which was adjudged to favour leiomyosarcoma of the prostate gland. Immunohistochemichal staining had shown that the spindle cell proliferation was negatively stained for PSA, S100, pancytokeratin, CD117, and CD34. Immunohistochemical staining had shown that the tumour was strongly positively stained for smooth muscle actin, calponin, and CD44 and focally positive for desmin. His perineal pain deteriorated subsequently and he developed urinary retention which required insertion of suprapubic cystostomy. The case was discussed at a multidisciplinary team meeting which concluded that the lesion was leiomyosarcoma of prostate and the treatment would require surgery which should involve total pelvic exenteration or if the tumour was bulky then neoadjuvant chemotherapy with or without radiotherapy, followed by surgery. His hyponatraemia resolved and his mentation had improved; however, with his low performance status, he was adjudged unsuitable to undergo surgical operation as well as not fit to receive chemotherapy. He developed persistent haematuria for which he was able to tolerate a single high dose 8-gray radiotherapy out of the 30 Gy/10 fractions which was planned. His bleeding had stopped in a few weeks, but he had severe pelvic pain which was not controlled by regular narcotics and he required palliative care and he received methadone but died of his disease after two weeks.

Chen et al. [15] reported a 27-year-old man who had had difficulty with voiding. He developed acute retention of urine and was catheterized and one week later was referred to a different institution. He had rectal examination which revealed a solid mass of approximately 11 cm × 8 cm × 7 cm with a smooth surface and elastic consistency. His serum PSA level was 4.8 ng/mL. But his urine analysis and his blood biochemistry were on the whole normal otherwise. He had transrectal ultrasound scan-guided biopsy of prostate and histological examination of the specimen revealed features consistent with spindle cell sarcoma. He had a chest X-ray which was normal. He also had intravenous urography which had shown an atonic urinary bladder with marked residual urine volume after voiding. He had magnetic resonance imaging (MRI) scan of pelvis which showed a large lesion in the pelvis arising from the prostate gland and which had invaded the urinary bladder. He underwent radical cystoprostatectomy and during the operation it was noted that there was involvement of the rectum by the tumour; therefore low anterior resection was undertaken with segmental resection of the rectum and construction of an ileal conduit. Microscopic examination of the tumour had revealed that the tumour had consisted of spindle cells with enlarged hyperchromatic nuclei as well as increased mitotic activity. Immunohistochemical staining of the tumour had shown positive staining for vimentin and weakly positive staining for actin as well as negative staining for desmin. The tumour was therefore adjudged to have illustrated leiomyosarcoma of the prostate gland with invasion of the urinary bladder and rectum. Furthermore, electron microscopic examination of the tumour revealed features of spindle cell sarcoma which established a definite pathological diagnosis of leiomyosarcoma of the prostate gland. He had remained alive for 48 months at the time of publication of the paper with no evidence of recurrence of his tumour. Lessons learnt from this case would indicate the following: leiomyosarcoma of the prostate gland could be locally advanced, but if radical surgery is undertaken and there is complete clearance of tumour without any evidence of residual disease even without adjuvant chemotherapy or radiotherapy some of the patients would tend to have a medium/long-term survival.

Vakilha et al. [29] reported a 72-year-old man who presented with urinary dribbling, hesitancy, and perineal pain. He had rectal examination which revealed a firm and immobile prostatic mass. He had CT scan which showed a nonhomogeneous prostatic mass which was confined to the prostate gland and not invading other organs and it also showed no evidence of lymph node involvement. He had CT scan of thorax and chest X-ray which were normal. His serum PSA level at presentation was 4.2 ng/mL. He had transrectal ultrasound-guided biopsy of prostate and histological examination of the specimen revealed features which were considered to be suspicious of malignancy and the patient underwent radical surgery (prostatectomy). Histological examination of the specimen showed a high-grade spindle cell sarcoma which was diagnosed as leiomyosarcoma of prostate with clear surgical margin. Immunohistological examination of the tumour showed that the tumour cells were weakly stained with desmin, but EMA staining was negative. This result was adjudged to be consistent with a diagnosis of leiomyosarcoma of prostate gland. He initially received one course of chemotherapy with three drug regimens which consisted of ifosfamide, dacarbazine, and farmorubicin. He did not want to continue having chemotherapy. He, therefore, received 4500 cGy of radiotherapy to the pelvis and 1500 cGy to the prostatic bed. He was initially well for 10 months; nevertheless, he represented with shortness of breath and he had CT scan of thorax which showed multiple lung metastases. He had a rectal examination which revealed a nontender firm nodule. He was started on chemotherapy with the MAID regimen (mesna, Adriamycin, ifosfamide, and dacarbazine). After he had received four courses of chemotherapy, a partial response was observed both in his radiological image findings and with regard to his symptoms. He was still receiving chemotherapy at the time of publication of the paper.

Horiguchi et al. [28] reported a 69-year-old man who had been diagnosed as having adenocarcinoma of prostate gland and who had been treated by means of brachytherapy. Six years after he had undergone brachytherapy, he developed dysuria and visible haematuria. He underwent urethroscopy which had shown a stenosis caused by a tumour at the level of the prostate. He underwent transurethral resection of the prostate and histological examination of the tumour showed features consistent with a diagnosis of leiomyosarcoma of the prostate gland. He was treated by means of three cycles of neoadjuvant chemotherapy which consisted of doxorubicin and ifosfamide. And this was followed by radical cystoprostatectomy and pelvic lymphadenectomy. It was found that the tumour originated from the prostate gland and had infiltrated the wall of the urinary bladder and serosa with lymphatic and venous invasion. The surgical margin was clear of tumour and there was no evidence of residual adenocarcinoma of the prostate gland on histological examination. Histological examination had also revealed that the proportion of necrotic tumour cells which had been induced by the chemotherapy was 50%. He was offered adjuvant chemotherapy later on, but he opted to be followed up without receiving any further chemotherapy. At three months pursuant to his surgical operation, he had a CT scan of abdomen, pelvis, and thorax which showed local recurrence and lung metastasis. He was then treated with ifosfamide; nevertheless, he did not respond to chemotherapy and he died six months after the operation. Horiguchi et al. [28] concluded that effective treatment strategy for sarcoma of the prostate gland should be developed in the near future, although the clinical features of sarcoma of the prostate gland remain unclear due to its rare incidence. The development of dedifferentiation of totipotential cells in the prostate gland following radiotherapy to the prostate gland or hormonal therapy for adenocarcinoma has been known.

Sastri et al. [14] reported a 60-year-old man who presented with dysuria, lower abdominal pain, and pain in his left lower limb. He had undergone open prostatectomy in another hospital from where he was referred. On examination he was found to have on palpation underneath his hypogastric surgical scar a 5 cm diameter, almost globular nontender, immobile mass. He had a rectal examination which revealed a large, hard growth anterior to his rectum with obliteration of the median sulcus of the prostate gland and the upper border of the prostate gland could not be reached. He had ultrasound scan of the abdomen and pelvis and this revealed a mass which measured 104 mm × 94 mm in the region of the prostate gland. He had transrectal ultrasound scan of the prostate which showed the mass to be predominantly echogenic in the central part of the prostate with compression of the peripheral zone. A provisional diagnosis of benign prostatic hyperplasia was made. His serum PSA was 3 ng/mL. He later on had open biopsy of the prostate gland and histological examination of the specimen showed diffusely infiltrating spindle cell tumour which was arranged in interlacing fascicles. There was also evidence of moderate to marked nuclear pleomorphism and high mitotic activity. But there was no evidence of epithelial elements. Immunohistochemical staining of the tumours showed positive staining for desmin and smooth muscle actin; however, immunohistochemistry was negative for cytokeratin and PSA. A diagnosis of primary leiomyosarcoma of the prostate gland was made. He received 30 Gy of palliative external beam radiotherapy in 10 fractions over two weeks. The patient was doing well at his six-month follow-up. This case had illustrated the use of external beam radiotherapy in the palliative treatment of primary leiomyosarcoma of prostate, but considering the fact that the case was reported after 6-month follow-up one cannot predict the medium-term and long-term outcome of the patient with regard to the effect of the radiotherapy alone as treatment.

Germiyanoglu et al. [9] reported a 2.5-year-old boy who had presented with difficulty in voiding. He had had urinary frequency for 7 days prior to the onset of his voiding difficulty. He had a rectal examination which revealed a mass which measured 6 cm × 4 cm × 2 cm in the prostatic fossa. His urine examination and blood biochemistry results were normal except for his serum urea nitrogen which was raised at 40 mg/dL. He had an X-ray of the chest which was normal. He also had a cystogram which had shown that the urinary bladder had been displaced superiorly. He had computed tomography (CT) scan which had shown a 51 mm diameter hypodense homogeneous mass within the location of the prostate gland. He had transrectal ultrasound-guided biopsy of the prostate gland and histological examination of the specimen had shown leiomyosarcoma of the prostate gland. The family of the patient did not accept the offer of radical surgical operation and in view of this a suprapubic cystostomy was carried out and chemotherapy and radiotherapy were planned. After the initial days of receiving chemotherapy, the patient was not brought back to complete the planned treatment. He died 4 months later. Germiyanoglu et al. [9] stated the following: Mottola et al. [50] had postulated that chronic inflammatory processes are responsible for causing leiomyosarcoma of the prostate gland in view of the fact that it had been known that hyperplasia had been observed in the smooth muscles of the prostate gland in chronic prostatitis; nevertheless, the reason behind the aetiology of leiomyosarcoma of the prostate has not been clarified; Palma et al. [39] had stated that leiomyosarcoma reaches a peak in childhood; however, leiomyosarcoma of the prostate gland is most often encountered in the 6th decade; the commonest manifestations tend to be symptoms associated with urinary obstruction and these include dysuria, nocturia, urinary frequency, or retention of urine; Barone and Joelson [36] had stated that leiomyosarcoma of the prostate gland should be differentiated from benign prostatic hyperplasia, carcinoma of the prostate gland, prostatic abscess, mullerian duct cysts, and retrovesical tumours [36].

Yee et al. [37] reported a 75-year-old man who presented with haematuria. He had rectal examination which had revealed a mass in the prostate. He had a history of having been diagnosed 8 years earlier with a stage T2b adenocarcinoma of the prostate gland which was treated by means of external beam radiotherapy and brachytherapy. Both his treatments had failed in that his serum prostate specific antigen (PSA) had been increasing. Four years subsequently he had undergone cryosurgical ablation for a poorly differentiated Gleason 4 + 5 = 9, adenocarcinoma of the prostate gland which was clinically staged as T2b. He had isotope bone scan and CT scan of abdomen and pelvis which showed absence of metastasis. His serum PSA prior to his cryosurgical ablation treatment was 11.4 μg/L and his prostate volume was 26 cc and his rectal examination had revealed a small irregular prostate with induration over both lobes of the prostate. Pursuant to his cryotherapy his serum PSA had decreased to 0.2. After the cryotherapy his serum PSA had increased to 1.5 after one year and 2.7 after two years and he was found to have a questionable induration at the base of the prostate. He had a CT scan which had shown a 2.3 cm mass anterior to the rectum behind the seminal vesicles. He was commenced on hormonal therapy and he received bicalutamide 50 mg orally daily and 30 mg leuprolide depot injections every 4 months and after 8 months his serum PSA had dropped to 0.1. Rectal examination then had revealed a small benign feeling prostate gland. The serum PSA had remained at 0.1 whilst he remained on hormonal therapy, but 2 years later he developed visible haematuria at which time his serum PSA had remained at 0.1 and his rectal examination had shown his prostate gland to be indurated and of about 30 grams. He underwent cystoscopy which had revealed an enlarged necrotic and bleeding median lobe of his prostate gland. He had CT scan which had shown an increase in the size of the prostatic neoplasm which had invaded the rectum, but it had not invaded the pelvic side wall and there was no lymph adenopathy. He had prostate biopsies and histological examination of the specimens showed infiltrative, interlacing fascicles of spindle cells which had eosinophilic cytoplasm and had exhibited high cellularity, marked nuclear atypia, and many atypical mitotic figures which were suggestive of sarcoma of the prostate gland. Immunohistochemical staining of the specimen revealed negative staining for PAS, PCA3, CK A1/A3, CK 903, PSA, and hormone receptor ER/PR which had ruled out any residual adenocarcinoma of the prostate gland. Immunohistochemichal stains for leiomyosarcoma were positive in that desmin and smooth muscle actin were weakly positive, and vimentin was strongly positive. He underwent radical cystoprostatectomy and bilateral pelvic lymph adenectomy, resection of sigmoid colon, and rectum, colostomy, and ileal conduit construction. Histopathological examination of the specimen had revealed features consistent with high-grade leiomyosarcoma of the prostate gland. Pathological examination had shown that the tumour had replaced the prostate gland completely and had extended into the periprostatic fat and the urinary bladder. There was evidence of perineural invasion but no evidence of angiolymphatic involvement. The tumour had also extended and involved the full thickness of the rectum. The tumour additionally had involved the posterior margin of the prostate gland and the deep margin of the rectum; therefore additional deep margins were excised which were free of the designated ink margin. The apex of the prostate was also positive for tumour. Pathological examination of the resected rectum had shown infiltration by high-grade leiomyosarcoma which had involved the full thickness of the bowel wall and numerous ulcerations of the bowel mucosa. There was no tumour in the sigmoid colon and the pelvic lymph nodes. Immunohistochemical staining was positive for desmin and smooth muscle actin which supported a diagnosis of leiomyosarcoma. With regard to the differential diagnosis of mesenchymal neoplasms and sarcomatoid carcinoma, these were ruled out by means of immunohistochemical staining which were negative for myogenin, S100, CD34, high molecular weight cytokeratin, and pancytokeratin. His tumour continued to progress and three months later there was evidence of a nodule in the middle lobe of the right lung and a lesion in the area of the prostatic bed as well as rectal stump which was adjudged to represent tumour recurrence and in view of this he received chemotherapy. Several months later he had CT scan which had shown that the tumour near the prostatic bed had increased in size and extended to involve the perineum and abdominal wall and this had resulted in a cutaneous fistula. It had also shown many new pulmonary metastases. Twenty-five months after the surgical operation and chemotherapy he had remained alive with adjudged poor prognosis. Yee et al. [37] stated the following:

(i) Leiomyosarcoma of the prostate gland is associated with poor prognosis in view of the aggressive biological behaviour of the tumour, lack of early symptoms, and late presentation; the rate of survival varies between 0% and 60% and the survival rates vary from months to years.

(ii) Miedler and MacLennan [51] had stated that 50% to 75% of patients die as a sequel of leiomyosarcoma of the prostate gland after 2.5 years.

(iii) Mondaini et al. [49] had recommended surgical treatment in the form of cystoprostatectomy followed by chemotherapy or radiotherapy for leiomyosarcoma of the prostate gland.

(iv) Surgical operation may give symptomatic relief and may be an option of palliation for patients rather than cure in view of the fact that development of local recurrence and metastasis tends to be common.

(v) There is no treatment option that has been regarded as optimum; nevertheless, Mansouri et al. [48] had iterated that radical surgery with complete resection of tumour is the therapeutic option which offers the chance of prolonged survival when the tumour has low mitotic activity.

(vi) Dotan et al. [30] had shown that complete surgical resection of tumour can lead to decreased local recurrence and decreased metastasis which prolongs survival. Nevertheless, leiomyosarcomas of the prostate are often diagnosed late in the process of the disease; in view of this the size of the tumour at the time of resection tends to be extensive.

(vii) Sexton et al. [32] did not find any association between survival and negative surgical margins, the tumour size, or stage of the tumour.

(viii) With regard to adjuvant treatment, Sexton et al. [32] and Janet et al. [52] had shown that survival advantage may exist for a combined multimodality therapeutic strategies to improve the outcome of leiomyosarcoma of the prostate gland. However, studies had revealed that uncommon carcinomas which develop pursuant to radiotherapy tend to be aggressive tumours which manifest with metastatic deposits, for which the prognosis tends to be poor irrespective of treatment.

(ix) In view of the fact that sarcomas tend to be associated with a high recurrence rate, it had been recommended that patients with leiomyosarcoma of the prostate gland should be monitored closely with imaging of the chest, abdomen, and pelvis. The reported sites of metastasis in leiomyosarcoma of the prostate gland in order of frequency include the lung, bone, lymph nodes, and brain [53].

(x) The exact aetiology of leiomyosarcoma of the prostate gland has not been ascertained and there has been an ongoing debate regarding whether radiotherapy to the prostate gland can induce a secondary cancer.

(xi) Moreira et al. [41] had postulated a causal effect of leiomyosarcoma of prostate pursuant to brachytherapy to the prostate gland. Moreira et al. [41] had discussed the complications of brachytherapy, in which 3 patients had developed carcinoma of the prostate gland after they had received brachytherapy. One of the patients had subsequently developed recurrence of adenocarcinoma of the prostate gland, another patient had developed subsequently neuroendocrine tumour of the rectum, and the third patient had subsequently developed leiomyosarcoma of the prostate gland.

(xii) McKenzie et al. [54] had reported three cases of postradiotherapy sarcoma which had developed in the pelvis, 8 years, 15 years, and 16 years, ensuing localized adenocarcinoma of the prostate gland.

(xiii) Mazzucchelli et al. [53] had undertaken a study on histological variants of carcinoma of the prostate gland and reported that half of the sarcomatous components (SC) and carcinosarcomas of the prostate gland had developed following hormonal treatment or radiotherapy treatment ensuing an initial diagnosis of acinar adenocarcinoma of the prostate gland. Nevertheless, Mazzucchelli et al. [53] stated that sarcomatous component of carcinosarcoma status of the prostate gland after radiotherapy is not necessarily the only cause of malignancy and that de novo carcinosarcoma of the prostate gland can also develop.

(xiv) Prevost et al. [55] had also reported a case of postradiotherapy sarcoma which did develop 8 years after the patient had received extended beam radiotherapy for adenocarcinoma of the prostate gland.

Talapatra et al. [31] reported a 67-year-old man who had presented with a history of recurrent episodes of haematuria and poor urinary stream. He had previously been diagnosed as having had a benign prostatic hypertrophy for which he had undergone transurethral resection of prostate (TURP) tumour elsewhere two years earlier. The histology slides had not been available for review. He had rectal examination which revealed an enlarged, hard prostate gland with obliteration of the median sulcus and the right lobe of the prostate gland was noted to be enlarged and abutting the rectum but not fixed to it. The examination also revealed a mass which had infiltrated the periprostatic tissue and extended to the pelvic side wall. His serum PSA level at presentation was normal. He had ultrasound scan of abdomen and pelvis which revealed a hypoechoic heterogeneous mass within the prostate gland and infiltrating the base of the urinary bladder and invading the lumen of the urinary bladder. The urinary bladder was noted to have a thick wall and it also contained blood clots. He had magnetic resonance imaging (MRI) scan of the pelvis which had revealed a 7.5 cm × 4.3 cm tumour mass in the right lobe of the prostate and which had distorted the capsule and had extended into the periprostatic fat, neurovascular bundle, and the base of the urinary bladder. He underwent cystoscopy which revealed a large fleshy growth in his prostatic urethra and within the lumen of the urinary bladder in association with blood clot in the urinary bladder. The right lobe of the prostate was enlarged especially at the apex. He had biopsy of the tumour mass and histological examination of the specimen had revealed spindle cell sarcoma which had destroyed the prostate gland with only the occasional benign prostatic gland entrapped within the tumour. With regard to the details of the microscopic features of the tumour, the tumour was laid out in intergrating fascicles. The spindle-shaped cells had elongated blunt ended cigar-shaped hyperchromatic nuclei and eosinophilic fibrillary cytoplasm which had the characteristics of leiomyosarcoma. Other characteristics of the tumour which confirmed the diagnosis include nuclear pleomorphism, raised mitotic activity, and areas of necrosis. He had metastatic work-up which showed no evidence of metastatic disease. He was adjudged to be unsuitable for curative surgery in view of the extent of the disease and the associated expected morbidity. He was treated by means of adjuvant chemotherapy which included ifosfamide and this was followed by external beam radiotherapy. Upon completion of the chemotherapy and radiotherapy treatments the patient's symptoms had resolved. At his six-month follow-up, he was asymptomatic in that he did not have any haematuria and his lower urinary tract symptoms had resolved. He had a CT scan which showed significant reduction in the size of the prostatic mass and minimal periprostatic stranding as well as normal looking urinary bladder. His serum PSA was normal. Talapatra et al. [31] stated the following: Limon et al. [16] had studied the cytogenetic analysis of primary leiomyosarcoma of the prostate and reported that their study had revealed clonal chromosomal rearrangement involving Chromosomes 2, 3, 9, 11, and 19; Cambronero et al. [42] reported a case of leiomyosarcoma of prostate which presented as an exophytic tumour mass in the rectum as a rare presentation of leiomyosarcoma of the prostate gland; Cuesta Alcaca et al. [43] reported leiomyosarcoma of the prostate gland which was detected in a patient who underwent TURP for lower urinary tract symptoms diagnosed as benign prostatic hypertrophy, but histological examination of the specimen had revealed leiomyosarcoma of the prostate gland; Chen et al. [44] had stated that rectal examination in leiomyosarcoma of the prostate gland generally tends to reveal a prostatic mass; however, biopsy of the prostatic mass is required for histological examination to confirm the diagnosis; Ahlering et al. [35] reported 11 patients who had leiomyosarcoma; of these 11 patients, 7 had leiomyosarcoma of the urinary bladder, and 4 patients had leiomyosarcoma of the prostate gland. They reported that the patients who did not have bulky tumours underwent surgical resection and they were observed as to if their operative surgical margins and lymph nodes were negative for tumour. The patients who were found to have surgical margins or lymph node positive for tumour received adjuvant external beam radiotherapy and chemotherapy. With regard to the patients who had bulky tumours, they received preoperative chemotherapy with or without radiotherapy which was followed by exenteration. With regard to the outcome, Ahlering et al. [35] reported that, out of the 11 patients, 9 patients did not have any evidence of disease after a mean follow-up of 61 months and the follow-up had ranged between 35 months and 96 months; Camuzzi et al. [45] had reported a patient with leiomyosarcoma of the prostate gland who was successfully treated by means of transperineal radon seed implantation and external beam radiotherapy; Kuroda et al. [46] had reported a case of leiomyosarcoma of the prostate gland which was accompanied by multiple hepatocellular carcinomas who had received combination chemotherapy that consisted of cyclophosphamide, vincristine, Adriamycin, and DTIC (CYDAVIC). He died one year and two months after his initial diagnosis as a result of liver failure. During postmortem examination it was revealed that the histology of the liver tumours was hepatocellular carcinoma and even though the leiomyosarcoma of the prostate gland had invaded the wall of the urinary bladder and the rectum, there was no obvious distant metastasis from the leiomyosarcoma of the prostate gland; Tazi et al. [47] stated the following: a number of treatment modalities had been adopted including radical surgery, radiotherapy, and chemotherapy for the treatment of primary leiomyosarcoma of the prostate gland, but in their opinion a successful outcome had not been achieved in any instance. Leiomyosarcoma of the prostate gland has a poor prognosis, even though the survival time is variable. In view of the aforementioned reasons, it is very important that leiomyosarcoma of the prostate gland is correctly identified and that occurrence of each case of the disease, type of treatment given, and response to treatment should be reported in order to enable the understanding of the natural history of the disease.

Russo et al. [34] reported a 57-year-old man who had a high-grade leiomyosarcoma of the prostate. MRI scan was used to define the extent of the tumour. He was treated by means of chemotherapy and he had a further MRI scan which had shown that the size of the tumour had reduced by 60% and based upon the MRI scan findings the tumour was adjudged to be clinically resectable. He underwent radical cystoprostatectomy but subsequently died of metastatic disease.

Dundore et al. [33] reviewed the notes and pathological findings of 21 cases of carcinosarcoma of the prostate in the Mayo Clinic and reported the results as follows: the mean age of the patients was 68 years and the ages had ranged between 50 years and 89 years; ten of the patients (48%) were previously diagnosed as having acinar adenocarcinoma of the prostate gland two to seventy-three months prior to the diagnosis of carcinosarcoma and the mean time of the diagnosis of acinar adenocarcinoma prior to the diagnosis of carcinosarcoma was 33 months. Eight of the patients, meanwhile, had received androgen deprivation treatment and/or radiotherapy; the Gleason scores of the adenocarcinomas had ranged from Gleason 7 to Gleason 10 and the mean Gleason score was 9 and, furthermore, the median Gleason score was also 9; the various types of sarcomas which were diagnosed were as follows: 13 cases of osteosarcoma, 5 cases of leiomyosarcoma, 1 case of fibrosarcoma, 1 case of malignant fibrous histiocytoma, and 1 case of rhabdomyosarcoma. The grades of the sarcoma components of the tumours had ranged from 2 to 4 and the mean grade was 4. The median grade of the sarcomatous components of the tumour was 4; with regard to the dominant component of the tumours, adenocarcinoma was the dominant histological pattern in 7 cases and sarcoma was the dominant component in 14 cases; with regard to the immunohistochemistry of the tumours, positive immunohistochemical staining cytoplasmic reactivity was revealed for prostate specific antigen or keratin in 16 of 16 cases in the adenocarcinoma component. The sarcoma component exhibited positive staining: in 16 out of 16 cases for vimentin, in 8 out of 16 cases of which 2 were focally positive, in 2 out of 16 cases for S-100 protein, and in 1 out of 16 for desmin; at the time of the initial diagnosis of carcinosarcoma, 11 of the patients were found to have had metastases and of these patients 4 had had metastatic adenocarcinoma prior to the diagnosis of adenocarcinoma; the patients had undergone various types of treatment and they had found that nonsurgical treatment was ineffective; the sites of the metastatic lesions included the lung in 10 cases, bone in 7 cases, brain in 4 cases, liver in 1 case, and the peritoneum in 1 case; with regard to the follow-up of patients, this had ranged between 1 month and 107 months pursuant to the diagnosis of carcinosarcoma and the mean follow-up was 34 months, but the median follow-up was 10 months; with regard to outcome, the mean time to progression of tumour was 23 months, but this had ranged between 1 month and 96 months and the median time to progression was 18 months. Eighteen of the patients had died of carcinosarcoma from 2 months to 107 months following their diagnosis, but the mean and median times of their deaths pursuant to their diagnosis were 34 months and 9.5 months, respectively. The 5-year survival was 41% and the 7-year survival was 14%. The progression and survival of the patients were observed not to be affected by the histological pattern of the carcinosarcomas. Dundore et al. [33] concluded that carcinosarcoma of the prostate gland is an aggressive malignancy, irrespective of the histological type of the carcinosarcoma of the prostate gland.

Globally, a large number of patients undergo treatment for adenocarcinoma of the prostate gland with curative intent in the form of radiotherapy (external beam radiotherapy or brachytherapy) plus or minus adjuvant hormonal therapy and out of these patients a number of patients subsequently develop relapse or progress of their tumours. What is not known globally is the percentage of patients who were initially diagnosed as having adenocarcinoma of prostate who subsequently develop either de novo carcinosarcoma including leiomyosarcoma of the prostate or dedifferentiated carcinoma of the prostate gland including leiomyosarcoma of the prostate. Perhaps the reason behind the lack of information regarding the percentage of patients globally who develop carcinosarcoma alone or in association with adenocarcinoma may be due to the fact that globally routine rebiopsies are not generally undertaken in the majority of patients who are treated globally for adenocarcinoma of prostate gland in the form of radiotherapy plus or minus hormonal therapy. It would be argued perhaps if all patients who develop relapse after radiotherapy/hormonal treatment for adenocarcinoma of the prostate gland undergo rebiopsies of the prostate a number of cases of dedifferentiated carcinomas would be found alone or in association with adenocarcinoma. In view of the finding that carcinosarcomas have been found to be aggressive tumours that would require aggressive treatment with curative intent in the form multimodal treatment including radical surgery, chemotherapy, and radiotherapy in cases of patients who are fit to undergo aggressive treatment, it would be argued that a global multicentre study should be undertaken in which patients whose adenocarcinomas have relapsed given the chance to undergo rebiopsies of their prostates to see if their carcinomas remain the same or they have subsequently developed different types of prostate cancers. If a pilot study shows a high percentage of patients developing other types of prostate cancers, then perhaps new guidelines could be formulated globally for the follow-up of patients with adenocarcinoma of the prostate. Finally, it is conjectural, but it may be that the percentage of other types of carcinomas of the prostate that are reported globally is higher than is believed and this would hopefully be known in the future if lots of patients undergo rebiopsies of their prostatic lesions for histological examination.

Lida et al. [38] in 1998 reported two patients with PLSOPs. The first patient was a 45-year-old man who presented with lower urinary tract symptoms. He had ultrasound scan and CT scan which revealed a tumour in his prostate gland. He had ultrasound-guided biopsy of the prostatic lesion and histological examination of the specimen revealed leiomyosarcoma of the prostate gland. He underwent radical cystoprostatectomy. He was alive at the time of publication of the paper 12 months after his operation. The second patient was a 63-year-old man who was admitted for the treatment of lung and colon cancers. He had CT scan which had shown multiple tumours in the lung, in the liver, and bilaterally in the kidney as well as prostate gland. Histological examination of biopsies from the prostate gland had confirmed the presence of leiomyosarcoma of the prostate. Lida et al. [38] also reviewed 57 cases of primary leiomyosarcoma of the prostate gland which had been reported in the Japanese literature.

Palma et al. [39] reported a case of leiomyosarcoma of the prostate gland in association with an incidental adenocarcinoma of the prostate gland in 1983 and in 1997 Stallwood and Davidson [40] reported leiomyosarcoma of the rectum and prostate gland.

Mansouri et al. [48] reported a 14-year-old boy who presented with perineal pain on voiding and during defecation as well as dysuria and haematuria. His rectal examination revealed an indurated left lobe of the prostate gland. He had intravenous urography and CT scan of abdomen and pelvis which showed the urinary bladder displaced anteriorly compressed by a large pelvic mass, 15 cm × 11 cm, multiseptated pelvic mass with thickened irregular walls which had displaced the urinary bladder and rectum. He had surgical biopsy of the mass elsewhere and histological examination of the specimen had shown a smooth muscle neoplasm which did not have any features that would exclude leiomyosarcoma. He underwent radical cystoprostatectomy and pelvic lymph node dissection. The radical prostatectomy specimen contained a tumour on the left side which was not circumscribed and the tumour had extended from the apex to the base. Histological examination of the tumour had shown an infiltrative tumour that had invaded and displaced the normal prostate stroma of glands and these tumours had abnormal mitotic figures and giant cells. Necrosis was observed and a high mitotic count of 14 per 10 high-power fields was also observed. Immunohistochemical staining of the tumour revealed strong cytoplasmic positive staining for actin, desmin, and vimentin, but there was negative staining for keratin and S-100 protein. The surgical margin at the resection site was involved by tumour as well as extraprostatic extension. Three left iliac nodes contained metastatic tumour. He was treated by means of adjuvant radiotherapy and received 46 Gy of therapy, but he died as a result of metastases in the lung, liver, and bone as well as gross local recurrence 4 months following his initial diagnosis.

All the aforementioned information could be confusing to a clinician who is faced with a patient who is diagnosed with PLSOP. One of the questions that would be on the mind of the clinician is what is the best treatment option for the disease (PLSOP) Sexton et al. [32] had recommended that multimodality treatment include surgery, radiotherapy, and chemotherapy. Some authors [2, 11, 26, 32] had iterated that the overall outcome for PLSOPs is not good, and 50% to 75% of patients tend to die of their leiomyosarcoma between 3 months and 72 months. Sexton et al. [32] stated that the outcome of PLSOPs tends to improve in patients who do not have evidence of distant metastasis at initial manifestation and in those patients who have localized disease in whom complete resection of the tumour can be undertaken with histological evidence of negative surgical margins.

4. Conclusions

Leiomyosarcoma of the prostate gland is a rare tumour which can afflict children and adults. On the whole the prognosis is poor. Surgery with or without chemotherapy/radiotherapy would appear to be the mainstay of treatment for leiomyosarcoma of the prostate for operable cases, but generally there is no consensus opinion on the best therapeutic approach. Most cases of PLSOP at the time of initial presentation tend to be diagnosed in an advanced stage of the disease. There is the need for all cases of PLSOP diagnosed to be entered into a global multicentre trial in order to find therapeutic modalities that would improve the prognosis of this aggressive disease. Perhaps if all patients who have developed progressive disease or relapse of local disease in cases of adenocarcinoma prostate undergo repeat prostate biopsies early, some cases of dedifferentiated leiomyosarcomas of the prostate may be diagnosed early.

Acknowledgment

Sarcoma is acknowledged for granting copyright permission for contents of the articles to be reproduced under the Creative Commons Attribution License: Copyright © 2008 Gerasimos P. Vandoros et al.

References

[1] S. C. Quay and K. H. Proppe, "Carcinosarcoma of the prostate: case report and review of the literature," *Journal of Urology*, vol. 125, no. 3, pp. 436–438, 1981.

[2] J. C. Cheville, P. A. Dundore, A. G. Nascimento et al., "Leiomyosarcoma of the prostate. Report of 23 cases," *Cancer*, vol. 76, no. 8, pp. 1422–1427, 1995.

[3] B. H. Smith and L. P. Dehner, "Sarcoma of the prostate gland," *American Journal of Clinical Pathology*, vol. 58, no. 1, pp. 43–50, 1972.

[4] L. W. Riba and M. C. Wheelock, "Leiomyosarcoma of the prostate," *The Journal of Urology*, vol. 63, no. 1, pp. 162–164, 1950.

[5] K. Arora, "Prostate Leiomyosarcoma Pathology Outlines," Pathology Outlines, http://www.Pathologyoutlines.com/topic/prostatelms.html.

[6] Prostate sarcoma Oral B Official Website, http://www.urology-textbook.com/.

[7] Li-Fraumeni Syndrome—Genetics Home Reference, http://ghr.nlm.nih.gov/condition/li-fraumeni-syndrome .

[8] Prostate Sarcoma Oral B, http://www.urology-textbook.com/.

[9] C. Germiyanoglu, H. Özkardes, Ü. Kurt, A. Öztokatli, and D. Erol, "Leiomyosarcoma of the prostate. A case report," *International Urology and Nephrology*, vol. 26, no. 2, pp. 189–191, 1994.

[10] J. P. Singh, D. Chakraborty, M. K. Bera, and D. Pal, "Leiomyosarcoma of prostate: a rare aggressive tumor," *Journal of Cancer Research and Therapeutics*, vol. 9, no. 4, pp. 743–745, 2013.

[11] A. Dubey, G. Sivananthan, T. Bradel, and R. Koul, "Prostatic leiomyosarcoma—a rare case report with review of literature," *The Internet Journal of Oncology*, vol. 8, no. 1, 2010, http://ispub.com/IJO/8/1/9519.

[12] K. Arora, "Prostate Benign lesions/conditions Leiomyoma," Pathology Outlines, 2014, http://www.pathologyoutlines.com/topicprostatelms.html.

[13] G. P. Vandoros, T. Manglidis, M. V. Karamouzis et al., "Leiomyosarcoma of the prostate: case report and review of 54 previously published cases," *Sarcoma*, vol. 2008, Article ID 458709, 5 pages, 2008.

[14] G. J. Sastri, S. K. Mohanty, A. Munshi, S. Ghosal, S. C. Sharma, and F. D. Patel, "Leiomyosarcoma of the prostate—a case report," *Indian Journal of Urology*, vol. 18, no. 2, pp. 171–172, 2002.

[15] K. C. Chen, C. M. Lin, T. S. Hsieh et al., "Leiomyosarcoma of the prostate," *The Journal of Urology*, vol. 11, pp. 39–42, 2000.

[16] J. Limon, P. Dal Cin, and A. A. Sandberg, "Cytogenetic findings in a primary leiomyosarcoma of the prostate," *Cancer Genetics and Cytogenetics*, vol. 22, no. 2, pp. 159–167, 1986.

[17] A. Amin, "Prostate Benign lesions/conditions. Nodularhyperplasia," PathologyOutlines.com, January 2012, http://www.pathologyoutlines.com/topicprostatelms.html.

[18] S. Tawfic, G. A. Niehans, and J. C. Manivel, "The pattern of CD10 expression in selected pathologic entities of the prostate gland," *Human Pathology*, vol. 34, no. 5, pp. 450–456, 2003.

[19] M. Roychowdhury, "Prostate Benign lesions/conditions Postoperative spindle cell nodules," Pathology Outlines, 2012, http://www.pathologyoutlines.com/topic/prostatepostop.html.

[20] H. Koruma, T. Ao, K. Suyama et al., "A case of gastrointestinal stromal tumor of rectum, difficult to differentiate from leiomyosarcoma of rectum," *Nihon Hinyokika Gakkai Zasshi*, vol. 92, no. 6, pp. 624–627, 2001.

[21] C. Singh, "Colon tumor Mesenchymal tumors Gastrointestinal stromal tumors (GIST) of colon Pathology," Pathology Outlines, 2014, http://pathologyoutlines.com/topic/colontumorgist.html.

[22] L. Insanato, D. Di Vizio, G. Ciancia, G. Pettinato, L. Tormillio, and L. Terracciano, "Malignant gastrointestinal leiomyosarcoma and gastrointestinal stromal tumor with prominent osteoclast-like giant cells," *Archives of Pathology & Laboratory Medicine*, vol. 128, no. 4, pp. 444–443, 2004.

[23] H. Yamazaki, T. Ohyama, T. Tsuboi et al., "Prostatic stromal sarcoma with neuroectodermal differentiation," *Diagnostic Pathology*, vol. 7, article 173, 2012.

[24] K. Arora, "Prostate Other carcinomas. Carcinosara," Pathology-Outlines.com, March 2012, http://www.pathologyoutlines.com/topic/prostatecarcinosarcoma.html.

[25] M. R. Wick, R. H. Young, R. Malvesta, D. S. Beebe, J. J. Hansen, and L. P. Dehner, "Prostatic carcinosarcomas. Clinical, histologic, and immunohistochemical data on two cases, with a review of the literature," *American Journal of Clinical Pathology*, vol. 92, no. 2, pp. 131–139, 1989.

[26] D. E. Hansel, M. Herawi, E. Montgomery, and J. I. Epstein, "Spindle cell lesions of the adult prostate," *Modern Pathology*, vol. 20, no. 1, pp. 148–158, 2007.

[27] D. Hossain, I. Meiers, J. Qian, G. T. MacLennan, and D. G. Bostwick, "Prostatic leiomyoma with atypia: follow-up study of 10 cases," *Annals of Diagnostic Pathology*, vol. 12, no. 5, pp. 328–332, 2008.

[28] H. Horiguchi, K. Tukada, R. Takimoto et al., "Radiation-induced leiomyosarcoma of the prostate after brachytherapy for prostatic adenocarcinoma," *Case Reports in Oncology*, vol. 7, no. 2, pp. 565–570, 2014.

[29] M. Vakilha, F. N. Dadgar, and T. Tuirgani, "Leiomyosarcoma of prostate: report of a case," *Iranian Journal of Radiation Research*, vol. 1, no. 4, pp. 229–231, 2004.

[30] Z. A. Dotan, R. Tal, D. Golijanin et al., "Adult genitourinary sarcoma: the 25-year Memorial Sloan-Kettering experience," *Journal of Urology*, vol. 176, no. 5, pp. 2033–2038, 2006.

[31] K. Talapatra, B. Nemade, R. Bhutani et al., "Recurrent episodes of hematuria: a rare presentation of leiomyosarcoma of prostate," *Journal of Cancer Research and Therapeutics*, vol. 2, no. 4, pp. 212–214, 2006.

[32] W. J. Sexton, R. E. Lance, A. O. Reyes, P. W. T. Pisters, S.-M. Tu, and L. L. Pisters, "Adult prostate sarcoma: the M. D. Anderson cancer center experience," *The Journal of Urology*, vol. 166, no. 2, pp. 521–525, 2001.

[33] P. A. Dundore, J. C. Cheville, A. G. Nascimento, G. M. Farrow, and D. G. Bostwick, "Carcinosarcoma of the prostate. Report of 21 cases," *Cancer*, vol. 76, no. 6, pp. 1035–1042, 1995.

[34] P. Russo, B. Demas, and V. Reuter, "Adult prostatic sarcoma," *Abdominal Imaging*, vol. 18, no. 4, pp. 399–401, 1993.

[35] T. E. Ahlering, P. Weintraub, and D. G. Skinner, "Management of adult sarcomas of the bladder and prostate," *The Journal of Urology*, vol. 140, no. 6, pp. 1397–1399, 1988.

[36] J. M. Barone and J. J. Joelson, "Leiomyosarcoma of the prostate: report of a case," *The Journal of Urology*, vol. 63, pp. 533–538, 1950.

[37] S. Yee, M. J. Goldfischer, R. J. Rosenbluth, D. A. McCain, I. Jackson, and I. S. Sawczuk, "Post radiotherapy leiomyosarcoma of the prostate: can radiation therapy induce a secondary cancer? A case report," *UroToday International Journal*, vol. 2, no. 3, 2009.

[38] K. Lida, M. Tanaka, S. Matsumoto et al., "Leiomyosarcoma of the prostate: report of two cases," *Hinyokika Kiyo*, vol. 44, no. 10, pp. 739–742, 1998.

[39] P. C. R. Palma, N. R. Netto Jr., O. Ikari, C. A. D'Ancona, and A. Billis, "Leiomyosarcoma in association with incidental adenocarcinoma of the prostate," *The Journal of Urology*, vol. 129, no. 1, pp. 156–157, 1983.

[40] G. Stallwood and J. W. Davidson, "Leiomyosarcoma of the rectum and prostate," *Canadian Journal of Surgery*, vol. 20, no. 5, pp. 446–449, 1977.

[41] S. G. Moreira Jr., J. D. Seigne, R. C. Ordorica, J. Marcet, J. M. Pow-Sang, and J. L. Lockhart, "Devastating complications after brachytherapy in the treatment of prostate adenocarcinoma," *BJU International*, vol. 93, no. 1, pp. 31–35, 2004.

[42] S. J. Cambronero, M. M. Martín, A. F. Villacampa, A. C. Hörndler, O. R. Espuela, and G. O. Leiva, "Prostate leiomyosarcoma with perineal exophytic mass," *Actas Urologicas Espanolas*, vol. 23, no. 9, pp. 797–800, 1999.

[43] J. A. Cuesta Alcaca, P. I. Pascual, J. L. Arrondo et al., "Stromal tumor of the rectum and leiomyosarcoma of the prostate as a cause of urinary syndrome attributable to BPH," *Archivos Españoles de Urología*, vol. 53, no. 9, pp. 763–768, 2000.

[44] H.-J. Chen, M. Xu, L. Zhang, Y.-K. Zhang, and G.-M. Wang, "Prostate sarcoma: a report of 14 cases," *Zhonghua Nan Ke Xue*, vol. 11, no. 9, pp. 683–685, 2005.

[45] F. A. Camuzzi, N. L. Block, K. Charyulu, S. Thomsen, and V. A. Politano, "Leiomyosarcoma of prostate gland," *Urology*, vol. 18, no. 3, pp. 295–297, 1981.

[46] H. Kuroda, Y. Yasunaga, H. Takatera, H. Fujioka, and M. Tsujimoto, "Leiomyosarcoma of the prostate accompanied by multiple hepatocellular carcinoma: report of a case," *Acta Urologica Japonica*, vol. 40, no. 2, pp. 147–149, 1994.

[47] K. Tazi, S. M. Moudouni, J. Elfassi et al., "Leiomyosarcoma of prostate: a study of two cases," *Annales d'Urologie. EMC-Urologie*, vol. 35, no. 1, pp. 56–59, 2001.

[48] H. Mansouri, L. Kanouni, T. Kebdani, K. Hassouni, H. Sifat, and B. El Gueddari, "Primary prostatic leiomyosarcoma," *Journal of Urology*, vol. 165, no. 5, p. 1676, 2001.

[49] N. Mondaini, D. Palli, C. Saieva et al., "Clinical characteristics and overall survival in genitourinary sarcomas treated with curative intent: a multicenter study," *European Urology*, vol. 47, no. 4, pp. 468–473, 2005.

[50] A. Mottola, C. Selli, M. Carini, A. Natali, and G. Gambacorta, "Leiomyosarcoma of the prostate," *European Urology*, vol. 11, no. 2, pp. 131–133, 1985.

[51] J. D. Miedler and G. T. MacLennan, "Leiomyosarcoma of the prostate," *Journal of Urology*, vol. 178, no. 2, p. 668, 2007.

[52] N. L. Janet, A.-W. May, and R. S. Akins, "Sarcoma of the prostate: a single institutional review," *American Journal of Clinical Oncology*, vol. 32, no. 1, pp. 27–29, 2009.

[53] R. Mazzucchelli, A. Lopez-Beltran, L. Cheng, M. Scarpelli, Z. Kirkali, and R. Montironi, "Rare and unusual histological variants of prostatic carcinoma: clinical significance," *BJU International*, vol. 102, no. 10, pp. 1369–1374, 2008.

[54] M. McKenzie, I. MacLennan, E. Kostashuk, and T. Bainbridge, "Postirradiation sarcoma after external beam radiation therapy for localized adenocarcinoma of the prostate: report of three cases," *Urology*, vol. 53, no. 6, p. 1228, 1999.

[55] J.-B. Prevost, A. Bossi, R. Sciot, and M. Debiec-Rychter, "Post-irradiation sarcoma after external beam radiation therapy for localized adenocarcinoma of the prostate," *Tumori*, vol. 90, no. 6, pp. 618–621, 2004.

Permissions

All chapters in this book were first published by Hindawi Publishing Corporation; hereby published with permission under the Creative Commons Attribution License or equivalent. Every chapter published in this book has been scrutinized by our experts. Their significance has been extensively debated. The topics covered herein carry significant findings which will fuel the growth of the discipline. They may even be implemented as practical applications or may be referred to as a beginning point for another development.

The contributors of this book come from diverse backgrounds, making this book a truly international effort. This book will bring forth new frontiers with its revolutionizing research information and detailed analysis of the nascent developments around the world.

We would like to thank all the contributing authors for lending their expertise to make the book truly unique. They have played a crucial role in the development of this book. Without their invaluable contributions this book wouldn't have been possible. They have made vital efforts to compile up to date information on the varied aspects of this subject to make this book a valuable addition to the collection of many professionals and students.

This book was conceptualized with the vision of imparting up-to-date information and advanced data in this field. To ensure the same, a matchless editorial board was set up. Every individual on the board went through rigorous rounds of assessment to prove their worth. After which they invested a large part of their time researching and compiling the most relevant data for our readers.

The editorial board has been involved in producing this book since its inception. They have spent rigorous hours researching and exploring the diverse topics which have resulted in the successful publishing of this book. They have passed on their knowledge of decades through this book. To expedite this challenging task, the publisher supported the team at every step. A small team of assistant editors was also appointed to further simplify the editing procedure and attain best results for the readers.

Apart from the editorial board, the designing team has also invested a significant amount of their time in understanding the subject and creating the most relevant covers. They scrutinized every image to scout for the most suitable representation of the subject and create an appropriate cover for the book.

The publishing team has been an ardent support to the editorial, designing and production team. Their endless efforts to recruit the best for this project, has resulted in the accomplishment of this book. They are a veteran in the field of academics and their pool of knowledge is as vast as their experience in printing. Their expertise and guidance has proved useful at every step. Their uncompromising quality standards have made this book an exceptional effort. Their encouragement from time to time has been an inspiration for everyone.

The publisher and the editorial board hope that this book will prove to be a valuable piece of knowledge for researchers, students, practitioners and scholars across the globe.

List of Contributors

Benoît Vogt
Department of Urology, Polyclinique De Blois, 1 Rue Robert Debré, 41260 La Chaussée Saint-Victor, France

Ilham Chokri
Laboratory of Anatomocytopathology, 1 Av Prof Alexandre Minkowski, 37170 Chambray-Lés-Tours, France

Diomidis Kozyrakis, Stefanos Perikleous and Anastasios Zarkadas
Department of Urology, "Achillopouleio" General Hospital of Volos, Magnesia, Greece

Dionyssios Paridis and Antonios Tsagkalis
Department of Orthopaedics, Animus-Kyanous Hospital, Larisa, Greece

Konstantinos Malizos
Department of Orthopaedics, Faculty of Medicine, School of Health Sciences, University of Thessaly, Larissa, Greece

Nikolaos Mertziotis, Andreas Konandreas and Christos Kyratsas
IASO General Hospital, Athens, Greece

Michael Kennelly
Department of Urology, Carolinas Medical Center, Charlotte, NC, USA

Nikesh Thiruchelvam
Department of Urology, Addenbrooke's Hospital, Cambridge, UK

Márcio Augusto Averbeck
Moinhos de Vento Hospital, Porto Alegre, Brazil

Charalampos Konstatinidis
Urology & Neuro-urology Unit, National Rehabilitation Center, Athens, Greece

Emmanuel Chartier-Kastler
Urology Clinic, Hôpital Raymond Poincaré, Paris, France

Pernille Trøjgaard and Rikke Vaabengaard
Coloplast A/S, Humlebaek, Denmark

Andrei Krassioukov
Division of Physical Medicine and Rehabilitation, Department of Medicine, Faculty of Medicine, University of British Columbia, Vancouver, British Columbia, Canada
G.F. Strong Rehabilitation Centre, Vancouver, British Columbia, Canada

Birte Petersen Jakobsen
Independent Medical Consultant, MD, MedDevHealth, Copenhagen, Denmark

Brian Ceballos, Charles U. Nottingham and Amy E. Krambeck
Indiana University School of Medicine, Department of Urology, 1801 Senate Blvd. Suite 220, Indianapolis, IN 46202, USA

Seth K. Bechis and Roger L. Sur
University of California San Diego School of Medicine, Department of Urology, 200 West Arbor Drive #8897, San Diego, CA 92103, USA

Brian R. Matlaga
Johns Hopkins University School of Medicine, James Buchanan Brady Urological Institute, 600 North Wolfe Street Park 2 Room 221, Baltimore, MD 21287, USA

Oumar Gaye, Mohamed Jalloh, Ngor M Thiam, Medina Ndoye, Youssef Bellamine, Mouhamadou M Mbodji, Ayun Cassell, Issa Labou, Lamine Niang and Serigne Gueye
Urology-andrology Department, Hôpital General Idrissa Pouye, Dakar, Senegal

Khadidiatou Dansokho and Cherif Dial
Pathological Anatomy Laboratory, Hôpital General Idrissa Pouye, Dakar, Senegal

Saint C. N Kouka
Urology-andrology Department, UFR Santé Université dé ies, Dakar, Senegal

Anthony Wanjala
Malava County Hospital, Kakamega, Bungoma, Kenya

Henry Mwangi
Moi Teaching and Referral Hospital, Eldoret, Kenya

Hillary Mabeya
Department of Reproductive Health, Moi University School of Medicine, Eldoret, Kenya

Elie Nemr, Elie El Helou, Georges Mjaess, Albert Semaan and Josselin Abi Chebel
Université Saint Joseph, Faculty of Medicine, Beirut, Lebanon

Raúl Vozmediano-Chicharro
Department of Urology, Hospital Regional de Málaga, Hospital Civil, University of Malaga, Plz Hospital Civil s/n, 29009 Malaga, Spain

Blanca Madurga
Department of Urology, Hospital Universitario Puerta del Mar, Av. Ana de Viya 21, 11009 Cadiz, Spain

Pedro Blasco
Department of Urology, Hospital Universitario de Valme, Ctra. de Cádiz Km. 548.9, 41014 Seville, Spain

Chi-Hang Yee, Peter Ka-Fung Chiu, Jeremy Yuen-Chun Teoh, Chi-Fai Ng, Chi-Kwok Chan, and See-Ming Hou
S. H. Ho Urology Centre, Department of Surgery, Prince of Wales Hospital, the Chinese University of Hong Kong, Hong Kong

Walid Shahrour and Hazem Elmansy
Thunder Bay Regional Health Sciences Center, Northern Ontario School of Medicine, Division of Clinical Sciences, Thunder Bay, Canada

Pankaj Joshi, Craig B. Hunter, Vikram S. Batra, Sandesh Surana and Sanjay Kulkarni
Kulkarni Reconstructive Urology Center, Pune, India

Stephen McGeorge
Department of Urology, Royal Brisbane and Women's Hospital, Butterfield St, Herston 4029, Queensland, Australia
Department of Urology, Redcliffe Hospital, Anzac Avenue, Redcliffe 4020, Queensland, Australia
Faculty of Medicine, the University of Queensland, Herston 4006, Queensland, Australia

Michael Kwok
Department of Urology, Redcliffe Hospital, Anzac Avenue, Redcliffe 4020, Queensland, Australia
Faculty of Medicine, the University of Queensland, Herston 4006, Queensland, Australia

Andrew Jiang
Faculty of Medicine, the University of Queensland, Herston 4006, Queensland, Australia

Louise Emmett
Department of theranostics and Nuclear Medicine, St. Vincent's Hospital Sydney, 390 Victoria St, Darlinghurst 2010, New South Wales, Australia
Garvan Institute of Medical Research, 384 Victoria St, Darlinghurst 2010, New South Wales, Australia

David A. Pattison and Paul A. Thomas
Faculty of Medicine, the University of Queensland, Herston 4006, Queensland, Australia
Department of Nuclear Medicine & Specialised PET Services, Royal Brisbane and Women's Hospital, Butterfield St, Herston 4029, Queensland, Australia

John W. Yaxley
Department of Urology, Royal Brisbane and Women's Hospital, Butterfield St, Herston 4029, Queensland, Australia
Faculty of Medicine, the University of Queensland, Herston 4006, Queensland, Australia
Wesley Urology Clinic, Wesley Hospital, 451 Coronation Dr, Auchenflower 4066, Queensland, Australia

Matthew J. Roberts
Department of Urology, Royal Brisbane and Women's Hospital, Butterfield St, Herston 4029, Queensland, Australia
Department of Urology, Redcliffe Hospital, Anzac Avenue, Redcliffe 4020, Queensland, Australia
Faculty of Medicine, the University of Queensland, Herston 4006, Queensland, Australia
University of Queensland Centre for Clinical Research, Faculty of Medicine, Building 71/918 RBWH, Butterfield St, Herston 4029, Queensland, Australiatt

Amanda F. Saltzman and Nicholas G. Cost
Department of Surgery, Division of Urology, University of Colorado School of Medicine and Children's Hospital Colorado, Aurora, CO, USA

Rahul Rajendran
University of Texas San Antonio, Department of Electrical and Computer Engineering, San Antonio, TX, USA

Kevan Iffrig, Deepak K Pruthi, Allison Wheeler and Brian Neuman
University of Texas Health San Antonio, Department of Urology, San Antonio, TX, USA

Karen Panetta
Tufts University, School of Engineering, Medford, MA, USA

Sos Agaian
College of Staten Island, &e City University of New York (CSI-CUNY), New York City, NY, USA

Elizabeth Mallam and Hilary Archer
Bristol Brain Centre, Southmead Hospital, Bristol, UK

Patrick Juliebø-Jones
Bristol Brain Centre, Southmead Hospital, Bristol, UK
Bristol Urological Institute, Southmead Hospital, Bristol, UK
University of Bristol, Bristol, UK

Elizabeth Coulthard
Bristol Brain Centre, Southmead Hospital, Bristol, UK
University of Bristol, Bristol, UK

Marcus J. Drake
Bristol Urological Institute, Southmead Hospital, Bristol, UK
University of Bristol, Bristol, UK

Joshua L. Pierce
Department of Pediatrics, University of Texas Southwestern Medical Center, Dallas, TX 75390, USA
Department of Molecular Biology, University of Texas Southwestern Medical Center, Dallas, TX 75390, USA

A. Lindsay Frazier
Department of Pediatric Oncology, Children's Hospital Dana-Farber Cancer Care, Boston, MA 02115, USA

James F. Amatruda
Department of Pediatrics, University of Texas Southwestern Medical Center, Dallas, TX 75390, USA
Department of Molecular Biology, University of Texas Southwestern Medical Center, Dallas, TX 75390, USA
Department of Internal Medicine, University of Texas Southwestern Medical Center, Dallas, TX 75390, USA

Adham Zaazaa, Ramzy Elnabarawy, Mahmoud Elbitar and Taymour Mostafa
Department of Andrology, Sexology & STIs, Faculty of Medicine, Cairo University, Cairo 11562, Egypt

Michaela Bayerle-Eder
Department of Endocrinology & Metabolism, Medical University of Vienna, W¨ahringer Gürtel 18–20, Vienna 1090, Austria

Travis K.Mann-Gow and Benjamin J. King
Department of Surgery, University of Vermont, Burlington, VT 05405, USA

Ahmed El-Ghannam
Department of Mechanical Engineering and Engineering Science, University of North Carolina at Charlotte, Charlotte, NC 28223, USA

Christine Knabe-Ducheyne
Department of Medicine, Philipps University of Marburg, 35039 Marburg, Germany

Masatoshi Kida
Department of Pathology and Laboratory Medicine, University of Vermont, Burlington, VT 05405, USA

OleM. Dall
TAK Biopharma, 2000 Frederiksberg, Denmark

Jan Krhut
Department of Surgical Sciences, Ostrava University, 703 00 Ostrava, Czech Republic

Peter Zvara
Department of Surgery, University of Vermont, Burlington, VT 05405, USA
Department of Surgical Sciences, Ostrava University, 703 00 Ostrava, Czech Republic
Department of Urology and Biomedical Laboratory, Clinical Institute, University of Southern Denmark, 5000 Odense, Denmark

Michal Mego
2nd Department of Oncology, Faculty of Medicine, Comenius University, National Cancer Institute, Bratislava, Slovakia

Michal Chovanec
2nd Department of Oncology, Faculty of Medicine, Comenius University, National Cancer Institute, Bratislava, Slovakia
Divison of Hematologya and Oncology, Indiana University Melvin and Bren Simon Cancer Center, Indianapolis, IN, USA

Ugo De Giorgi
Medical Oncology Department, Istituto Scientifico Romagnolo per lo Studio e la Cura dei Tumori (IRST), IRCCS, Via Piero Maroncelli 40, 47014 Meldola, Italy

Mohammed Akhtar, Sameera Rashid, Mohamed Ben Gashir, Noheir Mostafa Taha and Issam Al Bozom
Department of Laboratory Medicine and Pathology, Hamad Medical Corporation, Doha, Qatar

Ivan M. Petyaev, Nigel H. Kyle and Yuriy K. Bashmakov
Lycotec Ltd, Granta Park, Cambridge CB21 6GP, UK

Naylia A. Zigangirova, Elena Y. Morgunova and Elena D. Fedina
Department of Medical Microbiology, Gamaleya National Research Center of Epidemiology and Microbiology, Ministry of Health, 18 Gamaleya Str, Moscow 123098, Russia

Deaglan J. McHugh
Department of Medicine, Memorial Sloan Kettering Cancer Center, New York, NY, USA

Darren R. Feldman
Department of Medicine, Memorial Sloan Kettering Cancer Center, New York, NY, USA
Department of Medicine, Weill Medical College of Cornell University, New York, NY, USA

Fasèwindé Aristide Kabore, Stéphanie Dominique Amida Nama, Moussa Kabore and Brahima Kirakoya
Department of Urology and Andrology, University Hospital Yalgado Ouedraogo of Ouagadougou, Ouagadougou, Burkina Faso

Boureima Ouedraogo
Urology Department, University Hospital of Tingandogo, Tingandogo, Burkina Faso

Adama Ouattara
Urology Department, Souro Sanou University Hospital of Bobo-Dioulasso, Bobo-Dioulasso, Burkina Faso

Gilles Karsenty
Aix-Marseille Université, Marseille, France

Ajaydeep S. Sidhu, George Wayne, Elizabeth Nagoda, Akshay Bhandari and Alan M. Nieder
Columbia University Division of Urology, Mount Sinai Medical Center, Miami Beach 33140, FL, USA

Eric Marten and Nikita Bodoukhin
Herbert Wertheim College of Medicine, Florida International University, Miami 33199, FL, USA

Milap J. Shah, Mohan Amaresh, Padmaraj Hegde and Suraj Jayadeva
Department of Urology, Kasturba Medical College and Hospital, Manipal Academy of Higher Education, Manipal, India

B. M. Zeeshan Hameed
Department of Urology, Kasturba Medical College and Hospital, Manipal Academy of Higher Education, Manipal, India
Chief of Innovation Centre, Kasturba Medical College, Manipal Academy of Higher Education, Manipal, India

Nithesh Naik
Faculty of Engineering, Manipal Institute of Technology, Manipal Academy of Higher Education, Manipal, India

Rahil Hussein Beary
Kasturba Medical College, Manipal Academy of Higher Education, Manipal, India

Bhaskar K. Somani
Department of Urology, University Hospital Southampton NHS Trust, Southampton, UK

Jenniffer Puerta Suárez and Walter D. Cardona Maya
Reproduction Group, Department of Microbiology and Parasitology, School of Medicine, University of Antioquia-UdeA, Medellin, Colombia

Ali Bourgi, Rana Aoun, Elias Ayoub and Maroun Moukarzel
Department of Urology, Hotel-Dieu de France University Hospital, Boulevard Alfred Naccache, Achrafieh, Beirut, Lebanon

Elizabeth B. Roth, John V. Kryger, Charles T. Durkee, Melissa A. Lingongo, Ruth M. Swedler and Travis W. Groth
Division of Pediatric Urology, Department of Urology, Medical College of Wisconsin, Children's Hospital of Wisconsin, Milwaukee, WI, USA

Ronald Rodriguez, Hanzhang Wang, Ahmed Mansour and Dharam Kaushik
Department of Urology, University of Texas Health San Antonio, San Antonio, TX, USA

Deepak Pruthi
University of Texas Health San Antonio, Department of Urology, San Antonio, USA
Department of Urology, University of Texas Health San Antonio, San Antonio, TX, USA

Yidong Chen
Greehey Children's Cancer Research Institute, University of Texas Health San Antonio, San Antonio, TX, USA

Teresa Johnson-Pais
Department of Cell and Molecular Biology, University of Texas Health San Antonio, San Antonio, TX, USA

James R. White
Resphera Biosciences, Baltimore, MD, USA

Ghanendra Kumar Yadav, Mrinal Pahwa, Mahendra Singh, Vipin Tyagi and Sudhir Chadha
Department of Urology, Sir Ganga Ram Hospital, New Delhi, India

Keri Rowley and Osamah Al-Bayati
University of Texas Health San Antonio, Department of Urology, San Antonio, U

Joseph Basler
University of Texas Health San Antonio, Department of Urology, San Antonio, USA
University of Texas Health San Antonio Cancer Center, San Antonio, USA
South Texas Veterans Healthcare System, Department of Surgery, Division of Urology, San Antonio, USA

Michael A. Liss
University of Texas Health San Antonio, Department of Urology, San Antonio, USA
University of Texas Health San Antonio Cancer Center, San Antonio, USA
South Texas Veterans Healthcare System, Department of Surgery, Division of Urology, San Antonio, USA
University of Texas, College of Pharmacy, Austin, USA

Kaan Kaltalioglu
Espiye Vocational School, Giresun University, 28600 Giresun, Turkey

Fatmanur Tugcu-Demiroz and Fusun Acarturk
Pharmaceutical Technology Department, Pharmacy Faculty, Gazi University, 06330 Ankara, Turkey

Barbaros Balabanli and Sule Coskun-Cevher
Biology Department, Science Faculty, Gazi University, 06500 Ankara, Turkey

Anthony Kodzo-Grey Venyo
Department of Urology, North Manchester General Hospital, Delaunays Road, Manchester, UK

Index

www.ingramcontent.com/pod-product-compliance
Lightning Source LLC
LaVergne TN
LVHW082200200926
848484LV00008B/2192